New Challenges in Communication with Cancer Patients

Antonella Surbone · Matjaž Zwitter
Mirjana Rajer · Richard Stiefel
Editors

New Challenges in Communication with Cancer Patients

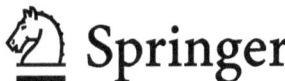
Springer

Editors
Antonella Surbone
Department of Medicine
New York University Medical School
New York, NY, USA

Mirjana Rajer
Institute of Oncology Ljubljana
Ljubljana, Slovenia

Matjaž Zwitter
Institute of Oncology Ljubljana
Ljubljana, Slovenia

Richard Stiefel
Hunter College of the University
　of the City of New York, and
　The New York Academy of Sciences (ret.)
New York, NY, USA

ISBN 978-1-4614-3368-2   ISBN 978-1-4614-3369-9 (eBook)
DOI 10.1007/978-1-4614-3369-9
Springer New York Heidelberg Dordrecht London

Library of Congress Control Number: 2012940534

© Springer Science+Business Media, LLC 2013
This work is subject to copyright. All rights are reserved by the Publisher, whether the whole or part of the material is concerned, specifically the rights of translation, reprinting, reuse of illustrations, recitation, broadcasting, reproduction on microfilms or in any other physical way, and transmission or information storage and retrieval, electronic adaptation, computer software, or by similar or dissimilar methodology now known or hereafter developed. Exempted from this legal reservation are brief excerpts in connection with reviews or scholarly analysis or material supplied specifically for the purpose of being entered and executed on a computer system, for exclusive use by the purchaser of the work. Duplication of this publication or parts thereof is permitted only under the provisions of the Copyright Law of the Publisher's location, in its current version, and permission for use must always be obtained from Springer. Permissions for use may be obtained through RightsLink at the Copyright Clearance Center. Violations are liable to prosecution under the respective Copyright Law.
The use of general descriptive names, registered names, trademarks, service marks, etc. in this publication does not imply, even in the absence of a specific statement, that such names are exempt from the relevant protective laws and regulations and therefore free for general use.
While the advice and information in this book are believed to be true and accurate at the date of publication, neither the authors nor the editors nor the publisher can accept any legal responsibility for any errors or omissions that may be made. The publisher makes no warranty, express or implied, with respect to the material contained herein.

Printed on acid-free paper

Springer is part of Springer Science+Business Media (www.springer.com)

Preface

> *The basis of any human coexistence is communication. Communication is also the basis of every therapeutic action. The more severe and threatening the illness is, the more important the communicative interaction between the affected persons ... and the medical professional or team.*

So write Drs. Klocker-Kaiser and Klocker in their chapter of this book. Their words go to the root of the book's subject. Communication between cancer patient and oncology professional is essential to the achievement of their common goal—bringing about the greatest length and quality of life for the patient. Such communication is a complex, evolving subject.

Communication with the Cancer Patient: Information and Truth (Annals of the New York Academy of Sciences, Vol. 809, Antonella Surbone and Matjaž Zwitter, eds.) was published in 1997 and offered a representative view of the field at that time. Since then much has changed in the content, methods, and circumstances of communication between cancer patients and their doctors—the growth of modern information technologies, to name just one. The editors believe the time is ripe to present a new picture of the field in its various aspects. Toward that end we have assembled 42 chapters by professionals in the field practicing in 22 countries throughout the world. No attempt has been made to be systematic or complete; the authors discuss a large range of issues of current interest and importance and offer a wealth of ideas for what is needed to improve communication between cancer patients and physicians.

Assembling this book has been an inspiring, rewarding task, but not an easy one. Oncologists tend to be very busy people, and writing tends to demand substantial time and effort. We are grateful to the authors who have been willing and able to offer us and you, the reader, their knowledge, experience, and wisdom; we hope their work will inspire you to communicate more effectively with your patients and to join the continuing discussion of this important topic.

We wish to thank Ms. Laura Walsh and Ms. Rachel Corsini, of Springer Science+Business Media, for their invaluable assistance in assembling and publishing this book.

New York, NY, USA   Antonella Surbone
Ljubljana, Slovenia   Matjaž Zwitter
Ljubljana, Slovenia   Mirjana Rajer
New York, NY, USA   Richard Stiefel

Introduction
Communication: Back to the Human Side of Medicine

Diagnostics, treatment, and communication are the three pillars of oncology. None of them can stand alone; even two of them are not enough, just as a table cannot stand on two legs. By definition, if all three are indispensable, no one is more important than the others. If one fails, the other two collapse, and the game is over.

None of us can imagine oncology without a laboratory. No one should ever say "I can't do anything for this patient," since our help is most needed precisely at the moment when the standard treatment guidelines are no longer enough to support our decisions. And no one should approach a cancer patient without a sincere, honest, humble desire to knock on the doors of a new world, of a new, unique person.

Until 100 years ago, medicine was an art, very close to philosophy, theology, and the other humanities. In the twentieth century, modern science came on the scene and, somehow, kidnapped medicine. The unbelievable progress of biology, natural sciences, and technology shifted our attention to precise diagnostics, often based on our increasingly deeper understanding of genetics, and to remarkable new possibilities of effective cancer treatment. By the end of the century, however, a second kidnapping of medicine came about more silently, without Nobel Prize laureates: this time money was responsible. Not all of us are fully aware of the dominant role of pharmaceutical companies, which are intruding into all our activities, including everyday medical decisions, medical research, medical conferences and journals, teaching, regulatory bodies, medical societies, the formulation of national and international guidelines, and the distribution of financial resources.

The time has come for medicine to reclaim its roots and its place among the humanistic sciences—fully scientific and fully humanistic. This is not a nostalgic desire for the "good old days," since none of us would wish for our cancer patients to be deprived of today's increasing chances of being cured or of living with cancer as a chronic long-term illness. Rather, it is becoming obvious that the spiral of progress, with its technical and biological discoveries and its unlimited self-confidence, is leaving aside an essential element of cure and care: the fragility and strength of the human soul. Medicine without a soul is a table on two legs, bound to collapse.

To restore the human dimension of medicine, communication is indispensable. This is even more true for oncology, a discipline that inevitably deals with patients harboring a serious, often incurable, illness pervaded with existential, physical, and psychosocial suffering.

This book offers a nonsystematic approach to the wide spectrum of opinions, ideas, and experiences around one central issue: bringing patient and physician together and helping them both cope with the illness in the most appropriate way. In this introductory chapter, we will briefly review the five sections of the book, which we call the five dimensions of communication:

- The illness: discovering its truths
- The patient and the family
- The physician
- The cultural and social context
- The contribution and interference of modern information technologies

The book's chapters are grouped in correspondingly titled sections and are presented in the order in which they are referred to here.

The Illness: Discovering Its Truths

Surbone
Aggarwal and Rowe
Schapira
Al-Amri
Stiefel and Krenz
Grassi, Caruso, and Nanni
Abrams
Norris, Walseman, and Puchalski
Thombre and Sherman

In spite of medical progress, talking about cancer is still, in its essence, talking about our own mortality. And when we speak about mortality we speak about values of life: death and mortality are what make our lives valuable. When we think about the end of life (or, some will say, the end of this life), we realize why we wish to live. Talking about life and death is talking about values. Once values have been introduced, truth is no longer a static object. Physician and patient discover truth as a unique meeting point of their values.

We are never really prepared for the shock of a diagnosis of cancer: denial, anxiety, depression, and fear are normal reactions. On the physician's side, trust and honesty are essential to building a sincere relationship with the patient. Quite often, the message of bad news is not a single event; rather, the sequence of fear, bad news, hope, and then bad news again may be a patient's and physician's companion from diagnosis until the end. As we do not live in isolation, the waves of concern, depression, hope, and irrational thoughts spread to family, friends, and even to unknown people or to self-proclaimed healers. Following the principles of integrative medicine, a physician restores the central position of the patient and assists him or her in resuming responsible decisions.

Yet, the earthquake in our soul also has a positive side. The experience of serious disease brings forward spiritual issues, and cancer can, indeed, turn out to be one of the most enriching experiences in life.

The Patient and the Family

Baider
Parikh, Prabhash, Bhattacharyya, and Ranade
Aljubran
Lascar, Alizade, and Diez
Balducci and Extermann
Husebø and Husebø
Biasco, Moroni, and De Panfilis
Carapetyan, Smith, and Muggia

Cancer does not affect a single individual, but also those around him or her. Virtually every text on communication with the cancer patient emphasizes the importance of establishing a sincere relationship with the patient's family, friends, and community. Most often, the family supports the patient, and experiencing the threat of a serious disease brings family members closer and helps reestablish broken relationships. Yet, the opposite reaction is not rare: family members may simply be unable to cope with such a stressful situation. In many cultures, the family tries to protect their sick relative by blocking all direct communication and insisting on withholding the truth about the malignant nature of their illness.

There is no doubt that cancer in a child affects the whole family. While parents are always involved, siblings also feel the shock of a new, extremely stressful situation. The emotional burden upon the siblings is often ignored: the "go and play" attitude is clearly inappropriate, as it leaves them hurt by their fears and without attention. Sincere talk not only to parents but also to a child with cancer and his or her siblings can remove much of the tension. Last, but not least, pediatric oncologists themselves need support for their exhaustive work and most often they get it from sincere communication with their little patients.

In this section on patients and family, we include also the other extreme: elderly patients and patients requiring palliative and end-of-life care. Here often it is not the presence, but the *absence,* of family that must be considered. Communication with elderly cancer patients and with those approaching the end of their life is all too often a pale substitute for what these patients really wish for and need: the caring presence of a close family member. Drugs can relieve pain, constipation, or insomnia; but no drug can relieve the feeling of abandonment. A sincere human relationship with a physician can restore dignity. And it must not be forgotten that a warm "thank you and good-bye" from a dying patient also has a powerful healing power for the oncologist and staff members of a palliative or geriatric unit.

The diagnosis of a hereditary cancer brings distinct issues into communication with a cancer patient. Even for the most individualistic patient, such cancer ceases to be only his or her own problem and becomes an issue that directly concerns other members of the family. For young patients, a diagnosis of hereditary cancer also opens questions of family planning, including the option of preimplantation genetic screening: genetic counseling thus requires special communication skills.

The Oncology Professional

Die Trill
Klocker-Kaiser and Klocker
Annunziata and Muzzatti
Lowenstein
Brook
Dikici, Yaris, and Artiran Igde
Baile
Travado
Fujimori, Shirai, and Uchitomi

The great majority of physicians of any specialty occasionally see, diagnose, or treat a patient with cancer. For some physicians, however, oncology is their only discipline.

We believe that experience in communication is among the most important reasons why cancer should be treated by oncologists. For physicians of other specialties, a cancer patient may be an unusual challenge or even an additional burden; oncologists, by contrast, choose to invest all their knowledge and empathy for the benefit of cancer patients. Good communication includes sharing knowledge as well as emotions, and listening to patients' narratives, by giving priority to subtle nuances rather than binary thinking. Careful listening to patients' complaints can also protect patient and physician from medical errors.

While stressing the importance of trained oncologists in cancer treatment, we do not underestimate the role of physicians of other specialties, who are indispensable in a multidisciplinary approach to cancer. A special place goes to practitioners of family medicine, who make invaluable contributions at both ends of the journey of most cancer patients—in finding the first suspicion of malignancy and in palliative treatment in the home setting. Hence, proper education of and support to family physicians are of utmost importance.

Can communication with the cancer patient be taught, or is it a talent that some physicians simply possess or acquire through experience? It seems that both answers are correct. Traditionally, there was no formal training in communication, a situation resulting in a wide spectrum of attitudes, ranging from physicians with deep empathy and excellent communication skills to others who seem totally unaware of the communication needs of their patients. However, there is now no doubt that inappropriate practices can be changed and that communication can be improved by proper teaching of communication skills.

The Cultural and Social Context

Cohen
Dolbeault and Brédart
Pavlovsky, Bertolino, Patxot, and Pavlovsky
Kagawa-Singer
Butow, Tattersall, Clayton, and Goldstein
Güven
Montazeri
Mehic
Schwartsmann and Brunetto
Demin and Gamaley
Ndlovu

The dependence of communication on cultural factors is increasingly being recognized and studied. The influence of culture on perceptions, beliefs, and reactions to a severe illness such as cancer is especially evident when one compares attitudes and practices in different countries where health care systems are also different. As most Western countries are becoming increasingly multiethnic and multicultural, cross-cultural medical encounters are becoming more frequent; they need to be approached with cultural competence: culturally sensitive communication with patients and families is necessary when patients and oncology professionals do not share the same culture. We are referring not only to differences in ethnicity, nationality, language, and religion, but also to such factors as gender, age, sexual orientation, disability, education, health literacy, and socioeconomic status.

As any clinical encounter is an encounter of different fellow human beings, oncology professionals should always practice sensitivity, humility, and curiosity in carefully exploring the patient's cultural and individual beliefs, preferences, and priorities. Listening and understanding comes as the first step of communication and is at its core, followed by a continuous sensitive reassessment of the patient's wishes, preferences, and needs, which evolve during the course of the illness. The oncologist should establish a trusting relationship with the patient and discuss with him or her the most appropriate plan of care, from both the medical and the patient's cultural perspectives. Psychosocial assistance is essential both in communicating the diagnosis and in formulating a realistic treatment plan. Good communication is of utmost importance for treatment compliance. Cultural sensitivity and competence comprise a set of knowledge, skills, and professional values that can and should be taught.

In many parts of the world and within some communities in multicultural countries, physicians' paternalism has deep and strong roots, to the extent that open discussion with a cancer patient is considered inappropriate and harmful to the patient. Despite a wealth of Western empiric studies showing that better-informed patients contribute more actively to their care plans and receive higher quality of care at medical and psychosocial levels, in many countries patients are still kept unaware of their cancer diagnosis and prognosis.

Economic inequalities and their influence upon medical decisions are rarely discussed, even in many democratic societies. Yet, low socioeconomic status has been confirmed as an independent unfavorable predictor of cancer survival. The difficult balance between the optimal treatment and the treatment that is realistically available is achieved largely through open communication between oncologists and their patients.

African countries appear to face a special blend of deeply rooted traditional beliefs regarding the origins and treatment of diseases, economic deprivation, a high prevalence of HIV infection, and the priority of the family over the individual in making decisions. In such a setting and until comprehensive cancer programs become available, communication with cancer patients is often limited to basic help and symptomatic relief.

The Contribution and Interference of Modern Information Technologies

Vasconcellos-Silva
Rajer
Zakotnik
Zhuang and Chou
Zwitter

The extent to which modern information technologies influence all our relations is enormous and rapidly growing. The information obtained through the Internet, albeit not always reliable, has already replaced in large part the direct flow of information from physician to patient. We as oncologists have no choice other than to be knowledgeable and proactive with regard to virtual medical information. Ignoring the importance of virtual global communication media would give even more power to those who see medicine exclusively as a profitable enterprise.

Even before the Internet, printed educational material was used to disseminate information about specific cancers, their early symptoms, diagnostics, and treatment. While this printed material can, indeed, spare some physician's time, it should not become a substitute for bidirectional talk with the patient.

The global presence of the Internet and related communication networks has dramatically changed the level of information available to patients. This, in turn, has generated a strong pressure upon health professionals and policy makers responsible for resource allocation and the organization of medical care. In China, until recently considered a developing country, most patients from urban areas consult the Internet even prior to their first visit to an oncologist.

Finally, we come to the question of communication in clinical research. As an activity directed to improving the efficacy of our treatments, research is not only ethically justified but, indeed, indispensable. Clinical research has brought significant progress in virtually all fields of oncology. Yet, ethical problems remain, and most of them are connected to communication: information for patients aims at protecting the sponsor, rather than informing the patient in support of his or her free decision-making. If we are sincere in our words about patients as partners in research, then we should offer them information that is accurate, simple, and understandable to each patient.

New York, NY, USA	Antonella Surbone
Ljubljana, Slovenia	Matjaž Zwitter
Ljubljana, Slovenia	Mirjana Rajer
New York, NY, USA	Richard Stiefel

Contents

Part I The Ilness: Discovering Its Truth

1. From Truth Telling to Truth in the Making: A Paradigm Shift in Communication with Cancer Patients 3
   Antonella Surbone

2. Denial in Patient–Physician Communication among Patients with Cancer 15
   Neil Aggarwal and Michael Rowe

3. Managing Uncertainty 27
   Lidia Schapira

4. Ethical Issues in Disclosing Bad News to Cancer Patients: Reflections of an Oncologist in Saudi Arabia 39
   Ali M. Al-Amri

5. Psychological Challenges for the Oncology Clinician Who Has to Break Bad News 51
   Friedrich Stiefel and Sonia Krenz

6. Dealing with Depression: Communicating with Cancer Patients and Grieving Relatives 63
   Luigi Grassi, Rosangela Caruso, and Maria Giulia Nanni

7. Communication Issues in Integrative Oncology 81
   Donald I. Abrams

8. Communicating about Spiritual Issues with Cancer Patients 91
   Lorenzo Norris, Kathryn Walseman, and Christina M. Puchalski

9. Understanding Perspective Transformation among Recently Diagnosed Cancer Patients in Western India 105
   Avinash Thombre and Allen C. Sherman

Part II The Patient and the Family

10 In the Pursuit of Meaning: Cancer and the Family 125
Lea Baider

11 The Patient's Personality as a Guide to Communication Strategy 137
Purvish M. Parikh, Kumar Prabhash, G.S. Bhattacharyya, and A.A. Ranade

12 Challenges to the Disclosure of Bad News to Cancer Patients in the Middle East: Saudi Arabia as an Example 145
Ali Aljubran

13 Talking to a Child with Cancer: Learning from the Experience 153
Eulalia Lascar, María Angelica Alizade, and Blanca Diez

14 Effective Communication with Older Cancer Patients 169
Lodovico Balducci and Martine Extermann

15 "I Never Died Before…": End-of-Life Communication with Elderly Cancer Patients 179
Stein B. Husebø and Bettina S. Husebø

16 Communication with Cancer Patients about Palliative and End-of-Life Care 191
Guido Biasco, Matteo Moroni, and Ludovica De Panfilis

17 Communication with Patients with Hereditary Cancer: Practical Considerations Focusing on Women's Cancers 207
Karen Carapetyan, Julia Smith, and Franco Muggia

Part III The Physician

18 Physicians' Emotions in the Cancer Setting: A Basic Guide to Improving Well-Being and Doctor–Patient Communication 217
Maria Die Trill

19 The Setting, the Truth, and the Dimensions of Communication with Cancer Patients 231
Ursula Klocker-Kaiser and Johann Klocker

20 Improving Communication Effectiveness in Oncology: The Role of Emotions 235
Maria Antonietta Annunziata and Barbara Muzzatti

21 Binary Thinking, Hope, and Realistic Expectations in Communication with Cancer Patients 247
Jerome Lowenstein

Contents

22	**A Physician's Personal Experiences as a Cancer-of-the-Neck Patient: Communication of Medical Errors to Cancer Patients and Their Families** .... Itzhak Brook	253
23	**Communication with Cancer Patients in Family Medicine** .... Mustafa Fevzi Dikici, Fusun Yaris, and Fusun Aysin Artiran Igde	263
24	**How to Train Teachers of Communication Skills: The Oncotalk Teach Model** .... Walter F. Baile	275
25	**Communication Skills Training of Physicians in Portugal** .... Luzia Travado	291
26	**Communication between Cancer Patients and Oncologists in Japan** .... Maiko Fujimori, Yuki Shirai, and Yosuke Uchitomi	301

Part IV Cultural and Social Context

27	**Multicultural Aspects of Care for Cancer Patients in Israel** .... Miri Cohen	317
28	**Cancer Diagnosis Disclosure: The French Experience** .... Sylvie Dolbeault and Anne Brédart	333
29	**Communication with Patients with Hematological Malignancies in Argentina** .... Astrid Pavlovsky, Lourdes Bertolino, Victoria Patxot, and Carolina Pavlovsky	349
30	**Teaching Culturally Competent Communication with Diverse Ethnic Patients and Families** .... Marjorie Kagawa-Singer	365
31	**Breaking Bad News and Truth Disclosure in Australia** .... Phyllis Butow, Martin H.N. Tattersall, Josephine Clayton, and David Goldstein	377
32	**Defining the Possible Barriers to Communication with Cancer Patients: A Critical Perspective from Turkey** .... Tolga Güven	389
33	**Cancer Disclosure, Health-Related Quality of Life, and Psychological Distress: An Iranian Perspective** .... Ali Montazeri	403

34	The Challenges in Communication with Cancer Patients in Contemporary Bosnia and Herzegovina Society 411
	Bakir Mehić

35	Evolution of Truth-Telling Practices in Brazil and South America 419
	Gilberto Schwartsmann and Andre T. Brunetto

36	Communication with Cancer Patients in Russia: Improving Patients' Participation and Motivation 429
	Eugeny Demin and Anastasia Gamaley

37	Communication with Cancer Patients in Zimbabwe 441
	Ntokozo Ndlovu

Part V The Contribution and Interference of Modern Information Technologies

38	The Dialectics of the Production of Printed Educational Material for Cancer Patients: Developing Communication Prostheses 453
	Paulo Roberto Vasconcellos-Silva

39	The Benefits and Pitfalls of the Internet in Communication with Cancer Patients 469
	Mirjana Rajer

40	To Tell or Not to Tell: No Longer a Question! Communication with Cancer Patients 479
	Branko Zakotnik

41	Impact of the Internet and the Economy on Cancer Communication in China 489
	Zhi-gang Zhuang and Jia-Ling Chou

42	Communication with Patients in Clinical Research 495
	Matjaž Zwitter

About the Authors 505

Index 519

Contributors

Donald I. Abrams Chief Hematology-Oncology San Francisco General Hospital, Integrative Oncology, UCSF Osher Center for Integrative Medicine, San Francisco, CA, USA

University of California San Francisco, UCSF Osher Center for Integrative Medicine, San Francisco, CA, USA

Neil Aggarwal Department of Psychiatry, Yale School of Medicine, New Haven, CT, USA

Connecticut Mental Health Center, New Haven, CT, USA

Ali M. Al-Amri Department of Internal Medicine and Oncology, King Fahd Hospital of the University, Al-Khobar, Saudi Arabia

María Angélica Alizade Buenos Aires Psychologists Association (APBA), Buenos Aires, Argentina

Ali Aljubran Medical Oncology, King Faisal Specialist Hospital and Research Center, Riyadh, Saudi Arabia

Maria Antonietta Annunziata Centro Di Riferimento Oncologico Aviano, National Cancer Institute, Unit of Oncological Phsychology, Aviano, PN, Italy

Fusun Aysin Artiran Igde Department of Family Medicine, Ondokuzmayis University School of Medicine, Samsun, Turkey

Lea Baider Sharett Institute of Oncology, Hadassah University Hospital, Jerusalem, Israel

Walter F. Baile Departments of Behavioral Science and Faculty Development, Program on Interpersonal Communication and Relationship Enhancement (I*CARE), The University of Texas MD Anderson Cancer Center, Houston, USA

Lodovico Balducci Senior Adult Oncology Program, Moffitt Cancer Center, Tampa, FL, USA

Lourdes Bertolino FUNDALEU, Psicologia, Caba, Buenos Aires, Argentina

G. S. Bhattacharyya AMRI, Kolkata, India

Guido Biasco Academy of the Science of Palliative Medicine, Bentivoglio-Bologna, Italy

Anne Brédart Supportive Care Department, Institut Curie, Paris, France

Psychology Institute, University Paris Descartes, Boulogne Billancourt, France

Itzhak Brook Department of Pediatrics, Georgetown University School of Medicine, Washington, DC, USA

Andre T. Brunetto Hospital de Clinicas, de Porto Alegre, Universidade Federal do Rio Grande do Sul, Porto Alegre, RS, Brazil

Phyllis Butow Centre for Medical Psychology and Evidence-based Medicine (CeMPED), School of Psychology and Department of Medicine, University of Sydney, Sydney, NSW, Australia

Psycho-Oncology Co-operative Research Group, University of Sydney, Sydney, NSW Australia

Karen Carapetyan Department of Medicine, New York University School of Medicine, New York, NY, USA

Rosangela Caruso Section of Psychiatry, Department of Biomedical and Specialty Surgical Siences, University of Ferrara, Ferrara, Italy

Jia-Ling Chou Department of Breast Surgery, Shanghai First Maternity and Infant Hospital, Tongji University School of Medicine, Shanghai, China

Josephine Clayton Centre for Medical Psychology and Evidence-based Medicine (CeMPED), School of Psychology and Department of Medicine, University of Sydney, Sydney, NSW, Australia

Hammond Care Palliative and Supportive Care Service, Greenwich Hospital, Sydney, NSW, Australia

Miri Cohen Department of Gerontology and School of Social Work, University of Haifa, Haifa, Israel

Eugeny Demin Department of Cancer Control, N.N. Petrov Research Institute of Oncology, Russia

Ludovica De Panfilis Academy of the Sciences of Palliative Medicine, Bentivoglio, Italy

Blanca Diez Fleni, Neuro-Oncology, Buenos Aires, Argentina

Mustafa Fevzi Dikici Department of Family Medicine, Ondokuzmayis University School of Medicine, Samsun, Turkey

Sylvie Dolbeault Supportive Care Department, Institut Curie, Paris, France
Inserm, Paris, France
Univ Paris-Sud and Univ Paris Descartes, Paris, France

Martine Extermann Senior Adult Oncology Program, Moffitt Cancer Center, Tampa, FL, USA

Maiko Fujimori Psycho-Oncology Division, National Cancer Center Hospital, Tokyo, Japan

Anastasia Gamaley Department of Cancer Control, N.N. Petrov Research Institute of Oncology, Russia

David Goldstein Department of Medical Oncology, Prince of Wales Hospital, Randwick Sydney, NSW, Australia

Luigi Grassi Section of Psychiatry, Department of Biomedical and Specialty Surgical Siences, University of Ferrara, Ferrara, Italy

Tolga Güven Department of Medical Ethics and History of Medicine, Marmara University, Istanbul, Turkey

Bettina S. Husebø Department of Public Health and Primary Healthcare, University of Bergen, Bergen, Norway

Stein B. Husebø Dignity Centre, Red Cross Nursing Home, Bergen, Norway

Marjorie Kagawa-Singer Department of Asian American Studies, UCLA School of Public Health, Los Angeles, CA, USA

Johann Klocker Klinikum Klagenfurt am Wörthersee, Klagenfurt, Austria

Ursula Klocker-Kaiser Klinikum Klagenfurt am Wörthersee, Klagenfurt, Austria

Sonia Krenz Psychiatric Liaison Service, University Hospital Center, Lausanne, Switzerland

Eulalia Lascar Hospital de Niños Dr. Ricardo Gutierrez, Buenos Aires, Argentina

Jerome Lowenstein Department of Medicine, NYU Langone Medical Center, New York, NY, USA

Bakir Mehić Clinical Center University of Sarajevo, Clinic of Lung Diseases and TB, Sarajevo, Bosnia and Herzegovina

Ali Montazeri Iranian Institute for Health Sciences Research, ACECR, Tehran, Iran

Matteo Moroni "Giorgio Prodi" Center of Cancer Research, University of Bologna, Academy of the Science of Palliative Medicine, Bentivoglio-Bologna, Italy

Franco Muggia Department of Medicine, New York University Langone Medical Center, New York University Medical Institute, New York, NY, USA

Barbara Muzzatti Centro Di Riferimento Oncologico Aviano, National Cancer Institute, Unit of Oncological Psychology, Aviano, PN, Italy

Maria Giulia Nanni Section of Psychiatry, Department of Biomedical and Specialty Surgical Siences, University of Ferrara, Ferrara, Italy

Ntokozo Ndlovu Department of Radiology, College of Health Sciences, University of Zimbabwe, Harare, Zimbabwe

Parirenyatwa Hospital, Harare, Zimbabwe

Lorenzo Norris Survivorship Center Psychiatric Services, The George Washington University, Washington, DC, USA

Purvish M. Parikh Indian Cooperative Oncology Network, Parel, Mumbai, India

Victoria Patxot Fundaleu, Psicologia, Caba, Buenos Aires, Argentina

Astrid Pavlovsky Department of Hematology, FUNDALEU, Centro de Hematologia, Buenos Aires, Argentina

Carolina Pavlovsky FUNDALEU, Hematology, Buenos Aires, Argentina

Kumar Prabhash Tata Memorial Hospital, Mumbai, India

Christina M. Puchalski George Washington Institute for Spirituality and Health (GWish) and The George Washington School of Medicine and Health Sciences, The George Washington University, Washington, DC, USA

Mirjana Rajer Institute of Oncology Ljubljana, Ljubljana, Slovenia

A. A. Ranade Sahyadri Hospital, Pune, India

Michael Rowe Connecticut Mental Health Center and Department of Psychiatry, Yale School of Medicine, New Haven, CT, USA

Lidia Schapira Harvard Medical School, Massachusetts General Hospital, Boston, MA, USA

Gilberto Schwartsmann Hospital de Clínicas de Porto Alegre, Universidade Federal do Rio Grande do Sul, Porto Alegre, RS, Brazil

Allen C. Sherman Behavioral Medicine Division, Winthrop P. Rockefeller Cancer Institute, University of Arkansas for Medical Sciences, Little Rock, AR, USA

Yuki Shirai Human Resource Development Plan for Cancer, Graduate School of Medicine, The University of Tokyo, Tokyo, Japan

Julia Smith Department of Medical Oncology, New York University Medical Center, New York, NY, USA

Friedrich Stiefel Psychiatric Liaison Service, University Hospital Center, Lausanne, Switzerland

Contributors

Antonella Surbone Department of Medicine, New York University Medical School, New York, NY, USA

Martin H.N. Tattersall Centre for Medical Psychology and Evidence-based Medicine (CeMPED), School of Psychology and Department of Medicine, University of Sydney, Sydney, NSW, Australia

Avinash Thombre Department of Speech Communication, University of Arkansas at Little Rock, Little Rock, AR, USA

Luzia Travado Clinical Psychology Unit, Central Lisbon Hospital Centre, Hospital de S. José, Rua José António Serrano, Lisboa, Portugal

Maria Die Trill Department of Oncology, Psycho-Oncology Unit, Hospital Universitario Gregorio Marañón, Madrid, Spain

Yosuke Uchitomi Department of Neuropsychiatry, Okayama University Graduate School of Medicine, Dentistry and Pharmaceutical Sciences, Okayama, Japan

Paulo Roberto Vasconcellos-Silva Oswaldo Cruz Foundation – IOC. Laboratory of Therapeutic Innovation, Education and Bioproducts—LITEB Federal university of the state of Rio de Janeiro; Gaffrée e Guinle School Hospital, Rio de Janeiro, Brazil

Kathryn Walseman Department of Psychiatry, George Washington University Hospital, Washington, DC, USA

Fusun Yaris Department of Family Medicine, Ondokuzmayis University School of Medicine, Samsun, Turkey

Branko Zakotnik Department of Medical Oncology, Institute of Oncology Ljubljana, Ljubljana, Slovenia

Zhi-gang Zhuang Department of Breast Surgery, Shanghai First Maternity and Infant Hospital, Tongji University School of Medicine, Shanghai, China

Matjaž Zwitter Institute of Oncology Ljubljana, Ljubljana, Slovenia

Part I
The Ilness: Discovering Its Truth

Chapter 1
From Truth Telling to Truth in the Making: A Paradigm Shift in Communication with Cancer Patients

Antonella Surbone

Abstract Direct observation shows how traditional narrow biomedical conceptions of truth in medicine, coupled with increasing technological sophistication and the consequent fragmentation of care practiced under major economic constraints, run parallel to a loss of humanism and of satisfaction for both partners in the patient–doctor relationship. A new conceptualization of truth in medicine, and of communication about it, is needed to restore the integrity of clinical practice, medical education, training, and health care policy. Multiple truths are at stake in clinical medicine, different and yet interrelated. These truths are shared by both partners within the patient–doctor relationship, rather than being simply discovered or imposed by health professionals. A nuanced understanding of the truths at stake in clinical medicine as essentially relational, dynamic, provisional, and situated gives raise to a paradigm shift from truth telling to truth making. This can not only improve communication between patients and their oncologists, but also affect perceptions, attitudes, and practices of education and training, as well as public perceptions of emerging aspects of cancer care and policy making with regard to minority cancer patients and survivors, elderly cancer patients, or mutation carriers.

Keywords Truth telling • Truth making • Patient-doctor relationship • Asymmetry • Trust

Introduction

My reflections on communication in oncology stem from over 20 years of practice of medical oncology, including designing, conducting, and reporting clinical trials and counseling underprivileged and minority women who undergo genetic testing

---

A. Surbone, MD, PhD, FACP (✉)
Department of Medicine, New York University Medical School,
New York, NY, USA
e-mail: antonella.surbone@gmail.com

for breast and ovarian cancer predisposition; as well as from my scholarly work in the philosophy of medicine and the ethical implications of clinical oncology. These have taught me that the essence of being an oncologist goes far beyond the increasingly possible therapeutic successes of cancer therapies and that it lies in the human connection between us and our patients [1–3]. This connection is built and maintained through communication with our patients—a bidirectional process that poses increasing challenges in today's multicultural, highly technological, and globalized world, where we need to disclose painful truths without destroying hope or discuss uncertainty without diminishing our patients' trust in our full commitment to care and be there for them even when cure is no longer possible [4–6].

The many challenges of communication with cancer patients are addressed in detail elsewhere in this book. My contribution aims rather at clarifying what is the subject of our communication with cancer patients: not a static, predetermined truth known only to us oncologists and waiting to be disclosed to our patients, but rather a "truth in the making," which emerges over time within and from each individual patient–doctor relationship, under the influence of many contextual, internal, and external factors [7].

While clinical medicine and oncology deal with many truths, the cancer patient and the oncologist engage in a reciprocal relationship in search for the unique truth of the particular patient's illness, with the specific therapeutic goal of curing the illness or alleviating its symptoms [7]. The notion of illness, in contrast to the more restrictive notion of disease, is a complex, multilayered one, encompassing objective, subjective, and intersubjective elements, including sociocultural ones [8–14]. Various methods of inquiry into the truth and various criteria of truth contribute to understanding the patient's cancer. The truth about its objective dimension may seem, at first glance, to be only the sum of pathologic, molecular, and genetic changes. These, however, occur in an embodied living subject, who experiences the symptoms and signs of cancer in a given context and manifests the discomfort or suffering associated with his or her illness according to socioculturally determined and accepted expressive means [4, 7, 15, 16]. Understanding and applying these concepts lead to a holistic view of illness and of cancer care that are necessarily based on open, effective communication.

Despite the increasingly recognized role of subjectivity and intersubjectivity, and of uncertainty, ambiguity, and vagueness in the contemporary philosophy of science, the strict biomedical view of disease, based and focused on objective quantifiable data obtained generally by ever-improving technological means, still pervades Western medicine and medical training [17–19]. When the subjective and intersubjective elements of illness are not taken into proper account, the illness is reified. Reification is a process that occurs when an object is posited as being given, rather than the result of human actions and interactions [20, 21]. Reification of an illness means that its truth is reduced to that of an external static object awaiting experts' unilateral discovery, description, and truth telling [4]. In such a perspective, the physician becomes increasingly dominant, while the patient is silenced.

On the contrary, the many interrelated truths of the patient's cancer are known by both the patient and the doctor together, albeit from different perspectives.

Objective and subjective dimensions give rise to the reality of a person's illness within the context of the patient–doctor relationship, in which the anonymous, ambiguous suffering of the patient is open to the rational scrutiny of the doctor, who interprets it and transposes it to a level of rationality and objectivity, where it can be more easily managed [22]. Such a process is the result of interactive, selective presentation and interpretation of multiple stories and multiple data by both parties [23].

The increased emphasis on personal self-governance in most Western countries is mirrored in the current model of the patient–doctor relationship, which includes the doctors' moral obligation to respect and foster their patients' autonomy and to develop equal partnerships with them, first and foremost through the practice of disclosure and informed consent [24]. The autonomy model is in sharp contradistinction to the formerly dominant paternalistic model of charismatic physicians who, at their discretion, maintain all power, including that of withholding the truth. Truth telling, however, has often been reduced to a matter of providing information, rather than sharing a truth in the making that emerges from the relationship itself [4].

The patient–doctor relationship is inherently asymmetrical at the existential, social, and epistemic levels. The ill person, by virtue of the illness, is in a "uniquely dependent state" [25]. Vulnerability limits the patient's autonomy and introduces an element of dependency on the physician, as the patient begins to relate the "truth" of his or her symptoms and the doctor elaborates and pronounces another "truth" in terms of diagnosis, prognosis, and risks [22, 26]. A nuanced conceptualization of truth in medicine as relational, dynamic, and provisional that takes into consideration the asymmetrical nature of the patient–doctor relationship and the specific knowledge of each partner can lead to true communication and advance the cancer patient's autonomous participation in his or her treatment and care.

Sensitive and effective communication also contributes to changes in the practice of clinical oncology and might have a "bottom up" influence on healthcare policy, through larger-scale changes in public and professional perceptions and attitudes toward cancer patients and survivors. Oncologists often struggle to maintain their allegiance to the individual patient in the midst of impossible institutional demands, and yet have some freedom to create positive policy changes in day-to-day practice, strategizing with their patients to provide the maximum quality and quantity of care within financial constraints and institutional demands [7].

For a shift from truth telling to truth making to occur, it would be necessary to introduce in medical school curricula a dynamic, evolutionary concept of truth in clinical medicine and of the social, scientific, technological, and economic forces that shape clinical practice. The development in medical students and oncology fellows of an appreciation of the interpersonal, social, and ethical issues of power, control, authority, dominance, dependency. and responsibility in the patient–doctor relationship, with attention to the current situation and the foreseeable changes in future clinical practice—such as those due to the aging of the worldwide population or the developments of genetics—is key to laying the foundations for open, effective communication with all cancer patients [27–29].

Understanding the Dynamic, Relational Nature of Communication with Cancer Patients

Each patient–physician interaction is inherently dynamic and relational in nature, expressed in a series of steps and occasional epiphanies that lead to a shared understanding of the patient's illness, made of multiple, particular, provisional, and often partial truths that encompass different elements and levels. These truths are also of different kinds: medical, clinical, therapeutic, as well as scientific; existential, practical, and moral, as well as objective; in the first as well as the third person; and about diagnosis as well as prognosis and cure (or lack of cure). These disparate truths rarely blend harmoniously into a single truth. Rather, there always seems to be a persistent gap, an unbridgeable distance between the subjective and objective elements of the illness [7, 30].

There is also a distance between the cancer patient and the oncologist, which is not merely existential, but primarily epistemic, as the patient and the doctor learn and know different aspects of the patient's illness and its treatments. The patient knows by direct personal and singular corporeal experience, the physician by generalization and abstraction [4]. Not only are they two different knowing subjects making use of the different cognitive categories of subjectivity vs. objectivity, but the objects of their knowledge and their interests are different. It is in this gap that the truths about the patient's illness are "in the making" [7].

Truth in the Making: A Paradigm Shift in Communication with Cancer Patients

Viewing truth as in the making leads to a paradigm shift in the traditional conception of truth telling to, and communication with, cancer patients. The conceptual framework necessary to support this shift can be summarized as follows:

1. Illness consists of more-or-less objectively quantifiable data that are subjectively lived, intersubjectively interpreted, and socially constructed. By contrast, the objective dimension of the person's illness, generally referred to as the "disease," consists of measurable anatomical, physiological, biochemical, molecular, and genetic changes that are independent of the patient's will [19]. The changes that make up the disease occur in a specific human being, where body, psyche, and mind are united as a whole. They impose a functional rigidity or limitation with respect to the homeostatic relationship of the person and its environment [31]. This rigidity results in a condition of discomfort and suffering of various kinds and degrees. The more-or-less ambiguous consciousness of this suffering constitutes the subjectively lived dimension of a person's illness [32].
2. The objective and subjective elements of each illness are interpreted within the context of the patient–doctor relationship, where the patient's experience of suffering is offered to the scrutiny and interpretation of another person—an expert, the

physician—who transposes a still anonymous, ambiguous, chaotic suffering onto a level of greater order and rational intelligibility [22]. The purpose of this transposition is to render the reality of the patient's illness more manageable and livable. For this transposition to take place in a sensitive and effective way, both the cancer patient and the oncologist must be engaged in open, honest reciprocal communication about the many truths contributing to the patient's illness and suffering.
3. To the patient, the illness is known by direct, unique perception of changes in body and self. The patient's corporeal experience is inevitably characterized by a certain degree of ambiguity [32]. The physician, on the contrary, must look for commonalities and applies to the individual patient a foreknowledge of the disease(s) that is obtained through the cognitive categories of objectivity, including universality, abstraction, and generalization [4]. Patient and doctor together, however, attain better, more complete, knowledge through the process of ongoing communication, where these truths are shared relationally and dynamically.
4. In the truth-making perspective, the patient–doctor relationship moves from an authoritarian relationship of unilateral power to an asymmetric, yet reciprocal, relationship of help delimited by intrinsic boundaries as well as by its inherent therapeutic *telos*. The patient–doctor relationship is at one and the same time a professional relationship of help based on a covenant sanctioned by a promise, generally in the form of a public oath, and a relationship of care based on the special and often intimate involvement of the caregiver (the physician) with a particular Other (the patient) [33–36]. The help requested by the patient and offered and provided by the physician is the first step in the establishment of a meaningful and effective therapeutic relationship. Such "priority of help" occurs at chronological, moral, and epistemic levels during the illness' trajectory, and it shapes the nature of the relationship and of the communication between oncologists and their patients.
5. The oncologist always acts both as a professional and as a caregiver [37]. The distinction between "professional" and "caregiver" stresses those formal, distanced aspects of clinical practice as opposed to the personal, close, human aspects of the caregiver side [38, 39]. Certain characteristics of clinical medicine make it a functionally specific professional activity, defined by clear boundaries that are recognized by society and by individual patients [39, 40]. For example, oncologists engage in extensive training that involves a significant intellectual component and leads to the acquisition of specific abilities that provide an important service to the community; they go through an extensive process of certification and recertification to become members of their countries' professional associations; and they acquire a set of ethical, professional, and practical responsibilities. By virtue of their credentials, they are called upon to exercise autonomous discretionary judgments, including those related to how, when, and to what degree they inform their cancer patients. Yet, being a clinical oncologist not only is a professional activity, but it also belongs to the realm of caregiving labor, deeply embedded in altruism and love, such as when the oncologist makes a nonrequested call or a house call to a patient at the end of life or sends a condolence note or attends the patient's funeral, or continues to care for the patient's children and spouse after the patient dies.

6. In recent years, the patient–doctor relationship has shifted from paternalism to contractualism, but the true essence of the partnership between patient and doctor lies in the asymmetry of help and is based on trust [26, 37]. The weight and the kind of responsibility borne by the two partners are quantitatively and qualitatively different, for the physician has the ability (and is entrusted with the responsibility) to affect the well-being of the patient [41]. The consequences of a possible breakdown of trust in a relationship of help are also quantitatively and qualitatively different. The uncertainty, fear of loss, and helplessness experienced by the patient elicit an empathic response in the oncologist, and the patient's suffering challenges him or her also at the emotional level [26]. Yet, even this sharing is asymmetric; the oncologist always carries particular responsibilities of care, trust, and justice toward his or her patients [42]. In analogy to other relationships of care that involve one partner's dependence on the other, the patient–doctor relationship is not characterized by "parity," as in a free exchange among peers, but rather by a "connection-based equality," where the different responsibilities of each partner arise from the relationship itself [39]. Such connection-based equality becomes a source of shared creativity between patient and doctors that is best expressed and conveyed when communication is based on a nuanced notion of dynamic, relational truth in the making.

The Need for a Paradigm Shift in Communication with Cancer Patients: Illustrations

The domain of cross-cultural differences in health care offers a compelling case for a truth-making approach, where truths are not imposed but shared. Jay Katz's 1984 book, *The Silent World of Doctor and Patient*, had an enormous influence on the current emphasis on truth telling and sharing information with patients [43]. Narrative and empirical publications on cultural differences in truth telling have had a visible impact on our understanding of the knowledge, skills, and sensitivity that true communication entails [45, 46]. In cross-culturally diverse medical encounters with cancer patients and their families, we encounter barriers of language and nonverbal means of communication, such as gestures, pauses, or silence; of health literacy and ability to navigate healthcare systems; and of different expectations and values regarding the reciprocal interaction between patients and physicians [45, 47, 48]. Cultural minority cancer patients in the United States and other Western countries face many structural difficulties of access, including lack of a fixed address or telephone number, transportation problems, or caregiving responsibilities that cannot be delegated by patients to others in order to make time for their own optimal cancer treatment [48, 49]. Sensitive, effective cultural communication can occur only when we are open to the notion of truth in the making that patient and doctor can share even beyond language and cultural barriers.

Learning about cross-cultural differences in patients' perceptions of cancer, modalities of relationships to oncologists and institutions, attitudes toward treatment and research, degree of family involvement in information and decision making, and preferences with regard to end-of-life matters requires basic virtues of humility, respect, and admiration for what each patient brings to the clinical encounter; these virtues should inform the process of communication with all cancer patients [48].

Genetic testing for cancer predisposition provides another illustration of the potential for truth making at work in today's clinical oncology. When genetic information is interpreted and applied within the strict biomedical model upon which unilateral truth telling is based, the carrier of a genetic mutation predisposing to a certain disease may find herself "asymptomatically ill" in the absence of, and/or prior to, "having" the disease, with potentially devastating medical, psychological, and social consequences [50]. As an example, a woman carrying a BRCA mutation predisposing her to a high risk of developing breast and/or ovarian cancer is likely to experience personal and social consequences of a potential cancer before it actually develops or manifests [51, 52]. By virtue of her carrier status, compounded with social perceptions and practices of subtle or overt discrimination, the BRCA-positive woman becomes "ill" whether or not she actually has cancer. First, the carrier woman enters the path of "medicalization," where innumerable medical tests and interventions are performed at substantial economic and emotional costs not only to her, but also to her family and community. Second, her individual psychological reactions can greatly influence the dynamics of her relationships with others. Third, her responsibility to family and community members may be enhanced by possessing specific genetic information that may benefit or harm others, with whom she might or might not feel like sharing it [54, 53].

The notion of a predisposing genetic illness can, however, be deconstructed in a truth-making perspective at the level of the patient–doctor relationship by approaching genetic predisposition as one of many life variables upon which the carrier, together with her oncologists and/or genetic counselor, can act, without interpreting genetic data as a form of genetic destiny [55]. Most diseases, including cancer, are, in fact, multigenic and multifactorial: the mutation carrier is thus predisposed to be more susceptible to the future development of cancer as a result of stable genetic and changing environmental factors [42].

Once our standards for normalcy and diversity are understood and communicated in light of the dynamic nature of the truths involved, the current culture of "medicalization" and stigmatization of mutation carriers may start changing toward acceptance of all forms of human diversity, including genetic [56, 57]. Each mutation carrier can, therefore, greatly benefit from communication based on conceiving truth as in the making, rather than in a deterministic way.

Conclusion

Cancer patients and their oncologists share the relational nature of the truth of the patient's illness within a relationship of care between "particular embodied unique others" that is ambiguous, dynamic, provisional, partial, and situated [7].

To the extent that scientific truths in oncology are constantly being revisited, they hold a degree of vagueness; the clinical context in which they are applied is subject to ambiguity and uncertainty. Uncertainty in clinical oncology is now recognized as an inherent and essential aspect of all communication between cancer patients and their oncologists. Yet, many oncologists are still unprepared for, and uncomfortable with, admitting or discussing medical uncertainty with their patients without undermining the patients' natural need and right to rely on the knowledge and expertise of the doctors to whom they have entrusted their care [58].

The truths in the making in the relationship between cancer patients and oncologists are dynamic, because they are forceful and emerging. These truths change as the cancer evolves, as the patient modifies his or her psychological attitude, as the relationship between patient and treating oncologist grows and becomes deeper, and under the influence of many external variables that must also be taken into account in communicating with cancer patients.

Communication, thus, has a provisional character, based on objective and subjective truths under constant redefinition. Communication is situated within a specific therapeutic purpose, as well as within the special circumstances of suffering of each individual and within each patient's familial, social, and cultural contexts. Finally, the truths that patient and doctor can make together are committed to a specific life project [7]. Great humility, creativity, and a great sense of responsibility are necessary for the oncologist engaged in communicating about a truth in the making with the aim of enhancing the patient's negative freedom from the impediments of the illness, while also contributing to the patient's positive freedom to "make sense" of life with cancer.

In recent years, there has been increased interest in the humanistic practice of clinical oncology and in the art and science of communication with cancer patients [59]. While many physicians, acutely aware of tensions in the patient–doctor relationship and shifting public attitudes toward physicians, are now cultivating the humanistic aspects of clinical medicine and developing better communication skills in the encounter with their patients even in the absence of institutional or insurance guidelines, rewards, or credits, there is also increasing focus on the humanistic areas of medicine in medical schools in many countries. In the United States, the Accreditation Council for Graduate Medical Education, for example, requires residency programs to teach six competencies, including interpersonal and communication skills and professionalism [60]. Bedside teaching and training of residents and oncologist fellows, as well as continuous medical education in communication with seriously ill patients of all cultures, are essential to maintaining one's awareness, knowledge, and abilities. The importance of role models can never be underscored enough, as most of what is learned in medical school and during specialty training is transmitted through hidden curricula, where the educational messages are not verbally transmitted, but rather acquired through observation and experience of how older physicians interact and communicate with their patients, colleagues, staff, and students [61].

Notwithstanding recent efforts to teach and practice patient-centered medicine, the patient–doctor relationship in Western countries is now troubled by a ubiquitous loss of patients' trust in individual physicians and institutions and by dissatisfaction of patients and doctors alike. To a certain extent, this has to do with a "pervasive suspicion about truth itself" [62]. Consequently, the practice of oncology has become progressively more defensive and less attentive to the interpersonal dimension. Both the old paternalism, which used to suppress the patient's wishes and active participation in the decision-making process, and today's dominant consumer-provider model, shaped in part upon the business-like contractual ethics of free-market relationships, obscure and fail to capture the asymmetry of help that characterizes the patient–doctor relationship. This asymmetry requires a high degree of reciprocal trust, which we need to establish and maintain through constant, conscious efforts. Trust, in turn, facilitates ongoing, open, sensitive, effective communication with all patients, especially those rendered more vulnerable by the physical, psychological, and existential pain of cancer.

Despite today's scientific understanding of truth as provisional, less certain, and more contextual than traditionally believed, communication with our patients must be based on truthfulness. Truthfulness, as Bernard Williams wrote in his last book, "implies a respect for truth," and this requires "two basic virtues of truth": accuracy in doing the best we can to acquire true information and beliefs, and sincerity in what we say to each other [62]. By sharing with our patients the path toward a truth in the making and by communicating truthfully with them, we may never reach a final truth, but we will help them make sense of their illness and suffering in a way that "will not leave everyone in despair" [62]. Communication, then, is in the service of hope for our patients and their loved ones, and for us as well.

References

1. Matthews DA, Suchman AL, Branch WT. Making connexions: enhancing the therapeutic potential of patient-clinician relationships. Ann Intern Med. 1993;118:973–7.
2. Spiro H. What is empathy and can it be taught? In Empathy and the practice of medicine. New Haven: Yale University Press; 1993.
3. Schroeder SA. Don't let medicine lose its soul. The Pharos. 2004;4:21–4.
4. Surbone A. Truth telling. In: Cohen-Almagor R, editor. Medical ethics at the dawn of the 21st century, vol. 913. New York: Annals of the New York Academy of Science; 2000. p. 52–62.
5. Surbone A. The information to the cancer patient: psychosocial and spiritual implications. Support Care Cancer. 1993;1:89–91.
6. Surbone A. Information, truth and communication: for an interpretation of truth-telling practices throughout the world. In: Surbone A, Zwitter M, editors. Communication with the cancer patient. Information and truth. New York: USA Annals of the New York Academy of Sciences; 1997. p. 7–16.
7. Surbone A. From truth telling to truth making. PhD unpublished dissertation. New York: Fordham University Press; 2004.
8. Engelhardt Jr HT. The concept of health and disease. In: Engelhardt Jr HT, Spicker SF, editors. Evaluation and explanation in the biomedical sciences. Dordrecht: Reidel; 1975. p. 125–41.
9. Boorse C. On the distinction between illness and disease. Philos Public Aff. 1975;5:49–68.
10. Callahan D. Concepts of disease and diagnosis. Perspect Biol Med. 1977;20:528–38.
11. Erde EL. Philosophical considerations regarding defining health, disease and their bearing on medical practice. Ethics Sci Med. 1979;6:31–48.

12. Rollin B. On the nature of illness. Man Med. 1979;4(3):157–72.
13. Miller-Brown W. On defining disease. J Med Philos. 1985;4:311–28.
14. Sontag S. Illness as a metaphor. New York: Farrar, Straus and Giroux; 1978.
15. Cattorini P. The many aspects of the therapeutic relationship for an epistemology of complexity in medicine. In: Galeazzi O, editor. Strategie della Guarigione (strategies of healing). Firenze: Leo S. Olschki; 1993.
16. Surbone A. Telling truth to patients with cancer: what is the truth? Lancet Oncol. 2006;7: 944–50.
17. Foucault M. Naissance De La Clinique. Une Archeologie Du Regard Medical. The Birth of the clinic. An Archeology of medical perception (Transl. by Sheridan AM, 1975). New York: Vintage Books; 1963.
18. Balestra DJ. Technology in a free society: the new Frankestein. Thought. 1990;65:154–68.
19. Code L. Taking subjectivity into account. In: Alcoff L, Potter E, editors. Feminist epistemology. New York: Routledge; 1993.
20. Lukacs G. History and class consciousness (Transl. by Livingston R, 1920). Perth: Merlin Press; 1967.
21. Habermas J. The theory of communicative action (Transl. by McCarthy TB). Boston: Beacon Press; 1987
22. Galeazzi G. Disease and prognosis an historical—anthropological analysis. In: Surbone A, Zwitter M, editors. Communication with the cancer patient. Information and truth, vol. 809. New York: USA Annals of the New York Academy of Sciences; 1997. p. 40–55.
23. Nelson HL. Stories and their limits. Narrative approaches to bioethics. New York: Routledge; 1997.
24. Beauchamp T, Childress JF. Principles of biomedical ethics. 4th ed. New York: Oxford University Press; 1994.
25. Pellegrino ED. Altruism, self interest, and medical ethics. JAMA. 1987;258:1939–40.
26. Surbone A, Lowenstein J. Exploring asymmetry in the relationship between patients and physicians. J Clin Ethics. 2003;14:183–8.
27. Herbert MS, Philip S, Danoff D, et al. Teaching professionalism in undergraduate medical education. JAMA. 1999;282:830–83.
28. American Society of Clinical Oncology. American society of clinical oncology policy statement update: genetic and genomic testing for cancer susceptibility. J Clin Oncol. 2010;28:893–901.
29. Institute of Medicine. Retooling for an aging America: building the health care workforce. New York: The National Academic Press; 2008.
30. Maguire P, Faulkner A. Communicate with cancer patients: handing uncertainty, collusion, denial. Brit Med J 1988;297:972–974.
31. Canguilhem G. Le normal et le pathologic (the normal and the pathologic). Paris: Press Universitaire Francaise; 1966.
32. Merleau-Ponty M. Phenomenologie de la Perception. Phenomenology of perception (Transl. by Smith C, 1995). London: Routledge and Kegan Paul; 1962.
33. Surbone A. Recognizing the patient as other (editorial). Support Care Cancer. 2005;13:2–4.
34. Peperzack AT, Critchely S, Bernasconi R. Basic philosophical writings. Indianapolis, IN: Indiana University Press; 1996.
35. Clifton-Soderstrom M. Levinas and the patient as other: the ethical foundation of medicine. J Med Philos. 2003;28:447–60.
36. Levinas E. Totality and infinity: an essay on exteriority. Pittsburg: Duquesne University Press; 1969.
37. Pellegrino ED, Thomasma DC. For the patient's good. The restoration of beneficence in health care. New York: Oxford University Press; 1988.
38. Bert G. Tra Realta' e Verita' (between reality and truth). In: Istituto change. Verita' e Rappresentazione (truth and representation). Napoli: CUEN; 1997.
39. Kittay EF. Love's labor. Essays on women, equality and dependency. New York: Routledge; 1999.

40. Parsons T. The professions and social structure. In: Parsons T, editor. Essays in sociological theory, pure and applied. Glencoe, IL: The Free Press; 1939.
41. Baier A. In: Moral prejudices. Essays on ethics. Cambridge, MA: Harvard University Press; 1994.
42. Mahowald MB, McKusick VA, Scheuerle AS, Aspinwall TJ, editors. Genetics in the clinic. St. Louis: Mosby; 2001.
43. Katz J. The silent world of doctor and patient. New York: The Free Press; 1984.
44. Carrese J, Rhodes L. Western Bioethics On The Navajo Reservation: Benefit Or Harm? JAMA 1995;274:826–829.
45. Authors Various. In: Surbone A, Zwitter M, editors. Communication with the cancer patient. Information and truth (vol. 809). New York: Annals of the New York Academy of Sciences; 1997.
46. Baider L, Surbone A. Cancer and the family: the silent words of truth. J Clin Oncol. 2010;28: 1269–72.
47. Surbone A. Cultural aspects of communication in cancer care. In: Stiefel F, editor. Communication in cancer care. Recent results in cancer research, vol. 168. Heidelberg: Springer; 2006. p. 91–104.
48. Kagawa-Singer M, Valdez A, Yu MC, Surbone A. Cancer, culture and health disparities: time to chart a new course? CA Cancer J Clin. 2010;60:12–39.
49. Institute of Medicine. Crossing the quality chasm: a new health system for the 21st century. Washington, DC: National Academy Press; 2001.
50. Billings PR, Kohn MA, deCuevas M, et al. Discrimination as a consequence of genetic testing. Am J Hum Genet. 1992;40:476–82.
51. Surbone A. Social and ethical implications of BRCA testing. Ann Oncol. 2011;22 Suppl 1:i60–6.
52. Pasacreta JV. Psychosocial issues associated with genetic testing for breast and ovarian cancer risk: an integrative review. Cancer Invest. 2003;21:588–623.
53. Lucassen A, Parker M. Confidentiality and sharing genetic information with relatives. Lancet. 2010;375:1508–9.
54. Nycum G, Avard D, Knoppers BM. Factors influencing intrafamilial communication of hereditary breast and ovarian cancer genetic information. Eur J Hum Genet. 2009;17:872–80.
55. Murray TH. Genetic exceptionalism and "future diaries": is genetic information different from other medical information? In: Rothstein MA, editor. Genetic secrets: protecting privacy and confidentiality in the genetic era. New Haven, CT: Yale University Press; 1997.
56. Wolf S. Beyond genetic discrimination: toward the broader harm of geneticism. J Law Med Ethics. 1995;23:345–53.
57. Billings PR. Genetic nondiscrimination. Nat Genet. 2005;37:559–60.
58. Kimberly S, Greene A, Bush JP. Preparing physicians for the 21st century: targeting communication skills and the promotion of health behavior change. Ann Behav Sci Med Educ. 2010;16:7–13.
59. Accreditation Council for Graduate Medical Education. Core competencies. By 2001 by Michael G. Stewart, MD, MPH. http://www.acgme.org/acwebsite/RRC_280/280_corecomp.asp. Accessed 25 Oct 2011.
60. Hafferty FW. Beyond curriculum reform: confronting medicine's hidden curriculum. Acad Med. 1988;73:403–7.
61. Williams B. Truth and truthfulness. An essay in genealogy. Princeton, NJ: Princeton University Press; 2002.
62. Billings PR. Genetic nondiscrimination. Nat Genet. 2005;37:559–60.

Chapter 2
Denial in Patient–Physician Communication among Patients with Cancer

Neil Aggarwal and Michael Rowe

Abstract In this chapter, we discuss the significance of the psychological mechanism of denial in cancer care. We review relevant research literature on the topic, supplemented by clinical literature and personal vignettes. We then discuss key themes in regard to denial in oncology care—the impact of denial on the patient–doctor relationship; denial as a mechanism that "hides" the reasons individuals employ it; denial as an entity with clinical, personal, social, and cultural complexity; physician denial; and physician and family member collusion in the patient's denial—and offer communication strategies to help address the challenge of denial in cancer care.

Keywords Denial • Oncology care • Patient–doctor communication • Social-cultural factors

Introduction

Denial belongs to a group of technical psychological terms—*closure* is another that comes to mind—that come into popular use and are then applied to explain individual and collective responses to situations and experiences that overwhelm their explanatory capacity. Thus, for example, within hours of a commercial airline disaster, we may hear a newscaster speak of the "closure" process for surviving family members. *Denial*, a clinical term coined a century ago, has suffered a similar fate in becoming popular parlance for another's failure to face a truth that we think they are not facing in the way we think we would, and they should.

The history and contemporary use of denial of illness is a good deal more complex than its popular use, even if the latter finds its way into clinical care at times. Kortte and Wegener's review article [18] gives us a good grounding in the term's origins. Sigmund Freud was the first to use it, describing denial as warding off the reality of a traumatic experience and of repressed thoughts related to that experience. Denial, in this and in Anna Freud's later designation of the term as a specific defense mechanism, involves keeping unwanted thoughts and facts unconscious, not a conscious choice to deny their existence. *Denial*, Kortte and Wegener write, is an "unawareness syndrome" generally seen as having a psychological source, while *anosognosia* is an unawareness syndrome related to neurological deficit.

Researchers and clinicians have long recognized that denial may have either beneficial or detrimental impacts on patients. Differentiating these impacts has been an arduous task, but it appears that these are related to stages of illness and treatment and can change over time. For example, during early stages of recovery, denial may support hope in patients. Later, though, it may have a negative impact on coping with the continuing effects of chronic illness.

Kortte and Wegener suggest that the definition of *denial* complicates efforts to determine its links to patient outcomes, and that this, in turn, suggests there are subtypes of illness behaviors or strategies for avoiding information related to the illness, leading either to maladaptive adjustment or to positive reframing or reinterpretation of the illness leading to more adaptive outcomes. Time is another critical factor, with the impact of denial changing during symptom identification, acute hospitalization/rehabilitation, and posthospitalization periods. They conclude their review by describing denial as a multidimensional construct that includes both adaptive and maladaptive behaviors and as a phenomenon that interacts with time to have a differential impact on outcomes.

We will turn shortly to the research literature on denial in cancer, but first we would like to offer two case vignettes from our own personal-family experiences. One of the two concerns denial in cancer; the other concerns denial related mainly to the results of surgical mishap. Both vignettes, however, may socially and clinically contextualize denial's applications and problems.

Aggarwal

How does cancer alter families? My psychiatric residency included a mandatory month of oncology, but the attending physicians excluded us interns from end-of-life or palliative-care discussions. On such occasions, the tense quietude of the waiting rooms shattered into the cries and wails of family members tortured by such information.

I received a distressing answer to my question—how does cancer alter families?—in 2011. I come from a family replete with physicians—my parents, my three maternal aunts, their husbands, and my two oldest cousins. Two years ago, I learned that a paternal cousin whom I shall call N, 17 years old, had been diagnosed with leukemia. N's father, an immensely successful bank manager in India, rushed throughout the country: "I went to over 50 physicians," he cried, "and they all told me the same thing—your son has a 40% chance of survival. Make your peace and prepare for the worst." Refusing to acknowledge the possibility of his son's death, he consulted physician after physician until he reached the best cancer institute in India. "They gave him two courses of chemotherapy, and he has been in remission for the past 3 months," he sobbed. "Not a day has passed since 2009 when I haven't cried. And not a day has passed when I've ever seen him cry," he added.

Intrigued about this discrepancy of coping mechanisms between father and son, I decided to ask each family member about their experiences with my cousin's illness. N's father lives in constant fear of a new focus of cancer: "I have given up everything—promotions, business trips, time with friends—to be with him. I don't care about anything else." N's mother worships at home for hours on end: "I used to go on pilgrimages and temples, crying in front of God until a priest once said, 'Ma'am, you're creating a scene.' I told him, 'If I can't cry in front of God, who can I cry in front of?' At that point, I decided to stay at home and pray." N's older brother, an engineering student in Bombay with whom I chat several times a week through the Internet, always changes the topic when I broach the issue. And my cousin N, an all-India top 100 high school student who has beaten hundreds of thousands of other academic all-stars, prefers not to dwell on his illness: "Every night, after I study, I go for a walk, play basketball or video games with my friends, or learn the guitar. If my days are numbered, why think about it? It only makes me sad and wastes the time I have now."

As a psychiatrist with an interest in patient communication, I have often wondered how I would handle this situation. How would I break this news? Would I stress the causes or focus on the treatment? Would I nervously recite statistics or sit silently in solidarity? Would I countenance forbearance or foster hope? How would patients and their families receive this information?

Rowe

As a medical sociologist with training in qualitative methods of inquiry, I've spent a good deal of time talking with people about their experiences with health care. As a family member, I've had experience with illness, too, and the issue of denial, with both my father, who died from metastatic prostate cancer, and my son, who died from complications of a liver transplant.

In my father's case, denial of the extent of his cancer and difficulty talking about his prospects seemed to fit the usual connotation of denial as inability or unwillingness to face the full extent of his illness and impending death. Denial was also an issue, or a question, in my son's case, but in a much more complicated manner, which involved his family members and doctors as well.

Jesse was a good candidate for success with a liver transplant. Following diagnosis of ulcerative colitis at age 15 and sclerosing cholangitis at age 16, he was diagnosed with "fibrosis transitioning to cirrhosis" during subtotal colectomy surgery at age 17. At the time of receiving a liver transplant at age 19, he was younger and healthier than most adult recipients and did not have complicating factors of drug or alcohol use. During transplant surgery, though, the task of cutting through abdominal adhesions secondary to his colitis surgery was difficult.

Four days following his transplant, Jesse was back in surgery for an intestinal perforation. He died 3 months later following a number of other surgeries, including a second liver transplant and a splenectomy. During this time, his condition worsened and improved, sometimes dramatically, several times. Jesse's doctors, including surgeons, gastroenterologists, and a number of other specialists, expressed a range of views that varied with the individual doctor and over time, with enough dismal news to puncture our hope (or our denial), but enough hope (or denial) to sustain us until near the end.

Jesse himself, although unable to speak during much of his hospitalization, communicated hope ("Will you take me home?") and despair ("I want to die.") through mouthing words at different times. Yet even in the latter case, we, his parents, could tell ourselves that his mood improved markedly when his pain medication was changed. Were we deluding ourselves, and Jesse, all along? Were Jesse's doctors deluding themselves, or erring on the side of hope in their conversations with us?

This chapter is written with these inquiries in mind.

Denial in Cancer: Current Understanding

Denial has generated tremendous interest in cancer studies. A March 2011 search for the terms *denial* and *cancer* in PubMed over all years resulted in over 500 articles. Here, we review major themes with implications for communication between patients and healthcare providers. Therefore, this review is more representative of this scholarship than exhaustive.

The earliest studies of denial in patients with cancer drew heavily from psychoanalysis. For example, Bahnson and Bahnson [2] used unstructured interviews, questionnaires, Rorschach tests, and projective checklists, concluding that cancer patients deny and repress contracontradictory impulses and emotions, leading to regressive anger and depression. They counseled researchers to "try to understand the formation of tumors as a determined psychobiological reaction rather than as an intrusion of a puzzling foreign matter" (p. 844). Henderson [16] interviewed 50 patients with a variety of cancers, finding that 57.8% of treatment delayers, in comparison to 33% of controls, exhibited a "hysterical personality," defined by being "emotionally labile" and predisposed to denial and repression. Wool [42] conducted a study of 20 patients with breast cancer under the assumption that denial reflects primitive ego development. Douglas and Druss [12] discussed two patients who postponed medical treatment for over a decade and contended that illness released them from the demands of daily life. They concluded that the physical defects of patients manifested internalized, defective processes of self-image and self-esteem. In a considerably different turn, Salander and Windahl [31] asked physicians to differentiate among three terms: conscious "avoidance," preconscious "disavowal" (representing the majority of health literature), and unconscious "denial," in which the patient rarely distorts reality completely.

In the past 2 decades, researchers have progressively turned to theories of denial from health psychology. Nelson et al. [25] attempted to correlate survival rates in breast cancer patients with coping attitudes of denial or "fighting spirit," but realized that denial is a difficult construct to measure. Exhaustive reviews have subsequently detailed the challenges of defining denial given discrepancies in the designs of research instruments [37]. These complex issues should be borne in mind when assessing the results of clinical trials. For example, 13 patients with interpersonal denial in terminal illness benefited from structured psychosocial interventions, as measured by pre- and posttest scores [7]. In a study of 30 breast cancer patients delaying treatment, Phelan et al. [26] found no demographic predictors, but each patient utilized denial as a defense mechanism as measured by physicians. Sharf et al. [32] conducted in-depth interviews with nine patients diagnosed with lung cancer who refused physician recommendations, discovering that the subjects emphasized autonomy, faith or fatalism, and distrust of medical authority, especially in communication with physicians. The multiplicity of approaches to studying denial has even caused some researchers to develop the semistructured Denial in Cancer Interview (DCI) [38].

Other researchers examined the role of denial in patient–physician communication. Hackett and Weisman [15] observed that physicians informed cancer patients less frequently compared to cardiac patients about diagnosis and prognosis out of frustration with their inability to provide cures. Cooperman [8] noted that patients who deny their illness and complain about physicians are typically unhappy about infrequent or abrupt communication. Medical staff may erroneously attribute the silence of patients upon hearing bad news to denial when patients may instead be maturely engaging in suppression of information to cope [10]. Cancer patients often want to make treatment decisions autonomously with providers who comprehend their emotional needs, not with providers who act paternalistically [9]. Disciplinary differences may further complicate approaches to denial. Physicians may withhold medical information with denying patients, whereas nurses tend to insist on complete openness [29]. Also, nurses frequently overgeneralize negative responses of the patient as "denial" without appreciating its adaptive value [36].

Social and demographic factors may predispose certain patients toward denial. In a study of 16 patients with leukemia, Spinetta and Maloney [34] found that children coped better when they could discuss diagnosis and prognosis openly with families. In another study of 100 consecutive outpatients undergoing radiation therapy, men wished for a greater sense of control and were more likely to minimize the seriousness of their illnesses than women, both initially and at 2-year follow-up [21]. Patients with psychiatric histories prior to cancer onset may develop organic causes of delirium, paranoia, and dementia, manifesting as treatment nonadherence, doctor shopping, and late presentations to oncologists [20]. There may be interethnic differences toward denial: Asian patients with cancer tend to explicitly deny illness and present with more depressive symptoms than Whites, who adapt to psychological pressures more successfully [30]. In a study of 195 patients diagnosed with lung cancer and serially administered the DCI, Vos et al. [39] found that male gender, older age, and lower levels of education predicted denial. In later analysis, Vos et al. (2009) noted that male patients with moderate denial displayed better overall perceptions of health and physical functioning, calling attention to positive coping strategies. Furthermore, patients with moderate denial over time reported better role transitions and social functioning, less anxiety and depression, and improved quality of life than patients with a low level of denial [41].

Consequently, many physicians and researchers have advised providers not to confront denial in cancer patients. Abrams [1] challenged healthcare providers to understand their own feelings of guilt and inadequacy, suggesting that cancer patients in denial may be responding maturely to preserve self-image and functioning. Providers should intervene only if the patient, not they, finds the course of illness intolerable. Similarly, Levine and Zigler [22] measured disparities in real and ideal senses of self through descriptive questionnaires, finding that denial is common to stroke, cancer, and cardiac patients (stroke>cancer>cardiac), performing a vital psychological function in protecting ill patients from frustration and despair. When patients live beyond the projected time of death, denial may allow for cooperation with treatment and adjustment to survival [11, 33]. Denial can relieve initial anxiety about diagnosis and terminal anxiety about death, but physicians must be vigilant about the middle phases of illness, when denial can delay treatment, affect interpersonal relations, and prevent assimilation of the event in one's life [19].

Some health professionals have offered recommendations on dealing with denial, arguing that physicians should not challenge defenses unless it causes problems for patients and families [24]. Greer [14] encourages providers to recognize three types of denial: (1) complete denial, (2) denial of the implications of a cancer diagnosis, and (3) denial of affect. Brock et al. [4] believe that most patients ultimately accept illness on their own terms, though physicians can expedite this process by asking patients about concerns in a caring, nonjudgmental way. Rabinowitz and Peirson [27] suggest that physicians divide denial into "maladaptive" and "adaptive" forms, with the former interfering with treatment and the latter allowing patients to integrate emotionally distressing information at an acceptable rate and intensity. Kallergis [17] recommends that physicians determine the extent to which denial is conscious or unconscious through subtle history taking. Charavel and Brémond [6] suggested that researchers altogether avoid the question of whether the denying patient is ill or healthy and instead inquire into how denial permits construction of a new postillness reality. Despite these suggestions, case reports abound of physicians perplexed by patients who deny their illnesses [5, 13, 28, 35].

Discussion and Recommendations

Clinical writings on patient–physician relationships have provided rich contextual perspectives on denial in cancer care. One clearly discernible trend is the changing role of the physician. No longer is the prototype that of an authoritative, charismatic, and (usually) male physician. Lowenstein [23] writes of a patient with lung cancer whose wife tells him not to disclose this fact to her husband since, she says, he will fare better without this knowledge. Lowenstein complies with her request, realizing that he has a responsibility to the wife, whom he believes has the patient's best interests at heart and knows him best, as well as an obligation to his patient. He also makes the provocative comment that "current strict norms regarding truth telling and disclosure reflect a breakdown in doc-pt relationship, when every doubt or possibility must be raised with the patient. Truth and facts are not discrete entities," he writes. "What is said should also reflect the doctor's understanding of the needs of the patient" (p. 80).

Brewin [3], writing at a time when physicians were, arguably, more protective of patient knowledge of dire prognosis, nonetheless makes important points regarding the complexity of communication in the case of serious illness and diagnosis, and of cancer as presenting additional difficulties due to fears not encountered with other diseases. The art of being a good doctor, he argues, involves knowing one's patient. "Telling the truth" bluntly may be the right path with one patient, but may destroy fragile defense mechanisms that another patient uses to cope with bad news. The act of truth telling in diagnosis, however, is not the end of the matter, Brewin writes:

> Communication of diagnosis and prognosis is not a dilemma to be faced once and then forgotten ... Sometimes a patient 'knows' [his prognosis] and sometimes he does not. Perhaps when he is with one person he seems to know; when he is with another he seems not to know. He may know; but not want to think about it. His mood changes. Perhaps he accepts probable death, but can still plan for possible recovery or remission (pp. 1624–1625).

Brewin also places the issue of denial in a larger social context. Suppose, he writes, we're asked to state in public our assessment of the odds of social chaos in the next 20 years due to nuclear or other disaster? We are likely, he writes, to shun the question based on the fact that there's nothing we can do about it, that it may not happen, and that our task is to live our lives now, while we can. Returning to cancer patients, he argues that insisting on the patient's knowledge and acceptance of his poor diagnosis is far too doctrinaire.

Denial of illness, then, is a topic that has gained the attention of clinicians as well as researchers, continuing to affect clinical care. Here, we would like merely to propose several principles, or conditions, related to denial in cancer care, with sample probe questions to illustrate our points.

1. Denial affects the patient–doctor relationship: Denial occurs in the context of the patient-relationship in cancer care. This statement implies questions regarding the length and intensity of the relationship; its connection to other treating physi-

cians (the internist, for example, and his or her relationship with the oncologist as well as with the patient); and the form of "truth telling" the oncologist practices. The closeness of the relationship and its character may support empathic truth telling or hinder it. In addition, the doctor's emotional investment in the patient may unleash strong, and sometimes contradictory, emotions in regard to truth telling. Physicians may vary in their degree of assertion and desire to confront the patient's denial.

Sample questions for physician introspection:

- How is the patient responding to this news?
- Why is the patient responding in this way?
- Has this response changed my relationship with the patient?

2. Denial is a mechanism that hides its reasons: If denial is a partly or largely unconscious mechanism, it stands to reason that it may be difficult to locate some of its sources. It might also be confused with other coping mechanisms. Physicians can further the process of healing by specifying the exact type of denial at play and by trying to figure out its sources. Gentle questions can shepherd the patient toward incorporating the experience of cancer in a way that helps them make meaning out of illness.

   Sample questions to the patient:

   - Could you tell me how you feel about the information that you've just heard?
   - Have you had experiences with cancer before? How have they been?
   - How do you think the cancer will take its course?
   - What kind of treatment do you think the cancer needs?
   - How will cancer affect your life?
   - What do you fear or worry most about the cancer?

3. Denial is an entity with clinical, personal, social, and cultural complexity: The clinical complexity of denial includes the lethality or treatability of the cancer, the stage of the cancer at diagnosis, and survival rates at various points in its course. Personal complexity includes the individual's age at diagnosis, preexisting mental conditions that may influence resort to denial as a defense mechanism, and the strength and form of denial manifested. Social-cultural complexities may include the cultural identity-related context of the cancer (breast cancer in females), social expectations of coping, and cultural practices of denial of cancer. We advise healthcare professionals, especially those in multicultural societies, to ascertain the cultural influence on coping styles by asking family members about the degree to which denial may be culturally syntonic and by turning to the medical, anthropological, and sociological literature for corroboration.

   Sample questions to the patient:

   - Did anyone in your family ever have cancer? If so, what happened and how did they react?
   - How do people where you're from typically respond to cancer? Are there particular beliefs or practices that may help or worsen the cancer?

- Do your relatives and friends have different expectations of you now that you have this diagnosis? If so, what are they and how have they changed?
- Do they think that you're making a big deal out of this? Or do they think that you're not making a big enough deal?

4. Physician denial can occur through various levels of fact vs. truth telling: Truth telling, like denial, occurs in the context of the patient–doctor relationship. Physicians may struggle to find their voice in attempting the tricky task of providing patients with information about cancer in a broader relationship that demands doing no harm. Some physicians may zealously demand that patients grapple with cancer, whereas other physicians may minimize information out of a desire to not hurt the patient at all. We advocate that physicians hone their sense of what we call "oncological countertransference," by which we mean the cognitive, emotional, and behavioral responses that a physician exhibits to a patient based on prior experiences with cancer.

    Sample questions for physician introspection:

- Am I feeling any strong responses to this patient or this diagnosis? If so, what are they and why?
- Have I told the patient what they need to know about cancer? Am I telling them too much or too little? Why?
- Am I speaking to this patient in the most sensitive way possible?
- How would my [nonphysician] mother or brother react to this question?
- Am I trying to convince this patient one way or another about their prognosis or treatment? Why?
- Are my personal experiences with cancer [self, family, or friends] hindering me from helping this patient?

5. Physicians and family members may collude in the patient's denial: Physicians, patients, or family members—indeed, all parties—may engage in denial based on multiple factors and multiple signals that each gives to others. Our literature review illustrates a subtle shift in framing denial: older papers squarely attributed denial to the patient, whereas newer papers concede that denial may be introduced, reinforced, and even extinguished in the interaction with physicians and family members. Healthcare providers can observe patients ecologically to see how denial is transacted among familial supports and stressors.

    Sample questions for physician introspection:

- Are there family or friends in the patient's life who are influencing the patient's responses?
- Does the patient tend to respond differently depending on the presence of particular individuals?
- Are these responses helpful or harmful?
- Do we need a family or group meeting to process the patient's condition and treatment?

In conclusion, we have presented a brief history of the scholarship on denial in cancer communication. We have delineated the various forms of denial and its complicated manifestations according to situation. We have also offered healthcare professionals basic ideas and questions to consider in their relationships with patients. While this chapter represents anything but the last word on this subject, we hope it will stimulate broader discussion on effective strategies for dealing with cancer in patient–physician communication.

References

1. Abrams RD. Denial and depression in the terminal cancer patient. A clue for management. Psychiatr Q. 1971;45:394–404.
2. Bahnson CB, Bahnson MB. Role of the ego defenses: denial and repression in the etiology of malignant neoplasm. Ann N Y Acad Sci. 1966;125:827–45.
3. Brewin TB. The cancer patient: communication and morale. Br Med J. 1977;2:1623–7.
4. Brock G, Gurekas V, Deom P. Denial among cancer patients. Tips and traps. Can Fam Physician. 1993;39:2581–4.
5. Carson HJ, Fiester R. Denial and avoidance in an unusual case of death from breast cancer. Can J Psychiatry. 2004;49:867.
6. Charavel M, Brémond A. Problem of perception and denial of illness by women who have had breast cancer. Eur J Cancer Prev. 1995;4:259–60.
7. Connor SR. Denial in terminal illness: to intervene or not to intervene. Hosp J. 1992;8:1–15.
8. Cooperman EM. Coping with cancer: denial and the need for a better bedside manner. Can Med Assoc J. 1977;117:1123–4.
9. Cousins N. Denial. Are sharper definitions needed? JAMA. 1982;248:210–2.
10. Dansak DA, Cordes RS. Cancer: denial or suppression? Int J Psychiatry Med. 1978–1979;9(3–4):257–62.
11. Detwiler DA. The positive function of denial. J Pediatr. 1981;99:401–2.
12. Douglas CJ, Druss R. Denial of illness: a reappraisal. Gen Hosp Psychiatry. 1987;9:53–7.
13. Flynn TC. Denial of illness: basal cell carcinoma. Dermatol Surg. 2004;30:1343–4.
14. Greer S. The management of denial in cancer patients. Oncology (Williston Park). 1992; 6:33–6.
15. Hackett TP, Weisman AD. Denial as a factor in patients with heart disease and cancer. Ann N Y Acad Sci. 1969;164:802–17.
16. Henderson JG. Denial and repression as factors in the delay of patients with cancer presenting themselves to the physician. Ann N Y Acad Sci. 1966;125:856–64.
17. Kallergis G. Using the denial mechanism to inform the cancer patient. J BUON. 2008;13:559–63.
18. Kortee KB, Wegener ST. Denial of illness in medical rehabilitation populations: theory, research, and definition. Rehabil Psychol. 2004;49(3):187–99.
19. Kreitler S. Denial in cancer patients. Cancer Invest. 1999;17:514–34.
20. Kunkel EJ, Woods CM, Rodgers C, Myers RE. Consultations for 'maladaptive denial of illness' in patients with cancer: psychiatric disorders that result in noncompliance. Psychooncology. 1997;6:139–49.
21. Leigh H, Ungerer J, Percarpio B. Denial and helplessness in cancer patients undergoing radiation therapy: sex differences and implications for prognosis. Cancer. 1980;45:3086–9.
22. Levine J, Zigler E. Denial and self-image in stroke, lung cancer, and heart disease patients. J Consult Clin Psychol. 1975;43:751–7.
23. Lowenstein J. The midnight meal and other essays about doctors, patients, and medicine. New Haven: Yale University Press; 1997.

24. Maguire P, Faulkner A. Communicate with cancer patients: 2. Handling uncertainty, collusion, and denial. BMJ. 1988;297:972–4.
25. Nelson DV, Friedman LC, Baer PE, Lane M, Smith FE. Attitudes of cancer: psychometric properties of fighting spirit and denial. J Behav Med. 1989;12:341–55.
26. Phelan M, Dobbs J, David AS. 'I thought it would go away': patient denial in breast cancer. J R Soc Med. 1992;85:206–7.
27. Rabinowitz T, Peirson R. "Nothing is wrong, doctor": understanding and managing denial in patients with cancer. Cancer Invest. 2006;24:68–76.
28. Reich M, Gaudron C, Penel N. When cancerophobia and denial lead to death. Palliat Support Care. 2009;7:253–5.
29. Ross DM, Peteet JR, Medeiros C, Walsh-Burke K, Rieker P. Difference between nurses' and physicians' approach to denial in oncology. Cancer Nurs. 1992;15:422–8.
30. Roy R, Symonds RP, Kumar DM, Ibrahim K, Mitchell A, Fallowfield L. The use of denial in an ethnically diverse British cancer population: a cross-sectional study. Br J Cancer. 2005;92:1393–7.
31. Salander P, Windahl G. Does 'denial' really cover our everyday experiences in clinical oncology? A critical view from a psychoanalytic perspective on the use of 'denial'. Br J Med Psychol. 1999;72:267–79.
32. Sharf BF, Stelljes LA, Gordon HS. 'A little bitty spot and I'm a big man': patients' perspectives on refusing diagnosis or treatment for lung cancer. Psychooncology. 2005;14:636–46.
33. Siemerink EJ, Jaspers JP, Plukker JT, Mulder NH, Hospers GA. Retrospective denial as a coping method. J Clin Psychol Med Settings. 2011;18:65–9.
34. Spinetta JJ, Maloney LJ. The child with cancer: patterns of communication and denial. J Consult Clin Psychol. 1978;46:1540–1.
35. Srivastava R. Denial. N Engl J Med. 2009;360:1174–7.
36. Stephenson PS. Understanding denial. Oncol Nurs Forum. 2004;31:985–8.
37. Vos MS, de Haes JC. Denial in cancer patients, an explorative review. Psychooncology. 2007;16:12–25.
38. Vos MS, Putter H, Leurs A, Rooijmans HG, de Haes HC, van Houwelingen HC. The denial of cancer interview: development and first assessment of psychometric properties in lung cancer patients. Patient Educ Couns. 2007;67:224–34.
39. Vos MS, Putter H, van Houwelingen HC, de Haes HC. Denial in lung cancer patients: a longitudinal study. Psychooncology. 2008;17:1163–71.
40. Vos MS, Putter H, van Houwelingen HC, de Haes HC. Denial and physical outcomes in lung cancer patients, a longitudinal study. Lung Cancer. 2010;67:237–43.
41. Vos MS, Putter H, van Houwelingen HC, de Haes HC. Denial and social and emotional outcomes in lung cancer patients: the protective effect of denial. Lung Cancer. 2011;72:119–24.
42. Wool MS. Extreme denial in breast cancer patients and capacity for object relations. Psychother Psychosom. 1986;46:196–204.

Chapter 3
Managing Uncertainty

Lidia Schapira

Abstract Handling and managing uncertainty provide an additional communication challenge for patients with cancer and their physicians. Addressing and treating not only physical symptoms but also distress, anxiety, and fear are vital to a good outcome. Doctors need to recognize the importance of providing structure and a safe relationship to facilitate coping and can do so through clear and supportive communication.

Keywords Communication • Uncertainty • Language • Framing • Empathy • Research

Therapeutic Value of Communication

A good therapeutic relationship begins when patient and doctor meet, typically face to face, and negotiate the nature of their partnership, including expectations and hopes for the future. From the patient's perspective, this is both meaningful and important, since it will serve as a source of solace and guidance as events unfold. Patients often remember the doctor's words verbatim as well as accompanying gestures and facial expressions years later.

It is during that first meeting that doctor and patient explore through verbal and nonverbal communication just how they will share both power and information, according to their individual style and preference and prevailing cultural norms. Patients bring their own agenda and worldview and vary greatly in their need for information and preference for involvement in decision making. When it comes to

---

L. Schapira, MD (✉)
Harvard Medical School, Massachusetts General Hospital,
55 Fruit Street, Boston, MA 02114, USA
e-mail: lschapira@partners.org

communication and relationships, one size certainly does not fit all. Some are unprepared to handle the complexity of diagnostic and treatment choices and to navigate the medical establishment. Others may be ready to address in detail and with expertise the pathophysiology of disease, to ask sophisticated questions about prognosis, and handle complicated statistical information. And yet, regardless of whether the patient is ready or not and whether he/she appears calm or overwhelmed, physicians know the first step is to build rapport, a requisite to establishing a trusting and therapeutic alliance. Surgeons called to relieve a bowel obstruction, oncologists attending a patient with acute leukemia, and radiation oncologists consulted on a patient with cord compression understand the importance of establishing instant rapport and trust.

If the patient does not trust the physician's expertise or if the relationship did not get off to a good start, any mention of uncertainty can be misunderstood as a personal admission of ignorance. As scientists and medical professionals, we are accustomed to dealing with uncertainty on many levels and accept both our personal capacity for error and also understand the limitations of our collective knowledge base. We are used to handling estimates of probabilities of treatment success or failure and to sort through options for treatment. We endorse the need for research and view it as a gateway to progress, even if it introduces additional uncertainty and complexity.

We cannot expect patients to understand our logic or share our enthusiasm for research. Many patients have a limited understanding of biology and scientific methods and may misinterpret any discussion of uncertain benefit or unpredictable outcome as an admission of ignorance. They may also harbor unrealistic expectations nurtured by media reports that exaggerate professional prowess and a popular culture of optimism that has little tolerance for ambiguity [1]. So if a physician explains there is no curative treatment or no established treatment and then says he will try one thing first and then another, the patient may get the erroneous impression that he is improvising or trivializing what is experienced as a personal disaster.

Oncologists and other specialist clinicians involved in the care of patients with cancer need to provide guidance to patients who find themselves facing new and threatening circumstances in an environment that is not always secure and where, despite best efforts, a good outcome cannot be guaranteed. This unpredictability is hard to accept even under the best of circumstances and much harder for somebody feeling anxious, overwhelmed, and terrified or devoid of social supports. The physician needs to create a platform of safety, a temporary "refuge" from the turbulence of diagnosis and from that vantage point begin the work of charting a path that eventually leads to the resolution of uncertainty.

Thus, the starting point for the clinician's work is to create a semblance of order and to provide guidance in a period of turbulence; to model for patient and family how to seek information, prioritize data, and make good decisions; and finally to offer an empathic and steadfast presence for the duration of the illness.

From Safety to Uncertainty

It may be a new cancer diagnosis or news of relapse or even a serious complication of treatment. Such bad and sad news disrupts routines with the fury of a natural disaster, at times accompanied by physical symptoms that demand immediate attention. Normalcy is interrupted, as patients and families face multiple threats and losses, while thrust into situations that require decisive actions and fortitude. Things previously taken for granted, such as health, employment, or the promise of a normal lifespan, are endangered. Some individuals cope by focusing their attention on matters at hand, while others find comfort in gathering information and planning for what lies ahead [2]. Under these circumstances, many doctors hesitate to discuss the ambiguity of a medical prognosis for fear of causing additional distress, which may decompensate a very precarious status quo [1]. Some respond by providing reassurance or adopting a paternalistic approach, perhaps an instinctive reaction intended to soothe. However, such paternalism could actually ricochet, causing harm if the patient is not given an opportunity to come to terms with the reality of the situation. Doctors often fear that mentioning the possibility of an untoward outcome or acknowledging uncertainty can increase the patient's anxiety and lead to distress. While it is true that anxiety can increase at first, most individuals with normal coping skills can and do find ways to move beyond the initial shock [3, 4]. This emotional work can be facilitated by supportive friends or relatives and by trained professionals and can be transformative.

Doctors and patients sometimes collude to avoid discussions of prognosis in ways that appear harmless at the outset, but lead to important misunderstandings and distortions of meaning as the situation unfolds and time runs out [5]. Talk of death used to be avoided by physicians or referred to indirectly and with intentional ambiguity. Instead of talking about death, loss, or disability, many doctors and patients prefer to talk about results of tests, medications, or options for further treatment [5]. Dodging conversations about death have been shown to lead to excessive technical interventions in the final days and hours of life [6]. It also leaves patients and families unprepared to handle emergencies or to have control over the final "chapter" of life, which many have described as a time for closure and peace [7]. Studies have documented that silence and evasion of frank discussions between doctor and patient have important consequences, such as late referral to hospice or the use of futile chemotherapy in the final days of life [6]. If doctor and patient cannot openly admit the gravity of the situation, they often resort to what is familiar to both: more treatment or more testing. This can even lead to iatrogenic complications, such as toxicity from treatment or harm caused by what turn out to be futile invasive procedures [8]. Avoidance leaves the patient at risk of learning vital information from a total stranger. It is not uncommon for patients with little insight or inadequate information to hear about the extent of their malignancy from an emergency room physician or a covering doctor called on a weekend. This can be construed as a form of abandonment and again lends support to the concept that having a difficult conversation is in fact kinder and more honest than avoidance and deceit [9].

What doctors say and what patients believe they heard are often quite different. Patients may not be able to process complex information either because they simply do not understand it or because they are too anxious to listen. Since doctors commonly use medical jargon and abbreviations that are incomprehensible even to an educated layperson, it is quite likely that during many consultations very little substantial information is actually understood [10]. A charismatic physician may have his patient's rapt attention, but that individual may just be comforted by listening to the "music" of the doctor's speech and nod appreciatively without fully understanding the message. Decisions are often made based on eagerness to follow the doctor's recommendation rather than through rational assessment of available information. The degree of patient involvement and participation in decision making varies considerably, and so does the level of satisfaction with consultations [11]. To ensure that a patient is truly informed, the doctor needs to check the patient's understanding by asking explicit questions and also by paying attention to casual remarks, which may give away hidden concerns or misconceptions. Simply put, doctor and patient need to be coeditors of a joint narrative in which goals are aligned and expectations conform to a realistic view of the future.

Individuals are unique in the way they experience the threat of illness and in how they come to terms with the anticipation of future loss. Clinicians cannot predict the level of existential distress a person feels by knowing only the medical diagnosis or the stage or type of a given cancer. One cannot make any assumptions about a patient's ability to bear a serious illness without a detailed exploratory interview. Recent research indicates that oncologists often miss important cues that reflect worry and concern [12, 13]. Audiotapes of clinic visits show doctors miss many opportunities to provide empathic and supportive comments, although the reasons cannot be properly surmised from such studies [12, 14]. It is quite likely that such failures to communicate verbal empathy stem from a variety of personal attributes and characteristics of the doctor and that they are influenced by context and environment. Time pressures can influence the doctor's demeanor, or worry about another sick patient may be temporarily distracting and cause the doctor to be inattentive. It is also important to recognize that empathy is conveyed not just verbally, but through facial expressions and body language; and these subtle but fundamental gestures can be missed in behavioral research that measures only the dialogue between patient and doctor [15].

Transforming a Threat into a Challenge

The medical culture values clarity and precision; and yet, surprisingly, there is no agreement on how best to convey prognostic information or how to discuss uncertain outcomes [1, 16, 17]. Each individual clinician is left to find expressions or statistics that best convey risk and orient a patient towards a particular treatment. Given the same medical scenario, one patient and doctor may opt for hospice care, another for intensive chemotherapy, and a third for an early-phase experimental treatment. How much depends on the physician's recommendation and how much reflects the patient's orientation and understanding is not adequately captured in medical records and has never been systematically addressed.

From a practical perspective, doctors work best when they have a clear concept of both task and process. One approach learned in communication workshops that I have found useful in practice is to encourage a patient to think of the existential and personal threat to his integrity and survival as a challenge. *While threats can be paralyzing and frightening, challenges typically can be met and resolved.* Interventions that bolster the patient's coping mechanisms, resources, and supportive relationships are then deployed to meet his or her needs. In getting to know a patient, it is very helpful to understand how he has met prior challenges and what he considers his sources of strength. Understanding what matters to an individual and where she feels comfortable asking for help is indispensable to assist her as the illness unfolds. New paradigms for cancer care now recognize the multidimensional aspects of the patient's experience and the importance of supporting the patient's psychological, emotional, and spiritual needs [18]. In addition to the medical staff, social workers and psychologists can provide expert evaluation and support for the patient and family unit and connect them to local resources available in the community.

Coaching interventions can be very helpful and lend themselves to creative adaptations designed to meet individual challenges [19]. A common technique involves the use of reflective language—reflecting back the patient's own words. Other techniques involve solution-focused approaches and problem solving, which may be very appealing to those looking for cognitive-based coping strategies [20, 21]. Goals first need to be defined in order to be met. Members of the multidisciplinary team can be trained to provide psychoeducation and encouragement in order to allow patients to deal with bothersome symptoms and better advocate for themselves. For instance, a nurse working in a chemotherapy infusion unit or in a radiation oncology department who has frequent contact with a patient can coach him to recognize certain symptoms and to deal with pain in an organized and effective manner and, in so doing, to become more involved in making decisions about his own care.

Providing information without guidance may actually increase anxiety. Patients need to have a certain amount of knowledge about their cancer, but also to learn how to communicate with their physician and to solve clinical problems [22]. If uncertainty is experienced as isolating, it can have profound consequences on mood and outlook. On the other hand, if patients are able to express their own fears openly and with clarity, then health professionals can provide useful information and perhaps assuage their concerns. Nurses and doctors can help patients by teaching them how to report and rate their pain and even their degree of emotional distress. Attending to quality of life requires a constant dialogue and partnership between patient and professional and a clear interchange of information that allows for a personalized and attentive treatment plan. Doctors can also point out natural landmarks in the disease trajectory and convey prognostic information in a way that is meaningful to each individual patient.

Family meetings can help mitigate conflict and mediate between relatives with very different values or perspectives. They serve as conduits for ensuring that everybody involved has access to the same information and provide face-to-face contact between professional staff and relatives. In situations where there is hostility or great tension within the family unit, a family meeting can help restore a semblance of order and establish clear goals of care based on realistic expectations of future recovery and function. Another useful aspect is simply to provide faces to professional caregivers, thus humanizing the experience and perhaps leading to greater confidence on the part of loving and fearful relatives. Parents of young children have expressed the view that it is important to them to have doctors ask about their family, and many feel it is important for their minor children to meet their professional caregivers.

It always helps to know the patient as a person and to have an understanding of her beliefs and values [23]. Providing specific examples of how other individuals and families have made important decisions can be useful, as well as helping patients understand the consequences of individual decisions and consider alternatives. It is essential to present choices, even if it entails drawing subtle distinctions between treatments or contrasting one to another. When patients are involved in decision making and feel they crafted their own plan of care, they are more likely to accept events with equanimity. Individuals sometimes bring complicated emotional baggage in addition to a medical diagnosis. Professional teams have no choice but to accept and deal with personal and family conflict and work towards a resolution that preserves the patient's integrity and conforms to her preferences for care.

Language and Framing

Medical oncologists confront uncertainty in every clinical encounter and become familiar with the nuances of not knowing. Yet the language they use to convey doubt and uncertainty with colleagues and at medical conferences is quite different from that which they use daily with patients and families. The greatest clinical challenge is to craft a relationship with each patient that feels safe and yet allows the expression of uncertainty without despair [16].

Medical jargon is full of qualifiers and expressions that may be confusing to patients [10]. For instance, a doctor will say a biopsy is "negative" and by that means there is no cancer or disease, which is good news for the patient [9]. Or a doctor may use a word such as "progress," typically associated with evolution and growth except when it refers to the advance of cancer and heralds a clinical deterioration. There is no quantitative linguistic research that captures the frequency with which doctors use words such as "possibly" and "maybe" in routine medical practice, although intelligent illness narratives provide insightful commentary [24].

Framing, on the other hand, has been studied extensively in medical contexts. Framing is about presenting an issue in a specific light and from a specific perspective and is a useful technique to mobilize the audience. Negative framing can work to motivate people to become active. A loss frame, such as presenting statistics for mortality from cancer, becomes a more urgent call to action and points out what can happen if no action is taken. Positive or gain frames point out the potential gain while emphasizing good things that will happen when something specific is done. Positive frames provide hope; negative frames are ideally suited to express the urgency and need of intervention. Physicians understand this and choose the way they express news and vital health information to influence patients [25]. Studies of conversations between doctors and patients with incurable cancer have shown that their dialogue often focuses on the generalities of treatment instead of the details of the disease itself and that indirect language is often used to buffer the bad news about the disease-related prognosis [26]. Given the reported variations in use of language and framing, it is not surprising that patients and doctors often give discordant accounts of what was actually communicated.

Awareness of simple communication principles can assist oncologists in finding the most appropriate and compassionate way of presenting complex and threatening information. Being mindful of language and the ambiguities inherent in communicating about prognosis and recognizing that the way information is framed is likely to have an impact on decision making can make an enormous difference in how much patients actually understand.

Dealing with Emotion

Patients with advanced cancer often experience intense emotions, such as sadness, fear, anxiety, or anger, that can impair function and impact negatively on their emotional well-being and quality of life [27–29]. Many patients find relief in discussing emotional concerns with their oncologists and prefer seeing physicians who are willing to address such concerns [13]. Studies have shown that very brief but genuine expressions of empathy and compassion provide reassurance and comfort and help patients bear the burden of negative emotions [30]. When oncologists recognize and attend to distress, patients report improved quality of life, are more likely to follow treatment plans, and seem more satisfied and willing to disclose future concerns [27, 31].

Doctors respond to emotion in a number of ways, ranging from detachment to genuine concern and engagement [32]. An empathic manner is no "quaint relic of the past" [15], but an invaluable skill that ensures trust and helps patients get through very difficult times. One legacy of medical education is overvaluing scientific measurement and undervaluing subjective experiences [15]. Fortunately, the study of empathy is no longer a soft science, but is increasingly grounded in empirical data [15]. Research indicates that patients and physicians are highly reactive to each other, producing physiological responses that can vary together in concordance or in discordance [15]. Fascinating advances in neuroscience provide a physiological model for understanding the brain activity that regulates behaviors and feelings [15]. Moreover, "feeling another's pain" is not just a figure of speech, because in fact people actually do feel it through neural pain representations in their own brain [15]. A trained observer of pain can experience it in such a way that it triggers an empathic response without overwhelming the professional with personal distress [15]. Empathy appears to be regulated by perspective taking and cognitive appraisal and is influenced by experience, training, and exposure. In fact, empathy research shows it is downregulated in those with constant exposure to others' pain and distress, likely a protective and unconscious mechanism, but nonetheless with alarming repercussions for patients. Lack of empathy can have profound clinical consequences and affect patient outcomes (Kenifer) [15].

Research shows that oncologists often ignore rather than address emotions and are more likely to respond to intense sadness than to fear or anger [12, 31, 33] (Kenifer). Perhaps this is because sadness draws more sympathy and does not present a personal challenge to the oncologist's competence. However, patients often include expressions of fear, which is not surprising in the context of uncertainty (Kenifer). In response to expressions of fear and anger, oncologists in one study often addressed the underlying biomedical cause of the emotion rather than the emotion itself (Kenifer) [14]. This is in keeping with the fact that most people avoid dealing with fear appeals and highlights the need for training physicians to respond appropriately to such important concerns [13, 34]. Interestingly, when oncologists responded to emotion with empathic responses, the discussions lasted 21 s on average before moving on to a different topic (Kenifer). If the oncologist ignored the emotion and moved to a factual topic, the majority of patients did not raise the same emotion again during the visit, having learned that it will not elicit any validation or reassurance (Kenifer).

Hiding from emotion or turning one's back on another's pain is experienced as uncaring. In sorting through the complex emotions that arise for patients facing a life-threatening illness, physicians need to understand their own feelings and deal with personal failure, frustration, or sadness before attending to others'. A useful analogy is that of a mother who, facing a change in cabin pressure during airplane travel, first places an oxygen mask on her own face before attending to her infant. Physicians working in emotionally charged disciplines such as oncology are constantly exposed to loss and suffering, and this can deplete their empathic abilities and the level of hopefulness they convey to patients and can lead to burnout. This factor needs to be considered in interpreting their poor performance in the research studies previously discussed.

Uncertainty and Medical Research

Managing uncertainty takes on a whole new dimension in medical research. Sources of uncertainty multiply and need to be addressed. In the setting of early-phase clinical trials, there is very little data to guide a conversation about likely benefits—both to the individual and to society. Physician-researchers need to provide a rationale for the study or treatment and describe how results might lead to future benefit for other cancer patients and, at the same time, provide reassurance to the individual that his needs will be met and he will be properly cared for. For studies of drug toxicity, this poses important ethical and communication challenges for the doctors who often "persuade" patients to enroll and provide an atmosphere of positivity and excitement that is based not on evidence but on hopefulness.

There is considerable literature supporting the notion that patients enrolled in early-phase clinical trials do not properly understand the intention of research and have inaccurate representations of possible personal benefit [35–39]. Healthcare professionals are sometimes confused themselves about the prospect of medical benefit to the individual participant [36, 40, 41]. To help patients better understand their own expectation of benefit can be quite challenging, especially if the physician and patient have already resolved to push ahead with enrollment into the study. Many patients decide to participate because they are drawn by the message of positivity, the promise of innovation, and the hope for a transformative result [11, 37, 38]. In a recent British study of the communication and informed consent process for phase I clinical trials, researchers found that in several key areas, information was either missing or had been explained but was interpreted incorrectly by patients [37]. They identified eight key issues that needed to be addressed: prognosis, other options for care, the aims of the trial, medical benefits, the extra effort involved, unknown adverse effects, the voluntary nature of participation, and the right to withdraw. Discussion of prognosis was a frequent omission [36]. This research points to common "gaps" in information and communication practices, and it is likely that they are indeed quite common.

Although less dramatic, patients enrolled in randomized clinical trials also accept an additional dimension of uncertainty. By choosing to be assigned by chance alone to a standard treatment or a new protocol, they are perhaps guided, too, by their doctor's persuasive recommendation or their own desire to contribute to medical progress. Many may not understand that the experimental treatment may, in fact, be less effective than the standard. Motivations vary, as do personal choices. It is to a certain extent quite remarkable that, under great personal stress, many individuals are able to make such complex and meaningful decisions. Others are almost paralyzed by indecision and may need a more directive approach in addition to emotional support. For the purpose of our discussion on uncertainty, suffice it to say that issues raised during conversations with patients considering treatment in a clinical trial will likely evoke additional questions and concerns regarding estimates of personal benefit or harm and pose intellectually and emotionally important new challenges.

Conclusion

Individuals vary in their capacity to bear uncertainty. Cancer patients express various emotions as they are confronted with complex decisions and receive important news that affect their life. Doctors need to work towards creating an atmosphere of safety that provides a refuge from the chaos and turbulence brought on by life-threatening illness. Conversations need to focus on the patient's needs for information and support and need to be structured in such a way as to convey information with clarity and precision. Negative and positive framing of health information has important behavioral consequences, and this needs to be used strategically by physicians when they convey complex information and present options for treatment. Finally, empathic and compassionate communication is not a cliché or a nostalgic appeal to a simpler era, but a *sine qua non* for an enduring and therapeutic relationship between patient and doctor.

Disclosure I have no disclosures regarding funding or sources of support.

References

1. Christakis NA. Death foretold. Prophecy and prognosis in medical care. Chicago, IL: The University of Chicago Press; 1999.
2. Spiegel D. A 43 year-old woman coping with cancer. JAMA. 1999;28(4):371–8.
3. Weisman AD, Worden JW. The existential plight in cancer: significance of the first 100 days. Int J Psychiatry Med. 1976–1977;7(1):1–15.
4. Weisman AD, Worden JW. The emotional impact of cancer recurrence. J Psychosoc Oncol. 1985;3:5–16.
5. The AM, Hak T, Koeter G, et al. Collusion in doctor-patient communication about imminent death: an ethnographic study. BMJ. 2000;321:1376-81.
6. Earle CC, Landrum MB, Souza JM, et al. Aggressiveness of cancer care near the end of life: is it a quality of care issue? J Clin Oncol. 2008;26(23):3860–6.
7. Block SD. Perspectives on care at the close of life. Psychological considerations, growth, and transcendence at the end of life: the art of the possible. JAMA. 2001;285(22):2898–905.
8. Gadgeel SM. Hope and realism: the perfect balance? J Clin Oncol. 2011;29(16):2291–2.
9. Fallowfield L. Truth sometimes hurts but deceit hurts more. In: Surbone A, Zwitter M, editors. Communication with the cancer patient, vol. 809. New York: The New York Academy of Sciences; 1997. p. 525–36.
10. Chapman K, Abraham C, Jenkins V, et al. Lay understanding of terms used in cancer consultations. Psychooncology. 2003;12:557–66.
11. Brown RF, Hill C, Burant CJ. Satisfaction of early breast cancer patients with discussions during initial consultations with a medical oncologist. Psychooncology. 2009;18(1):42–9.
12. Pollak KI, Arnold RM, Jeffreys AS. Oncologist communication about emotion during visits with patients with advanced cancer. J Clin Oncol. 2007;25:5748–52.
13. Kennifer SL, Alexander SC, Pollak KI, et al. Negative emotions in cancer care: do oncologists' responses depend on severity and type of emotion. Patient Educ Couns. 2009;76(1):51–6.
14. Levinson W, Gorawara-Bhat R, Lamb J. A study of patient clues and physician response in primary care and surgical settings. JAMA. 2000;284:1021–7.
15. Riess H. Empathy in medicine—a neurobiological perspective. JAMA. 2010;304(14):1604–5.
16. Schapira L, Butow P, Brown R. Pessimism is no poison. J Clin Oncol. 2010;28(4):705–7.
17. Schapira L. Shared uncertainty. J Support Oncol. 2004;2(1):14–8.
18. Institute of Medicine. Cancer care for the whole patient: meeting psychosocial health needs. Bethesda: The National Academies Press; 2007 http://www.iom.edu.
19. Kravitz RL, Tancredi DJ, Grennan T, et al. Cancer health empowerment for living without pain (Ca-HELP): effects of a tailored education and coaching intervention on pain and impairment. Pain. 2011;152(7):1572–82.

20. Cella DF. Health promotion in oncology: a cancer wellness doctrine. J Health Care Chaplain. 1992;4:87–101.
21. Yellen SB, Cella DF. Someone to live for: social well-being, parenthood status, and decision-making in oncology. J Clin Oncol. 1995;13:1255–64.
22. Mishel MH, Germino BB, Lin L, et al. Managing uncertainty about treatment decision making in early stage prostate cancer: a randomized clinical trial. Patient Educ Couns. 2009;77(3):349–59.
23. Kleinman A. What really matters. Living a moral life amidst uncertainty and danger. Oxford: Oxford University Press; 2006.
24. Diamond J. Because cowards get cancer too: a hypochondriac confronts his nemesis. New York: Crown; 1999.
25. Hilbig B. Sad, thus true: negativity bias in judgements of truth. J Exp Soc Psychol. 2009;45(4):983–6.
26. Rodriguez KL, Gambino F, Butow P, et al. It's going to shorten your life: framing of oncologist–patient communication about prognosis. Psychooncology. 2008;17(3):219–25.
27. Heaven CM, Maguire P. Disclosure of concerns by hospice patients and their identification by nurses. Palliat Med. 1997;11:283–90.
28. Parle M, Jones B, Maguire P. Maladaptive coping and affective disorders among cancer patients. Psychol Med. 1996;26:735–44.
29. Epstein RM, Street RL. Patient-centered communication in cancer care: promoting healing and reducing suffering. NIH Publication No 07-6225. Bethesda, MD: National Cancer Institute; 2007.
30. Fogarty LA, Curbow BA, Wingard JR, et al. Can 40 seconds of compassion reduce anxiety? J Clin Oncol. 1999;17:371–9.
31. Ford S, Fallowfield L, Lewis S. Can oncologists detect distress in their out-patients and how satisfied are they with their performance during bad news consultations? Br J Cancer. 1994;70:767–77.
32. Halpern J. From detached concern to empathy. Humanizing medical practice. New York: Oxford University Press; 2001.
33. Friedrichsen MJ, Strang PM. Doctors' strategies when breaking bad news to terminally ill patients. J Palliat Med. 2003;6:565–74.
34. Witte K, Allen M. A meta-analysis of fear appeals: implications for effective public health campaigns. Health Educ Behav. 2000;27:591–615.
35. Weinfurt KP, Seils DM, Tzeng JP, et al. Expectations of benefit in early-phase clinical trials: implications for assessing the adequacy of informed consent. Med Decis Making. 2008;28:575–81.
36. Miller FG, Joffe S. Benefit in phase I oncology trials: therapeutic misconception or reasonable treatment option? Clin Trials. 2008;5(6):617–23.
37. Jenkins V, Solis-Trapala I, Langridge C, et al. What oncologists believe they said and what patients believe they heard: an analysis of phase I trial discussions. J Clin Oncol. 2011;29(1):61–8.
38. Brown R, Bylund C, Siminoff LA, et al. Seeking informed consent to phase I cancer clinical trials: identifying oncologists' communication strategies. Psychooncology. 2011;20(4):361–8.
39. Albrecht TL, Eggly S, Gleason ME. Influence on clinical communication on patients' decision-making on participation in clinical trials. J Clin Oncol. 2008;26(16):2666–73.
40. Weinfurt KP. Varieties of uncertainty and the validity of informed consent. Clin Trials. 2008;5:624–5.
41. Kass NE. Early phase clinical trials: communicating the uncertainties of magnitude of benefit and likelihood of benefit. Clin Trials. 2008;5:627.

Chapter 4
Ethical Issues in Disclosing Bad News to Cancer Patients: Reflections of an Oncologist in Saudi Arabia

Ali M. Al-Amri

Abstract Cancer is a complicated illness, which for many decades and in many cultures has been perceived as an incurable and devastating disease. Patients who receive a diagnosis of cancer are in a position of extreme uncertainty and vulnerability. Breaking such bad news is not an easy task. Doctors face particular difficulties when breaking bad news to cancer patients especially at the time of disclosing or discussing the diagnosis. Sometimes doctors collude with the relatives of cancer patients to protect the patients from the bad news. Mutual trust and respect enable better management and implementation of the treatment plan. Since doctors expect patients to tell the truth, similarly, patients expect doctors to give truthful information about their illness. Therefore, the mutual relationship between cancer patients and doctors depends on the establishment of trust and honesty, which are strongly connected with truthful communication. Truth disclosure should be considered the first step toward a good doctor–patient relationship and the basis for any decision-making in treating cancer. Culture should not be a barrier to realistic, honest, good communication, which can reduce uncertainty and anxiety, improve compliance, and avoid false information. Uncertainty or doubts do not offer a better relationship. The patients' attitude and view about truth-telling, confidentiality, and autonomy should take precedence and be respected over and above anybody else's view. Choosing the right time and place and lending hope through successful therapy, pain relief, and emerging new drugs can lead to better outcomes. The aim of this chapter is to view the world as a single unit and all patients as one.

Keywords Truth • Cancer • Patients • Bad news • Relatives

A.M. Al-Amri (✉)
Department of Internal Medicine and Oncology, King Fahd Hospital of the University,
Makkah Street, P.O. Box 40182, Al-Khobar 31952, Saudi Arabia
e-mail: aliamri49@hotmail.com

Introduction

The basic four principles of ethics in medicine include autonomy, beneficence, nonmalfeasance, and justice [1, 2]. Factors that could affect the furthering of these principles during communication with cancer patients include the emotions of physicians and patients, religion, social and cultural factors, and, not least, the strength of the bond between family members.

Communicating bad news to cancer patients can be approached from three positions: First, the nondisclosure model (paternalism), in which the doctors decide what is best for the cancer patients. Second, the full-disclosure model (consumerism), in which the doctors give full information; this approach stresses the right of the cancer patient to know the truth and to take part in decision-making. Third, the flexible approach (the individualized disclosure model), in which the amount of information disclosed should be selected and tailored according to the preferences of each cancer patient [3].

There are no obvious, clear objective measures by which to select which approach is the best for patients, physicians, relatives of the patients, and the community as a whole. The truth may be brutal, but the telling of it should not be.

In this chapter, we will review seven issues: (1) truth-telling from the historical perspective; (2) tradition; (3) religion; (4) truth communication in relation to: (a) patients, (b) relatives, (c) physicians, (d) the community; (5) the importance of truth in ethics, (6) policy and law, and (7) prognosis. Finally, we have a summary.

The History of Breaking Bad News

Hippocrates, considered the father of medicine, advised that most information should be withheld from the patients, and that only what is necessary for the patients to know should be selected for them. The first code of ethics of the American Medical Association (1847) recommended that physicians should not discourage the patient and depress his/her spirits with gloomy prognostications. This was not different from Hippocrates's advice for physicians.

The Italian Medical Association code, written in 1989, stated that a bad prognosis can be hidden from the patients, but not from the relatives. It is similar to what has been mentioned above [4, 5].

The Lebanese Code of Medical Ethics, 1995, mandates that patients not be informed of their diagnosis if such disclosure would have a deleterious effect on their recovery. At the same time, the Lebanese law states that patients have the right to know their options for therapy and to refuse any of those options [6, 7].

Problems can arise if there are obscure statements, but many more problems can arise if there are discrepancies. More important, we have a dilemma if no clear code of medical ethics exists in the country or health care institution.

Tradition

In Saudi Arabia, the Arabic meaning of the word *cancer* is one of the following: (a) *warm* or *waram*, which means swelling, benign or malignant. However, when this word is used, it is frustrating; its meaning not clear. (b) In some regions, the question arises, Is this swelling male or female? This is to classify them as malignant or benign lesions, where a "male" tumor is malignant. (c) The word that is commonly used for malignant disease is *saratan*, the Arabic word for "crab." This word means, generally, bad prognosis, with no curative therapy and imminent death, because a crab has many claws, which can regenerate and grow. Since *saratan* is the most feared of all diseases, most physicians in Saudi Arabia avoid using this word in front of patients or their relatives.

Some Saudis believe there are mysterious causes of cancer. One of the common causes is *Al-Ain*. An *Al-Ain* in Arabic means a kind of miracle that relates to demons or bad spirits and inflicts diseases. Some patients describe this event as an electrical shot coming from an evil eye to cause cancer. Unfortunately, because of this belief, many patients waste a lot of time trying to heal *Al-Ain* with local healers and so arrive at the hospital with advanced cancer.

There is an impression that physicians will not tell the truth about cancer diagnosis and prognosis to patients or family members. Occasionally, this can lead to misunderstanding and mistrust, even though the patient has benign or curable cancer.

In this particular situation, as noted by Cabot [8], a true impression is not created in the mind of the patients.

This leads to mistrust, seeking a second opinion, irregular follow-up, and fear of therapy failure and the future. This is a result of not telling the truth and poor communication and affects the public confidence in the medical profession.

Furthermore, most female and elderly patients are considered "incompetent" persons, because in many cases they are neither financially independent nor educated; therefore, social power overruns patient autonomy.

Religion

False or misleading information is prohibited in all religions among normal and healthy people. How, then, can false information be given to weak and sick people? More important, how can true information about diagnosis, therapy options, and prognosis be replaced with false information?

The wise say the true path will lead to the best outcome.

The Torah says, Distance yourself from words of falsehood. The Safer Chassidim write that one who speaks only truth can actually change destiny; by decreeing something to happen, it will.

Ezekiel sanctioned the religious community because it did not meet its responsibility for truth-telling. Such lies, said Ezekiel, will lead to death.

Jesus said, I am the truth. He is teaching us to speak only truth; a lie is a sin against God.

In Buddhism, it was stated that one should utter the truth. In Hinduism as well, it is said, let your conduct be marked by truthfulness in word, deed, and thought.

In Confucianism, the Master said, Be loyal and true to your every word. Taoism advises that one should be honest like heaven in conducting one's affairs. In African traditional religions, Yoruba Proverbs say, If a lie runs for 20 years, it takes truth 1 day to catch up with it.

It is stated in the *Qur'an* that God instructs people to tell the truth as a sign of a person of faith, and whosoever tells lies is deprived of the luster and beauty of light upon their face.

Communication of the Truth

Patients

Patients from any area of the earth behave essentially the same. It is a misleading concept to divide human patients according to geographical area or cultural background. All patients have the same feelings and emotions. Studies in the West have shown that patients want the truth about the nature of their illness; there is no difference in that respect between Asians, Black, and White patients living in Western communities. Similar studies in other geographical areas showed almost identical results [9–18].

There were no significant differences between adult male, female, young, and elderly patients [13, 19, 20]. Furthermore, patients were dissatisfied with the level of information they generally received [21, 22].

Control of information is not the right way to preserve patients' hopefulness; lack of information increases the suspicion of serious disease, affecting patients' mood and consequently their ability to take decisions [17–21].

The patients' attitude toward the right to know their diagnosis has been constant over time: they want to be informed about their condition [13, 17, 18, 20–23].

However, the physicians' attitude has changed from not disclosing the truth to cancer patients (90%) in 1961 to disclosing it (97%) in 1987 [24–26]. This shift indicates "doing the right thing"; patients were right and have the right to be informed. The psychological well-being of the patients will never be optimized while they continue suffering from symptoms of which they do not know the causes.

The attitudes about disclosure of information on cancer are undergoing slow change in Saudi Arabia due to a communication revolution and globalization. However, studies have shown that 50% of cancer patients were informed that they had either "cancer" or a "tumor" [27]. A survey in Turkey showed similar findings: 52% of cancer patients did not know their diagnosis [28]. The majority of Saudi physicians preferred to talk with and inform close family members rather than the patients directly [29, 30]. Bedikian and Saleh interviewed 100 Saudi patients with malignant diseases and reported that the reaction of the patients to the diagnosis was distressing in 93% of them. He found that only 50% of the patients were told that they had either cancer or a tumor.

The first survey that was conducted to assess Saudi patients' preference toward disclosure of information on cancer found that 99% wished to know all the information about their cancer, and 100% rejected the idea of withholding any information. Most of the patients (77%) wanted their family to know the diagnosis, but a few (17%) wanted their friends to be informed. Almost all patients wanted to know both the benefits and adverse effects of therapy (98 and 99%, respectively). All patients wanted to be informed about the prognosis of their disease [12].

Relatives

Family members' attitude toward truth-telling to patients is variable, depending on differences in background, sex, age, strength of their relationship to the patient, and different interests. In general, they claim that they have known the patients for a long time and want to protect them. However, patients can say, We know ourselves better than they do.

One study in the West (United Kingdom) showed that all patients wished doctors to respect their views rather than those of their family members. Another study from the East (Taiwan) showed that cancer patients strongly proclaimed their superior rights over their family members and preferred their doctors to inform them before releasing any information to their relatives [31]. Furthermore, the attitude of family members toward disclosure of the patients' condition may differ [32]. Confidentiality is broken when information is given to family members rather than patients, and therefore patients' autonomy becomes at risk.

The information should be revealed to patients because it belongs to the patients, not their relatives. The best way to get out of this dilemma is to include as part of informed consent one more section: ask patients to indicate their preference about information disclosure with respect to their family members. Otherwise, the principle of informed consent will be violated.

Saudi cancer patients' family members trust and rely on health professionals as authority figures who will do what is best for their patients; but they need education about the benefits of truth-telling regarding cancer diagnosis disclosure—reducing uncertainty, avoiding deception, and providing a basis for action [33].

Saudi female cancer patients have some power but are offered much less autonomy than males. Most decisions concerning females are made by males, for the following reasons:

(a) Males consider females weak and vulnerable.
(b) The female is not independent financially.
(c) Women are housebound; they are not allowed to travel alone, or at least their mobility is restricted.

(d) Men want to minimize exposure of their female relatives to other males as much as possible (according to some religious interpretations).
(e) Women are afraid to defend themselves because of fear of forfeiting their relatives' protection.
(f) Women have no independent houses in which to live; they are not allowed to live alone; if they fail to obey, where they can go? (Women should not be left alone.)
(g) Absence of foundations to defend women's rights and of education to clarify women's rights; it is difficult to distinguish between a supportive attitude and a dominant attitude.

All of the above diminish female patients' right of knowledge and decision-making.

Physicians

Until 50 years ago, the majority of American physicians usually did not tell cancer patients their diagnosis. Nowadays, the debate in the USA is not whether cancer patients should be told the truth, but how and when to inform them of the truth. Physicians from many other countries still do not tell patients the full truth about the diagnosis and prognosis of their malignant diseases.

Four terms should be discussed in these issues: (1) the right to know; (2) the right not to know; (3) the right not to tell; and (4) the right to tell. It is important not to forget that physicians should do the right thing for the best interests of their patients. This should be the basis when breaking bad news. Studies have shown that patients can cope with disclosure of bad news related to their condition [34, 35]. However, patients may not cope well if they discover that they had been deceived.

If a patient comes to hospital complaining of symptoms, signs the informed consent to be informed and treated, is it right for the physician to withhold information? If the patient comes to the hospital to find out the causes of his symptoms, would it be valid to ask him/her to agree to not being told the truth? It is clear that patients have the right to know the cause of their symptoms; it is logical that no patient comes to a hospital not to know what is the cause of his/her condition. Otherwise, why come to the hospital? The consent form is just a validation of the patients' intent to know about their condition.

Asking physicians to decide whether or not to inform patients of their malignant diseases could affect their responsibility toward their patients, help physicians avoid the risks of telling bad news, and force their patients to seek information from different sources. This would mean decreasing the burden on physicians but increasing it on patients. It is evident that the vast majority of patients with cancer want disclosure of cancer diagnosis, irrespective of geography, ethnicity, or cultural background [12, 13, 17, 19, 20, 22, 23].

However, there is evidence that doctors fail to inform patients of their diagnosis of cancer [10, 23, 36, 37]. In Saudi Arabia, one study showed that only 47% of physicians provided information on the diagnosis and prognosis of a serious illness. The majority (75%) preferred to discuss this information with close relatives rather than patients, even when the patients were competent [29]. In a similar study, of cases of incurable cancer, 67% of doctors indicated that they would inform the patients of the diagnosis rather than the relatives [30]. In Kuwait, the great majority of physicians (79%) would withhold the truth if the patients' relative requested them to do so [38].

Community

Two studies interviewed adult healthy Saudi on their attitude and knowledge of cancer. These studies showed a high level of anxiety, fear, and misperception. The authors of these studies recommended health education for the general public and for them to be made aware that cancer is a treatable disease [27, 39].

Nowadays, in the era of the Internet, faxing reports for a second opinion, and increased level of education and awareness, information is not limited to the physician. Relatives of patients and patients themselves have a lot of information prior to, at the time of, and after diagnosis. The patient–doctor relationship is broken or weakened if the information provided by the doctor is untrue or inconsistent.

More important, patients or their relatives are more likely to ask for their medical report so that they may obtain a second opinion. There will be confusion if what they learn is different than what is written in the medical report. Patients may feel that the trust they placed in their physicians was misplaced if they discover or perceive a lack of honesty and candor by the physician if the information they had been given is inconsistent or untrue.

Not telling patients the truth about their medical condition probably entails deceiving them. All relatives and friends who know the story feel they could be deceived, too. In time, the community will come to disbelieve and disregard information from that physician or group of physicians. Therefore, lack of honesty or giving false information can undermine the public's confidence in the medical profession [40, 41]. Even if information about the illness of an individual patient is not considered to belong to the patient, the majority of respondents are in favor of disclosure of diagnosis and prognosis [28, 42–44].

The Importance of Truth

Ethics

The first book dedicated to medical ethics is *The Conduct of Physician*, by Ishag Bin Ali Rahawi. Thomas Percival wrote about medical jurisprudence and reportedly coined the phrase *medical ethics*. His work became the basis for the American

Medical Association Code of Ethics. Currently, the principles of medical ethics include:

(a) Autonomy. The right of the individual patient to know and make an informed decision either to refuse or accept the physician's recommendation. The decision will be inaccurate if information is withheld or false.
(b) Beneficence. To make the best effort for the best outcome for the patient. "Always do good."
(c) Nonmalfeasance. To make the best effort to avoid undesirable outcomes. "First do no harm." Violation of this term may result in malpractice.
(d) Justice. To treat all patients equally, irrespective of geography, religion, culture, and social class.
(e) Truthfullness and honesty. The concept of informed consent reconfirms the autonomy of the individual patient.

Inaccurate or false information will not enable patients to make the right choices about their illness and other aspects of their lives. Therefore, truth-telling becomes the cornerstone of the ethics of the medical profession: truth-telling is the preferred option; deception needs justification [45].

Policy and Law

The first thing patients do is sign an informed consent agreement, since no medical therapy may be undertaken unless the appropriate consent form has been signed and duly witnessed. It is recommended that if for any reason the patient is unable to sign the consent form, it should be signed by relatives on the patient's behalf. Informed consent includes the provision that all medical therapy and surgical procedures be fully explained to patients, including possible risks, complications, and alternative treatment. The patients should understand and have complete knowledge of all relevant facts. The explanation is to be given prior to giving informed consent.

All Saudi patients have the right to request at very short notice a medical report in either Arabic or English for obtaining a second opinion. False information can be difficult in practice, where it can create mistrust and break the doctor–patient relationship if what the patient hears is different from what is written in the medical report. More important, patients feel and understand that truth-telling is one of the physicians' responsibilities regarding informing patients about their condition [46, 47].

Saudi patients have no right of access to, nor are they allowed to see, their own medical records. However, as mentioned above, they have the right to get a medical report and get copies of all relevant investigations.

In our hospital, it is stated that medical records are the property of the hospital and shall not be removed without permission from the administration. Furthermore, the information contained in the medical records is confidential and will not be released to anyone without clearance from the administration. Requests from patients or their relatives for medical reports or copies of investigations will clear the above-mentioned restrictions, but patients may not see their own charts.

Prognosis

It is important to define the term *prognosis*. Prognosis can mean: (a) how a disease behaves and progresses in time; (b) when the patient will die; (c) both (a) and (b), without accounting for the activity of the patient's immune system or the emergence of new medications.

The definition of *qualitative prognosis*: the disease will lead to the death of the patient along with other causes; or the disease will be the only cause of the death of the patient.

The definition of *quantitative prognosis*: the length of time before the patient will die; the time of death, which may be caused by things not related to the current clinical condition. Considerable inaccuracy in doctors' prediction of the survival of an individual patient with incurable disease has been documented [48, 49].

It is important that when physicians communicate with patients, they be honest and limit their discussion to the diagnosis, options of therapy, and therapy complications, but not to reveal the cancer patient's gloomy future or to prophesy death unless the patient so desires.

Prognosis should be separated from consideration of death, since prognosis does not mean or equal death. Avoiding discussion of life expectancy or mention of death is an important way to foster trust and show respect for the patients. Patients place a great deal of trust in their physician's ability to diagnose and treat disease, not to talk about death.

Because of advances in cancer therapy and new emerging drugs, and because the causes of death are not limited to cancer per se, disclosing true information of cancer diagnosis and prognosis does not indicate imminent death. Studies have shown that patients want to be given prognostic information, in the form of chance of a cure, extent of the disease, and possible effects of therapy. Patients rate this information as important to them and necessary, even though they do not want to be told a bad prognosis or want their physicians to be specific about their prognosis [14, 16, 20, 23, 50–53]. These studies confirm the need to inform patients about their disease, not about death

Research on the relationship between truth disclosure and quality of life are limited. The available studies suggest that disclosure of cancer information does not affect the quality of the patient's life, at least not conclusively. However, other studies have shown that control of information is not necessarily effective in preserving patient hopefulness [17, 28, 54, 55]. In the presence of evidence that patients prefer truth-telling and the absence of obvious harm to their quality of life, it is deception that needs justification; truth-telling should be considered universally good for patients, family members, physicians, and the community.

Summary

The golden rule is to do the right thing. Breaking bad news of a cancer diagnosis will never be pleasant. Living with suspicions of a lethal condition and suffering from unrelieved symptoms without good news, while being surrounded by anxious friends and relatives, may make death happen even sooner. Unless withholding information is requested by the patient, it is unpleasant to demean and undermine patients' autonomy, since the information belongs to them. All patients everywhere should be treated equally and according to principles of medical ethics without exclusion if they can understand and sign informed consent. Patients are unable to take charge of their own care and make the right decision without awareness of and appropriate information about their condition.

References

1. Devita VT, Hellmon S, Rosenberg SA. Cancer principles and practice of oncology. 6th ed. Philadelphia: Lippincott Williams and Wilkins; 2001. p. 3126–7.
2. Engelhardt HT. The foundations of bioethics. 2nd ed. New York: Oxford University Press; 1996. p. 330.
3. De valck C, Bensing J, Bruynooghe R. Medical student's attitudes towards breaking bad news: an empirical test of the world health organization model. Psychooncology. 2001;10:398–409.
4. Hippocrates. Decorum. Jones W (Trans.). Hippocrates. Cambridge: Harvard University Press; 1967. p. 297.
5. Surbone A. Truth telling to the patients-letter from Italy. JAMA. 1992;268(13):1661–2.
6. Lebanese code of medical ethics. Decree 24. Journal Official Lebanais 1995 May.
7. Adib SM, Hamadeh GN. Attitudes of the Lebanese public regarding disclosure of serious illness. J Med Ethics. 1999;25:399–403.
8. Cabot RC. The use of truth and falsehood in medicine: an experimental study. Am Med. 1903;5:344–9.
9. Young HY, Chang L, Si-young K, Sang-wook L, Dae Seong H, et al. The attitudes of cancer patients and their family toward the disclosure of terminal illness. J Clin Oncol. 1995;22(2):307–14.
10. Muthu K, Symonds RP, Sunder S, Ibrahim K, Savelyich BSP, Miller E. Information needs for Asians and white British cancer patients and their families in Leicesterstershire: a cross sectional survey. Br J Cancer. 2004;90:1474–8.
11. Blackhall LJ, Murphy ST, Frank G, Michel V, Azen S. Ethnicity and attitudes toward patient autonomy. JAMA. 1995;274(10):820–5.
12. Al-Amri AM. Cancer patients desire for information: a study in a teaching hospital in Saudi Arabia. East Mediterr Health J. 2009;5(1):19–24.
13. Hagerty RG, Butow PN, Ellis PA, Lobb EA, Pendlebury S, Leighl N, et al. Cancer patient preferences for communication of prognosis in metastatic setting. J Clin Oncol. 2004;22:1721–30.
14. Meredith C, Symonds P, Webster L, Lamont D, Pyper E, Gillis CR, et al. Information needs of cancer patients in West Scotland: cross-sectional survey of patients views. BMJ. 1996;313:724–6.
15. Hari D, Mark Z, Bharati D, Khadka P. Patients' attitudes toward concept of right to know. Kathmandu Univ Med J. 2007;5(4):591–5.

16. Merriman L, Perez DJ, McGee R, Campbell AV. Receiving a diagnosis of cancer: the perceptions of patients. N Z Med J. 1997;110:297–8.
17. Cassileth BR, Zupkis RV, Sutton-Smith K, March V. Information and participation preference among cancer patients. Ann Intern Med. 1980;92:832–6.
18. Masood J, Beenish Q, Zubia M, Shaukat A. Disclosure of cancer diagnosis: Pakistani patient's perspective. Middle East J Cancer. 2010;1(2):89–94.
19. Ajaj A, Singh P, Abdulla J. Should elderly patients be told they have cancer? Questionnaire survey of older people. BMJ. 2001;323:1160–3.
20. Lobb EA, Kenny DT, Butow PN, Tattersall MH. Women's preferences for discussion of prognosis in early breast cancer. Health Expect. 2001;4:48–57.
21. Slevin ML. Talking about cancer: how much is too much. Br J Hosp Med. 1987;38:56–9.
22. Sapir R, Catane R, Kaufman B, Isacson R, Segal A, Wein S, et al. Cancer patients expectation of and communication with oncologists and oncology nurses: the experiences of an integrated oncology and palliative care service. Support Care Cancer. 2000;8:458–63.
23. Jenkine V, Fallowfield L, Saul J. Information needs for patients with cancer: results from a large study in UK cancer center. Br J Cancer. 2001;84:48–51.
24. Oken D. What to tell cancer patients. JAMA. 1961;175:1120–8.
25. Novack DH, Plumer R, Smith RL, Ochitill H, Morrow GR, Bennett JM. Changes in physician's attitudes toward telling the cancer patients. JAMA. 1979;241:897–900.
26. Holland JC, Geary N, Marchini A, Tross S. An international survey of physician's attitudes and practice in regard to revealing the diagnosis of cancer. Cancer Invest. 1987;5(2):151–4.
27. Bedikian AY, Saleh V, Ibrahim S. Saudi patients and companion attitudes toward cancer. King Faisal Spec Hosp Med J. 1985;5:17–25.
28. Bozcuk H, Erdoğan V, Eken C, Ciplak E, Samur M, Ozdoğan M, et al. Does awareness of diagnosis make any difference in quality of life? Determinant of emotional functioning in group of cancer patients in Turkey. Support Care Cancer. 2002;10(1):51–7.
29. Mobeireek AF, Al-Kassimi FA, Al-Majid SA, Al-Shimemry A. Communication with the seriously ill: physicians attitudes in Saudi Arabia. J Med Ethics. 1996;22:282–5.
30. Mobeireek AF, Al-Kassimi F, Al-Zahrani K, Al-Shimemeri A, Al-Damegh S, Al-Amoudi O, et al. Information disclosure and decision-making: the middle east versus far east and the west. J Med Ethics. 2008;34:225–9.
31. John B, Nicky B. Respecting the autonomy of cancer patients when talking with their families: qualitative analysis of semistructrured interviews with patients. BMJ. 1996;313:729–31.
32. Young Ho Y, Chang Geol L, Si-Young K, Sang-Wook L, Dae Seog H, Kim JS, et al. The attitude of cancer patients and their families toward the disclosure of terminal illness. J Clin Oncol. 2004;22(2):307–14.
33. Erlen JA. Should the nurse participate in planned deception? Orthop Nurs. 1995;14(2):62–6.
34. Lazarus RS. Positive denial: the care for not facing reality. Psychol Today. 1979;13:44–5.
35. Atiken-Swan J, Easson EC. Reactions of cancer patients on being told their diagnosis. Br Med J. 1959;1:779–83.
36. Mosconi P, Meyerowitz BE, Liberati MC, Liberati A. GIVIO. Disclosure of breast cancer diagnosis, patients and physicians reports. Ann Oncol. 1991;2:273–80.
37. Thompsen OO, Wulff HR, Martin A, Singer PA. What do gasteroenterologists in Europe tell cancer patients? Lancet. 1993;341:473–6.
38. Qasem AA, Ashour TH, Al-Abdulrazzaq HK, Ismail ZA. Disclosure of cancer diagnosis and prognosis by physicians in Kuwait. Int J Clin Pract. 2002;56(3):215–8.
39. Ibrahim EM, Al-Muhanna FA, Saied I, Al-Jishi FM, Al-Idrissi HY, Al-Khadra AH, et al. Public knowledge: misperceptions and attitudes about cancer in Saudi Arabia. Ann Saudi Med. 1991;11:518–23.
40. Bok S. Lying: moral choice in public and private life. New York: Vintage Books; 1997. p. 14.
41. Hoppy V. Lepp. 1980 SCR: 192.
42. Elger BS, Harding TW. Should cancer patients be informed about their diagnosis and prognosis? Future doctors and lawyers differ. J Med Ethics. 2002;28:258–65.

43. Miyata H, Tachimori H, Takahashi M, Saito T, Kai I. Disclosure of cancer diagnosis and prognosis: a survey of the general public attitudes toward doctors and family holding discretionary powers. BMC Med Ethics. 2004;5:E7.
44. Baile WF, Lenzi R, Parker PA, Buckman R, Cohen L. Oncologists' attitudes toward and practices in giving bad news: an exploratory study. J Clin Oncol. 2002;20:2189–96.
45. Cassel C. The patient-physicain covenant: an affirmation Asklepios. Ann Intern Med. 1996;124:604–6.
46. Girgis A, Sanson-Fisher RW. Breaking bad news: consensus guidelines for medical practitioners. J Clin Oncol. 1995;13:2449–56.
47. Schattner A, Tal M. Truth telling and patient's autonomy: the patient's points of view. Am J Med. 2002;113:66–9.
48. Mackillop WJ, Quirt CF. Measuring the accuracy of prognostic judgments in oncology. J Clin Epidemiol. 1997;50:21–9.
49. Christakis NA, Lamont EB. Extents and determinants of errors in doctors' prognoses in terminally ill patients: prospective cohort study. BMJ. 2000;320:469–73.
50. Reynolds PM, Sanson-Fisher RW, Poole ED, Harker J, Byrne MJ. Cancer and communication: information given in an oncology clinic. Br Med J. 1981;282:1449–51.
51. Davey HM, Butow PN, Armstrong BK. Patients' preferences for written prognostic information. Br J Cancer. 2003;89:1450–6.
52. Kaplowitz SA, Campo S, Chui WT. Cancer patients' desire for communication of prognosis information. Health Commun. 2002;14:221–41.
53. Benson J, Britten N. Respecting the autonomy of cancer patients when talking with their families: qualitative analysis of semistructured interviews with patients. Br Med J. 1996;313: 729–31.
54. Aaron N, Steven J. Disclosing the cancer diagnosis procedures that influence patient hopefulness. Cancer. 1993;72:3355–65.
55. Montazeri A. Does knowledge of cancer diagnosis affect quality of life? A methodological challenge. BMC Cancer. 2004;4(1):21–6.

Chapter 5
Psychological Challenges for the Oncology Clinician Who Has to Break Bad News

Friedrich Stiefel and Sonia Krenz

Abstract Work-related stress of the oncology clinician is not only due to heavy clinical and administrative duties, but also arises when breaking bad news. However, there is important interindividual variation in stress levels during patient encounters, mainly due to the significance the situation represents for the oncologist. A reflection on his own development, his professional identity, and ways of dealing with the patient's suffering can reduce his levels of stress and distress and prevent burnout and other psychiatric disturbances. This chapter summarizes the psychological challenges the oncology clinician is facing when he announces the diagnosis of cancer, deals with the deception of relapse, discusses the transition to palliative care, copes with progression of the disease and uncertainty, and cares for the dying who is facing the unknown. Ways of reflecting on and dealing with these situations from a psychological and communicational perspective are described and illustrated by case vignettes.

Keywords Physician–patient communication • Cancer • Psycho-oncology • Physicians' defense mechanisms • Relapse • Death • Breaking bad news

Up to 30% of oncologists suffer from psychiatric morbidity and report high levels of emotional exhaustion and professional demotivation and low levels of personal achievement, indicating burnout [1]. Work-related stress in cancer care is related to heavy clinical and administrative duties, unpredictable work schedules, and exposure to suffering and death [2]. While patient volume, administration, and organization of work can be influenced only on an institutional level, the oncology clinician

F. Stiefel (✉) • S. Krenz
Psychiatric Liaison Service, University Hospital Center and University of Lausanne,
Rue du Bugnon 44, Lausanne, 1011, Switzerland
e-mail: Frederic.Stiefel@chuv.ch; Sonia.Krenz@chuv.ch

can reflect on his way of facing suffering and death and try to cope with it more adequately, thus reducing his stress in the patient encounter.

Indeed, patient interviews are stressful, especially for oncologists who have to break bad news, communicate about end-of-life issues, or disclose errors [3–5]. While these tasks are difficult, level of stress and subsequent distress for the clinician are highly individual, depending not only on the task to be performed, but also on the anxiety induced by the task. This is illustrated by a recent study by Bernard et al. [6], who showed that a 15-min (simulated) patient interview in communication skills training (CST) is associated with a high number and variety of defense mechanisms in oncology clinicians. Operating without consciousness and triggered by anxiety-provoking situations, defense mechanisms contribute to the individual's adaptation to stress [6]. Usually described in patients—for example, denial when facing cancer—defense mechanisms also operate in clinicians and may therefore be considered as an indicator for stress. The following consultation by an oncologist illustrates how defenses are triggered and how they operate (type of defense mechanism shown in parentheses):

> The patient, a 45-year-old man suffering from incurable stomach cancer, responds to the proposition of chemotherapy with palliative intent by sighing and states, "… and my kids are still in school and …"; before letting the patient end his sentence, the oncologist interrupts him: "we will be able to control the situation, at least for a while" (denial of the patient's concerns, rationalization by focusing on medical aspects) and continues, "I do understand that the treatment may worry you (projection), but according to the studies we have at hand, the positive effects clearly outweigh the potential side effects" (intellectualization).

This example illustrates that the clinicians feels threatened by the (emotional) reaction of his patient, but his defensive attitude is more related to his own than to the patient's anxiety; consequently the patient may feel misunderstood and perceive the physician as being detached and unable to provide empathic support.

While reacting with defenses, especially immature defenses, such as projection and denial, the clinician may avoid and temporarily reduce his own threatening and painful emotions, but he also (1) diminishes his capacity to integrate all aspects of a given situation, (2) weakens the working alliance with the patient, and (3) fails to respond to the patient's needs, which sooner or later complicates his relationship with the patient and thus increases his stress. In addition, it remains doubtful that a defensive attitude is really protective, since it seems to contribute in the long run to psychological distress and disturbance [7, 8].

Effective communication, on the other hand, is known to contribute not only to the patient's psychological adjustment, quality of life [9–11], and satisfaction [10, 12], but also to the clinician's satisfaction by reducing his levels of professional stress [9]. In addition, effective training in communication skills seems to reduce anxiety, as has been demonstrated in the above-mentioned study [6]: clinicians who participate in CST show an increase in mature defenses after training, indicating lower levels of anxiety. However, anxiety during patient encounters is related not only to the clinician's skills, but also to the significance the situation has for the oncologist, as illustrated by a case vignette from a CST [13]:

> Dr. H, a 35-year-old oncologist, reported during an individual supervision a very stressful situation while she was on duty during the weekend. Called to an elderly lady who was suffering from pain due to bone metastases of a breast cancer, she proposed to prescribe a stronger analgesic, but it was refused by the patient. This irritated the oncologist to such a degree that she started to shout at the patient, telling her that "she has to decide whether to stop complaining or to take the medication." Realizing that the elderly woman was moved to tears, the oncologist immediately excused herself, feeling ashamed. After having explored how to understand the situation (the patient's ambivalence towards morphium and her struggle for autonomy), the oncologist was invited to speak about her feelings when facing the patient. She reported that she not only felt angry, but also very anxious "because the lady did not follow the doctor's advice." She then paused and linked her anxiety to her own medical history of melanoma, diagnosed three years previously, which she still experienced as a very traumatic event; she concluded: "If I hadn't followed the doctor's advice, I wouldn't be sitting here in front of you ... ."

This example illustrates that an external event becomes stressful because of the meaning it has for the clinician. In other words, stress arises when the "outer" world meets the "inner" world of the clinician. While there are situations that are stressful for most clinicians (e.g., cardiac resuscitation), "everyday stress" is individual due to the "intrapsychic echo" the external event triggers in the clinician. This echo depends not only on the professional identity he has acquired over his career, but also on life events and his personal identity developed since childhood. However, professional and personal identity are interwoven, as illustrated by studies assessing childhood development and career choices. Eliott and Guy [14], for example, found that women choosing to become psychiatrists report higher prevalence of physical abuse, psychiatric hospitalization of their parents, or death of a family member. Paris and Frank [15], who compared law students with medical students, found more reports of illness in the family of medical students, even after excluding students who chose the same profession as their parents. These studies illustrate that the choice of a "caring" profession may—at least in some cases—be directly related to childhood experiences: parentified children who have internalized their role as a carer might choose their profession in an attempt to experience emotional closeness that was lacking in their childhood, thus providing to others what they have missed [14]. While it may be quite obvious that some clinicians choose their career because of disturbances during their development, for others their development may have been less dramatic and its influence therefore more subtle. However, there is no doubt that biographical elements also operate in oncology clinicians and play a role in the practice of the profession. The existence of such biographical and life trajectory elements in themselves is not problematic as long as these elements are conscious and the physician is able to reflect on them. On the other hand, if they remain unidentified, unreflected and unresolved, the physician might be subjected to these dynamics, pushing him into an impossible mission by trying to resolve issues of the past by acting in the present. Emotional exhaustion might be the price the clinician pays.

These studies and our clinical experiences working with clinicians during CST, individual supervisions, or psychotherapeutic treatments confirm that the inner world of physicians is often affected by the patient's suffering, which may trigger strong emotions such as anxiety, rage, or sadness. Some situations are emotionally loaded not only because of their individual significance, but because they represent a kind of "archetypical" situations that constantly provoke stress in physicians. These situations will be discussed below, with special emphasis on their psychological and communicational challenges for the oncology clinician.

Trying Not to Hurt: Announcing a Diagnosis of Cancer

Announcing the diagnosis of a life-threatening disease is one of the most challenging and stressful tasks for an oncology clinician. Knowing that not only the bad news will hurt the patient, but also that the subsequent treatments will harm him without providing a guarantee for cure, is the contrary of what the clinicians would like to have happen, having chosen the caring profession supposed to heal and diminish suffering caused by disease. The temptation, therefore, is to avoid this uncomfortable role by trying to deny the threat of the disease or the side effects of the treatments or—as a kind of counterphobic reaction—to deliver the bad news as quickly and straightforwardly as possible.

On the other hand, if the physician is able to assume the responsibility that he sometimes has to harm in order to help the patient and recognizes that this task challenges his professional identity and provokes feelings of anxiety, guilt, isolation, and insecurity, he is better prepared to face these situations. The following sentences by a neuro-oncologist working with patients with brain tumors illustrate this point:

> When I have to announce a diagnosis of a malignant brain tumor, I already see the miserable future of the patient; and at the same time I perceive his unrealistic expectations. And I can't share with him what I feel; that would not be appropriate. I can't share it with colleagues; they have their own sorrows. And I don't want my family to be confronted with the hard sides of my professional life. It then happens that for a short moment I cry in my office and quickly focus again on my work. I can't stand to cry alone; it makes me feel even more lonely and miserable. Sometimes I also dare to make some cynical jokes, but that also provokes bad feelings, mainly guilt. I often feel inadequate.

This physician felt very relieved to have been able to communicate about these issues and was motivated, as a first step, to try to share his experiences in a more adequate way with his colleagues. Shame or guilt about feelings are counterproductive and produce an isolating silence, which is the first problem to overcome. They act like a censor, blocking the clinician's access to his own experiences and emotions, and thus depriving him of important information. Emotions, especially uncomfortable emotions, should be perceived not just as "negative side effects" of daily clinical work, but as a valuable source of information, revealing important aspects of the patient–physician relationship. However, emotions are often suppressed because of a confusion between "feelings," "thoughts," and "deeds"; while there are clear differences between them, on an intrapsychic level they may be treated as being the same and are therefore censored. As Holmes [16] stated in an article in the *British*

Medical Journal: "Have we not all sometimes felt bored and irritated by certain patients, longing for the consultation to end? Can any doctor honestly say that he or she has never felt a flicker of sexual interest in a patient? Have we never imagined the death of a certain patient and the relief that would bring, not just to them but to us, their impotent carers?"

The less we are able to identify our emotions, the more power they have to guide our behavior. This is especially true for the stressful task of announcing the diagnosis of cancer. Anxiety and guilt, which are associated with announcing a cancer diagnosis, are understandable reactions that indicate that the clinician is exposed to a threat (anxiety) and is performing a task (do harm) that he perceives as being aggressive (guilt). Anxiety should not be suppressed, but should guide the oncologist to identify the source of the threat: is he anxious about the psychological impact the information has on the patient, or is he anxious about his own capacities to communicate bad news? Is he anxious about the reactions of the patient or about how to face them? Is he anxious about what the patient might want to ask, or is he anxious about how to respond? Depending on the source of the anxiety, the ways to react and cope with it are different. To identify his feelings, to think about them, and to share them with others is therefore essential for the clinician in order to understand the challenges arising in patient encounters, to prevent stress, and to react adequately.

Dealing with Deception: Relapse

Relapse of cancer is associated with deception, both on the side of the patient, who has suffered to overcome the disease, and on the side of the clinician, who has hoped to cure the patient. Unidentified and unreflected feelings of deception may mislead the treating physician to provide an optimistic outlook and to rapidly propose additional treatments without giving the patient an opportunity to express his emotions. Some patients may react by stating that they thought they were cured or by refusing further treatments because of the unsatisfactory results; physicians may then feel criticized and respond with scientific-medical arguments, thus denying the patient's experience [17], or feel threatened and react with anger, as illustrated by statements such as, "but I have told you that cure might not be possible" or "what do you think, that I have a magic wand?"

When facing relapse, it is important first to carefully explore what the patient has to say and to let him express his deception and worry. Meanwhile, the clinician should try to listen to his own feelings; and if guilt, anger, or anxiety is perceived, he might question these feelings and try to understand why he takes the patient's reaction so personally. The following case vignette, reported by a patient, illustrates this issue:

> The patient, a 60-year-old woman with breast cancer, described that when she expressed disappointment after relapse was diagnosed, her oncologist answered: "I always told you that you should never feel totally cured; you have to face it, the disease will always be stronger than we are... ."

This example illustrates that the physician has taken the remark of his patient very personally ("… always be stronger than we are…") and reacted with anger ("you have to face it…"). The patient reported that these sentences left her in a state of hopelessness that was very difficult to overcome. As she put it, "I knew he was right, but his reaction hurt me terribly… ."

If the physician is able to accept that communicating the relapse of cancer is a difficult but inevitable task of his professional life that will induce a variety of feelings and reactions in both the patient and himself, he will be more able to understand and adequately respond to the patient's emotions and/or transitory feelings of ambivalence with regard to future treatment options. It is only after having given room to the patient's views and feelings that a "new contract" can be established, based on the choice by the informed patient to accept or refuse further treatment. On the other hand, unexpressed or suppressed emotions in either or both patient and physician produce a situation of "business as usual," which is inadequate, complicates the physician–patient relationship, and contaminates future encounters. Instead of denying deception, the clinician is better advised to recognize it: "Yes, this is disappointing. I can understand that you're sad or even angry, with all that effort you have undertaken to get rid of the cancer; and I can understand that after having hoped to be cured, you might have mixed feelings about new treatments… ." In moments of pressure, the clinician should explore the patient's point of view and let him express his feelings instead of defending himself, as if he were being accused [18]. If the clinician is able to do this, the patient feels understood and the working alliance is fostered, which is an important condition for future treatment that will again demand a lot of effort from the patient.

Coping with Limits: Transition from Curative to Palliative Care

Another challenging and distressing situation for oncology clinicians is facing the limits of medicine and communicating the impossibility of cure. Such situations frequently occur in clinical practice and may even be a major aspect of the work in some settings—for example, in the treatment of patients with brain tumors. For some clinicians, facing the limits of treatment and guiding the patient through the transition to palliative care is extremely stressful. This is especially so for oncologists who make very high demands on themselves and have great difficulty respecting their own limitations. Facing the limits may then trigger feelings such as guilt or rage, reactions such as denial of the patient's suffering, or acting out by pursuing treatments that do more harm than good.

To be able to recognize and respect limits, which are part of life and of the medical profession, requires that the oncology clinician reflect on (1) his attitude toward limits, (2) his personal and professional experiences with limits, and (3) his professional identity. How did and does he experience and react to limits in child- and adulthood? How does he understand his professional duties? How does he deal with the fact that not all cancer patients can be cured? How important such reflections can be is illustrated by a case vignette of an individual supervision of a 30-year-old oncologist who participated in a CST:

> Reviewing his video-taped consultations, he recognized that he often acted like a "salesman" when proposing chemotherapy with palliative intent, focusing on the possible positive impact and minimizing the associated side effects. Questioned about this attitude, he very honestly "confessed" that he feels somehow anxious in such situations, "like in an exam," and then freely associated that he is always concerned with his image and how he is perceived by others. He then continued that he often had the impression that his school performances were not sufficient and that, despite a quite successful medical career, he felt that his parents were not satisfied. He also reported that he often daydreamed during his childhood—for example, of coming upon an accident where some of his peers were injured and saving them heroically. Linking these different elements, he was able to recognize that he still experiences fantasies of unlimited power and projects on patients that they have (unrealistic) expectations towards him.

Winnicott [19] describes in his concept of the "good enough mother" that we cannot ask for and do not have to be "perfect mothers": it is sufficient to be a good enough mother, who provides adequate care and is sensitive to the infant's needs. In health care, an oncologist's duty is to cure patients and to care for those he cannot cure. If he denies or ignores the limits of curative power, he might expose his patients to a danger illustrated by a citation attributed to Hannah Arendt: "It seems that we are subjected to a magic formula, which provides us with the capacity to do the impossible under the condition to lose the capacity to do the possible" [14]. In other words, if limits are ignored, the clinician loses the patient and becomes "a bad mother" and a bad doctor.

Continuous reflection on the personal way of facing limits and on how the institutional and cultural context of his professional environment deals with limits is therefore an important task of the oncology clinician in order to be able to adequately care for the patients for whom curative treatment is no longer possible. Such reflection is not only important for the patient, but also for the clinician's psychological well-being. Feeling constantly pressured by situations of transition to palliative care may induce feelings such as helplessness, impotence, guilt, or rage, which are difficult to endure and lead to high levels of stress and distress. These feelings may ultimately end in professional burnout and/or psychiatric disorders, such as depression or substance abuse. On the other hand, if a clinician is able to accept the limits of medicine, he will diminish work-related stress, increase his job satisfaction, and be more effective in the care of the palliative patient. In many cancer centers, these issues are not reflected upon despite the fact that they could play an important role in reducing professional stress. Creating an environment that allows open discussion of these issues and provides access for their clinicians to collective and/or individual supervision would therefore be most beneficial, for patients and physicians.

From a communicational point of view, the challenge for the oncology clinician is how to address the medical limits and to guide the patient in this transition. For the patient, such bad news is not only a "piece of information," but also a highly emotional and threatening moment. While the informational part of the message may not be too difficult to convey (there are reasons why one has to change the perspective and do not just "what is possible," but "what makes sense"), the emotions evoked in the patient call for an empathic attitude and the containing of painful emotions.

While empathy towards the patient does not require specific skills or interview techniques, it requires a "containing capacity" similar to a mother's capacity to take the crying child in her arms. Such a containing capacity demands from the clinician the ability to stop acting and to remain actively engaged in the relationship with the patient, which in turn demands that he is able to bear his own emotions. If he is unable to experience moments of sadness or anxiety triggered by the transition to palliative care, he will not be able to face the patient's emotions. Physicians who cannot contain their own emotions utilize so-called blocking behaviors [20], which are unconscious communication strategies aimed at suppressing the patient's emotional expression. Blocking behaviors are operating, for example, in unbalanced interviews with an overwhelming speaking time of the physician, a focus on the biomedical aspects of the situation, abrupt transition from emotions to medical information, cynical remarks, nonverbal behavior indicating time pressure, or a distant attitude. As a senior oncology staff member, looking at his video-taped (simulated) patient interview, stated: "This is incredible, it seems as if I am playing chess, everything seems under control; I provide all the information, step by step, letting no chance for doubt or questions, with the effect that the patient just doesn't exist... ."

Depending on individual development, there may be important interindividual differences with regard to the clinician's capacities to contain the patient's emotions. However, being able to recognize limits and to accept them as a natural part of life and medicine is a first step in diminishing the clinician's own stress and to have more intrapsychic "room" for his patient. If the limits of medical power, so frequently encountered in daily oncological practice—often in alternation with enormous medical power in situations of cure—are preoccupying the physician, he is absorbed by his inner world and unable to open up to the patient. For example, some of the psychiatric consultation requests for cancer patients are directly linked to the physician's incapacity to tolerate his own painful preoccupations. To introduce a third person, a psychiatrist or psychologist, in the dyadic relationship with the patient may be adequate, but it may also be an expression of the physician's incapacity to tolerate his own emotions and contain the patient's emotions. This is illustrated during CST, when the simulated patient sighs, saying that he has young children: some clinicians immediately respond by stating that there are psycho-oncologists who might be of help, even before exploring the patient's concerns and clarifying whether he really needs and wants help. We observe important differences with regard to the containing capacity between physicians and nurses, and also between men and women. Nurses and women seem more able to tolerate their own and patients' painful emotions; this may be due to the different individual and professional socialization, but also to the differences of the tasks between the professions [21].

Based on our experience, clinicians can improve their capacity to contain emotions if they are motivated to reflect on these issues and to encounter their own emotions. As with other tasks, constant exposure and training can enhance one's capacity to contain an emotional situation; exchange with peers about difficult tasks and/or individual supervisions with a psycho-oncologist can also be of great help.

Facing Uncertainty: Progression of Disease

Progression of disease represents a considerable psychological distress, also for the physician, especially when he faces patients who are desperately searching for new treatments and innovative drugs, who are in denial or feeling hopeless; or when he meets family members who may put considerable pressure on the patient and/or the health care providers. Progression of disease challenges not only the capacities of the physician's "ego" by demanding from him medical, psychological, and human experience and competence, but also his "ego ideal." From the ego ideal, a strong motivation for professional engagement and achievements, originate our wishes of how we would like to be. If there is a gap between how we are and how we wish to be, distress arises. Unreflected ego ideals may create psychological tensions that may lead not only to physician burnout, but also to inadequate or aggressive treatments in the last months of a patient's life. During a professional career, the process of deconstructing ego ideals without becoming resigned or cynical is an important process, one that is rarely discussed within oncology and in some settings is even avoided by creating an institutional illusion of "winning the war on cancer." On the other hand, physicians who have been able to mourn their ego ideals and who are satisfied with their actual capacities and competences, experience less pressure, and are more capable of establishing a trustful and supporting relationship with the patient, which is the most important aspect of palliative care. As a senior oncologist has stated:

> It was quite sad for me to slowly adjust my ambitions to the reality of what we can do in oncology. Of course we are constantly shifting between potence and impotence and of course we should never give up; but to strive for pushing the edges should be restricted to the research and not occur in the clinical treatment of far advanced cancer. And during the adjustment between my expectations and reality, I also felt liberated by the idea that I no longer feel that I have to do more than I can; I felt more comfortable talking with patients whose disease progresses despite my efforts, and I became able to listen to them. And that's what counts in these situations.

The Unknown: Death as Man's Destiny

Communication with dying patients is often limited to short conversations, since patients are exhausted or present a certain relational withdrawal when facing the end of their life. Therefore, nonverbal communication and attitudes of the physician, directly influenced by his emotional state, become crucial. Death and dying is associated with strong emotions, and various phenomena, not only empathy, may arise in the physician. Empathy, which can be defined as "understanding, being aware of, being sensitive to, and experiencing the feelings and thoughts of another" [14], implies not only closeness to the patient, but also the ability to distance oneself again and concentrate on oneself. If adequate distance is lacking, "identification" may occur, with the consequence that there is no distinction between the roles of the physician and the patient: the physician experiences "being the patient," and the patient has the impression of not being able to count anymore on a competent, professional health care provider.

Empathy has to be distinguished not only from identification, but also from "counter-transference," defined as an interpersonal experience with roots in the clinician's own biography. Counter-transference, colored by positive or negative emotions, may occur when features of the patient remind the physician of persons of the past who were important to him. Such counter-transferential reactions, especially frequent in emotionally loaded situations, such as the end of life, may influence the physician's attitude—for example, leading him to avoid a dying patient (negative counter-transference) or to favor a dying patient excessively compared to other patients in need (positive counter-transference).

Finally, the phenomenon of "collusion" also has to be distinguished from empathy. Collusion, often perceived as extremely strong emotional experiences of anxiety or anger, occurs when patient and physician are both struggling with the same unconscious and unresolved problems. This may involve unresolved losses in the past leading to highly emotional reactions—for example, with regard to a request for assisted suicide: due to his own unresolved issues concerning loss, symbolically represented by the wish for anticipating the loss of life by the patient, the physician, without an in-depth analysis of the situation, immediately complies with the request, or, due again to the same unresolved problem, reacts in an aggressive way, refusing even to discuss what might have caused such a request.

In conclusion, facing the dying patient often mobilizes very strong emotions within the physician, which should be recognized as empathy or distinguished from identification, counter-transference, or collusion.

The way the oncology clinician faces the dying patient is also influenced by his own representation of death. Without a reflection on his own death and on the meaning of death, the oncologist is not able to accompany the dying patient, since he will be guided more by his own representation of death than by what the patient actually experiences. A discussion with an oncology team about how death is perceived illustrates this point:

> Medical oncologist: "for me, death represents a crevice; there is nothing more after death, just a dark and lonely hole... ."
> Oncology nurse: "I think that after the patient has died, he will be gone for an eternal trip in the galaxy... ."
> Psychiatrist: "How do you separate from dying patients?"
> Medical oncologist: "I never say good-bye to them; I try to avoid this topic, and I sometimes even avoid the patient."
> Oncology nurse: "When I feel that my patient might pass away while I'm off duty, I tell him that I hope he will have a peaceful journey."

This vignette illustrates how important the clinicians' representations of death are for daily clinical work and how confusing and distressing it might be for a patient to be subjected to a variety of attitudes by his caregivers. On the contrary, the oncologist who is aware of and able to question his own representations of death and his attitudes toward the dying patient is more able not to confuse his own ideas with the patient's and can join him in the way the patients feels and not the way he imagines or wants him to feel.

This will provide him the opportunity to realize that patients have a variety of feelings and thoughts about death and dying; and many of them face this situation without fear, but with a feeling of inner peace. He will also realize that there is no "good" death with universal meaning for everyone. Some patients may want to settle things, others may not; some patients may want to solve conflicts, and others may not; some may want to say good-bye to loved ones, and others may not. It might be important to question the patient's attitudes, even or especially at the end of life; but no patient should be burdened with the carer's own wishes and needs, and everyone should have the right to die his own death. The fact that the oncologist opens up to the patient's experience in terminal illness will ultimately help him to reduce his own fears about death and thus reduce the stress evoked by the encounter with a dying patient.

Conclusions

Communication skills can be effectively taught, if the minimal standards with regard to the time investment, content, and pedagogic qualities of the training programs are respected [22]. While CST improves clinicians' communication behaviors [18], decreases anxiety related to patient interviews [6], and thus reduces levels of stress and distress in both patients and clinicians, some aspects of the physician–patient encounter call for additional reflection. This concerns the psychological challenges the oncology clinician faces when meeting patients to whom he has to convey threatening and painful truths. These psychological challenges, which have a strong impact on the quality of the relationship and therefore on communication with the patient, are also a potential source of suffering for the physician. Closely related to the personal and professional development and biography and the subsequent professional identity, these psychological aspects of the physician–patient encounter are at the same time universal and individual; they therefore call for a reflective, psychological approach—usually based on collective or individual supervision with a liaison psychiatrist or psychologist—that should be encouraged on an institutional level.

References

1. Ramirez AJ, Graham J, Richards MA, Cull A, Gregory WM. Mental health of hospital consultants: the effects of stress and satisfaction at work. Lancet. 1996;347:724–8.
2. Shanafelt T, Chung H, White H, Lyckholm LJ. Shaping your career to maximize personal satisfaction in the practice of oncology. J Clin Oncol. 2006;24:4020–6.
3. Ptacek JT, Fries EA, Eberhardt TL. Breaking bad news to patients: physicians' perceptions of the process. Support Care Cancer. 1999;7:113–20.

4. Fallowfield L, Jenkins V. Communicating sad, bad and difficult news in medicine. Lancet. 2004;363:312–9.
5. Fallowfield L, Jenkins V. Effective communication skills are the key to good cancer care. Eur J Cancer. 1999;35:1592–7.
6. Bernard M, de Roten Y, Despland JN, Stiefel F. Communication skills training and clinicians' defences in oncology: an exploratory, controlled study. Psychooncology. 2010;19:209–15.
7. Greenberg JR, Mitchell SA. Object relations in psychoanalytic theory. Cambridge: Harvard University Press; 1983.
8. Gabbard GO. Psychodynamic psychiatry in clinical practice. Washington, DC: American Psychiatric Press; 1994.
9. Lernan C, Daly M, Walsh WP, et al. Communication between patients with breast cancer and health care providers: determinants and implications. Cancer. 1993;72:2612–20.
10. Ford S, Fallowfield L, Lewis S. Doctor-patient interactions in oncology. Soc Sci Med. 1996;42:1511–9.
11. Razavi D, Delvaux N, Marchal S, De Cock M, Farvacques C, Slachmuylder JL. Testing health care professionals' communication skills: the usefulness of highly emotional standardized role-playing sessions with simulators. Psychooncology. 2000;9:293–302.
12. Loge JH, Kaasa S, Hytten K. Disclosing the cancer diagnosis: the patients' experiences. Eur J Cancer. 1997;33:878–82.
13. Stiefel F. Support of the supporters. Support Care Cancer. 2008;16:123–6.
14. Eliott DM, Guy JD. Mental health professionals versus nonmental health professional: childhood trauma and adult functioning. Prof Psychol Res Pract. 1993;24:83–90.
15. Paris J, Frank H. Psychological determinants of a medical career. Can J Psychiatry. 1983;28:354–7.
16. Holmes J. Good doctor, bad doctor. BMJ. 2002;325:722–3.
17. Despland JN, Bernard M, Favre DM, De Roten Y, Stiefel F. Clinicians' defences: an empirical study. Psychol Psychother Theory Res Pract. 2009;82:73–81.
18. Stiefel F. Communication in cancer care. Berlin: Springer; 2006.
19. Winnicott DW. Winnicott on the child. Cambridge: Cambridge University Press; 2002.
20. Maguire P. Communication skills for doctors: a guide to effective communication with patients and families. Oxford: Oxford University Press; 2001.
21. Stiefel F, Bernhard J, Bianchi G, et al. The Swiss model. In: Kissane D, Bultz B, Phyllis Butow P, Finlay I, editors. Handbook of communication in oncology and palliative care. Oxford: Oxford University Press; 2010. p. 642–8.
22. Stiefel F, Barth J, Bensing J, Fallowfield L, Jost L, Razavi D, Kiss A. Communication skills training in oncology: a position paper based on a consensus meeting among European experts in 2009. Ann Oncol. 2009;21:204–7.

Chapter 6
Dealing with Depression: Communicating with Cancer Patients and Grieving Relatives

Luigi Grassi, Rosangela Caruso, and Maria Giulia Nanni

Abstract Cancer is an extremely stressful event for both the patients and their families, potentially leading to the development of depression, which has been shown to have a general prevalence of 15–25%. When left unaddressed, depression has a great negative influence on quality of life, coping strategies, and active participation in medical care of both patient and caregivers. The relational components of effective communication with depressed cancer patients and their family members include the clinician's availability for listening, exploring emotions, identifying affective problems, and providing empathic responses, in order to promote reciprocal trust and consolidate the therapeutic alliance. Of first importance is correct assessment of the symptoms (e.g., cognitive-affective dimensions with/without exclusion of neurovegetative symptoms), for a correct diagnosis (e.g., differentiating major depression from minor depression, adjustment disorder, demoralization). Suicide assessment is extremely important in the context of cancer care. A second aspect is intervention, at the counseling level or more specific psychotherapeutic treatment. Several types of psychological therapy have been proved to be effective in treating depression of cancer patients and family members (e.g., cognitive-behavior therapy, supportive-expressive group psychotherapy, interpersonal psychotherapy, complicated grief therapy, family-focused grief therapy). A sensitive, collaborative, comprehensive approach to the diagnosis and treatment of depression is the cornerstone of communication. Clinical education and training of cancer care professionals and integration with psychooncologists are mandatory for providing adequate care to cancer patients and their families with depression.

Keywords Depression • Communication • Counseling • Psychotherapy • Oncology

L. Grassi (✉) • R. Caruso • M.G. Nanni
Section of Psychiatry, Department of Biomedical and Specialty Surgical Siences,
University of Ferrara, Corso Giovecca 203, Ferrara 4410, Italy
e-mail: luigi.grassi@unife.it; rosangela.caruso@unife.it; mariagiulia.nanni@unife.it

The Problem of Depression in Cancer Care

Being confronted with the trauma of a diagnosis of cancer and consequent treatment is extremely stressful for both the patients and their families and can lead to the development of psychosocial and psychiatric disorders [27]. In fact, during the several phases of the illness, cancer patients and their caregivers often experience intense and difficult emotions, such as fear, sadness, uncertainty, helplessness, guilt, and anger. Symptoms such as sleep problems, anxiety, irritability, loss of interests, ruminating thoughts, and concerns about the future may occur; and patients' and caregivers' functioning may become impaired. Usually, this adjustment phase has a limited duration; most people, especially if adequate social support is provided, manage to adapt successfully to the new condition [5, 31]. In some cases, however, cancer patients and their relatives continue to show high levels of distress far beyond the normal adjustment period, and clinically significant emotional disorders may occur [28, 31], of which depression is one of the most frequent [26].

During the last decades, a considerable number of studies have investigated the epidemiology of depression in cancer patients, reporting significant variability in prevalence rates due to the use of different assessment measures, the populations examined, and the methodological approaches [10, 15]. A review based on 31 studies examining depression in cancer patients estimated prevalence rates of major depression as high as 10.8% [54]. A more recent meta-analysis indicated that the prevalence of major depression—as defined by the *Diagnostic and Statistical Manual of Mental Disorders* (DSM)—in palliative and active care settings was about 14%. When DSM-defined minor depression was explored, observed prevalence rates were 9.6 and 19.2% for, respectively, palliative and active care settings examined [52]. Moreover, other psychosocial dimensions related to affective disorders, such as demoralization and health anxiety, as assessed by other systems, such as the Diagnostic Criteria for Psychosomatic Research (DCPR), can affect a further 20% of cancer patients [23].

The prevalence of depression has shown important variations depending on cancer sites: the highest prevalence rates having been reported in oropharyngeal (22–57%), pancreatic (33–50%), breast (1.5–46%), and lung (11–44%) cancers; while a lower association has been found for colon (13–25%), gynecological (12–23%) cancer, and lymphoma (8–19%) [11, 50, 88].

Significant levels of emotional distress have also been reported to affect family members equally or even more than cancer patients [21], and there is evidence that unrecognized and unmet psychosocial needs are important predictors of psychological morbidity in caregivers [6, 58]. Moreover, a recent study exploring caregivers' distress in the early phases of cancer showed that high levels of depression affected nearly a quarter of the subjects studied [57]. Again, emotional disorders, especially depression, can be shown among cancer patients' caregivers in every phase of the illness, even though most literature has concentrated on grief and bereavement [22]. Although so largely represented, psychosocial comorbidity, especially depression, is often undetected in cancer care, both among patients and their caregivers [18, 19, 27, 33, 67].

One reason is that depressive-spectrum syndromes represent one of the most difficult psychiatric diagnoses in oncology settings, in terms of semiology, screening, prognosis factors, and treatment. A large pivotal study demonstrated that emotional distress was recognized by physicians in only 29% of affected cancer patients [18]. On the other hand, when left unaddressed, depression has a great negative influence on quality of life, coping strategies, and active participation in medical care both of the patient and caregivers [19, 27, 33].

In light of these considerations, physicians should be able to communicate in a way that facilitates the assessment and recognition of depression in oncology settings, and improves referral to interventions, including psychotherapy and psychopharmacology, when appropriate.

In this chapter the relevance and implications of communication with depressed cancer patients and their caregivers will be discussed in terms of diagnostic, relational, and therapeutic issues—specifically psychological intervention; psychopharmacotherapy of depression is described elsewhere [25, 34].

Communicating with Depressed Cancer Patients

Assessment and Diagnostic Issues

Communicating with depressed cancer patients poses numerous challenges and represents an important and complex facet of care.

In a true patient-centered relationship of care, identifying the presence of psychological symptoms, specifically depression, is one of the first aims of communication in oncology. A challenging issue is that depression in cancer patients can have many different phenomenological expressions. Some depressed patients may soon verbalize feelings such as sadness, anger, inappropriate guilt, or high levels of anxiety; others may appear withdrawn and reluctant to express emotions. In a number of cases "negative" symptoms, such as loss of initiative, inability to feel pleasure or to make decisions may be predominant; while in others mainly somatic complaints, such as pain, loss of appetite and weight, sleep disturbances, fatigue, and poor concentration emerge. This may make it difficult to discriminate between the neurovegetative and somatic component of depression and cancer or treatment-derived somatic symptoms [54]. These diagnostic problems have been extensively discussed in order to clarify whether depression in cancer patients should be diagnosed by taking into account all the symptoms, both somatic and cognitive-affective, irrespective of whether they are determined by depression or cancer or both (inclusive approach); by replacing somatic symptoms with cognitive-affective items (substitute approach); by adding some new affective symptoms to the original criteria (alternative approach); by completely excluding somatic symptoms and using only affective symptoms (exclusive approach) [27, 54, 56, 63].

Table 6.1 Risk factors related to development of depression in cancer patients (from Grassi and Riba [26] mod.)

Personal or family history of depression/suicide attempts
Personality factors (e.g., external locus of control, emotional repression)
Concomitant stressful events
Poor social support and isolation
Unrelieved pain
Serious physical impairment consequent to cancer

Recently two clusters, one including "somatic" specifiers (e.g., functional somatic symptoms, persistent somatization) and the other including anxious/irritable symptoms, were reported in a large sample of depressed medically ill patients [32].

Furthermore, both in medical illness in general and cancer in particular, depression should be differentiated from demoralization, as assessed by using the DCPR [49] or other diagnostic tools [4, 12]. Demoralization is characterized by loss of control, loss of hope, anger/bitterness, sense of failure, feeling life is a burden, loss of meaning, and a belief that life's meaning is dependent on health, rather than anhedonia and guilty feelings [51]. Even though a considerable overlap between the two diagnoses may exist, almost half of patients with major depression are not classified as demoralized, and almost two-thirds of demoralized patients do not satisfy the criteria for major depression [49].

These issues can be particularly challenging in palliative-care settings, where the advanced stage of cancer, with possible effects on the central nervous system, and, at the same time, the hopeless and futureless situation may render the differentiation between normal sadness and clinical depression extremely difficult [62, 80].

In communicating with cancer patients, the risk factors for depression should be also scrutinized and carefully analyzed. A sensitive, skillful exploration is thus a crucial point in the diagnostic phase of communication, as summarized in Table 6.1, which indicates the most common areas to be explored when dealing with depression in cancer patients, including the presence of other stressful life events and a previous personal and family history of psychosocial disorders [26]. Thus, from the relational point of view, good communication skills, the amount and quality of received information, and patient participation in the consultation are extremely important, since it is associated with better outcomes and increased adherence to cancer treatment [16], as well as with lower levels of depression and better quality of life over time [77].

The relational components of an effective communication include the clinician's availability for listening, exploring emotions, identifying affective problems, and providing empathic responses, as repeatedly suggested by many authors [17, 47, 48] (Table 6.2).

In a therapeutic relationship with depressed cancer patients, communication tasks should include (1) promoting reciprocal trust; (2) encouraging patients' emotional expression; (3) fostering shared decision-making; (4) achieving early detection and treatment; (5) providing support; (6) consolidating the therapeutic alliance.

Table 6.2 Examples of statements and questions with a relational focus

How are the symptoms you mentioned affecting your daily life?—Open-ended question (encourages a full description; communicates availability to listen)
When exactly has this happened?—Clarifying question (helps comprehension; communicates interest in what is being told)
It must be very hard for you to deal with this sense of helplessness—Emotion acknowledgment (communicates emotional participation; facilitates further emotional expression) and empathy
Many patients feel the same when diagnosis is communicated—Normalization (lets the person know that the feelings he/she is experiencing are normal and understandable)
Would you like to tell me more about how you are feeling?—Invitation to continue (encourages a full description; communicates availability to listen)

Table 6.3 Some suggestions related to communication skills in dealing with suicidal patients

Be calm and supportive and encourage disclosure
Allow the patient time to talk and be available (by being listened to and shown interest and concern, patients feel understood and not alone)
Carefully assess suicide ideation and the motive for suicide (what they have done? for how long they have considered suicide? why do they want to die? what advantages are there in dying?)
Educate about depression and instill hope (hopelessness predicts suicide, and it is important to reassure the patient that people with depression can get better, particularly if they are given professional help)

In pursuing these goals, communication with depressed cancer patients needs to be founded on cooperation, and the clinician has to be aware that what originates from the relationship with the patient is the result of the coparticipation of two active counterparts. Unlike simple information exchange, this has therapeutic value and requires from the clinician the ability to reflect about him/herself, about his/her relational styles and personal emotions. In some cases physicians may find it uncomfortable to delve into patients' feelings, because they are concerned that depressive symptoms, once elicited, would be too difficult to manage. As a reaction it may be tempting, for instance, to adopt a paternalistic attitude, avoiding discussions with an emotional focus, offering inappropriately early reassurance, using ambiguous terms, or giving in to the temptation of communicating false hope. In other cases, patients may evoke in clinicians frustrating emotions, such as sadness, anger, boredom, and sense of failure. Nevertheless, when recognized and tolerated, these emotions can represent an important "diagnostic clue." Indeed, by mirroring the patient's own experience, they may reveal extremely useful information and become, if considered among other signs, a valuable relational indicator of depression in the cancer patient.

A major challenge of communication with depressed cancer patients regards the assessment and evaluation of the possibility of suicide. Suicide is, in fact, a major complication of depression, including depression related to cancer [64]. From the most important recommendations and guidelines in psychiatry [3, 53], some suggestions in communication should be taken into account when dealing with suicidal cancer patients, as indicated in Table 6.3.

Psychological Intervention Issues

Psychological intervention is a special form of communication in which the dialogue between the doctor and the patient has the specific aim of helping the patient overcome possible emotional, behavioral, and interpersonal problems. The most important communication and relational factors associated with psychological intervention, both in psychiatric settings and oncology, can be summarized as the following: (1) therapeutic alliance (i.e., an agreement between therapist and patient on the goals of treatment, the tasks needed to accomplish those goals, and a sense of a personal bond between therapist and patient); (2) empathy (i.e., the therapist's sensitive ability and willingness to understand the client's thoughts, feelings, and struggles from the client's point of view based on accurate recognition of the client's experience, the ability to share the client's feelings, and the capacity to express empathy with the client); (3) goal consensus (i.e., the patient–therapist agreement on the therapeutic goals and the expectations for therapy); and (4) collaboration (i.e., a mutual involvement by patient and therapist in the helping relationship, including patient cooperation, patient resistance, homework completion, hostility, defensive styles, or involvement in the patient role) [65]. In the last 20 years, psychological intervention in oncology has been the object of intense research [81]. This has been particularly evident for cancer patients reporting psychosocial disorders, especially depression, for which there is agreement confirming the benefit of treatment in reducing the level of depressive symptoms, irrespective of the stage of cancer [1, 36, 55, 85]. As for psychotherapy for people with depression in the general population, psychotherapy for depression in oncology has several aims, such as to understand one's own behavior, emotions, and thoughts that contribute to the depressed state; to understand the specific role of stressful events in the development and maintenance of depression and how to work through or solve them; to regain a sense of control of one's own life by learning coping and problem-solving strategies. Several forms of psychotherapy for depression exist [40], including cognitive-behavior therapy (based on the assumption that depression is related to the inaccurate perception people have of themselves and the world around them and to automatic thoughts that should be modified and replaced by more adaptive ones during therapy); psychodynamic therapy (based on the assumption that a person is depressed because of unresolved, unconscious conflicts, reenacted by a stressful event, such as cancer); interpersonal psychotherapy (IPT) (based on the assumption that depression is related to interpersonal variables and that working on interpersonal disputes, role transitions, grief, or interpersonal deficits helps in reducing symptoms and improving social functioning).

Alongside these models, existentially oriented group therapies have also been shown to be important in depressed cancer patients. Supportive-expressive psychotherapy is an example of such a therapy, with the main goals of building bonds, expressing emotions, "detoxifying" death and dying, redefining life's priorities, fortifying families and friends, enhancing doctor–patient relationships, and improving coping [71]. The role of the therapist is to create a high level of group cohesion and a supportive environment in which participants are encouraged to confront their problems, strengthen their relationships, and find enhanced meaning in their lives. Some specific aims for depressed cancer patients are facilitating the expression of depressive feelings (e.g., despair, hopelessness–helplessness, guilt); confronting fears (e.g., death and dying, being a burden to caregivers, fears of abandonment and stigmatization); building new bonds of social support in order to counteract loneliness and receive help; learning and finding more effective and active coping strategies. In a recent study involving breast cancer patients with an ICD-10 diagnosis of affective syndromes (mainly major depression, adjustment disorders with depressed mood), supportive-expressive group psychotherapy was effective in reducing depressive symptoms, as well as hopelessness and anxious preoccupation, with results that were maintained at 6-month follow-up [29]. Interestingly, breast cancer patients whose depression did not improve after supportive-expressive group psychotherapy had shorter survival than those whose depression did improve [20]. Furthermore, the positive effects of psychological intervention on several symptoms, including depression, pain, and fatigue, determined a reduction of inflammation markers among cancer patients [74].

Communicating with Depressed and Grieving Relatives

As mentioned, caregivers of cancer patients frequently report symptoms indicating emotional problems, including depression [21, 57]. Usually, a family approach to cancer allows clinicians to assess the level of psychosocial distress of family members, too, helping the whole family unit—not only the person affected by cancer—to adjust to the situation [6].

A special area of interest that should be examined is the grieving process and the possible development of depression among family members after the loss of their loved one. During this phase, physicians are confronted with major challenges, such as the wide range of grieving symptoms and reactions, and the difficult separation between normal and abnormal symptoms and behaviors; these should be recognized by knowing the boundary between "normal" grief and complicated ("abnormal") grief, including clinical depression, as summarized in the following paragraphs.

Assessment and Diagnostic Issues

At the death of cancer patient, the whole family enters the process of grief, which is a human, universal, and healthy psychological response to the loss of a loved one. It has specific aims, such as realizing gradually the reality and the meaning of the death; adapting to the absence of the loved one; coming to terms with the changes that the loss has brought about in the image of self, world, and future of the bereaved person; and reorganizing his/her own internal models [22].

Table 6.4 Possible forms of complicated (pathological) grief

Psychiatric disorders following bereavement (exaggerated grief)
Major depression
Anxiety disorders
Eating disorders
Substance abuse disorders
Brief psychotic reactions

Avoidance of grief
Mummification, with prolonged treasuring of objects and a tendency to leave everything (e.g., the person's room, personal objects, clothing) as immediately before death
Idealization of the quality of the deceased person and magnification of the loss
Persistent anger or guilt response rather than acceptance of death

Chronic grief (or prolonged grief)
Excessive duration of grief response, with difficulty in speaking about the death without intense overwhelming several years after the loss
Themes of loss coming out during daily conversation
Inability to resume one's own life and adjusting to new roles

Delayed grief
Reexperience of excessive grief reactions secondary to new stressful events or losses and reemergence of symptoms linked to the past loss

Inhibited grief (or masked grief)
Onset of physical complaints resembling the physical illness of the deceased ("facsimile illness")
Physical symptoms (e.g., pain)
Behavioral problems (e.g., impulsive decisions, poor health care, promiscuity, acting out)

A number of authors have attempted to define the stages and tasks of grief, including an initial period of numbness, leading to a depressive phase, and finally to reorganization and recovery. More recently the variability and fluidity of grief experiences, which differ considerably in intensity of the symptoms and duration among cultural groups and from person to person [8, 46, 61], have been recognized.

Besides data on normal experiences after the death of a loved one, a large amount of data over the last 40 years have indicated that in 15–25% of cases the process of grief can be complicated in several possible phenomenological forms, such as "chronic grief," "delayed grief," "inhibited grief," "masked grief," "avoidance of grief," "hypertrophied grief," or "exaggerated grief" [70, 73, 90], the latter characterized by psychiatric disorders including clinical depression (Table 6.4). Furthermore, by taking into account the traumatic effect of the death of a loved one, the concept of "traumatic grief," more recently defined as "prolonged grief disorder," has been proposed as a distinct form of pathological/complicated grief [30, 59, 60, 70]. Even if these different forms of clinical disturbances related to bereavement can also include depressive symptoms, it has been demonstrated that all of them—in particular traumatic (prolonged) grief—have their own specificity and phenomenological expression and that they should be considered different from grief-related major depression [7, 35, 91], also defined as "complicated bereavement-triggered depression" [70]. DSM-5 will take into consideration that bereavement, in its pathological form, can present as an "adjustment disorder related to bereavement," for which 12 months of symptoms are needed after the death of a close relative or friend before the diagnosis may be employed; and will leave the depressed form as occurring within major depressive episodes[1].

In normal grief, bereaved individuals often describe grief as a painful experience characterized by symptoms (such as shock, yearning, anguish, anger, anxiety, fear, loneliness, depression, intrusive images of the deceased, and others) that typically seem acute and persistent in the period that immediately follows the death of the loved one; but which assume, in the first few months, a trend with waves or fluctuations, initially unprovoked and later brought on by specific reminders of the deceased person [91]. Furthermore, in an uncomplicated grief process, these symptoms are usually mixed with positive feelings (e.g., relief, joy, peace) [9], which may immediately after the loss elicit negative emotions of disloyalty and guilt in the bereaved person. Even if the duration of grief is highly variable, the reality and meaning of the death are gradually faced, and cognitive and behavioral adjustments are progressively made until the bereaved can hold the deceased in a comfortable place in the memory and finally resume a fulfilling life [69].

---

[1] In DSM-5 the criteria for adjustment disorder related to bereavement are that for at least 12 months following the death of a close relative or friend, the individual experiences on more days than not intense yearning/longing for the deceased, intense sorrow and emotional pain, or preoccupation with the deceased or the circumstances of the death. The person may also display difficulty accepting the death, intense anger over the loss, a diminished sense of self, a feeling that life is empty, or difficulty planning for the future or engaging in activities or relationships. Mourning shows substantial cultural variation; the bereavement reaction must be out of proportion or inconsistent with cultural or religious norms. However, the DSM-5 work group is also proposing a specific bereavement-related disorder characterized by the following criteria: (a) the experience of death of a close relative or friend at least 12 months earlier; (b) the onset of symptoms on more days than not and to a clinically significant degree, including persistent yearning/longing for the deceased, intense sorrow and emotional pain because of the death, preoccupation with the deceased person, preoccupation with the circumstances of the death; (c) the experience of at least six specific symptoms since the death, on more days than not and to a clinically significant degree, such as for *reactive distress to the death*, marked difficulty accepting the death, feeling shocked, stunned, or emotionally numb over the loss, difficulty in positive reminiscing about the deceased, bitterness or anger related to the loss, maladaptive appraisals about oneself in relation to the deceased or the death (e.g., self-blame), excessive avoidance of reminders of the loss (e.g., avoiding places or people associated with the deceased); for *social/identity disruption*, the desire not to live in order to be with the deceased, difficulty trusting other people since the death, feeling alone or detached from other people since the death, feeling that life is meaningless or empty without the deceased, or the belief that one cannot function without the deceased, confusion about one's role in life or a diminished sense of one's identity (e.g., feeling that a part of oneself died with the deceased), difficulty or reluctance to pursue interests since the loss or to plan for the future (e.g., friendships, activities); (d) the disturbance causes clinically significant distress or impairment in social, occupational, or other important areas of functioning; (e) mourning shows substantial cultural variation; the bereavement reaction must be out of proportion or inconsistent with cultural or religious norms. It is also necessary to specify if, *with traumatic bereavement* is applicable, in which, following a death that occurred under traumatic circumstances (e.g., homicide, suicide, disaster, or accident), there are persistent, frequent distressing thoughts, images or feelings related to traumatic features of the death (e.g., the deceased's degree of suffering, gruesome injury, blame of self or others for the death), including in response to reminders of the loss.

In contrast, depression tends to be more pervasive and persistent and includes a recognizable cluster of disabling symptoms, accompanied by an enduring low mood. The diagnosis of clinical depression is generally given if the symptoms are still present 2 months after the loss. The depressed bereaved relatives reported significant difficulty in experiencing self-validating and positive feelings, while they show the presence of clinical characteristics that are similar to those of other, non-bereavement-related major depression [38]. Moreover, certain symptoms that are not present in a normal grief reaction can be helpful in diagnosing a clinical depression state. These may include (1) guilt, usually associated with some specific aspects of the loss rather than a general, overall sense of culpability; (2) thoughts of death other than the survivor's feeling that he/she would be better off dead or should have died with the deceased person; (3) preoccupation with worthlessness and hopelessness; (4) marked psychomotor retardation; (5) prolonged and marked functional impairment; (6) hallucinatory experience other than thinking to hear the voice or transiently sees the image of the deceased person [22].

Research carried out in the last 5 years has also shown that it is incorrect to exclude by definition bereavement symptomatology from major depression, since bereavement-excluded subjects may be more severely depressed than patients with major depression without bereavement, or as depressed as patients with major depression with bereavement [13]. The need to be more specific and to evaluate the symptoms by taking into consideration individuals that had to cope with bereavement, as well as other stressful events, has been also confirmed in a large study of 8,098 persons aged 15–54 years representative of the US population (National Comorbidity Survey [NCS]) [38, 78, 79].

The negative consequences of bereavement-related major depression are documented and include impaired psychosocial functioning, increased adrenocortical activity and impaired immunological function, increased physical illness and mortality, higher risk of suicide [43, 72].

For all these reasons, it is extremely important to explore the problems of the family members who have undergone bereavement, to respond to doubts and questions, and to offer practical support and counseling, or referral to mental health services when needed [22, 42, 84]. Empathic and reassuring communication, active listening, a nonjudgmental attitude, provision of encouragement, facilitation of emotional expression, validation of the grief reactions ("It is not unusual that people have such feelings and responses after the loss of a loved one…"; "Many bereaved people say their thinking is very confused…"; "It is a human and inevitable experience, just because we love someone so much, that we feel depressed or despair if we lose this person…") are the skills to be regularly used in the relationship with bereaved family members [45]. Furthermore, the therapist should encourage the description of depressive symptoms and facilitate the recognition of symptoms (including suicidal ideation) and dysfunctional thoughts and feelings. Automatic and persistent negative thoughts result, in fact, in intense feelings of guilt, anger, and irrational fears ("I should have taken my wife to the doctor sooner. If I had, she might be still alive today"; "It is doctors' and nurses' fault, because they didn't do everything possible"; "If I do not stay attached to my pain, I am afraid I might forget my loved one"; "I would rather die in his/her place"). Speaking openly and directly about these issues with the physician can help the bereaved relative revisit these thoughts in a more rational way and alleviate the intensity of the distressed symptoms. Exploring and taking into account some other important factors is also important, including personality variables, the nature of the relationship between the deceased person and the bereaved relative [75], the personal historical antecedents of significant loss [76] and other depressive episodes, family and social support, possible concurrent stressful life events [91].

It is also important to explain to depressed relatives that the symptoms he/she reports are caused by a depressive disorder, which can significantly improve with existing appropriate treatments [89].

Psychological Intervention Issues

The models of psychological intervention for families of cancer patients are numerous and have the general aim not to leave caregivers alone in the process of their relatives' illness and helping them adjust to the several challenges brought about by cancer. A recent meta-analysis of intervention studies from 1983 to 2009 indicated that psychosocial treatment significantly reduces caregiver burden; improves caregivers' ability to cope, increasing their self-efficacy; and ameliorates their quality of life [86]. The efficacy of psychological intervention during grief has been examined. Data indicate that grief counseling is not helpful for all families; that if grief counseling is applied to prevent complicated grief, the results are poor [2, 14, 86]. A consensus indicates that generic interventions delivered to the broad population of the bereaved are unnecessary and that preventive interventions should target high-risk caregivers and mourners [14, 66].

However, the efficacy of psychological intervention with family members with abnormal grief reactions, particularly depression, has been confirmed by a number of authors [34, 86]. While the goal of grief counseling in "normal" grief is to facilitate the process of mourning, psychotherapy for pathological grief has the aim of identifying and resolving the conflicts of separation that prevent the mourning tasks to be completed and that are at the basis of psychopathology [87]. Some communication and relational techniques of grief therapy for depressed family members are indicated in Table 6.5. To summarize, as recommended by Greer [30], a first important aspect is to be thoroughly acquainted with the details of the deceased's illness and treatment; to ask the bereaved person to give a detailed account of the months and weeks leading to the death of the deceased and its impact on his or her life; then to take a complete personal and psychiatric history, including any evidence of childhood separation anxiety.

In IPT, a 16-session focused intervention, education about depression is associated with an interpersonal reformulation of the causes of depression, specifically the events that occurred in the interpersonal realm, such as grief, role transition, interpersonal disputes, or interpersonal deficits [82, 83]. Bereavement-related depression

Table 6.5 Some suggestions and procedures for working with depressed grieving family members (from Worden [87] and Greer [30], mod.)

Relational techniques
- Rule out possible physical disease of the family members (in case of presentation of somatic symptoms, including vegetative symptoms of depression)
- Set up the contract and establish an alliance (clear definition with the bereaved of the aims of therapy)
- Revive memories of the deceased
- Assess which tasks of grief are not completed
- Deal with affects or lack of affects stimulated by memories (including unjustified guilt, self-criticism, "should" statements and "all or nothing" thinking, negative predictions, suicidal thoughts)
- Explore and defuse linking objects
- Acknowledge the finality of the loss
- Deal with the fantasy of ending grieving
- Help the patient say a final good-bye

Behavioral techniques
- Setting attainable, jointly agreed-upon goals that give a sense of pleasure (e.g., going out with friends, gardening, settling financial affairs arising from the partner's death)
- Recording daily activity schedules
- Encouraging emotional expression of grief

is one of the focuses of IPT, with data showing its efficacy in improving mood [44]; while it is less efficacious when dealing with complicated traumatic-like grief, for which a specific form of psychotherapy (complicated grief therapy [CGT]), using procedures for retelling the story of the death and exercises entailing confrontation with avoided situations, modified from in vivo exposure used for PTSD, was more effective [68].

Interesting data have also been reported on the efficacy of a family-focused grief therapy (FFGT) approach [39]. FFGT is a brief, focused, time-limited intervention (4–8 90-min sessions) with the aim of preventing complications of bereavement by enhancing the functioning of the family through exploration of its cohesion, communication (of thoughts and feelings), and handling of conflict. FFGT consists of three phases, of which the first (assessment, 1–2 sessions) concentrates on identifying issues and concerns relevant to the specific family and on devising a plan to deal with them; the second (intervention, 2–4 sessions) focuses on the agreed concerns; and the last (termination, 1–2 sessions) consolidates gains and confronts the end of therapy. Kissane et al. [41] showed that significant improvements in distress and depression occurred among individuals with high scores on depression at baseline and in *sullen families* (moderate levels of conflict, poor cohesion, poor expressiveness, muted anger, and high rate of psychosocial morbidity, including clinical depression) and *intermediate families* (moderate cohesiveness but still prone to psychosocial morbidity, with functioning tending to deteriorate under the strain of death and bereavement).

Conclusions

Depression among cancer patients and grieving family members is quite common. Empathic communication, as the expression of a relational and transactional interpersonal exchange, is the main instrument by which to evaluate the psychological impact of the disease-related events (diagnosis, treatment, outcome) for both the patient and his/her family. Careful examination and detailed review of the symptoms, including thoughts, feelings, and behaviors, are the first steps in diagnosing depression according to the most commonly used taxonomic systems (e.g., DSM and ICD). Useful information can come from other systems (e.g., DCPR) and from data derived from research studies on depression in the medically ill and/or family members (e.g., demoralization, bereavement-related depression). The assessment of suicidal ideation is particularly important when dealing with depressed cancer patients as well as depressed family members during their mourning.

The role of specific forms of psychological therapy, including cognitive-behavioral, interpersonal, existentially oriented, or family-centered, and based on specific communication techniques and therapeutic strategies should also be known by physicians dealing with cancer patients and their families. The efficacy of psychotherapy in treating depression in oncology, especially when associated with correct use of psychotropic antidepressant drugs, has been demonstrated by a number of studies showing the benefit that psychotherapy can provide in terms of quality of life and coping.

Since cancer is a bio-psycho-existential-social disease, which afflicts all aspects of life, a whole-person and family-centered approach is mandatory in all cancer settings, from outpatient clinics to palliative-care units, in order to detect as soon as possible depression and properly treat it, because of its negative consequences on the patients and their relatives. As internationally indicated and agreed upon [37], people with cancer should be offered a range of physical, emotional, spiritual, and social support in all the phases of illness through specific services, including psychooncology services, available to help both people living with the after-effects of cancer and those with advanced cancer or dying from cancer. Furthermore, the needs of families and other carers of people with cancer should be met, especially in phases of major suffering, such as grief and bereavement.

For these reasons, a more sensitive, collaborative, and comprehensive approach to the diagnosis and treatment of depression, including clinical education, enhanced role of nurses, and integrating oncology and specialist care, is the only way to provide adequate care in the clinical setting [24].

References

1. Akechi T, Okuyama T, Onishi J, Morita T, Furukawa TA. Psychotherapy for depression among incurable cancer patients. Cochrane Database Syst Rev. 2008;(2):CD005537.
2. Allumbaugh DL, Hoyt W. Effectiveness of grief therapy: a meta-analysis. J Couns Psychol. 1999;46:370–80.

3. American Psychiatric Association. Practice guideline for the assessment and treatment of patients with suicidal behaviors. Washington: American Psychiatric Association; 2003.
4. Angelino AF, Treisman GJ. Major depression and demoralization in cancer patients: diagnostic and treatment considerations. Support Care Cancer. 2001;9:344–9.
5. Arora NK, Finney Rutten LJ, Gustafson DH, Moser R, Hawkins RP. Perceived helpfulness and impact of social support provided by family, friends, and health care providers to women newly diagnosed with breast cancer. Psychooncology. 2007;16(5):474–86.
6. Baider L, Cooper CL, De-Nour K, editors. Cancer and the family. 2nd ed. Sussex, UK: Wiley; 2000.
7. Boelen PA, Van Den Bout J. Complicated grief, depression and anxiety as distinct postloss syndromes: a confirmatory factor analysis study. Am J Psychiatry. 2005;162(11):2175–7.
8. Bonanno GA, Boerner K. The stage theory of grief. JAMA. 2007;297:2693.
9. Bonanno GA, Wortman CB, Nesse RM. Prospective patterns of resilience and maladjustment during widowhood. Psychol Aging. 2004;19(2):260–71.
10. Bottomley A. Depression in cancer patients: a literature review. Eur J Cancer Care (Engl). 1998;7(3):181–91.
11. Brintzenhofe-Szoc KM, Levin TT, Li Y, Kissane DW, Zabora JR. Mixed anxiety/depression symptoms in a large cancer cohort: prevalence by cancer type. Psychosomatics. 2009;50: 383–91.
12. Cockram CA, Doros G, de Figueiredo JM. Diagnosis and measurement of subjective incompetence: the clinical hallmark of demoralization. Psychother Psychosom. 2009;78:342–5.
13. Corruble E, Chouinard VA, Letierce A, Gorwood PA, Chouinard G. Is DSM-IV bereavement exclusion for major depressive episode relevant to severity and pattern of symptoms? A case-control, cross-sectional study. J Clin Psychiatry. 2009;70:1091–7.
14. Currier JM, Neimeyer RA, Berman JS. The effectiveness of psychotherapeutic interventions for bereaved persons: a comprehensive quantitative review. Psychol Bull. 2008;134:648–61.
15. Derogatis LR, Morrow GR, Fetting J, Penman D, Piasetsky S, Schmale AM, et al. The prevalence of psychiatric disorders among cancer patients. JAMA. 1983;249:751–7.
16. Epstein RM, Street RL Jr. Patient-centered communication in cancer care: promoting healing and reducing suffering. NIH Publication No. 07-6225. Bethesda: National Cancer Institute; 2007.
17. Fallowfield L, Jenkins V. Effective communication skills are the key to good cancer care. Eur J Cancer. 1999;35:1592–7.
18. Fallowfield L, Ratcliffe D, Jenkins V, Saul J. Psychiatric morbidity and its recognition by doctors in patients with cancer. Br J Cancer. 2001;84(8):1011–5.
19. Friðriksdóttir N, Saevarsdóttir T, Halfdánardóttir SÍ, Jónsdóttir A, Magnúsdóttir H, Olafsdóttir KL, et al. Family members of cancer patients: needs, quality of life and symptoms of anxiety and depression. Acta Oncol. 2011;50:252–8.
20. Giese-Davis J, Collie K, Rancourt KM, Neri E, Kraemer HC, Spiegel D. Decrease in depression symptoms is associated with longer survival in patients with metastatic breast cancer: a secondary analysis. J Clin Oncol. 2011;29:413–20.
21. Goebel S, von Harscher M, Mehdorn HM. Comorbid mental disorders and psychosocial distress in patients with brain tumours and their spouses in the early treatment phase. Support Care Cancer. 2011;19(11):1797–805.
22. Grassi L. Bereavement in families with relative dying of cancer. Curr Opin Support Palliat Care. 2007;1:43–9.
23. Grassi L, Biancosino B, Marmai L, Rossi E, Sabato S. Psychological factors affecting oncology conditions. In: Porcelli P, Sonino N, editors. Psychological factors affecting medical conditions. A new classification for DSM-V, vol. 28. Basel: Karger; 2007.
24. Grassi L, Holland JC, Johansen C, Koch U, Fawzy F. Psychiatric concomitants of cancer, screening procedures, and training of health care professionals in oncology: The paradigms of psycho-oncology in the psychiatry field. In: Christodoulou GN, editor. Advances in psychiatry, vol. 2. Athens: World Psychiatric Association; 2005.
25. Grassi L, Nanni MG, Uchitomi Y, Riba M. Pharmacotherapy of depression in people with cancer. In: Kissane D, Maj M, Sartorius N, editors. Depression and cancer. London: Wiley; 2011.

26. Grassi L, Riba M. Depressive disorders in oncology. In: Riba M, Grassi L, editors. WPA educational programme on depressive disorders, vol II: physical illness and depression. Geneva: World Psychiatric Association; 2008.
27. Grassi L, Riba M. New frontiers and challenges of psychiatry in oncology and palliative care. In: Christodoulou GN, Mezzich JE, editors. Advances in psychiatry, vol. III. Athens: World Psychiatric Association; 2009.
28. Grassi L, Rossi E, Caruso R, Nanni MG, Pedrazzi S, Sofritti S, et al. Educational intervention in cancer outpatient clinics on routine screening for emotional distress: an observational study. Psychooncology. 2011;20:669–74.
29. Grassi L, Sabato S, Rossi E, Marmai L, Biancosino B. Effects of supportive-expressive group therapy in breast cancer patients with affective disorders: a pilot study. Psychother Psychosom. 2010;79:39–47.
30. Greer S. Bereavement care: some clinical observations. Psychooncology. 2010;19:1156–60.
31. Gregurek R, Bras M, Dordević V, Ratković AS, Brajković L. Psychological problems of patients with cancer. Psychiatr Danub. 2010;22(2):227–30.
32. Guidi J, Fava GA, Picardi A, Porcelli P, Bellomo A, Grandi S, et al. Subtyping depression in the medically ill by cluster analysis. J Affect Disord. 2011;132(3):383–8.
33. Hamer M, Chida Y, Molloy GJ. Psychological distress and cancer mortality. J Psychosom Res. 2009;66:255–8.
34. Hensley PL. Treatment of bereavement-related depression and traumatic grief. J Affect Disord. 2006;92:117–24.
35. Holtslander LF, McMillan SC. Depressive symptoms, grief, and complicated grief among family caregivers of patients with advanced cancer three months into bereavement. Oncol Nurs Forum. 2011;38(1):60–5.
36. Jacobsen PB, Jim HS. Psychosocial interventions for anxiety and depression in adult cancer patients: achievements and challenges. CA Cancer J Clin. 2008;58:214–30.
37. Johansen C, Grassi L. International psycho-oncology: present and future directions. In: Holland JC, editor. Handbook of psycho-oncology. New York: Oxford University Press; 2010.
38. Kendler K, Myers J, Zisook S. Does bereavement-related major depression differ from major depression associated with other stressful life events? Am J Psychiatry. 2008;165:1449–55.
39. Kissane DW, Bloch S. Family focused grief therapy: a model of family-centred care during palliative care and bereavement. Buckingham: Open University Press; 2002.
40. Kissane DW, Levin T, Hales S, Lo C, Rodin G. Psychotherapy for depression in cancer and palliative care. In: Kissane DW, Maj M, Sartorius N, editors. Depression and cancer. Chichester: Wiley; 2011.
41. Kissane DW, McKenzie M, Bloch S, Moskowitz C, McKenzie DP, O'Neill I. Family focused grief therapy: a randomized, controlled trial in palliative care and bereavement. Am J Psychiatry. 2006;163:1208–18.
42. Kutner JS, Kilbourn KM. Bereavement: addressing challenges faced by advanced cancer patients, their caregivers, and their physicians. Prim Care. 2009;36(4):825–44.
43. Lannen PK, Wolfe J, Prigerson HG, Onelov E, Kreicbergs UC. Unresolved grief in a national sample of bereaved parents: impaired mental and physical health 4 to 9 years later. J Clin Oncol. 2008;26(36):5870–6.
44. Levenson JC, Frank E, Cheng Y, Rucci P, Janney CA, Houck P, et al. Comparative outcomes among the problem areas of interpersonal psychotherapy for depression. Depress Anxiety. 2010;27:434–40.
45. Love AW. Progress in understanding grief, complicated grief, and caring for the bereaved. Contemp Nurse. 2007;27(1):73–83.
46. Maciejewski PK, Zhang B, Block SD, Prigerson HG. An empirical examination of the stage theory of grief. JAMA. 2007;297(7):716–23.
47. Maguire P. Improving the recognition of concerns and affective disorders in cancer patients. Ann Oncol. 2002;13 Suppl 4:177–81.
48. Maguire P, Pitceathly C. Key communication skills and how to acquire them. BMJ. 2002;325:697–700.

49. Mangelli L, Fava GA, Grandi S, Grassi L, Ottolini F, Porcelli P, et al. Assessing demoralization and depression in the setting of medical disease. J Clin Psychiatry. 2005;66:391–4.
50. Massie MJ. Prevalence of depression in patients with cancer. J Natl Cancer Inst Monogr. 2004;32:57–71.
51. Mehnert A, Vehling S. Cancer patients: loss of meaning, demoralization and embitterment. In: Maercker A, Linden M, editors. Embitterment: societal, psychological, and clinical perspectives. Berlin: Springer; 2010.
52. Mitchell AJ, Chan M, Bhatti H, Halton M, Grassi L, Johansen C, et al. Prevalence of depression, anxiety, and adjustment disorder in oncological, haematological, and palliative-care settings: a meta-analysis of 94 interview-based studies. Lancet Oncol. 2011;12(2):160–74.
53. National Institute for Clinical Excellence. Self-harm — the short-term physical and psychological management and secondary prevention of self-harm in primary and secondary care. London: National Institute for Clinical Excellence; 2004.
54. Ng CG, Boks MP, Zainal NZ, de Wit NJ. The prevalence and pharmacotherapy of depression in cancer patients. J Affect Disord. 2011;131(1–3):1–7.
55. Osborn RL, Demoncada AC, Feuerstein M. Psychosocial interventions for depression, anxiety, and quality of life in cancer survivors: meta-analyses. Int J Psychiatry Med. 2006;36:13–34.
56. Pasquini M, Biondi M. Depression in cancer patients: a critical review. Clin Pract Epidemiol Ment Health. 2007;3:1–9.
57. Pellegrino R, Formica V, Portarena I, Mariotti S, Grenga I, Del Monte G, et al. Caregiver distress in the early phases of cancer. Anticancer Res. 2010;30(11):4657–63.
58. Pitceathly C, Maguire P. The psychological impact of cancer on patients' partners and other key relatives: a review. Eur J Cancer. 2003;39:1517–24.
59. Priegerson HG, Horowitz MJ, Jacobs SC, Parkes CM, Aslan M, Goodkin K, et al. Prolonged grief disorder: psychometric validation of criteria proposed for DSM-IV and ICD-11. PLoS Med. 2009;6(8):e100121.
60. Priegerson HG, Vanderwerker LC, Maciejewski PK. Prolonged grief disorder: a case for inclusion in DSM-IV. In: Stroebe M, Hansson R, Schut H, Stroebe W, editors. Handbook of bereavement research and practice: 21st-century perspective, chapter 8. Washington: Psychological Press; 2008. p. 165–86.
61. Prigerson HG, Maciejewski PK. Grief and acceptance as opposite sides of the same coin: setting a research agenda to study peaceful acceptance of loss. Br J Psychiatry. 2008;193(6):435–7.
62. Reeve JL, Lloyd-Williams M, Dowrick C. Revisiting depression in palliative care settings: the need to focus on clinical utility over validity. Palliat Med. 2008;22:383–91.
63. Reich M. Depression and cancer: recent data on clinical issues, research challenges and treatment approaches. Curr Opin Oncol. 2008;20:353–9.
64. Robson A, Scrutton F, Wilkinson L, MacLeod F. The risk of suicide in cancer patients: a review of the literature. Psychooncology. 2010;19:1250–8.
65. Schnur JB, Montgomery GH. A systematic review of therapeutic alliance, group cohesion, empathy, and goal consensus/collaboration in psychotherapeutic interventions in cancer: uncommon factors? Clin Psychol Rev. 2010;30:238–47.
66. Schut H, Stroebe M, Van Den Bout J, Terheggen M. The efficacy of bereavement interventions: who benefits? In: Stroebe MS, Hansson RO, Stroebe W, Schut H, editors. Handbook of bereavement research. Washington, DC: American Psychological Association; 2001.
67. Sharpe M, Strong V, Allen K, Rush R, Postma K, Tulloh A, et al. Major depression in outpatients attending a regional cancer centre: screening and unmet treatment needs. Br J Cancer. 2004;90:314–20.
68. Shear K, Frank E, Houck PR, Reynolds III CF. Treatment of complicated grief: a randomized controlled trial. JAMA. 2005;293:2601–8.
69. Shear K, Mulhare E. Attachment, loss and complicated grief. Dev Psychobiol. 2005;47:253–67.
70. Shear MK, Simon N, Wall M, Zisook S, Neimeyer R, Duan N, et al. Complicated grief and related bereavement issues for DSM-5. Depress Anxiety. 2011;28:103–17.

71. Spiegel D, Classen C. Group therapy for cancer patients: a research-based handbook of psychosocial care. New York: Basic Books; 2000.
72. Stroebe M, Schut H, Stroebe W. Health outcomes of bereavement. Lancet. 2007;370:1960–73.
73. Stroebe M, Van Son M, Stroebe W, Kleber R, Schut H, Van den Bout J. On the classification and diagnosis of pathological grief. Clin Psychol Rev. 2000;20(1):57–75.
74. Thornton LM, Andersen BL, Schuler TA, Carson III WE. A psychological intervention reduces inflammatory markers by alleviating depressive symptoms: secondary analysis of a randomized controlled trial. Psychosom Med. 2009;71:715–24.
75. Tomarken A, Holland J, Schachter S, Vanderwerker L, Zuckerman E, Nelson C, et al. Factors of complicated grief pre-death in caregivers of cancer patients. Psychooncology. 2007;17:105–11.
76. Vanderwerker LC, Jacobs SC, Parkes CM, Priegerson HG. An exploration of associations between separation anxiety in childhood and complicated grief in later life. J Nerv Ment Dis. 2006;194:1–3.
77. Vogel BA, Leonhart R, Helmes AW. Communication matters: the impact of communication and participation in decision making on breast cancer patients' depression and quality of life. Patient Educ Couns. 2009;77:391–7.
78. Wakefield JC, Schmitz MF, Baer JC. Did narrowing the major depression bereavement exclusion from DSM-III-R to DSM-IV increase validity? Evidence from the National Comorbidity Survey. J Nerv Ment Dis. 2011;199:66–73.
79. Wakefield JC, Schmitz MF, First MB, Horwitz AV. Extending the bereavement exclusion for major depression to other losses: evidence from the National Comorbidity Survey. Arch Gen Psychiatry. 2007;64:433–40.
80. Wasteson E, Brenne E, Higginson IJ, Hotopf M, Lloyd-Williams M, Kaasa S, et al. European Palliative Care Research Collaborative (EPCRC). Depression assessment and classification in palliative cancer patients: a systematic literature review. Palliat Med. 2009;23:739–53.
81. Watson M, Kissane D, editors. The international psycho-oncology society's training guide for psychological therapies with cancer patients. London: Wiley; 2011.
82. Weissman M, Markowitz J, Klerman G. Comprehensive guide to interpersonal psychotherapy. New York: Basic Books; 2000.
83. Weissman MM, Markowitz JC, Klerman GL. Clinician's quick guide to interpersonal psychotherapy. New York: Oxford University Press; 2007.
84. Wellish DK. Family issues in palliative care. In: Chochinov HM, Breitbart W, editors. Handbook of psychiatry in palliative medicine. New York: Oxford University Press; 2000.
85. Williams S, Dale J. The effectiveness of treatment for depression/depressive symptoms in adults with cancer: a systematic review. Br J Cancer. 2006;94:372–90.
86. Wittouck C, Van Autreve S, De Jaegere E, Portzky G, van Heeringen K. The prevention and treatment of complicated grief: a meta-analysis. Clin Psychol Rev. 2011;31:69–78.
87. Worden JW. Grief counseling and grief therapy. A handbook for the mental health practitioner. 4th ed. New York: Springer; 2008.
88. Zabora J, Brintzenhofe-Szoc K, Curbow B, Hooker C, Piantadosi S. The prevalence of psychological distress by cancer site. Psychooncology. 2001;10:19–28.
89. Zaider T, Kissane D. The assessment and management of family distress during palliative care. Curr Opin Support Palliat Care. 2009;3:67–71.
90. Zeitlin SV. Grief and bereavement. Prim Care. 2001;28(2):415–25.
91. Zisook S, Shear K. Grief and bereavement: what psychiatrists need to know. World Psychiatry. 2009;8:67–74.

Chapter 7
Communication Issues in Integrative Oncology

Donald I. Abrams

Abstract Integrative oncology is an emerging subspecialty in oncology practice that engages the whole patient—body, mind, spirit, and community. In integrative medicine, the patient and the practitioner are partners in the healing process, with the relationship being a centerpiece of the paradigm. Integrative oncologists strive to combine the best of conventional interventions with evidence-based (as much as possible) complementary therapies into a personalized treatment regimen. Open and honest bidirectional communication that establishes a mutually respectful trusting relationship is a key component of the integrative oncology consultation. Whereas integration of complementary therapies is widely sought by patients living with and beyond malignant diagnoses, special communication issues are presented by patients choosing to pursue solely alternative therapeutic pathways. Attempting to understand patient motivations and fears fosters a greater potential that they may deflect potentially useless or harmful "treatments."

Keywords Integrative medicine • Complementary therapies • Alternative therapies

> His condition was rendered worse by the fact that he read medical books and consulted with doctors. The progress of his disease was so gradual that he could deceive himself when comparing one day with another—the difference was so slight. But when he consulted the doctors, it seemed to him that he was getting worse, and even very rapidly. Yet despite this, he was continually consulting them.
> That month he went to see another celebrity, who told him almost the same as the first had done but put his questions rather differently, and the interview with this celebrity only increased Ivan Ilych's doubts and fears. A friend of a friend of his, a very good doctor,

---

D.I. Abrams, MD (✉)
Chief, Hematology-Oncology, San Francisco General Hospital, Integrative Oncology, UCSF Osher Center for Integrative Medicine, San Francisco, CA 94115, USA

University of California San Francisco, UCSF Osher Center for Integrative Medicine, 1545 Divisadero Street, 4th Floor, San Francisco, CA 94115, USA
e-mail: dabrams@hemeonc.ucsf.edu

diagnosed his illness again, quite differently from the others; and though he predicted recovery, his questions and suppositions bewildered Ivan Ilych still more and increased his doubts. A homeopath diagnosed the disease in yet another way and prescribed medicine, which Ivan Ilych took secretly for a week. But after a week, not feeling any improvement and having lost confidence in the former doctor's treatment and in this one's, he became still more despondent. One day a lady acquaintance mentioned a cure effected by a wonder-working icon. Ivan Ilych caught himself listening attentively and beginning to believe that it had occurred. The incident alarmed him. "Has my mind really weakened to such an extent?" he asked himself. "Nonsense! It's all rubbish. I mustn't give way to nervous fears but, having chosen a doctor, must keep strictly to his treatment. That is what I will do. Now it's all settled. I won't think about it but will follow the treatment seriously till summer, and then we shall see. From now on there must be no more of this wavering!" This was easy to say but impossible to carry out [1].

The dilemma of Ivan Ilych summarized by Tolstoy in 1874 eloquently portrays the universality and timelessness of the issues facing patients with malignant disease today. Although the actual diagnosis is never confirmed in the fictional account, the congruence of Ilych's experience with that of modern cancer patients is quite remarkable, considering how far medicine has advanced in the last 130 years. The passage is particularly poignant in its presentation of so many of the issues relevant to the emerging field of integrative oncology—optimizing communication, disclosing use of complementary therapies, being attracted to alternative interventions, coping with fear and loss of control [2, 3]. Perhaps if Ilych had had access to an integrative oncologist, some of the angst expressed in the above passage could have been assuaged.

Integrative medicine provides relationship-centered care with an emphasis on addressing the needs of the whole person—body, mind, spirit, and community. The Consortium of Academic Health Centers for Integrative Medicine defines it as "the practice of medicine that reaffirms the importance of the relationship between practitioner and patient, focuses on the whole person, is informed by evidence, and makes use of all appropriate therapeutic approaches, healthcare professionals, and disciplines to achieve optimal health and healing" [4]. With a focus on wellness and prevention, integrative medicine aims to activate the body's innate healing response, using natural, less-invasive interventions than conventional medicine whenever possible. Integrative medicine, however, does not eschew conventional allopathic medicine. Quite the contrary, it supports the rational evidence-based combination of conventional and complementary therapies into an individualized therapeutic regimen that addresses the whole person. Integrative oncology, then, is the application of the principles of integrative medicine in the care of people living with and beyond malignant diagnoses.

Many equate integrative medicine with complementary and alternative medicine (CAM). CAM is a term that would best fall into disuse. The whole concept is a bit of an oxymoron. *Complementary therapies* suggest that they are being used *in conjunction with* conventional care. *Alternative therapies* implies that these interventions are used *instead of* conventional interventions. So how something can be both complementary and alternative, as CAM implies, becomes a bit difficult to grasp. *Integrative* gives a much clearer picture that these interventions are being used in conjunction with conventional treatment options.

Rather than a homeopathic remedy or a wonder-working icon, it is communication that the integrative oncologist uses as the main tool in caring for the cancer patient [5].

By the time patients are first seen in consultation by integrative medicine practitioners, they have usually had a significant amount of interaction with a medical system that they may never had had occasion to interact with previously. After a number of diagnostic studies, most often involving an invasive tissue sampling, the patient may have already seen a surgeon, a radiation oncologist, and perhaps a medical oncologist. Each of these specialists has likely focused on the piece of the patient that they needed to be concerned with, often overlooking the actual whole person with the disease. The integrative oncologist follows the words of Maimonides, repeated by Osler, that "it is more important to know what sort of patient has a disease than what disease a patient has."

To learn about the patient, the integrative oncologist may open the consultation by asking, "Tell me your story." The response to this simple query conveys a lot about the patient being seen. Some may say, "Which story?" Others will hand over a sheaf of papers—copies of X-ray and laboratory reports, a myriad of laboratory tests—and expect one to believe that this tells their story. A spouse may begin to answer, which can also be quite telling in itself. The patient may wander back 20 or 30 years and begin there. Often there is a remembered time of great stress that antedated the symptom that first alerted him or her that something was amiss. In any case, it is best for the integrative oncologist to listen without the interruption that patients have come to expect from their physician, and allow the individual to recreate how their cancer diagnosis has affected their life. Daniel Siegel, in his book *The Mindful Therapist*, reminds us that "research suggests that our presence as medical or mental health clinicians, the way we bring ourselves fully into connection with those for whom we care, is one of the most crucial factors supporting how people heal—how they respond to our therapeutic efforts" [6]. For many, this may be the first occasion they have had to verbalize the effect of their diagnosis on their life.

Three questions are worth asking during the family and social history after inquiring about religious beliefs and spirituality: "What brings you joy? What are your hopes? From where does your strength come?" are queries that allow the patient to reflect on topics that may have slipped from the forefront of their minds. Just formulating responses is often distressing and can produce tears. On the other hand, it is amazing how even patients struggling with a life-threatening diagnosis can still list joys, hopes, and strengths. Reminding the patient of these answers is often an excellent way to close the consultation.

Challenges in Communication about Complementary Therapies in Integrative Oncology

One of the original definitions of *alternative therapies* was "medical interventions not taught widely at U.S. medical schools or generally available in U.S. hospitals" [7, 8]. This is something of a moving target, though. For example, massage and acupuncture would have been considered alternative back then, but are now increasingly available in hospitals, and perhaps even taught to some degree at some medical schools. Hence, they have now become therapies that may be used to complement conventional interventions. The role of the integrative oncologist becomes that of assisting the patient in creating a treatment regimen that safely incorporates complementary therapies with their conventional treatment, using evidence-based information whenever possible. One could wonder why an integrative oncologist is necessary; cannot the conventional oncologist do the same? In these days of the exploding knowledge base in cancer therapeutics, it is easy to understand the increased specialization of the oncology professional. It is hard enough to keep up with all of the treatment algorithms and interventions for breast cancer. The general oncologist caring for patients with breast, lung, gastrointestinal malignancies, lymphomas, gynecologic cancers, head and neck, etc. has a daunting task to stay up to date on all the advances in this enormous field. To expect any of these practitioners to follow the expanding field of integrative oncology in addition would be asking too much.

The conventional oncologist—surgical, medical, or radiation—may also not embrace integrative interventions, particularly complementary therapies. Many have negative impressions of these interventions, either from personal experiences with patients or from reading the medical literature. Most will assume a "Don't ask, don't tell" position, choosing not even to inquire about the patient's use of complementary therapies for fear of opening a Pandora's box. Or if they do ask, the patient might inquire in return, assuming that the physician has knowledge of the field, potentially exposing the physician's actual ignorance. Research has demonstrated that during the short interview time the conventional oncologist has to care for his or her patient, questions about use of complementary therapies are not generally asked [9–11].

A study in Australia and New Zealand analyzed audiotapes of initial consultations of women with stage I–II breast cancer meeting with their oncologists to discuss treatment options [12]. Reference to use of complementary therapies was identified in 24 of 102 (24%) consultations analyzed. Of these discussions, nearly three-quarters (73%) were initiated by the patient, one-quarter by the doctor, and one by a family member. The most common complementary interventions discussed were vitamins and antioxidants (23%), positive thinking/stress-reduction techniques (20%), and dietary changes (18%). In this study, oncologists encouraged the use of the complementary intervention in 38% of the cases. In 23% of the instances, however, the oncologist discouraged the use of the complementary therapies, most often citing the lack of evidence for either safety or efficacy. Surprisingly, in 20% of the recorded conversations in which the patient initiated a discussion of complementary therapies, the physician ignored it altogether.

The Australian study focused on women with breast cancer and their rate of discussion of complementary therapies at their initial consultation. A larger body of publications addresses the question of how frequently patients divulge their use of complementary therapies while receiving their conventional cancer care. Estimates of the use of complementary therapies in cancer patients range from 7 to 82% [13, 14]. The truth likely lies somewhere within that wide range. It is clear, however, that the percentage who divulge their use of these interventions to their traditional cancer care providers is low, averaging about 33%. These findings are quite consistent with the figures regarding disclosure among 1,013 noncancer patients as well, which were derived from an October 2010 survey of consumer use of CAM conducted by the American Association of Retired People (AARP) and the National Center for Complementary and Alternative Medicine (NCCAM) [15]. Of 539 survey respondents who said they used complementary therapies and were also being seen by a conventional physician, only 33% reported discussing their complementary therapy with their physician. The participants who had not discussed this information were asked why they had not. The most frequent responses were that the physician never asked (42%), the respondents did not know they should (30%), there was not enough time during the office visit (17%), the respondent did not think that the physician was knowledgeable about the topic (17%), and the respondent thought the physician would be dismissive or advise them not to do it (12%). In an earlier study of cancer patients specifically, three barriers to discussion were identified as being the most common reasons for nondisclosure of complementary therapy: the physician's indifference or opposition, the physician's emphasis on scientific evidence, and the patient's anticipation of a negative response from the physician [16]. The study also involved direct observation of patient–physician interactions and demonstrated that prompting physicians merely to ask a direct question regarding use of complementary interventions during their history taking increased disclosure from 7 to 43%. The US National Center for Complementary and Alternative Medicine ultimately launched a "Time to Talk: Ask, Tell" campaign, encouraging physicians to inquire about their patients' use of these interventions while also encouraging patients to offer this information spontaneously to their healthcare providers [17].

Fear of being dismissed for lack of scientific evidence is one of the main reasons identified for why cancer patients do not spontaneously disclose their use of complementary interventions to their conventional caregivers. A small study of 34 men with prostate cancer using complementary therapies in the UK sought to define which factors most influence the men's choices of interventions [18, 19]. The investigators determined that the most important determinant of use of a therapy was personal testimonials of people who believed they had been helped by the therapy. This was followed by the long history and enduring popularity of the treatment, the plausibility of the mechanism of action, a belief or trust in the individual therapies or their providers, and, last, the scientific evidence. The investigators concluded that it is important to acknowledge the different standards of evidence used by patients and clinicians to evaluate the benefits or lack thereof of complementary interventions. Clinicians should be aware of these conflicting metrics when counseling patients on whether or not it is advisable to incorporate a particular therapy into their integrative regimen. Being judgmental about or belittling the patient's choice of a potential intervention is not likely to engender honest future discussions about the patient's use of complementary therapies.

In addition to the lack of evidence regarding the safety and effectiveness of particular therapies, the clinician likely also has other concerns. Worry about possible CAM–drug interactions that may decrease the efficacy or increase the toxicity of conventional cancer therapies are a real concern to the conventional oncologist [20]. Such interactions could be mediated through the cytochrome p450 hepatic enzyme system. It is known that some complementary therapies, such as St. John's wort, used in the treatment of mild-to-moderate depression, may induce the enzymes responsible for metabolism of cytotoxic chemotherapy agents as well as targeted therapies. Hence, if a patient is using St. John's wort, he or she may be decreasing the effective concentration of the conventional cancer therapy, jeopardizing its effectiveness.

This potential underscores the need for open and honest communication between patient and conventional cancer care provider about the use of all ingested complementary therapies. The other interaction that is greatly feared by the conventional oncologist and radiation therapist is the possibility that antioxidant supplements, or perhaps even an antioxidant-rich diet, may interfere with the efficacy of radiation and chemotherapeutic agents that damage malignant cells by way of oxidative stress [21]. Undisclosed use of antioxidants during active chemotherapy may negate the potential benefits of treatment. On the other side of the argument are those who suggest that no such clinically significant interference has ever been demonstrated and that antioxidants may protect normal tissues from the ravages of chemoradiation.

So wherein lies the truth? The reality is that very few of the hundreds, perhaps thousands, of botanical–chemotherapy pharmacokinetic interaction studies that need to be done to generate the evidence we all desire have ever been done, or will likely ever be done. Similarly, randomized placebo-controlled trials of antioxidants in patients undergoing radiation or chemotherapy are difficult to design and perhaps even more difficult to get approved by institutional review boards. With such uncertainty, the conventional radiation or medical oncologist will take the conservative approach and suggest that patients cease and avoid any such interventions while they are receiving conventional therapy. Such an approach may be stressed particularly in patients being treated with curative intent or those receiving adjuvant interventions. In patients with incurable conditions where palliation is the goal, the demand to avoid all such potential for theoretical interaction may be less strongly enforced.

An interesting conundrum arises in the setting of the patient with advanced disease who elects to participate in early-phase clinical trials. Such trials, usually of small size, are designed to collect information in a controlled setting where the only unknown variable is expected to be the phase I agent. These trials are particularly sensitive to the issue of concurrent use of biologically based orally ingested complementary therapies that may obfuscate the ability accurately to determine the safety profile of the experimental intervention. The difficulty studying this issue is demonstrated in a study where the investigators did not actually ask the 212 phase I study subjects if they were using biologically based interventions or planning to while actually enrolled in the study as "they had all been instructed specifically not to take them, and we were concerned that patients still taking CAM might not honestly reveal their consumption [22]."

What is the role of the integrative oncologist in counseling the patient who comes seeking information and advice as to whether it is okay to continue their fish oil and vitamin D during their chemotherapy? Although clinical trial-generated evidence is lacking, the integrative oncologist cannot just sit with a patient during a consultation repeating "I don't know, I don't know" in response to their queries about this supplement and that botanical. A recent e-mail from a meticulous 53-year-old woman with metastatic endometrial cancer illustrates the point well.

> I have been researching turmeric to try and determine:
>
> 1. How much one should ingest every day for maximum effect.
> 2. The proper ratio of black pepper to turmeric.
> 3. Whether olive oil has to be mixed with the turmeric and pepper. How much?
> 4. Whether turmeric tablets are a proper substitute for turmeric powder.

There is a lot of conflicting information even among major players in the field. I've finally connected with some other cancer patients who are practicing complimentary therapies like I am. I AM SO CONFUSED. Can you please clarify?

Responding emphatically to such queries may place the integrative practitioner in a somewhat awkward position, as any information communicated as truth is not likely to have the degree of supporting data that one usually demands. Similarly, when the patient comes with questions about an intervention that the integrative practitioner believes is a scam or hoax, the recommendation to discontinue or not consider it is also often communicated on the basis of intuition or gestalt, rather than any available hard evidence. Fortunately, resources to help the integrative oncologist make informed recommendations are becoming increasingly available [23–30].

The Patient Seeking Alternative Cancer Care

Seen as one who is willing to consider, if not embrace, complementary therapies, the integrative oncologist may be approached by patients seeking unconventional unproved therapies to assist either in obtaining such treatments or for advice on a particular intervention [31]. Patients seeking alternatives have generally bought in to some degree to the "slash, burn, and poison" concept of traditional cancer care and desire to avoid surgery, radiation, and chemotherapy at all costs. Try as one might, it is often quite difficult to dissuade such patients from their alternative paths. Many conventional oncologists at my institution, faced with "refusnik" patients, will refer them for an integrative oncology consultation in the hope that if anyone could convince them to change their mind, it would be their fellow oncologist with expertise in integrating complementary modalities into a rationale treatment program. These patients are often extremely intelligent and very Web savvy, having downloaded reams of information on their alternative of choice. It is important in these situations to get as complete an understanding as possible of what has led the patient away from conventional interventions and to share one's stories of the success of traditional interventions. Often, but by no means always, these patients have not accepted the reality of their diagnosis or have created a well-defended denial system. Sometimes referral to a psychooncology colleague can be useful if the patient does not see this in a threatening light.

There are, of course, cases of patients who have been seemingly successful following alternative pathways, just as there are isolated reports of spontaneous remissions of any presumed chronic, irreversible disease processes.

A 52-year-old previously healthy innovative and successful businessman with newly diagnosed Philadelphia-positive chronic myelogenous leukemia has normalized his complete blood count from a baseline of 90,900 white blood cells/mm^3 with 33% immature forms by a carefully concocted regimen of botanicals and supplements. Although he was presented with the remarkable survival data associated with the current oral targeted therapy interventions for CML, the patient opted to give his self-designed regimen a few months' trial before reconsidering standard treatment and is quite elated at his response to date.

A recent e-mail from a 42-year-old attorney demonstrates another positive outcome in a patient choosing a strictly alternative path. The patient had been diagnosed 3 years earlier with biopsy-confirmed invasive breast cancer presenting as a 2-cm mass in the right breast.

> You told me I was crazy for going on alternative plant-based protocols (no chemo, no radiation, no surgery). Well, I just wanted you to know that I'm doing fabulous! The last MRI in 2010 showed next to nothing active left. I'm going in for another soon, but in the meantime, my tumor markers have bottomed out on the normal range. At some point, there won't be any sign of anything left! And I'll live to 95 without any drug side effects!

Although calling any patient crazy is not recommended, particularly a lawyer, the frustration evoked by dealing with such a highly functional patient who refused to see it my way is easy to recall. Her apparent success may or may not be related to her "plant-based protocols," but her sense of empowerment in controlling her own destiny is certainly a boon to her health and well-being.

In both of the examples above, the patients had devised their own alternative regimens. Many, however, are steered to "alternative" practitioners by family, friends, popular books, or Internet links. Often visits to these providers are not covered by insurance companies, and cash up front, usually large sums, is required. Desperate patients, especially those who may have run out of options, are often willing to make a financial sacrifice for the hope of prolonged survival.

A 78-year-old widow from out of state was referred for consultation by her son, a physician living closer to the Bay Area. After 3 years of back-to-back regimens, she had come to the end of the line of sequenced chemotherapies for her advanced ovarian cancer. She sought recommendations for alternative interventions. Focusing instead on nutrition, physical activity, stress reduction, traditional Chinese medicine, mind–body interventions, and spirituality, we developed a program to see if we could slow her disease progression. The need to get her affairs in order was also discussed. I was surprised to see her again 18 months later. She reported that she had followed most of the protocol we had developed, but then she heard of a clinician who used to practice in the United States but had been "wrongly accused," had lost his medical license, and then regained it, afterwards deciding to continue to base his practice in South America. She and a cousin, also diagnosed with an incurable cancer, had both flown down for this physician's special alternative cancer care. When asked, she reported that the total cost for the two of them combined, including the travel, had amounted to only $36,000.

On return from her treatment in South America, she had a PET/CT scan to ascertain the effect of the treatment. The scan suggested progressive disease. The patient sent the results to her alternative practitioner and shared his e-mail response.

> I read what they reported from the scan. I have seen this so many times before. The (sic) call any growth anywhere in your body a cancer tumor since you have a history of cancer. There is absolutely no cancer cell frequencies, but there is Candida that looks like cancer cells on the scans and if they were to treat you they would treat you with a protocol for cancer and it absolutely would do no good as the chemo will not touch the Candida yeast fungus. Like the (sic) say on Fox News, I report and you decide what to believe.
>
> It would be a very good idea to go to the health food store and buy Candidase caps or whatever brand they would happen to have and start taking it three times a day plus Arm & Hamar (sic) baking soda (half teaspoon) in a glass of water three times a day. Put your efforts to fight the fungus as there are no cancer cells.

We are leaving Friday for a vacation and will return to the office the middle of Jan because there is (sic) a lot of patients coming to start the new year.

Looking into the eyes of a cachectic woman with tense ascites and pedal edema, I took her hands and assured her that this was not a fungus, but terminal cancer; she had fought the good fight, but I feared her time had come. I pleaded with her not to spend any more of her estate traveling worldwide for bogus cures and suggested instead that she spend time with her son and the rest of her family who loved and cherished her, as she was now terminal. She thanked me for being honest with her, said none of her other providers could do that, and remarked that she now fully understood why her son had suggested that she come back to see me for a second visit.

The effective practice of integrative oncology requires a communication skill set that many busy practitioners just do not find the time to use during a short clinical encounter, in which so many details concerning conventional cancer care need to be addressed. There are some practicing oncologists who attempt to treat the cancer as well as addressing the patient's other needs. More frequently, patients see an integrative care provider in addition to their conventional oncologist. In my consultative practice I explain to patients that cancer is like a weed. Others are working on their weed—the surgeon, radiation oncologist, and medical oncologist. My job is to work with the garden, making sure that the soil is inhospitable to growth and spread of the weed. The analogy is relevant for those undergoing acute treatment as well as cancer survivors and seems to resonate with most everyone. Offering the patient advice on nutrition, physical activity, mind–body interventions, and stress reduction and helping them to reengage with their long-standing religious or spiritual beliefs provide them with their own toolbox, which they can integrate with their conventional therapies, enhancing their sense of empowerment, further decreasing their stress, increasing their hope, and perhaps even adding quantity as well as quality to their lives. Integrative oncology is not just about complementary therapies or lifestyle modification—it is a field based on communicating in a meaningful way with the whole person living with the disease and not just targeting their cancer.

References

1. Tolstoy L. The death of Ivan Ilyich. Seattle: CreateSpace; 2009.
2. Abrams DI. An overview of integrative oncology. Clin Adv Hematol Oncol. 2007;5:45–7.
3. Deng G, Frenkel M, Cohen L, et al. Society for Integrative Oncology evidence-based clinical practice guidelines for clinical oncology: complementary therapies and botanicals. J Soc Integr Oncol. 2009;7:85–120.
4. www.imconsortium.org
5. Surbone A. Truth and truth-telling in integrative oncology. In: Abrams D, Weil A, editors. Integrative oncology. New York: Oxford University Press; 2009.
6. Siegal DJ. The mindful therapist. New York: W.W. Norton & Company; 2010.
7. Eisenberg DM, Kessler RC, Foster C, Norlock FE, Calkins DR, Delbanco TL. Unconventional medicine in the United States—prevalence, costs, and patterns of use. N Engl J Med. 1993; 328:246–52.
8. Eisenberg DM, Davis RB, Ettner SL, Appel S, Wilkey S, Van Rompey M, et al. Trends in alternative medicine use in the United States 1990–1997: results of a follow-up national survey. JAMA. 1998;280:1569–75.

9. Frenkel M, Ben-Ayre E, Baldwin CD, Sierpina V. Approach to communicating with patients about the use of nutritional supplements in cancer care. South Med J. 2005;98:289–94.
10. Frenkel M, Ben-Ayre E, Geva H, Klein A. Educating CAM practitioners about integrative medicine: an approach to overcoming the communication gap with conventional health care providers. J Complement Altern Med. 2007;13:387–91. doi:19.1089/acm.2006.6293.
11. Frenkl M, Ben-Ayre E, Cohen L. Communication in cancer care: discussing complementary and alternative medicine. Integr Cancer Ther. 2010;9:177–85. doi:10.1177/1534735410363706.
12. Juraskova I, Hegedus L, Butow P, Smith A, Schofield P. Discussing complementary therapy use with early-stage breast cancer patients: exploring the communication gap. Integr Cancer Ther. 2010;9:168–76. doi:10.1177/1534735410365712.
13. Boon HS, Olatunde F, Zick SM. Trends in complementary/alternative medicine use by breast cancer survivors: comparing survey data from 1998 and 2005. BMC Womens Health. 2007;7:4. doi:10.1186/1472-6874/7/4.
14. Goldstein MS, Lee JH, Ballard-Barbash R, Brown ER. The use and perceived benefit of complementary and alternative medicine among Californians with cancer. Psychooncology. 2008;17(1):19–25. doi:10.1002/pon.1193.
15. U.S. Department of Health and Human Services. AARP and National Center for Complementary and Alternative Medicine Survey Report. Complementary and alternative: what people aged 50 and older discuss with their health care providers. April 2011. http://nccam.nih.gov/news/camstats/2010/NCCAM_aarp%20survey.pdf
16. Richardson MA, Masse LC, Nanny K, Sanders C. Discrepant views of oncologists and cancer patients on complementary/alternative medicine. Support Care Cancer. 2004;12:797–804. doi:10.1007/s00520-004-0677-3.
17. http://nccam.nih.gov/timetotalk/
18. Evans MA, Shaw ARG, Sharp DJ, et al. Men with cancer: is their use of complementary and alternative medicine a response to needs unmet by conventional care? Eur J Cancer Care. 2007;16:517–25. doi:10.1111/j.1365-2354.2007.00786.x.
19. Evans M, Shaw A, Thompson EA, Falk S, Turton P, Thompson T, et al. Decisions to use complementary and alternative medicine (CAM) by male cancer patients: information-seeking roles and types of evidence used. BMC Complement Altern Med. 2007;7:25. doi:10.186/1472-6882-7-251.
20. Spaareboom A. CAM-chemo interactions: what is known. In: Abrams D, Weil A, editors. Integrative oncology. New York: Oxford University Press; 2009.
21. Kelly K. The antioxidant debate. In: Abrams D, Weil A, editors. Integrative oncology. New York: Oxford University Press; 2009.
22. Hlubocky FJ, Ratain MJ, Wen M, Daugherty CK. Complementary and alternative medicine among advanced cancer patients enrolled on phase I trials: a study of prognosis, quality of life, and preferences for decision making. J Clin Oncol. 2007;25:548–54. doi:10.1200/JCO.2005.03.9800.
23. http://www.integrativeonc.org/
24. http://www.cancer.gov/cancertopics/pdq/cam
25. http://www.mskcc.org/mskcc/html/11570.cfm
26. Abrams D, Weil A. Integrative oncology. New York: Oxford University Press; 2009.
27. Alschuler LN, Gazella KA. The definitive guide to cancer, 3rd edition: an integrative approach to prevention, treatment and healing. Berkeley: Celestial Arts; 2010.
28. Block K. Life over cancer: The Block Center program for integrative cancer treatment. New York: Bantam; 2009.
29. Servan-Schreiber D. Anticancer, a new way of life. New York: Viking Adult; 2009.
30. Integrative Cancer Therapies. SAGE Publications, http://intl-ict.sagepub.com
31. Jacobson GM, Cain MC. Ethical issues related to patient use of complementary and alternative medicine. J Oncol Pract. 2009;5:124–5.

Chapter 8
Communicating about Spiritual Issues with Cancer Patients

Lorenzo Norris, Kathryn Walseman, and Christina M. Puchalski

Abstract Many patients have expressed the importance of spirituality in their life and the wish that clinicians would discuss this topic with them and have it integrated into their health care. Clinicians also have noted the importance of spirituality, but have struggled with ways to address spiritual issues in a medical setting. Barriers to effective communication include: lack of knowledge, physician time, and fear of causing a negative reaction in patients. Understanding these barriers and developing an open-ended systematic approach is one key to starting the spiritual dialogue with patients. These dialogues are best conducted in some framework or spiritual care model. The current spiritual care models are derived from Engel's biopsychosocial model that places an emphasis on understanding and appreciating the patients' unique story but with the addition of a spiritual domain. Care models that are multidisciplinary can take advantage of each care team member's strength and provide a more opportune setting to appreciate the patient story from multiple perspectives.

Tools that aid clinicians in screening for spiritual distress include the FICA. The FICA tool provides a way for healthcare providers to use open-ended questions to assess the four domains of a patient's spirituality. While useful, these tools are meant to open the discussion that the clinician can then use to further appreciate the patient's

---

L. Norris, MD
Survivorship Center Psychiatric Services,
The George Washington University, Washington, DC, USA
e-mail: lnorris@mfa.gwu.edu

K. Walseman, MD
Department of Psychiatry, George Washington University
Hospital, Washington, DC, USA
e-mail: kjw27@gwu.edu

C.M. Puchalski, MD, MS, FACP (✉)
George Washington Institute for Spirituality and Health (GWish),
The George Washington School of Medicine and Health Sciences,
The George Washington University, 2030 M Street NW, Suite 4014, Washington, DC 20052, USA
e-mail: cpuchals@gwu.edu

life and any potential spiritual crisis. Points of concern detected by a spiritual screening can indicate a potential referral for a formal spiritual assessment. Formal spiritual assessment is usually done by a board-certified chaplain or spiritual care expert with the intent of forming a spiritual care plan. A spiritual care plan is ideally formed in a multidisciplinary framework, in which the patients' spiritual needs can be incorporated into their current medical treatment. The care plan can then be used to further inform targeted spiritual interventions such as meaning-centered group psychotherapy or the short-term life review. Entering into a dialogue about spirituality can give a sense of meaning and hope, as well as open up treatment opportunities. Approaches and models exist to help clinicians enter into this dialogue and deliver spiritually informed care.

Key words Spirituality • Religion • Cancer • Communication • Health • Spirituality and health • Spiritual issues • Spiritual history

Why Spirituality Is Important

Spirituality, referring to the way people express meaning and purpose, how they experience their interconnectedness with others, the self, the moment or the significant or sacred, is a fundamental aspect of personhood. All people seek meaning and connection to something greater than themselves. In general, spirituality is considered a universal human characteristic [1]. In his book, *The Rebirth of the Clinic: An Introduction to Spirituality in Health Care*, Daniel Sulmasy views spirituality as one's relationship with the transcendent, oftentimes expressed through one's attitudes, habits, and practices. Religion, a type of spirituality, is a set of organized beliefs about the transcendent shared by a group of people [2]. An individual may experience the transcendent through religion, but one may be spiritual without necessarily being religious. Spirituality also embraces humanism and the arts. People may derive meaning and purpose in life through their relationship with this transcendent dimension, however, a person understands that in his/her life. Spirituality can be seen as the inner life of people.

Having a strong sense of spirituality helps patients to adjust to illness [3]. Brady and colleagues assessed over 1,000 cancer patients and found that patients with high levels of spiritual well-being reported more life enjoyment, even in the presence of pain or fatigue. Specifically, for those patients in pain, 47.8% of patients who reported high levels of meaning and peace "enjoyed life very much," whereas only 9.3% patients who reported low levels of meaning and peace "enjoyed life very much" [4]. Other studies have shown that spiritual well-being in cancer patients has been associated with lower levels of depression, better quality of life near death, and protection against end-of-life despair and desire for hastened death [3, 5, 6].

Spirituality promotes adjustment to illness by providing a context in which to derive hope and meaning. An individual diagnosed with cancer will inevitably be plagued by profound transcendent questions: Why did this happen to me? Why would God allow me to suffer this way? What will happen to me after I die? [7, 8]. Answers to these questions are often guided by spiritual beliefs that allow one to reframe a negative experience into one with a potentially positive meaning. For instance, spiritual individuals may see their situation as a blessing or an opportunity to grow and experience life in a different, perhaps fuller, way. Religious people may see suffering as part of God's plan, ask how God may be trying to strengthen them in this situation, or feel that the event may bring them closer to God [9, 10]. Religion helps to answer these questions by connecting one with the transcendent, or God, by way of a recognized language, text, community, and set of practices. When questioning the meaning of suffering, many Christians find positive meaning by relating their suffering to that of Jesus Christ. Christians may derive meaning from death with the belief that death serves as a passage from this life to an eternal life with God. Muslims believe in life after death and see death not as an end, but as a transition from this life to the next [8]. Nonreligious patients may find their meaning through philosophical ideologies or may experience the transcendent in nature, other people, or in acts of kindness.

Numerous studies have reported that spirituality and/or religion may be important to cancer patients in part because they provide answers to transcendent questions, but also offer inner support or guidance and, therefore, influence important medical decisions. In a study of 100 patients with advanced lung cancer, the two most important factors that influenced treatment decisions were oncologists' recommendations and faith in God [11]. This religious influence is particularly important with end-of-life decisions that include the role of life support, artificially assisted nutrition and hydration, pain medication, advance directives, organ transplantation, hospice care, and involvement of religious leaders. For example, in Judaism life is viewed as sacred and a person should be kept on life support until they will inevitably die without it [1]. Although there is great variability within the Jewish faith, the strictest position holds that life-sustaining treatment may be withdrawn only when a person has lost the swallowing reflex and will likely die within 72 h [12]. On the other hand, for many Muslims it is inappropriate to use life support to prolong life when an illness is incurable, so that the withdrawal of life-sustaining treatments is seen as "allowing death to take its natural course" [13]. In contrast to Judaism, where the rabbi plays a critical role as to when life support should be withdrawn, in Islam the decision to withdrawal life support is largely dependent on the beliefs of a person's family and community and less on religious leaders [1]. Personal philosophies may also impact decision-making. For example, a naturalist my decline medications in favor of dietary and other interventions. Patients may also delay treatment choices in order to participate in spiritual rituals such as celebration of the solstice in the woods, or participation in a religious ceremony.

Finding positive meaning in suffering and death is a great source of comfort for many people as they face the uncertainties of cancer. Not surprisingly, the majority of patients want medical professionals to ask them about their spiritual concerns; unfortunately, few medical professionals do [14, 15]. If medical professionals are not aware of a patient's spiritual beliefs and values, particularly regarding end-of-life care, they risk recommending care that may not be congruent with the patient's beliefs, leading to treatment dissatisfaction and noncompliance. Moreover, without acknowledging a patient's spiritual beliefs, medical professionals overlook a vital coping mechanism for many individuals and consequently provide incomplete care by failing to assess the needs of the whole person.

While the literature varies on the utility of asking patients about their spirituality during routine outpatient office visits, research has found that the majority of individuals want their physicians to address their spiritual beliefs if they become gravely ill [16]. While most medical professionals agree that spirituality is an important piece of the biopsychosocialspiritual model of care, not all clinicians are asking patients about their spiritual beliefs [17]. Astrow and colleagues surveyed 369 patients in an outpatient cancer clinic and found that only 6% of patients had been asked about their spiritual needs by any staff member and only 0.9% of these inquires were by physicians [14]. A number of barriers to discussing spirituality have been identified in the literature and include physician discomfort, fears of negative patient reactions, and insufficient time to address spirituality during office visits [18]. This paper will present models of communicating with cancer patients about spiritual issues relevant to their care.

Barriers to Communication of Spiritual Issues

Part of what drives physician discomfort with spiritual discussions is the concern that they may not share the same spiritual point of view as the patient and consequently may not be able to answer the patient's questions appropriately, or risk projecting their own beliefs onto the patient [18, 19]. In part, this concern is justified. Ellis and colleagues found that when physicians and patients share spiritual beliefs, there is a common vocabulary and framework for understanding spiritual questions such that there are fewer barriers to discussing spiritual issues. While this may be true in some cases, the majority of patients are not looking for medical providers to "hold all the answers," but rather they are primarily looking for understanding, compassion, and hope [16]. Oftentimes, how a physician approaches a situation is more significant than the content of the spiritual assessment. For instance, qualities such as respect, caring, and openness, along with an emphasis on spirituality rather than religious or cultural doctrines help to facilitate a spiritual discussion even across different belief systems [19].

Traditionally, medical schools viewed spirituality as potentially detrimental to objective medical care [20]. In 1992, only 2% of US medical schools offered coursework in spirituality; however, as the literature began to emphasize the importance of spirituality in medical care, more schools began to realize the importance of spiritual issues so that by 2008, 67% of medical schools were teaching courses on spirituality [21]. Although each school varies, in general students learn how to lead a discussion about spiritual beliefs in a respectful, nonjudgmental, and nonimposing manner. They also learn how to communicate effectively and compassionately with chronically ill and end-of-life patients about their suffering, beliefs, and choices for therapy and care [22, 23]. The more schools incorporate spirituality into their curricula, the more physicians will possess the qualities necessary to conduct an unbiased spiritual interview and enhance a person's care.

Some physicians are hesitant to ask about spirituality because they fear a negative patient reaction [20]. In part, this is because physicians are unsure which patients would benefit from such questions, and at what point in the illness it is appropriate to ask about spirituality without implying a poor prognosis. Overall, the majority of Americans are not offended when they are asked about their spiritual beliefs. Qualitative data suggest that both patients and physicians prefer that spirituality be assessed early in the relationship and then as needed during crisis [17, 24]. Consequently, when faced with a diagnosis of cancer, spiritual beliefs should be discussed with all patients regardless of the stage of disease.

Spiritual discussions are distinct from end-of-life discussions. Spirituality should be addressed earlier than end-of-life issues particularly because spirituality can offer hope and meaning to patients. There may, however, be overlap especially in terminally ill cancer patients who may use their spiritual or religious beliefs to guide their decisions about life-sustaining interventions [25]. Although there is no clear consensus on when to address end-of-life concerns, the literature suggests that physicians are not adequately addressing end-of-life issues [14, 26, 27]. Quill's article *Initiating End-of-Life Discussions With Seriously Ill Patients* proposes that end-of-life concerns should be discussed when discussing prognosis, when discussing treatment with low probability of success, when discussing hopes and fears, and when the physician would not be surprised if the patient died in 6–12 months [28, 29].

Even when given the tools and guidelines to appropriately address spirituality, some medical providers feel they do not have enough time in an office visit to address all of a person's medical needs as well as their spiritual needs. While this is a valid concern especially among managed care practitioners, even a single question such as, "Is spirituality important to you, or do you have spiritual beliefs that might affect your care?" will acknowledge that spirituality is an important topic that the clinician is willing to discuss [30]. If time is limited, the discussion may be spread out over multiple visits. Furthermore, if a patient requires in-depth spiritual counseling, a patient should be referred to spiritual care professionals [25]. Finding the balance between neglecting and intruding on a patient's spiritual beliefs is challenging, but patients want their spiritual concerns to be acknowledged. While there are more barriers identified in the literature, the major ones were discussed above. What all the barriers have in common, however, is the ability to overcome barriers when spirituality is acknowledged as a key component to patient care.

Spirituality in the Clinical Setting: Models of Spiritual Care

The biopsychosocialspiritual model is an elaboration of the Engel biopsychosocial model that includes spirituality. This model places emphasis on understanding and appreciating the unique spiritual story of every patient. By doing this, the clinician will be better able to support and understand patients' various levels of relationships and meaning. This model is the basis of the field of Palliative Care, in which all four dimensions of care are required for quality palliative care. The 2004 National

Consensus Project for Quality Palliative Care (NCP), funded by the Foundation, brought together stakeholders to define required domains of care in the field of Palliative Medicine, creating spiritual, existential, and religious issues as a required domain of care. The 2009 National Consensus Conference (NCC), funded by the Archstone Foundation, and co-led by The City of Hope and The George Washington Institute for Spirituality and Health (GWish) took the findings of the NCP and other organizations, such as the National Quality Forum (NQF) and the National Comprehensive Cancer Network (NCCN), and developed care guidelines, interprofessional spiritual care models, and recommendations that integrate spiritual care as a component of professional development [31]. The NCC also expanded the definition of palliative care to include care from diagnosis of serious or chronic illnesses to death [31]. This definition is very applicable to patients with cancer, as well as other serious and/or chronic illnesses.

Interprofessional Spiritual Care Model

Interprofessional spiritual care is a relational model that places an emphasis on collaboration and shared effort between the patient and multiple clinicians. Due to the emphasis on collaboration and specialization, this model readily extends itself to being used in inpatient, outpatient, and multidisciplinary clinic settings [31].

In this model, a nurse, social worker, or other staff member screens the patient for spiritual distress and refers to a board-certified chaplain if the patient is identified as having a spiritual crisis or requests to see a chaplain. The spiritual history is obtained by a clinician on the team as part of the total clinical history, where clinicians may identify spiritual distress or other spiritual issues relevant to the clinical situation. In addition, it should be pointed out that the full spiritual history should be obtained for all patients even if they have screened "negative" for spiritual distress. Obtaining the full history allows the team to assess for patient strengths and meaning or to diagnose spiritual distress if this was not earlier identified.

The patient's case is presented in interdisciplinary team rounds where the patient's spiritual concerns are discussed in a multidisciplinary framework. Based on this discussion, a formal treatment plan is produced that incorporates a spiritual care plan. This model works well in a multidisciplinary setting, particularly if all staff are trained to screen for spiritual distress. Patients can form relationships with different staff members. If all staff are viewed as open and willing to speak about issues of spirituality, then this enhances patients' chances to discuss their spirituality. The multidisciplinary team conference allows for ideas to be exchanged in an interaction that can be transformative for the patient as well as the team. In many clinical settings, there are no interdisciplinary teams. In these settings, clinicians should work with board-certified chaplains, pastoral counselors, spiritual directors, or faith community nurses. Whether the interprofessional team is inpatient or outpatient, the core theme is that all members are committed to providing compassionate care that encourages and incorporates the topic of spirituality.

Communicating with Patients about Spiritual Issues

Most patients wish to have their clinicians communicate with them about their spiritual needs. In this communication, three broad themes should be considered. The first is the style of communication most suitable for the interaction. Next would be the stated purpose or goal of the interaction. Thirdly, clinicians should examine their own personal views and biases about spirituality [25, 32–34].

The communication style will depend on the setting and the amount of time available. There are currently a number of evidence-based methods that can be utilized to assess the spiritual needs of patients. Based on current research, these methods can be broken down into three broad categories: brief, semi-structured, and fully structured.

These three categories also roughly correspond with the suggested elements of a spiritual assessment. The elements of spiritual assessment were recently formulated at a consensus conference, involving leaders in palliative care and spirituality [31]. The main goal of the conference was to improve the quality of spiritual care delivered to patients in a palliative care setting. Among other recommendations, the group formally defined the components of a spiritual assessment. The model in Figure 8.1 shows were each of the three types of assessment–screening, history, and formal assessment–take place in a clinical setting along with the formation of the treatment plan. Due to the spiritual assessment's core role in the eliciting and understanding of existential issues, we will elaborate on each component in greater depth.

Spiritual Assessment

Spiritual Screening

The purpose of the spiritual screening is to look for spiritual "red flags" that could signal a spiritual crisis, and consequently, a patient in need of further assessment and treatment by a board-certified chaplain or other spiritual care professional. The spiritual screening is vitally important as it frequently serves as the gateway to the discussion of spiritual issues. As mentioned in the barrier section, many clinicians choose not to discuss issues of spirituality due to discomfort, lack of training, or perceived lack of time. A good spiritual screening is ideally suited to confront these obstacles, as it involves very little additional training beyond what most healthcare professionals receive. The screening is meant to be brief. It utilizes only a few questions, and is usually done by the nurse who does the intake interview.

One key to an optimal screening is the preparation that has already been put into place. It is helpful to already have information and staff available to aid patients in need of a referral. In addition to staff, a calm environment also greatly helps set the stage for patients to openly express their spiritual concerns. With these preparations, patient's concerns about their spiritual needs not being met can be significantly alleviated.

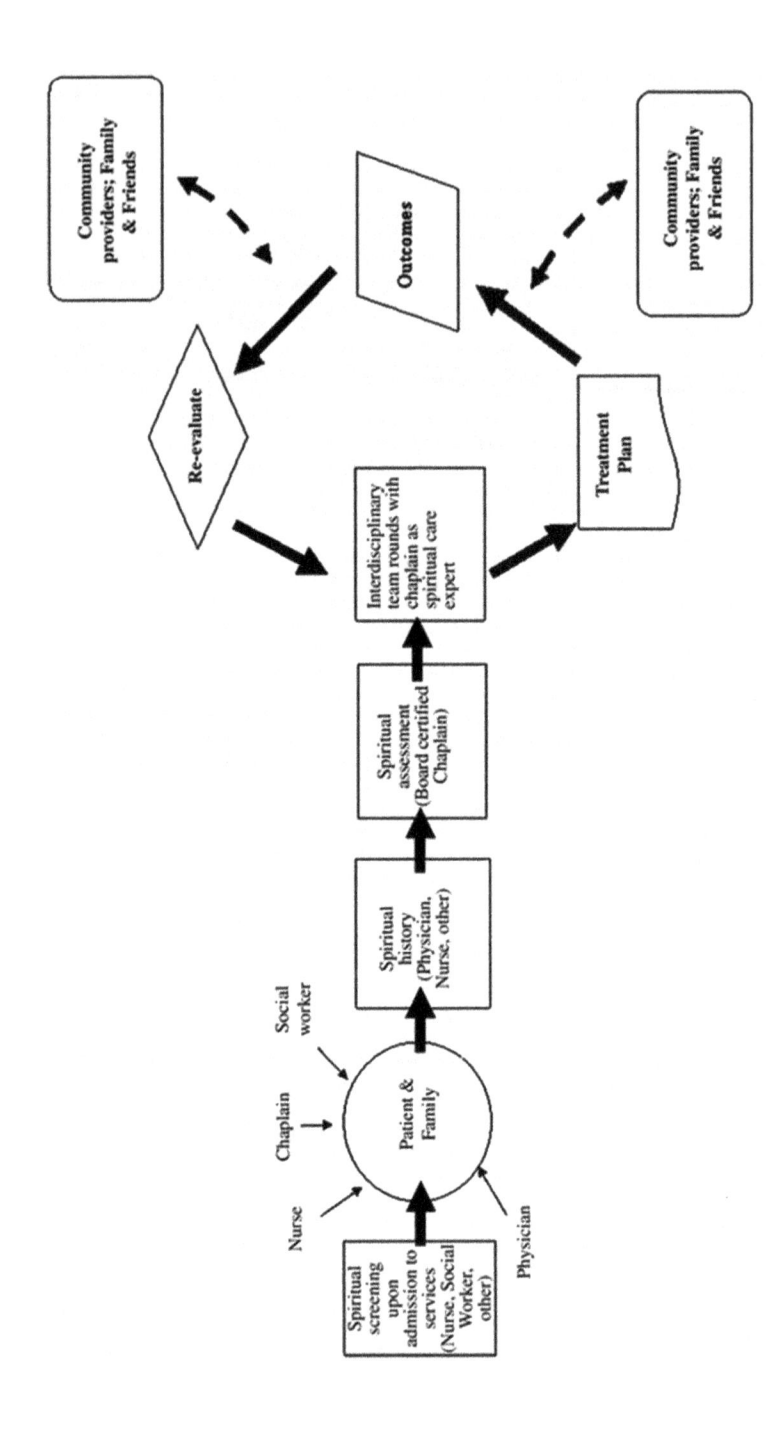

Fig. 8.1 Inpatient spiritual care implementation model (adapted from [31])

The actual screening is usually a brief question asked in the context of a focused triage interview. In the authors' experience, it is useful to have one standard screening question, with another follow-up question ready depending on the response to the initial inquiry. Fitchett developed an effective two-question screening; these two questions, asked at different times and in different ways, can form a very effective opening platform in which to screen for spiritual issues [35].

Spiritual History

The next phase of the spiritual assessment is taking a spiritual history. The goal of the spiritual history is to invite the patient to talk about spiritual issues if that patient wishes, to help the clinician diagnose spiritual distress, and to identify the patient's spiritual resources of strength. Clinicians who develop the patient's treatment or care plan do the spiritual history. In comparison to spiritual screening, it has been recommended that clinicians have some formal training in taking a spiritual history [31, 36]. Formal training would include instruction in the use of a standardized clinical tool. A number of these tools exist such as the FICA, SPIRIT, and HOPE.

The key to communicating with patients about their spiritual beliefs, or inner life, is to provide an atmosphere where patients feel they can trust the clinicians, as with any other part of the clinical encounter. Thus, clinicians should practice attentive listening skills, as well as being fully present to the patient. Letting go of a specific clinical agenda (e.g., need to fill out a checklist of responses) helps clinicians provide an open space for patients to share deeply what is most meaningful to them. Evidence suggests that when clinicians ask patients about their spiritual beliefs, patients feel an increased trust in their clinicians. We feel this may be because asking about spiritual beliefs, values, or what gives meaning to a person signals the clinician's interest in the patient beyond the disease diagnosis. If patients trust their clinicians, they are more likely to be more open about all of their issues and share openly about their symptoms and concerns. This enables clinicians to provide better care. Thus, taking a spiritual history serves to strengthen the sensitivity of other elements of the entire biopsychosocialspiritual history and enhances patient-centered care.

Formal Spiritual Assessment

Formal spiritual assessment is usually done by a board-certified chaplain or spiritual care expert. The key purposes of this level assessment are to have a formulation of the patient's spiritual needs and resources and to produce a spiritual care plan. This care plan should be discussed with other members of the treating team, with clear objectives that take into account all aspects of the patient's care.

With the use of semi-structured interview tools, this model can be readily adapted into the standard history. Since this model can place an emphasis on narrative, it lends itself well to a more advanced interaction style that might be used by a chaplain, or those specifically trained in the treatment of spiritual issues.

Spiritual History Tools

The HOPE questions developed by Anadarajah and Hight were originally developed as a teaching tool to help clinicians obtain a spiritual history [33]. This tool uses open-ended questions in a semi-structured format to focus on basic areas of spirituality and religion. The developers of the HOPE questions chose to not immediately focus on the use of the terms *spirituality* or *religion*. It was felt that limiting the use of these terms would eliminate barriers to discussion that could arise secondary to differences in use of language. The authors of the HOPE articulate three prerequisites to the use of the tool. They encourage clinicians using the tool to actually ask themselves the questions. This allows clinicians to better understand their own spirituality and potential biases. The authors also state the clinician should have a good patient relationship, and that the timing of the discussion should be appropriate. The HOPE questions give the clinician the option of starting with an open-ended question such as "What are your sources of hope, strength, comfort, and peace?" Clinicians can also opt for a more directed question, such as "For some people their religious or spiritual beliefs act as a source of comfort and strength in dealing with life's ups and downs. Is this true for you?" The HOPE questions can be used at various times during the interview depending on the examiners' interpretation of the situation. For instance, the questions can be asked in the spiritual portion of the social history, or alternatively, they can be woven into the interview at appropriate times based on patient response. The flexible utility of the HOPE questions lends itself to spiritual screening and serves as a useful template for gathering critical elements of a patient's spiritual history.

The FICA tool developed by Puchalski in collaboration with three other primary care clinicians provides a way for healthcare providers to use open-ended questions to assess the four domains of a patient's spirituality [32]. The FICA is designed to be taught to clinicians, who can then teach future users of the instrument. The FICA tool has undergone qualitative data analysis in order to test its psychometric properties. This analysis showed that the FICA tool was able to assess several dimensions of spirituality based on its correlations with spirituality subscales of the *COH-QOL tool*. The FICA tool was made with the intent to focus on a patient's spirituality, as opposed to strictly religious practices. It tends to place less emphasis on assessing coping with stress and more on understanding the patient's underlying structure for defining meaning in various relationships. The open-ended approach of the FICA tool can lay the groundwork for formal spiritual assessment and spiritual care planning by a spiritual care specialist. As a result of a spiritual history, if a clinician identifies spiritual distress, then the clinician should refer to the chaplain for further assessment and treatment. The FICA tool is the only clinical spiritual history tool that has been validated [32].

Both instruments give clinicians valuable questions to start the discussion of spirituality with patients. These questions are meant primarily to open a dialogue with patients. As mentioned earlier, the key to communicating with patients is to provide an atmosphere where patients feel safe as well as heard. One underappreciated aspect of discussing spirituality is that some patients also wish to feel connected to their clinician in a meaningful way other than medical treatment. Usual medical history places an emphasis on closure. The idea behind the use of a spiritual tool is to make sure the patient is aware that spirituality will be taken into account throughout the interview and that the door is always open for further discussion. This stance can strengthen and solidify the doctor–patient dialogue.

Spiritual Care Treatment Models

In recent years, a number of interventions have been developed to address patients in various states of spiritual distress. Ando has assessed the efficacy of a 1-week Short Term Life Review (STLR) to improve spiritual well-being in terminally ill cancer patients [37, 38]. The STLR is divided into four parts. During the first session, patients review their lives, with a focus on identifying key periods such as the most important moment, most important role, or most impressive memory. In the next three sessions, patients reevaluate, reconstruct, and appreciate their life. The short-term life review was found to significantly increase spirituality and reduce depression and anxiety. The authors postulated that the efficacy of the intervention arose from giving patients the ability to reframe life goals and purpose based on their current state.

Brietbart and colleagues have developed meaning-centered group psychotherapy as spiritual intervention for advanced cancer patients. MCGP is based on the work of Viktor Frankl's logotherapy [6]. The developers of MCGP focused on four main concepts of Frankl's work while developing MCGP:

1. Meaning of life
2. Will to meaning
3. Freedom of will
4. Creativity, experience, and attitude as the three main sources of meaning in life.

MCGP develops these themes over eight 1.5-h sessions. These sessions utilize a combination of discussion, didactics, homework, and experiential exercises to help patients establish peace, meaning, and purpose as they cope with cancer. Both MCGP and the STLR illustrate how concepts of a spiritual assessment can be translated into an effective intervention to help patients sustain and find new sources of spirituality.

Conclusion

The evidence is clear that patients desire to have spirituality incorporated into their care. Furthermore, most patients wish for clinicians to be actively attuned to their spiritual issues and receptive to making changes in the care plan based on how a patient defines meaning and value. The barriers to communicating about spirituality can be overcome through preparation and use of evidence-based models that take into account the demands of a time-constrained clinician. A number of tools that vary from brief to fully structured can be used to help the clinician engage in a spiritual dialogue with the patient. The board-certified chaplain in these models of care is recognized as the spiritual expert. This dialogue is but one example of the core idea of the doctor–patient relationship. By discussing the spiritual, clinicians not only uncover what is meaningful to the patient, they add an additional level of meaning to the doctor–patient relationship, which is one of the foundations of compassionate care.

References

1. Woll ML, Hinshaw DB, Pawlik TM. Spirituality and religion in the care of surgical oncology patients with life-threatening or advanced illnesses. Ann Surg Oncol. 2008;15(11):3048–57.
2. Sulmasy DP. Spiritual issues in the care of dying patients: "… it's okay between me and god". JAMA. 2006;296(11):1385–92.
3. McClain CS, Rosenfeld B, Breitbart W. Effect of spiritual well-being on end-of-life despair in terminally-ill cancer patients. Lancet. 2003;361(9369):1603–7.
4. Brady MJ, Peterman AH, Fitchett G, Mo M, Cella D. A case for including spirituality in quality of life measurement in oncology. Psychooncology. 1999;8(5):417–28.
5. Breitbart W. Spirituality and meaning in supportive care: spirituality- and meaning-centered group psychotherapy interventions in advanced cancer. Support Care Cancer. 2002;10(4): 272–80.
6. Greenstein M, Breitbart W. Cancer and the experience of meaning: a group psychotherapy program for people with cancer. Am J Psychother. 2000;54(4):486–500.
7. Puchalski CM. Spirituality and end-of-life care: a time for listening and caring. J Palliat Med. 2002;5(2):289–94.
8. Puchalski CM, Dorff RE, Hendi IY. Spirituality, religion, and healing in palliative care. Clin Geriatr Med. 2004;20(4):689–714, vi–vii.
9. Pargament KI, Zinnbauer BJ, Scott AB, et al. Red flags and religious coping: identifying some religious warning signs among people in crisis. J Clin Psychol. 1998;54(1):77–89.
10. Pargament KI, Koenig HG, Perez LM. The many methods of religious coping: development and initial validation of the RCOPE. J Clin Psychol. 2000;56(4):519–43.
11. Silvestri GA, Knittig S, Zoller JS, Nietert PJ. Importance of faith on medical decisions regarding cancer care. J Clin Oncol. 2003;21(7):1379–82.
12. Dorff EN. End-of-life: Jewish perspectives. Lancet. 2005;366(9488):862–5.
13. Sachedina A. End-of-life: the Islamic view. Lancet. 2005;366(9487):774–9.
14. Astrow AB, Wexler A, Texeira K, He MK, Sulmasy DP. Is failure to meet spiritual needs associated with cancer patients' perceptions of quality of care and their satisfaction with care? J Clin Oncol. 2007;25(36):5753–7.
15. Puchalski CM. The role of spirituality in health care. Proc (Bayl Univ Med Cent). 2001;14(4): 352–7.
16. McCord G, Gilchrist VJ, Grossman SD, et al. Discussing spirituality with patients: a rational and ethical approach. Ann Fam Med. 2004;2(4):356–61.
17. Ellis MR, Campbell JD, Detwiler-Breidenbach A, Hubbard DK. What do family physicians think about spirituality in clinical practice? J Fam Pract. 2002;51(3):249–54.
18. Ellis MR, Vinson DC, Ewigman B. Addressing spiritual concerns of patients: family physicians' attitudes and practices. J Fam Pract. 1999;48(2):105–9.

19. Ellis MR, Campbell JD. Concordant spiritual orientations as a factor in physician-patient spiritual discussions: a qualitative study. J Relig Health. 2005;44(1):39–53.
20. Chibnall JT, Bennett ML, Videen SD, Duckro PN, Miller DK. Identifying barriers to psychosocial spiritual care at the end of life: a physician group study. Am J Hosp Palliat Care. 2004;21(6):419–26.
21. Koenig HG, Hooten EG, Lindsay-Calkins E, Meador KG. Spirituality in medical school curricula: findings from a national survey. Int J Psychiatry Med. 2010;40(4):391–8.
22. Puchalski CM, Larson DB. Developing curricula in spirituality and medicine. Acad Med. 1998;73(9):970–4.
23. Puchalski CM. Spirituality and medicine: curricula in medical education. J Cancer Educ. 2006;21(1):14–8.
24. Ellis MR, Campbell JD. Patients' views about discussing spiritual issues with primary care physicians. South Med J. 2004;97(12):1158–64.
25. Lo B, Ruston D, Kates LW, et al. Discussing religious and spiritual issues at the end of life: a practical guide for physicians. JAMA. 2002;287(6):749–54.
26. Mystakidou K, Tsilika E, Parpa E, et al. Demographic and clinical predictors of spirituality in advanced cancer patients: a randomized control study. J Clin Nurs. 2008;17(13):1779–85.
27. Hampton DM, Hollis DE, Lloyd DA, Taylor J, McMillan SC. Spiritual needs of persons with advanced cancer. Am J Hosp Palliat Care. 2007;24(1):42–8.
28. Quill TE. Perspectives on care at the close of life. Initiating end-of-life discussions with seriously ill patients: addressing the "elephant in the room". JAMA. 2000;284(19):2502–7.
29. Quill T, Byock I. Responding to intractable terminal suffering. Ann Intern Med. 2000;133(7):561–2.
30. Koenig HG. Religion, spirituality, and medicine: research findings and implications for clinical practice. South Med J. 2004;97(12):1194–200.
31. Puchalski CM, Ferrell B, Virani R, et al. Improving the quality of spiritual care as a dimension of palliative care: the report of the consensus conference. J Palliat Med. 2009;12(10):885–904.
32. Borneman T, Ferrell B, Puchalski CM. Evaluation of the FICA tool for spiritual assessment. J Pain Symptom Manage. 2010;40(2):163–73.
33. Anandarajah G, Hight E. Spirituality and medical practice: using the HOPE questions as a practical tool for spiritual assessment. Am Fam Physician. 2001;63(1):81–9.
34. Puchalski C, Larson D, Post S. Physicians and patient spirituality. Ann Intern Med. 2000;133(9):748–9.
35. Peterman AH, Fitchett G, Brady MJ, Hernandez L, Cella D. Measuring spiritual well-being in people with cancer: the functional assessment of chronic illness therapy—spiritual Well-being Scale (FACIT-Sp). Ann Behav Med. 2002;24(1):49–58.
36. Puchalski C. Spiritual assessment in clinical practice. Psychiatr Ann. 2006;36(3).
37. Ando M, Morita T, Akechi T, Okamoto T. Japanese Task Force for Spiritual Care. Efficacy of short-term life-review interviews on the spiritual well-being of terminally ill cancer patients. J Pain Symptom Manage. 2010;39(6):993–1002.
38. Ando M, Morita T, Okamoto T, Ninosaka Y. One-week short-term life review interview can improve spiritual well-being of terminally ill cancer patients. Psychooncology. 2008;17(9):885–90.

Chapter 9
Understanding Perspective Transformation among Recently Diagnosed Cancer Patients in Western India

Avinash Thombre and Allen C. Sherman

Abstract Accumulating evidence indicates that some patients perceive positive life changes in the aftermath of serious illness. Construed as perspective transformation or posttraumatic growth, these health outcomes have received increasing attention from investigators. However, little is known about these outcomes in cultural settings outside of Western developed societies or the basic processes that contribute to positive changes. The current study examined communicative dimensions and cultural representations of perspective transformation among cancer patients receiving active treatment in Western India. Specific dimensions of perspective transformation, processes of change, and associated features were explored using narrative data. Individuals high in perspective transformation described changes in life review, life satisfaction, forgiveness, spirituality, and altruism. Among the factors associated with perceived growth was purposeful reflection and efforts to make sense of illness, to find benefits, and to use social support. Results provide an initial picture of perspective transformation among Indian cancer patients and point the way toward further research.

Keywords Culture and cancer • Intrapersonal communication • Perspective transformation • Trauma and growth • Indian cancer coping

A. Thombre, PhD (✉)
Department of Speech Communication, University of Arkansas at Little Rock,
2801 South University Avenue, Little Rock, AR 72204, USA
e-mail: axthombre@ualr.edu

A.C. Sherman, PhD
Behavioral Medicine Division, Winthrop P. Rockefeller Cancer Institute,
University of Arkansas for Medical Sciences, 4301 W. Markham Street, #765,
Little Rock, AR 72205, USA
e-mail: ShermanAllenC@uams.edu

There has been growing recognition among health investigators that the stressful, debilitating aspects of serious illness are sometimes accompanied by unexpected positive outcomes as well. Studies have noted perceptions of positive life changes among individuals with cancer [3, 10], as well as rheumatoid arthritis [39], HIV infection [5, 27], and heart disease [2]. Of course, these investigations do not negate the serious burdens and disruptions that patients encounter; however, they do point to potential health outcomes that until recently received little empirical attention. Understanding these experiences may have important public health and clinical implications as the population ages, and as growing numbers of individuals are confronted by debilitating illnesses and the complexities of long-term survivorship.

In this chapter, we examine the communicative dimensions and cultural representations of perspective transformation among cancer patients receiving active treatment in Western India. First, we provide a theoretical framework related to perspective transformation and factors influencing it, including cultural dimensions of communication and meaning-making. Then we present findings from a qualitative study with Indian cancer patients.

Perspective Transformation

Among the early investigators of positive life transitions were adult education specialists, such as Mezirow [24], who studied healthy individuals undergoing major transformations, a process he referred to as "perspective transformation." Mezirow [25] and Mezirow et al. [26] described perspective transformation as a shift in worldview that may result from a crisis or "disorienting dilemma," as individuals are pressed to reevaluate their assumptions about life and ultimately to arrive at "a new or revised interpretation of the meaning of one's experience in order to guide future action" [25, p. 163]. Theoretically, perspective transformation involves critical reflection [16], a means by which we work through beliefs and assumptions, assessing their validity in the light of new experiences or knowledge, considering their sources, and examining underlying premises. This process is thought to be facilitated by interpersonal communication—exchanging opinions and ideas, receiving support and encouragement, and engaging in discourse where alternatives are seriously weighed [17, 20, 33].

Subsequent investigators extended this inquiry to individuals with medical illness, such as HIV disease [6, 11, 27], focusing in particular on patients' narratives as a means of exploring positive life changes. These studies began to examine some of the self and interpersonal dimensions of communicative processes through which individuals wrestle with existential threats, seek or avoid health information, narrate their experience to others, and develop new roles, beliefs, and health behaviors.

Mohammed and Thombre [27], for example, examined evidence for transformative experience among 164 narratives posted on the World Wide Web by individuals with HIV or AIDS. Results pointed to salutary changes in participants' health behaviors, sensitivity to life, and desire for service to others—changes that seemed to reflect more fundamental shifts in their identities and goals, and in their patterns of communication with others in the HIV community.

Closely akin to the concept of perspective transformation are constructs such as posttraumatic growth [8, 19, 36], stress-related growth [31], and benefit-finding [39] that have emerged within the health literature. These constructs focus on adaptive changes in the aftermath of adverse or traumatic events. Tedeschi and Calhoun's [36] model of posttraumatic growth addresses beneficial changes in a number of specific domains, including increased appreciation for life, stronger relationships with others, an enhanced sense of personal strength, awareness of new goals, and deeper spirituality.

Several studies have documented these [36] and other types of perceived change [4] among diverse populations recovering from stressful events—findings that seem to resonate with investigations regarding perspective transformation [27]. Thus, although research on perspective transformation has been pursued in the fields of communication and education largely independently of the work on posttraumatic growth undertaken by other health investigators, there may be value in efforts to integrate insights from these separate lines of inquiry.

Factors Influencing Perspective Transformation

Despite accumulating evidence regarding the prevalence of perspective transformation among individuals facing serious illness, fundamental questions remain regarding the basic processes that underlie these changes. Further work is needed to explore the intrapersonal communicative or cognitive factors associated with these experiences (e.g., intrusive ideation or unwelcome thoughts, purposeful self-reflection, meaning-making), or their interpersonal communicative/relational dimensions (e.g., sharing and elaborating personal narratives with family and friends). For example, although both the perspective transformation and posttraumatic growth models [26, 36] emphasize the role of cognitive processing in promoting growth or transformation, these mechanisms have received relatively little study [34].

Coping responses, involving efforts to find personal meaning in adversity, may also influence perspective transformation or posttraumatic growth. Davis et al. [14] distinguished between two responses to crisis (bereavement): (1) making sense of the experience and (2) finding benefit in it (see also Thombre and Rogers [40] for parallel constructs). *Sense-making* involves attempts to understand the crisis, such as a life-threatening illness, by assimilating it into existing schemas or, if necessary, by reconstructing one's fundamental assumptions. *Benefit-finding* involves efforts to invest the experience with value or purpose, to discern positive implications (e.g., "I'm a stronger person now"). Evidence suggests that various dimensions of meaning-making are differentially related to mental health outcomes [14], but little is known about their associations with perspective transformation [41].

Cultural Influences

An additional issue in need of study involves the manner in which perspective transformation may be shaped by cultural context. Research in this area has been limited [23, 30]. Some investigators [23] have suggested that narratives steeped in positive outcomes or overcoming adversity may derive from a uniquely American sensibility. Clearly, additional work is needed to examine the prevalence, domains, and processes of perspective transformation in more diverse cultural settings (e.g., [1]). Cancer treatment centers in India offer a compelling setting in which to pursue this research, since cultural perceptions regarding illness and mortality, existential meaning, spiritual practices, and family ties may differ notably from those prevailing in much of the United States. Patterns of communication and disclosure about illness differ as well. To date, we are aware of no research that has examined perspective transformation among cancer patients in India.

The current study was designed to further examine the structure and process of perspective transformation, using in-depth interviews with cancer patients in the state of Maharashtra in Western India. Specific guiding research questions included:

RQ1: Are there indications of perspective transformation (i.e., perceptions of positive life transitions) among recently diagnosed cancer patients in Western India and, if so, what domains or growth areas seem most salient?

RQ2: What are some of the factors that might be associated with this process? In particular, we examined (1) intrusive vs. deliberative thinking, and (2) efforts to find meaning via sense-making and benefit-finding. In addition, we assessed other factors that have been linked with perspective transformation in earlier theoretical or empirical work, including (3) subjective appraisals of illness (e.g., perceived stressfulness and threat to life); (4) social support; and (5) coping efforts.

RQ3: To what extent is the process of change experienced as effortful and deliberative vs. automatic and undirected? Are these changes perceived as emerging in a gradual, linear fashion or in an abrupt, discontinuous manner?

RQ4: In what ways does Indian culture appear to influence perspective transformation?

Method

Participants

Participants in this qualitative study included 14 patients with recently diagnosed cancer receiving care at a cancer treatment center in Pune, Maharashtra state in Western India. Sixteen patients were invited to participate, of whom one declined due to feeling too ill, 15 consented, and one consented, but was subsequently called away to a medical appointment shortly after starting the interview. Inclusion criteria included receiving active medical treatment; there were no restrictions for site or stage of disease at this early phase of research. The sample was composed predominantly of participants with early-stage, recently diagnosed disease.

Procedures

The study was approved by the Institutional Review Board and the research director of the Morbai Naraindas Budhrani Cancer Institute, Pune. Patients completed a consent form and a demographic form, and then participated in 60–90 min interviews at the cancer center, which were administered individually, tape-recorded, and transcribed. Interviews were conducted by the first author, a health communications researcher who is highly experienced in qualitative interview studies with medical patients. The interviews followed a protocol designed to elicit narratives from interviewees about their perceptions of illness, communicative experiences, and coping mechanisms. The interviews further were designed to elicit the insider's perspective of a relationship that drew on *being in, being for, and being with* [28]. Essentially, "being in" involves immersing oneself in another's world; "being for" concerns taking a stand in support of the other person; and finally "being with" relates to bringing one's own knowledge and experience to the interview process. We sought to address investigator influence on the content of the narratives by establishing an accepting environment, conveying respect for all responses, and sequencing questions so that open-ended inquiries preceded more specific probes, and reserving questions about positive changes to the end of the encounter.

The first set of questions elicited narratives regarding the immediate aftermath of diagnosis; the second set focused on their current experiences over the past month. Participants were asked to describe their encounter with the illness ("What has this experience been like for you?"). As needed, subsequent open-ended questions and probes examined: (a) personal appraisals of the illness (i.e., the experience of being diagnosed with cancer; level of stress; concern about survival); (b) family context of cancer diagnosis (i.e., impact on the family); (c) social support (e.g., confiding in others, perceived support or constraints); (d) coping efforts; and (e) intrusive ideation; search for meaning via efforts to make sense of the illness or to find benefits; extent to which these responses seemed automatic/reflexive vs. deliberative/purposeful.

The final set of questions focused on participants' experience of perspective transformation or growth. The inquiry began with open-ended questions about any perceived changes (i.e., "Sometimes people who have been through very difficult circumstances discover that their lives have changed in some ways; they may feel that there are positive as well as negative changes. Have you found anything positive in this experience? [If yes] Can you tell me about that?"). These were followed at the end of the interview by more specific questions, if needed, about particular domains of growth, drawing in part on the framework developed by Tedeschi and Calhoun [36] and expanded by the investigators (appreciation of life, altered priorities, changes in relationships, personal strength, new opportunities, spirituality, life review, life satisfaction/integrity, forgiveness [self, others, God], personal control, sense of purpose/goals, sense of coherence/order, helping others with illness, generativity/altruism more generally, and health behavior changes). For those who reported a sense of growth, process questions inquired about temporal characteristics (i.e., whether positive changes were perceived to have emerged gradually or more abruptly) and effort (i.e., whether they seemed automatic/reflexive vs. deliberate/purposeful).

Data Analysis

Open-ended questions generated rich narrative responses and were analyzed using analytic coding [21]. Transcripts were read independently by both investigators to familiarize themselves with the data, and then were coded for themes in accord with established procedures. The investigators then met to discuss themes, add, condense, and refine codes, and resolve discrepancies until the point of data saturation. In addition to thematic codes that emerged from open-ended narratives, attempts were made to recognize specific domains of perspective transformation (e.g., altered health behaviors) and factors that might be related to it (e.g., disclosure of illness to others), to set the stage for future research. The coders were careful to try to distinguish accounts of positive changes in response to illness from reports of preexisting qualities (e.g., general optimism, well-being) or coping (e.g., fighting spirit, seeking support).

As always, the personal, cultural, and theoretical biases of the investigators must be acknowledged; efforts were made to account for these by seeking concordance in coding and interpretation from investigators across different academic disciplines (health communications, clinical psychology) and cultural backgrounds (India, US). There was no opportunity to conduct follow-up interviews with participants to further authenticate our interpretations, and this is a limitation of the study.

Results

The interviews produced a wealth of data, which were organized into themes regarding specific domains of perspective transformation, factors associated with transformation, process dimensions, and the sociocultural meaning of these experiences.

Based on the analysis of the extended interview data as a whole, we get a sense that participants demonstrated widely varying levels of perspective transformation. Some narratives provided clear descriptions of perceived positive changes in the aftermath of illness, while others did not. That is, some individuals (5) vividly depicted altered perspectives or favorable sequelae in response to their experience with cancer; some (5) provided no indications of such changes; and some (4) portrayed changes that seemed modest or intermediate (i.e., characterized by less elaboration, complexity, or integration with the rest of the narrative account). These distinct sets of narratives provide interesting illustrations of divergent responses to

Table 9.1 Domains of change described by patients with high-transformation perspective

Highly characteristic of transformation perspective	Modestly characteristic of transformation perspective	Not uniquely associated with transformation perspective
Life satisfaction	Perceived personal control	New opportunities
Life review	Sense of purpose in life	Appreciation for life
Forgiveness (self/others)	Sense that life is coherent/orderly	Altered priorities
Spirituality		Change in relationships
Helping others with cancer		Personal strength
Generativity/altruism		
Positive health behaviors		

the crisis of cancer. In the following pages, we draw comments from the "high growth" set and the "no change" set to exemplify important themes. Importantly, participants who provided clear descriptions of perspective transformation did not appear to deny or minimize the debilitating aspects of their illness; rather, they perceived both adversity and growth. For instance, one of the participants, Kiran (the names of all participants were changed to protect their identity), who was diagnosed with a brain tumor, said:

> I have found a lot of positive things. Yes, I agree the pain is very bad, almost unbearable at times that I almost want to die, and the process is not good, but going through all of this gives a different meaning to life itself. It is very challenging…. I have become very strong mentally and feel that I am ready for any kind of other challenges.

Hameed, who comes from a rural area, shared a similar perception:

> Right now my family and myself are in a very bad situation. I am merely 22 an only male in my family. We have lots of debts, only a small piece of land and basically very little hope. But I only rely on my confidence, stay very strong now and very positive about things that might happen. I need to pull out of this what ever it takes. It has given a sense of confidence and sometimes I feel I am a special person in many ways.

Domains of Perspective Transformation

The study sought to determine what specific domains of perspective transformation might emerge among recently diagnosed cancer patients in Western India (RQ1). Is the experience of growth uniform across all domains, or is it characterized by perceived changes in some domains more than others? Results suggested more marked shifts in some areas than in others (see Table 9.1). Patients who seemed high in perspective transformation (i.e., those whose narratives as a whole included clear depictions of positive sequelae) related personal changes in several areas that their counterparts did not include. These domains included life satisfaction, life review, forgiveness, spirituality, interest in helping others with illness, generativity, and health behaviors. In the following paragraphs, we consider some of these domains.

Life satisfaction: When discussing how they perceived their lives, those in the high-perspective transformation group expressed a new sense of fulfillment regarding the decisions they had made in the past, the paths their lives had taken, and their accomplishments. Said Kiran, who had a malignant brain tumor:

> I could not have asked for more. I have lived my life full and have no regrets. I would go very happily if death comes to me tomorrow. I am very happy to be a teacher and an administrator and enjoy it very well. I am happy about the life I led so far. More importantly, I am proud that my sons are doing well and we had a good life.

In contrast, those in the low-perspective transformation group were less apt to convey a sense of satisfaction and integrity. When asked about life satisfaction, Neelam, after a long silence, replied:

> Not much. I look back and there is nothing much to be good about. I wish things in my past were different, but sadly they are not and I don't know if I can do anything about it now. And now the present is no good, I don't want to think about it but I keep thinking about it. I think about life and things that I always wanted to do. I wanted to write but that did not happen as my family was not supportive. I also wanted to learn painting but did not get an opportunity. I regret all of that and much more.

Life review: A similar pattern emerged when participants were asked the extent to which they found themselves pausing to review life, to reflect on past experiences, or to consider the future (either in this life or the next). Those in the high-perspective transformation group uniformly expressed a sense of optimism or preparedness for challenges that may lie ahead. Surjeet said:

> I do that all the time and take time to reflect on things. That gives me a sense of hope and sense of strength somehow and feels like I am prepared for any stage of life now. I think about life and think that I have lived my life as best can be possible. I don't know what is in store for me but I feel hopeful.

Again, in contrast, those in the low-perspective transformation group reported being less reflective or optimistic. Neelam said:

> No time for that. I am so involved with dealing with the immediate pain that I do not want to think that I have cancer. Even if I think about how the future will look like, I get scared as I don't know if it will be any better.

Forgiveness: For patients in the high-perspective transformation group, changes in forgiveness included both forgiveness of self and of others. Interestingly, some patients had struggled with guilt that they had neglected to seek medical care, perhaps resulting in delayed diagnosis; these individuals had come to forgive themselves. For example, retired teacher Gouri regretted that she had neglected her initial symptoms related to nipple discharge:

> I should have told the doctor about my white discharge earlier, but I did not do so. I am a little angry with myself. But now I have learnt a lesson. Had I visited the doctor sooner I would have been diagnosed with more earlier stage. I need to take care of myself. So I feel it but I have forgiven myself.

Changes in forgiveness of self or others were not evident in the low-transformation perspective narratives. Few participants in either group reported forgiveness toward God. Most did not hold God accountable for their illness (e.g., Gajanan noted, "I do not blame God, so why forgive him?"). However, one patient in the high-perspective transformation group struggled with spiritual ambivalence and had not reconciled her religious faith with her anger (e.g., "I am angry with God. Why did You do this to me? Why does God give problems to poor people?").

Spirituality: With respect to spiritual changes, a few patients in the high-perspective transformation group reported increased spiritual practices, despite still being in the midst of active medical treatment. Surjeet said:

> I go to the temple now very often. I am there at 5 in the morning for the prayers and then back in the evenings as they have regular prayers every hour. I get very involved with everything they do and help with the arrangements till the last prayer, which is at 10 PM. It helps me to forget what I am going through and think about the larger aspects of our being alive.

More typically, patients in the high-perspective transformation group pointed to an internalized sense of spiritual identity or connection rather than changes in practices or institutional involvement (e.g., Hameed noted that "I don't get enough time to pray, but I am more spiritual now").

Themes Associated with Perspective Transformation

Participants were asked about a number of factors that might relate or contribute to the process of perspective transformation, such as their personal appraisals of the illness, coping efforts, cognitive responses, support systems, and concomitant stressors (RQ2). The high-perspective transformation group differed from the low-perspective transformation group most clearly in their efforts to find meaning in the illness experience.

Meaning-making: The high-perspective transformation participants reported striving to make sense of their experience—to understand the causes or implications of their disease (i.e., "sense-seeking"). They also sought to find benefits or positive changes (e.g., "benefit-seeking"). They regarded these efforts as deliberative, not automatic or conditioned. Notably, they were not always successful in their efforts—for most patients, coherent explanations or causes were elusive, and potential benefits were not always clear; but they grappled with these issues more actively and overtly than their low-perspective transformation counterparts. Efforts to make sense of the experience, with divergent levels of success, were reflected in comments by participants. Kanchan noted:

> As I said, God does everything for a purpose. It is how we take it that matters. The doctors and nurses have given me a lot of information about what is happening to my body and I try to also study about the disease as much as possible. So I am trying to understand aspects of it.

In contrast, those in the low-perspective transformation group were much less concerned with efforts to understand the reasons for or implications of their disease. Some had ready answers, some did not; but they did not devote much time to these questions. Ketaki said:

> I am a very positive person and so I thought it is a temporary problem and it will go away. I understand at my age there are health problems and I did not think much about this problem too until this happened to me. I now deeply regret it.

Efforts to find benefits in the crisis of illness followed a similar pattern. Patients in the high-perspective transformation group shared comments similar to those of Kanchan. Those in the low-perspective transformation group were less absorbed by efforts to find benefits. Whether they were faring well or poorly, they did not place much emphasis on seeking positive changes. Roma said:

> I thought I will go to the doctors a few times and it will be resolved like a normal problem. I really don't want to think much of this, as the more I think the more I get scared.

Kumar was very short but firm.

> I feel very apprehensive about cancer. I feel like a sword is dangling over my neck. The treatment is very expensive and financially it is unaffordable and thus problematic even though my brothers support me a lot. I don't know any positive thing that will come out of this.

Illness appraisals: Illness appraisals appeared to differ for the high- and low-perspective transformation groups. While most participants reported very high levels of stress and strong concern for survival in the immediate aftermath of diagnosis, these appraisals had become less pronounced in the current time period (past month) for those in the high-perspective transformation group. Their perceptions of the illness became less threatening.

Seeking support outside the family: The groups differed as well in their use of support outside the family. Those in the high-perspective transformation group talked about their illness to friends, coworkers, and others; while those in the low-perspective transformation growth group reported very limited disclosure. This difference was most evident within the past month. For example, after much hesitation Mohan explained that he willingly revealed that he was struggling with cancer and that actually helped relieve the burden. Ketaki was not very sure of telling anybody other than close family members about her cancer. She felt scared that a lot of questions would be asked and people would talk about her.

Process Dimensions of Perspective Transformation

When asked about the process of change (RQ3), the high-perspective transformation group uniformly reported that their experience of growth had emerged slowly and gradually rather than abruptly. All but one indicated that positive changes had been the result of deliberative effort. Thus, for these patients, perspective transformation required conscious intention or "work"; it did not "just seem to happen." Manjari replied instantly:

> For me, as I talked to myself in moments of silence as I was getting my chemo or radiation and thought about the situation I was in, it started making sense. It did take a lot of time but it surely was a very gradual process in the beginning I was very disturbed and negative but soon, as I reflected a lot, I started seeing positive things.

Cultural Context of Perspective Transformation

Participants' narratives about the poignant changes they had experienced reflected the influence of their Indian beliefs, customs, and cultural upbringing (RQ4). After an initial period of disequilibrium, participants responded to the complex challenges of their illness by drawing on their cultural beliefs, at times invoking religious resources. These convictions were particularly evident as participants shared their struggles to find meaning in the face of serious existential challenges. One particular theme that emerged repeatedly in the narratives related to the Indian notion of life as a continuum. The participants believed in reincarnation and viewed illness as part of the constant cycle of birth, death, and rebirth. They reasoned that it is very natural to have a health issue in life and they have to gather courage to face it. They coped in part by recalling how heroic figures in Hinduism, Islam, and Christianity handled life crises by being stoic and positive in outlook. Those who were diagnosed earlier were also more likely to share their illness with neighbors, friends, or other patients diagnosed with cancer.

We see in our data that social support in the Indian context is largely family-based, with fewer institutional resources available outside the family to help manage cancer. Initially, participants were uncomfortable disclosing that they had cancer, due to shame, stigma, or fear of burdening the family. Eventually, however, they sought assistance from kinship relationships, including adult children, siblings, in-laws, uncles, aunts, and sometime close friends. Most participants reported receiving unconditional emotional and financial support. However, many recounted their families being forced to delve into meager savings, take out huge loans, or sell property to help pay for the medical expenses of their cancer treatment in the absence of any governmental medical program.

Another striking cultural aspect was the level of patient concern for their families after their death. A major preoccupation both for the younger and older participants (including those with highly favorable prognoses) was centered on what would happen to family members. It is considered an individual's *dharma*—a central obligation—to take care of parents, children, and grandchildren. A common narrative was "my family members will suffer as a result of my being gone." That was a poignant struggle and hard to accept. Participants worried that they would not be able to fulfill role responsibilities, such as arranging marriage for their young adult children and guiding them as they start successful families of their own. Said Padmavati:

> I am in the last phase of my life and very realistic about the end of my life.
> I am prepared for the worst that can happen to me, but what I am not prepared for, and that is on my back all the time, is the fact that when I am gone, what is going to happen to my daughter? She is having a baby and I wanted to help her after her pregnancy to take care of her child.

Much like the older participants, two young participants, both in their 20s, were concerned that as a result of their cancer and disabilities they will not be able to take care of their parents, in accord with the norms of Indian culture. Thus, the trauma of cancer for our Indian participants disrupted collectivistic priorities (e.g., kinship obligations) that were central to their social roles and identities.

Discussion

Despite the growing research regarding perspective transformation in the aftermath of serious illness, there have been few attempts to study these phenomena in cultural settings outside of North America and western Europe (e.g., [34]). Moreover, much has yet to be learned about the important communicative factors, cognitive processes, and coping responses that might be related to perspective transformation. This study is the first we are aware of to characterize perspective transformation in an Indian sample of cancer patients.

Processes of Perspective Transformation

Results suggest that a number of patients perceived positive life changes in the aftermath of cancer diagnosis. Notably, these individuals did not appear to dismiss or avoid the debilitating aspects of their illness. Rather, they identified positive changes in conjunction with more harrowing ones, providing a picture that was complex and multifaceted. There has been limited research about the process characteristics of perspective transformation—the extent to which it is gradual or discontinuous, effortful or automatic [37]; prospective longitudinal studies are needed to address these questions. In the current investigation, patients experienced growth as gradual and deliberative, something they struggled toward, not as a more abrupt, discontinuous alteration that was somehow visited upon them. As defined by patients, positive life changes were substantive and effortful.

Domains of Perspective Transformation

Some domains appeared to be more characteristic of high-perspective transformation than others. Patients who demonstrated high levels of growth were more likely to engage in life review—to find a sense of fulfillment in the course their lives had taken, to feel reconciled to the choices they had made, and to look to the future with a sense of hopefulness. These findings are reminiscent of what Erikson [15] described as "integrity vs. despair," though his work focused on developmental rather than stress-related changes.

Patients with high-perspective transformation were also more likely to report forgiving themselves and others, to note a deeper spirituality and to express a greater interest in helping others. Positive changes in other domains were less distinctive. Recognition of new opportunities (for example, engaging in volunteering) was rarely reported by patients in either the high- or low-perspective transformation groups. Given that they were all in the midst of active medical treatment and had more pressing priorities, this result does not seem surprising.

On the other hand, almost all participants, even those classified as demonstrating "low perspective transformation," reported beneficial changes in their sense of personal strength, their appreciation for life, and the significance of their relationships. These changes were important to participants, but they did not seem uniquely characteristic of high-perspective transformation. Prior investigations have often focused on these domains, and thus future studies might benefit from casting a broader net, examining areas that have been less well scrutinized, particularly in culturally diverse settings [29].

Indian Culture and Perspective Transformation

These findings suggest that domains of growth may be influenced by participants' cultural and developmental context. Indian cancer patients from lower- to middle-class backgrounds in the second half of life generally found little relevance in seeking new opportunities or new paths in life. Instead, relational changes (e.g. forgiveness, altruism) and existential changes (e.g., life review, spirituality) were more resonant, reflecting values and narratives that are deeply woven into Indian society. At their phase in the life cycle, many participants perceived that they were moving closer to the end of their life journey and were mentally prepared for a decline in health. (For a majority of Indians, "advanced age" is viewed quite differently from the way it is in Western societies. Most Indian participants who were in their 40s and 50s regarded themselves as aged.) For those who were diagnosed in their late 40s, a central concern related to the developmental task of tending to adult children who were not married or did not have jobs and thus needed them.

Interestingly, studies undertaken in European American cancer samples have sometimes noted changes related to advocacy or a survivorship mission, such as volunteering, influencing policy, or being engaged in civic groups, health education, or religious ministry. In contrast, Indian participants with high levels of perspective transformation did not seem drawn to these types of activities. In part, this difference may reflect the fact that our participants were still engaged in active treatment rather than long-term survivorship (i.e., too ill or preoccupied to consider advocacy); however, it may also reflect cultural differences regarding opportunities for and the value of this type of health advocacy. Additional research in this area is warranted.

Pathways to Perspective Transformation

Within this cultural framework, this study offers insight regarding factors that might be strongly tied to perspective transformation. Transformation was related to efforts to find meaning. These attempts reflected a deeply self-communicative process that was characterized as deliberative and effortful, not reflexive. They were reported both in the early aftermath of diagnosis, as well as currently. What seemed most distinctive about the process of meaning-making was not the outcome (most patients continued to struggle without clear answers), but rather the effort and the process itself. As suggested by Davis et al. [14], meaning-making was evident both in attempts to make sense of the illness (i.e., to understand causes or reasons) and in efforts to find benefits.

In contrast to active efforts at meaning-making, ruminative self-communication was not associated with perceived growth in our study. In Tedeschi and Calhoun's [36] model, intrusive, ruminative thinking is believed to contribute to growth. It is thought to signify intensive engagement with the life-changing event (which is a prerequisite for growth) and to reflect a preliminary form of cognitive processing, which is eventually replaced by more deliberative cognitions. In our patient narratives, we did not find a consistent relationship between perceived growth and intrusive thoughts, either initially after diagnosis or currently. Null results were also reported in studies with breast cancer patients (e.g., Cordova et al. [10]; see also Helgeson et al. [18] for a meta-analytic review). For individuals facing serious illness, perhaps growth is rooted more firmly in deliberative, reflective self-communication than in a preliminary phase of intrusive rumination (see refs. [9, 34]). Longitudinal studies would help clarify this issue.

In the current study, perspective transformation was also associated with differences in illness appraisals. Although most patients reported similarly jarring perceptions of their ordeal in the immediate aftermath of diagnosis (i.e., highly stressful and life-threatening), over time those in the high-perspective transformation group viewed their illness in less threatening terms. This finding did not seem to be fully accounted for by differences in tumor stage or prognosis. Consistent with Tedeschi and Calhoun's [36] model, which posits that the crisis must be sufficiently intense to dislodge previously held worldviews, several studies have affirmed that growth is related to more stressful appraisals of the illness (e.g., [10, 42]). However, little research has focused on changes in these appraisals over time. In the current study, it appears that as individuals in the high-growth group successfully integrated the crisis of illness, their initial appraisals shifted, becoming less daunting and overwhelming. (Of course, these retrospective reflections will need to be further explored in longitudinal investigations.)

Current findings may help clinicians better appreciate the complexity of responses to cancer, which for some patients embody perceptions of growth as well as adversity. Some investigators have begun to develop interventions to enhance growth among cancer patients [12, 13]. Considerable care is required, however, because facile admonitions or exhortations in this area can be experienced by patients as offensive or insensitive to their struggles.

Limitations and Future Research

This preliminary study has a number of limitations. The extent to which self-reported perspective transformation reflects genuine life changes as opposed to self-protective illusions has been the subject of much debate [7, 22, 35]. Recollections of positive change may be influenced by self-enhancement processes or other forms of recall bias [22, 42], and thus one might question the veracity of these reports. In our view, the facts that data were derived from intensive interviews and that patients indicated negative as well as positive changes in specific areas lend partial credence to these reports [43]. Efforts were made to establish rapport and to use sensitive interview techniques in order to reduce demand characteristics. Moreover, in a few investigations, informants have corroborated participants' reports of growth [31]. Nevertheless, the extent to which the narratives in this study represent genuine "transformation" remains unknown. Clearly, future studies would benefit by obtaining repeated assessments of perspective transformation prospectively [38] and by inclusion of informant interviews or behavioral observations among patients at specific phases of illness to enhance confidence in the veracity of self-reported growth.

This qualitative study provides vivid descriptions of how some patients perceive important changes in their lives, but of course it does not allow causal interpretations. Moreover, in the absence of longitudinal data we have no information about how these experiences change over time. Longitudinal research is needed to provide a clearer picture of perspective transformation over the trajectory of treatment and long-term recovery (e.g., [32]). Finally, the sample in the current study was small and medically heterogeneous. All participants were at a similar phase of treatment; but they varied in disease site, stage, and type of treatment, and these differences may have influenced the findings. Inclusion of medically diverse patients was useful at this preliminary phase of research, but it would be helpful for future investigations to focus on more homogenous patient groups.

Conclusion

Despite these limitations, the current study offers a rich window into the experience of perspective transformation within a cultural context that has rarely been studied—cancer patients in Western India. Findings suggest that some patients perceive positive life changes as well as more harrowing ones; these changes seem rooted in a fairly effortful, deliberative self-communicative process. These narratives also suggest the value of reaching beyond domains of perspective transformation or growth that traditionally have been studied to examine additional areas of change (e.g., forgiveness, existential life review, altruism, generativity).

Acknowledgements The authors would like to thank Dr. (Brig) C.H. Gidvani, director (academics) Sadhu Vaswani Mission's Medical Complex, Pune, India for his generous support in counducting this study. Thanks are also due to surgical oncologist Dr. Manish Bhatia and the radiation center staff at the hospital.

References

1. Abraido-Lanza AF, Guier C, Colon RM. Psychological thriving among Latinas with chronic illness. J Soc Issues. 1998;54:405–24.
2. Affleck G, Tennen H, Croog S, Levine S. Causal attrition, perceived benefits, and morbidity following a heart attack: an eight-year study. J Consult Clin Psychol. 1987;55:29–35.

3. Anderson JO, Martin PG. Narratives and healing: exploring one family's stories of cancer survivorship. Health Commun. 2003;15:133–43.
4. Armeli S, Guntbert KC, Cohen LH. Stressor appraisals, coping, and post-event outcomes: the dimensionality and antecedents of stress-related growth. J Soc Clin Psychol. 2001;20: 366–95.
5. Baumgarther LM. Living and learning with HIV/AIDS: transformational tale continued. Adult Educ Quart. 2002;53(1):44–59.
6. Baumgautner LM. HIV-positive adults' meaning making over time. New Dir Adult Cont Educ. 2005;105:11–20.
7. Calhoun LG, Tedeschi RG. Posttraumatic growth: future directions. In: Tedeschi RG, Park CL, Calhoun LG, editors. Posttraumatic growth: positive changes in the aftermath of crisis. Mahwah: Lawrence Erlbaum Associates; 1998. p. 211–38.
8. Calhoun LG, Tedeschi RG. The foundations of posttraumatic growth: new considerations. Psychol Inq. 2004;15:93–102.
9. Cann A, Calhoun LG, Tedeschi RG, Kilmer RP, Gil-Rivas V, Vishnevsky T, Danhauer SC. The core beliefs inventory: a brief measure of disruption in the assumptive world. Anxiety Stress Coping. 2010;23:19–34.
10. Cordova MJ, Cunningham LLC, Carlson CR, Andrykowski MA. Posttraumatic growth following breast cancer. A controlled comparison study. Health Psychol. 2001;20:176–85.
11. Courtenay BC, Merriam SB, Reeves PM. The centrality of meaning-making in transformational learning: how HIV-positive adults make sense of their lives. Adult Educ Quart. 1998;48(2):65–84.
12. Coward DD. Facilitation of self-transcendence in a breast cancer support group: II. Oncol Nurs Forum. 2003;30:291–300.
13. Dann NJ, Mertens WC. Taking a "leap of faith": acceptance and value of a cancer program-sponsored spiritual event. Cancer Nurs. 2004;27:134–41.
14. Davis CG, Nolen-Hoeksema S, Larson J. Making sense of loss and benefiting from the experience: two construals of meaning. J Pers Soc Psychol. 1998;75:561–74.
15. Erikson EH. Childhood and society. 2nd ed. New York: Norton; 1950.
16. Frankl VE. Man's search for meaning. New York: Washington Square Press; 1959.
17. Garro LC, Mattingly C. Narrative as a construct and construction. In: Mattingly C, Garro LC, editors. Narrative and the cultural construction of illness and healing. Berkeley: University of California Press; 2000. p. 1–49.
18. Helgeson VS, Reynolds KA, Tomich PL. A meta-analytic review of benefit finding and growth. J Consult Clin Psychol. 2006;74:797–816.
19. Janoff-Bulman R. Shattered assumptions. New York: Free Press; 1992.
20. Janoff-Bulman R, Frantz CM. The impact of trauma on meaning: from meaningless world to meaningful life. In: Power M, Brewin CR, editors. The transformation of meaning in psychological therapies. New York: Wiley; 1997. p. 91–106.
21. Lindlof TR, Taylor BC. Qualitative communication research methods. 2nd ed. Thousand Oaks: Sage; 2002.
22. McFarland C, Alvaro C. The impact of motivation on temporal comparisons: coping with traumatic events by perceiving persona growth. J Pers Soc Psychol. 2000;79:327–43.
23. McMillan JC. Posttraumatic growth: what's it all about? Psychol Inq. 2004;15:48–52.
24. Mezirow J. Education for perspective transformation: women's re-entry programs in community colleges. New York: Columbia University, Teachers College, Center for Adult Education; 1978.
25. Mezirow J. Contemporary paradigms of learning. Adult Educ Quart. 1996;46(3):58–173.
26. Mezirow J, et al. Learning as transformation: critical perspectives on a theory in progress. San Francisco: Jossey-Bass; 2000.
27. Mohammed SN, Thombre A. HIV/AIDS stories on the World Wide Web and transformative perspective. J Health Commun. 2005;10(4):347–60.
28. Moustakas C. Being in, being-for, being-with. Northvale: Jason Aronson; 1995.
29. Pals JL, McAdams DP. The transformed self: a narrative understanding of posttraumatic growth. Psychol Inq. 2004;115:65–9.

30. Park CL. The notion of growth following stressful life experiences: problems and prospects. Psychol Inq. 2004;115:69–76.
31. Park CL, Cohen L, Murch R. Assessment and prediction of stress-related growth. J Pers. 1996;64:71–105.
32. Schwarzer R, Luszczynska A, Boehmer S, Taubert S, Knoll N. Changes in benefit finding after cancer surgery and the prediction of well-being one year later. Soc Sci Med. 2006;63: 1614–24.
33. Sharf BF, Vanderford ML. Illness narratives and the social construction of health. In: Thompson TL, Dorsey AM, Miller KL, Parrott R, editors. Handbook of health communication. Mahwah: Lawrence Erlbaum Associates; 2003.
34. Taku K, Calhoun LG, Cann A, Tedeschi RG. The role of rumination in the coexistennce of distress and posttraumatic growth among bereaved Japanese university students. Death Stud. 2008;32:428–44.
35. Taylor SE, Armor DA. Positive illusions and coping with adversity. J Pers. 1996;64:873–98.
36. Tedeschi RG, Calhoun LG. Posttraumatic growth: conceptual foundations and empirical evidence. Psychol Inq. 2004;15(1):1–18.
37. Tennen H, Affleck G. Personality and transformation in the face of adversity. In: Tedeschi RG, Park CL, Calhoun LG, editors. Posttraumatic growth: positive changes in the aftermath of crisis. Mahwah: Erlbaum; 1998. p. 65–98.
38. Tennen H, Affleck G. Assessing positive life change: in search of new methodologies. In: Park CL, Lechner SC, Antoni MH, Stanton AI, editors. Medical illness and positive life change. Washington, DC: American Psychological Association; 2009. p. 31–49.
39. Tennen H, Affleck G, Urrows S, Higgins P, Mendola R. Perceiving control, construing benefits, and daily processes in rheumatoid arthritis. Can J Behav Sci. 1992;24:186–203.
40. Thombre A, Rogers EM. Transformative experiences of cancer survivors. In: Wills M, editor. Communicating spirituality in health care. Cresskill: Hampton Press; 2009.
41. Thombre A, Sherman AC, Simonton S. Posttraumatic growth among cancer patients in India. J Behav Med. 2010;33:15–23.
42. Widows MR, Jacobsen PB, Booth-Jones M, Fields KK. Predictors of posttraumatic growth following bone marrow transplantation for cancer. Health Psychol. 2005;24:266–73.
43. Wong PTP, Wong LCJ, Lonner WJ. Handbook of multicultural perspectives on stress and coping. New York: Springer; 2006.

Part II
The Patient and the Family

Chapter 10
In the Pursuit of Meaning: Cancer and the Family

Lea Baider

Abstract When cancer strikes, the belief system that once provided a sense of stability, familiarity, and security is shattered by reflection and inquiry. Families and caregivers help give meaning to life by the act of consistently dispensing their love, care, and hope. The psychodynamics of hope and meaning challenge professionals to step beyond the dichotomy of traditionally defined notions of health, stress, and disorder and to see people in distress as unique, competent, and capable of constructing their own meanings within their cultural and family settings. These challenges provide the potential for generating alternative options to adequately address familial cognitive and coherent behaviors. Clinical and empirical evidence is rapidly emerging to suggest that meaning and coping are critical mediators between cancer-related distress and psychological well-being and may be possible mechanisms to explain the coexistence of alternative psychological states following cancer diagnosis.

Keywords Search for meaning • Family experiences • Cancer • Death • Family members' narrative

Introduction

> …This is a shared story of a family confronting the sudden catastrophic illness of one member. It recounts the experience as the family tries to find new ways of holding on to each other, of sharing the fears and frustration while trying to stay connected, and of fully embracing whatever time they have—amidst the stress—to laugh and love.

L. Baider, PhD (✉)
Sharett Institute of Oncology, Hadassah University Hospital, Jerusalem, Israel
e-mail: baider@cc.huji.ac.il

> ...The challenges were overwhelming for each of us separately and for us as a family. How would we come together and encourage each other, while simultaneously needing so much support ourselves? How would each of us manage the challenges of our individual lives while trying to pull together as a family? And how would we go on without him if we had to?...
>
> It is ultimately not about cancer or death. It is about the meaning of living as well as one can with the sharp, sudden awareness of an everyday fact: we are all living on borrowed time. It is our way to make meaning of a situation we face. This is not unique. It is the human condition, simply intensified by the circumstance. We all live on the knife's edge. It is the meaning we convey to our family experience with illness and death...
>
> —DK Treadway [35]

Hermeneutics: Exploration of Meaning

Hermes was born inside a cave on Mount Cyliene in Arcadia (Peloponnese) as the son of Zeus, the King of the Gods, and the mountain Nymph Maea, who was a daughter of the Titan Atlas.

The basic meaning of the word *hermeneutics* is to express, to assert, to communicate, to interpret a hidden meaning. Significantly, Hermes is associated with the function of transmuting what is beyond human understanding into a form that human intelligence can grasp. The various forms of the word suggest the process of bringing a thing or situation from unintelligibility to understanding. The Greeks credited Hermes with the discovery of language and writing—the tools that human understanding employs to grasp meaning and to convey this meaning to others [32].

Ricoeur [31] attempts to encompass the rationality of doubt and the faith of retrospective interpretation in a reflective philosophy that does not retreat into abstractions or degenerate into the simple exercise of doubt, a philosophy that takes up the hermeneutic challenge in myths and symbols and reflectively thematizes the reality behind language, symbol, and meaning [28].

Witness: On a Search for Meaning and Hope

> We must never forget that we may also find meaning in life even when confronted with a hopeless situation, when we are facing a fate that cannot be changed. For then what matters is to bear witness to the uniquely human potential at its best, which is to transform a personal tragedy into a triumph, to turn one's predicament into a human achievement. When we are no longer able to change a situation—just think of an incurable disease such as inoperable cancer—we are challenged to change ourselves.
>
> —V. Frankl [14]

One of the common tasks in comprehending theoretical concepts of family experience is to examine the narrative of life review. Inherent in this undertaking is the search for meaning—in the individual's life, as it has been lived. Meaning includes the reason for an event or events, the purpose of life in the most mundane tasks, and the belief in an irreversible force of life. For some people, meaning may be found through a retrospective view of external or subjective achievements. More frequently, the search is a moral or spiritual one, often dwelling on mistakes and inadequacies with the hope for something more desirable and suitable. However, there is more to this query into meaning than a simple search through the past or projection into the future. Meaning may also be implanted in the meaning of a process of loss, dying, grief, suffering, and of the remaining days of life and its accomplishments [17]. Contrarily, the absence of meaning in one's life—meaninglessness—is often expressed through hopelessness, despair, and emptiness.

Families and caregivers help give meaning to life by the act of consistently dispensing their love, care, and hope. It is, in fact, here, in the "eclipse" of meaning and hope, that strong faith has proved to many to be the most essential factor during the extended process of illness and dying [33].

Yalom [37] used common sense in distinguishing between searching for the meaning of life on the abstract cosmic scale—who made the stars?—and the meaning of common terrestrial life. Three questions are proposed to explore the meaning of meanings: Why does man have a need for meaning? What are the symptoms of losing meaning? How does meaning weave its therapeutic web?

Meaning occurs passively, as an afterthought of human activity or as a by-product of engagement in life. Meaning exists in the present, the here-and-now, and is not a cognitive process; it is an essential sense of coherence.

Three Categories of Life Meaning

Though Frankl [13] stressed that each individual has a meaning that no one else can fulfill, these unique meanings fall into three general categories: (1) what one accomplishes or gives to the world in terms of one's creations; (2) what one takes from the world in terms of encounters and experiences; and (3) one's stand toward suffering, toward a fate that one cannot change.

Yalom [37] classified the means of restoring meaning into the following domains: altruism, creativity, hedonism, self-actualization, and self-transcendence:

- *Altruism*—the world as a better place to live, serving, giving, opening the eyes of another to dignity, freedom, and blessed despair.
- *Creativity*—dedication to a cause that provides a sense of meaning, bringing something new to life in the other as part of mature loving and of the creative process as well.
- *Hedonism*—to live fully, to retain one's sense of astonishment at the miracle of life; life is a gift, enjoy it!
- *Self-actualization*—strive to actualize oneself. The aim of each human being is to come to fruition and to realize his/her own being. Maslow [24] presents a

hierarchy of built-in motives. Once the basic physiological needs are satisfied, the individual turns to security, love, belongingness, identity, self-esteem.
- *Self-transcendence*—though human beings should begin with themselves, they should not end with themselves (Hasidic thought). Self-actualized individuals dedicate themselves to self-transcendent goals.

The psychodynamics of hope and meaning challenge professionals to step beyond the dichotomy of traditionally defined notions of health, stress, and disorder and to see people in distress as unique, competent, and capable of constructing their own meanings within their cultural and family settings. These challenges provide the potential for generating alternative options to adequately address familial cognitive and coherent behaviors.

Furthermore, in their role as mediator, families have the capability to construe the meaning of illness in ways that can promote or inhibit healthy responses among their members. Families can mediate the context by (1) integrating multiple perspectives generated within and across the interactive triad; (2) providing or requesting environments that reframe or ease illness experience and behavior; and (3) coordinating key players to construct congruent themes aimed at defining and managing perceived or real illness. Families continually recycle through phases of development represented by internal meaning and meaning processes and degrees of internal and external permeability. These phases are system exploration, consolidation, enhancement, and transformation across the dimensions of illness, death, and loss [8].

Marris [23] tried to understand severe illness and grief by suggesting that, for some people, loss of a loved one can be equivalent to loss of all hope, meaning, and sense in the world. In such cases, the loved person serves not just as an attachment figure but also as a carrier of that which contains and structures life. Loss is thus experienced as falling through space, without purpose in the universe.

Although the psychodynamics of hope and meaning are distinct, the narrative interpretation of illness and impending loss is similar. When hope and meaning are absent, both independently cause a fractured, unfocused, unraveled burst of emotions and an incongruent process of thoughts. Conversely, when meaning and/or hope are restored, thinking becomes focused, organized, directed, and effective [18].

> I felt that the ground on which I stood was crumbling, that there was nothing for me to stand on, that what I had been living for was nothing, that I had no reason for living... The truth was that life was meaningless. Every day of life—every step in it—brought me nearer to the precipice, and I saw clearly that there was nothing but ruin [34].

Meaning provides a sense of one's life having made a difference, of one's having mattered, of one's having left part of oneself for posterity. It seems derivative of the wish not to perish and an expression of an effort to transcend the fear of death. When Tolstoy lamented that there was no meaning in his life that would not be destroyed by the inevitable death awaiting him, he was stating not that death destroyed meaning but that, as a person, he had failed to find a powerful meaning that would destroy death [37].

Family Meaning of Illness: A Bounded Universe

> ...We cannot find our way home to life as it was before the illness...
> ...Perhaps, we can never more find our way to feeling at home again...
> And we search for meaning and transcendent understanding...
> But life seems drained of meaning...
> The act of living is different all through. Her absence is like the sky, spread over everything... [21]

Clinical and empirical evidence is rapidly emerging to suggest that meaning and coping are critical mediators between cancer-related distress and psychological well-being and may be possible mechanisms to explain the coexistence of alternative psychological states following cancer diagnosis [19, 20, 25].

Park and Folkman [30] described a theoretical model of stress and coping by making more explicit the roles of belief and goals and the functions of meaning in the processes through which people appraise and cope with stressful events and circumstances. This model highlights the central role of reappraisal and the importance of achieving agreement and coherence between the individual's global meaning and the appraised meaning of a particular event.

The conceptualization of meaning posits that people hold a "global meaning" that is a personalized life schema built upon a set of beliefs and assumptions that provide a sense of order and purpose in life [38]. Global meaning allows individuals to get up in the morning, go about a daily routine, and strive for long-term goals. This overall global meaning is based on a set of illusions that are characteristic and essential for normal mental health. Such illusions include overpositive beliefs about the self and expectations that there will always be tomorrow, that good people deserve good things to happen to them, that it is possible to plan ahead into the future, and that the future looks bright. This set of positive illusions generally remains unexamined until something goes wrong, such as being diagnosed with cancer [5].

When cancer strikes, the belief system that once provided a sense of stability, familiarity, and security is shattered by reflection and inquiry. Family goals that were set out for a secure future may no longer appear realistic or attainable. The "existential plight of cancer" may refer to what is now known in the current literature as the "search for meaning"—a normative but distressing psychological process in which the individual attempts to appraise the impact of an event such as cancer on his/her life and understanding of the world encapsulated within the family. This is the process by which families and patients struggle to retain what is personally meaningful when virtually every aspect of their life will be threatened by changes imposed by the cancer illness and its unpredictable outcomes [20].

Family members strive to make sense of unforeseen illness and its intrusion by enduring and reinterpreting the meaning of each other's experience. Family researchers refer to "shared" meaning within the private family culture [12, 27]. Cultural expectations also regulate and influence basic meanings in the course of the socialization process and the roles that each member might assume. They need to make sense of their experience by either interacting with each other, embracing their silent grief, or withdrawing into an illusory space of denial and rationalization [3].

An important consideration in reorganizing family meanings is the relationship between meaning and family structure. A given family's openness or critical evasiveness to each other's meanings should be perceived in terms of family interaction, flexibility, and adaptability or unyielding distancing from the illness event [26].

The family constitutes a world in itself. It determines when to close itself off from everything else and when to admit parts of the external world. The family maps out its domain of acceptable and desirable experiences—its life space. As new and uninvited experiences occur, new feelings, narratives, and meanings invade the guarded boundaries of the family space. Meanings of narratives assume that family members have incorporated ways of thinking and expressing dilemmas brought on by the illness experience. Narratives provide clues to alternative resources of thoughts—through private or collective meanings—that affect patient and family communication. Each family member devises his/her own private script—recorded from personal emotions, experiences, and social appraisals—concerning the common family life [10].

Nonetheless, in their mutual interaction, family members develop an acceptable common meaning of one another, collaborating to establish consensus and to negotiate uncertainty. The family's life together is an endless process of movement in and around understanding one another, from attachment, conflict, withdrawal, and over again. Separateness and connectedness are the underlying conditions of a family's life, and its common task is to give form to both. Although this dual manifestation of the ties that bind and the barriers that separate are part of the family process of adapting to illness and of self-protection, neither one is an adequate indicator of the family's function and adaptation to the encounter with illness. Multiple external and internal connection points, at which feelings are concentrated and unmasked, are possible paths for probing the family's adaptability to the unpredictable course of the illness [1].

A number of concepts and ways of thinking about families are useful in describing family meaning and its interaction with family communication and family dynamics. The systems framework provides the concepts necessary for describing the structural changes that occur in the family following illness and death, changes in roles, communication, rules, boundaries, and the dynamic of the space between them.

The basic conditions characterizing the family are that its members are connected to one another and are also separate from one another. Every family gives shape to these conditions in its own way. Values and social norms provide greater emphasis on the one or the other, yet both constitute family life. This fundamental duality is of considerable significance across the illness trajectory. It is this matrix of interaction that allows the family to develop a new language and new meanings of illness. From the illness experience, a concept emerges of the "other person"— the patient—serving to direct and shape each member's actions towards the other and form what becomes the dynamic interpersonal relationship of the family [4].

In studying a family, then, it is necessary to investigate both the images that the members hold of one another and the meanings in which these images are interrelated. It is necessary to understand how the interaction of the members derives from and contributes to this interrelation of their visual impressions. The implication of this viewpoint is that interaction cannot be fully understood in its own terms, and that, instead, it must be viewed in the context of how the members define one another as relevant participants in perceiving the illness. From this experience, family members and the patient arrive at expressing new meanings of relationship and shifting life priorities [7].

Meaning: A Quantifiable Challenge

A patient diagnosed with advanced metastatic cancer, a 43-year-old male mathematician, spoke as follows (recorded and translated from Hebrew with his signed consent):

> …Meaning?… What is meaning? How can anyone measure the meaning of a person?… Much before cancer had invaded my lungs, I was able to describe—without any doubt or hesitation—the total, absolute meaning of my life—the smiles of my children, the smell of freshly ground coffee in the mornings, the furtive inquiries into the algebraic universe, the hope for drops of rain in the sands of the desert, the festival of lights, the taste of food and wine… Now, I am confined within windowless plastic walls…white, everything sounding white, everything smelling white… My blood has turned into white numbers… And meaning has become an empty, abstract measure of indecipherable numbers… They asked me to fill out a questionnaire about "meaning" … I read it, I squeezed it, I memorized it. I tried to understand each noun…nouns without verbs… How can a dying person measure the meaning of "his meaning?" By the smell of chloroform, alcohol, or by the silent scream of drops of morphine punching my brain?… Life has absolute, unconditional meaning. Death cannot restore the burning light of hope!… What is left is only the enduring memory of past life…

During different periods of research, a number of studies have focused on the methodological strictness of measuring family parameters during the illness process. There is an underlying thread of continuity woven through these various queries, the nature of the forces that link family members to one another, when confronted with illness, being cognizant that these forces are embedded into a larger structure of cultural and social norms [15].

Since the 1970s, researchers have convincingly argued that existing theories—despite their differences—essentially agree on four major psychological issues. When patients and families state that their lives are meaningful, this may imply that (1) they are positively committed to some formulation of the meaning of life; (2) this notion provides them with some framework or goal from which to organize and appreciate their lives; (3) they perceive their lives as related to or fulfilling some part of this general notion; and (4) they experience this fulfillment as an appraisal of worth, self-esteem, and family significance. This perspective, in contrast to other approaches, acknowledges that diverse ways (e.g., theistic, atheistic, humanistic) of developing meaning in life can coexist. This view also respects the fact that people have derived a sense of meaningfulness from various sources that do not appear to be reducible to one fundamental meaning system [36].

A qualitative study of patients' and nonpatients' sources of meaning in life was designed from this theoretical perspective. First, the most significant sources of meaning were explored in the healthy and patient groups of subjects and discriminative domains of correspondence and disparity. In this exploration, notions were considered that the onset of severe psychological confrontation with illness may, on one hand, obscure persons' values and personal meanings in life but, on the other hand, initiate a renewed search for what really matters in their lives. Findings hold that not so much the specific content of participants' personal meanings as the extent of their commitment to those particular personal meanings is the crucial factor in their deriving a sense of meaning in life [9].

Lee et al. [19] analyzed and synthesized the published literature related to the construct of meaning in families coping with cancer. Most studies alluded to the threat of cancer. It was identified in some studies as a confrontation with the possibility of death and a heightened level of awareness about one's mortality. Other studies focused on both the threatening and growth-enhancing aspects of the cancer experience. The results of their review convey that although cancer can profoundly disturb one's sense of global meaning—enough to instigate a search for meaning—a successfully completed search for meaning appears to confer positive effects, such as enhanced self-esteem, greater life satisfaction, and less distress, despite the uncertain and unpredictable nature of cancer.

In a qualitative study of 12 survivors of hematological malignancies, McGrath [25] described that confrontation with death resulted in spiritual meaning-making that helped patients make sense of their illness and led to personal growth and a reprioritizing of their values. Through such a framework, individuals can come to feel fortunate at having been forced to undertake the "journey" despite its difficulties. Similarly, the well-being of middle-aged and older persons with spinal cord injuries was positively related to their religiosity and a favorable appraisal of their disability.

Although cancer patients may be in total remission for a long time, being diagnosed with cancer forces most human beings to face their own death. Suddenly, any comfort of invulnerability or immortality is shattered, and the patient becomes profoundly aware of life's limitations. Cancer patients search for meaning in their lives and often reevaluate their own priorities, appraising physical, psychological, social, and spiritual needs and their place within the family space [11].

Ardelt et al. [1] presented a qualitative analysis of two focus-group interviews with cancer survivors, aged 39–60, with one focus group comprising seriously ill females (aged 66–78). The analysis indicated that religion and spirituality become more prevalent in meaning-making after diagnosis. The findings of the study confirm Pargament and Mahoney's [29] observation that "one way to maintain beliefs in a just, loving God in the midst of trauma and loss is to see a larger, benign, spiritual purpose behind the negative event. This is a form of reframing in which crises become spiritually meaningful, or even opportunities for growth."

For the middle-aged and "young old" cancer survivors, death approached before the end of their expected and desired life span. Hence, the meaning of their life-threatening illness had to be found elsewhere. The group of older patients, by contrast, had already reached or even exceeded their expected life span. Intellectually, they knew that they would die soon and that a life-threatening illness was almost an expected occurrence at their stage of life. The terminal illness and looming death were not meaningless, as they were for the younger patients. They were meaningful as an integral part of the life cycle and in the context of their own family life.

There was broad consensus among scattered studies that finding meaning is related to less intense grief, higher subjective well-being, more positive immune system functioning, lower mental distress, higher family satisfaction, and better physical health [8, 16].

> ...In the Pursuit of Meaning...
> What profit has man in all his toil that he toils under the sun?
> A generation goes and a generation comes, but the earth endures forever...
> All things are weariness; no man can utter it.
> That which has been is that which will be...
> And there is nothing new under the sun...
>
> —King Solomon, Ecclesiastes (Kohelet) 1:8–9

Patients and families revert to experiences and actions that are embedded in meanings. They attempt to accommodate the illness process by reorganizing, deepening, and expanding their beliefs and by creating a novel narrative to embrace the reality of impending loss. While not all family life experiences are predictable or controllable, families may come to appreciate their personal growth in the hidden meanings that these experiences may reveal [6].

Families return to familiar hopes, dreams, fantasies, and expectations. They revive what still works in themselves and in the recollection of memories and narratives. They draw nourishment and meaning from roots already planted within the family space. They discover and recover among them meanings that still sustain new and old family anticipations. Families struggle along a path of soulful reflection, learning about themselves within a collective interaction of meanings. They become aware of and accept meanings that seem to arise spontaneously in the unpredictable shapes of suffering. They find the way home within surroundings filled with well-established meanings. They learn to trust elements of daily life patterns that remain viable—to find that some long-held hopes and aspirations still move down familiar life paths. They recognize meaningful continuity in their life narratives and the characters that are embodied in their skin and in their silent words. And they often deepen the appreciation of understandings of the familiar place in the larger scheme of universal life [2, 22].

Families are absorbed in weaving and reweaving the webs of connections and patterns of caring as they search, explore, and pursue boundless meanings of family care, compassion, and love.

References

1. Ardelt M, Ai AL, Eichenberg SE. In search of meaning: the differential role of religion for middle-aged and older persons diagnosed with a life-threatening illness. J Relig Spiritual Aging. 2008;20:288–312.
2. Atting T. The heart of grief: death and the search for lasting love. New York: Oxford University Press; 2000.
3. Baider L. Communication about illness. Support Care Cancer. 2008;16:607–11.
4. Ballard-Reisch DS, Letner JA. Centering families in cancer communication. Patient Educ Couns. 2003;50:61–6.
5. Battista J, Almond R. The development of meaning in life. Psychiatry. 1983;36:409–27.
6. Calhoun L, Tedeschi RG, editors. Handbook of posttraumatic growth. Mahwah, NJ: Lawrence Erlbaum; 2006.
7. Charon R. Narrative medicine XII. Oxford, UK: Oxford University Press; 2006.
8. Davis CG, Wohl M, Verberg N. Profiles of posttraumatic growth following an unjust loss. Death Stud. 2007;31:693–712.
9. Debats DL. Source of meaning: an investigation of significant commitments in life. J Humanist Psychol. 2000;40:30–57.
10. Driskill GW, Brinton AL. Organizational culture in action: a cultural analysis workbook. Thousand Oaks, CA: Sage; 2005.
11. Efficace F, Marrone R. Spiritual issues and quality of life assessment in cancer care. Death Stud. 2002;26:743–56.
12. Fegg MJ, Brandstätter M, Kramer M, Kogler M, Doetkotte SH, Borasio GD. Meaning in life in palliative care patients. J Pain Symptom Manage. 2010;40:502–9.
13. Frankl V. The will to meaning. New York: World; 1969.
14. Frankl V. Man's search for meaning. New York: Simon and Schuster; 1984.
15. Jim HS, Purnell JQ, Richardson SA, Golden-Kreutz D, Andersen BL. Measuring meaning in life following cancer. Qual Life Res. 2006;15(8):1355–71.
16. Keesee NJ, Currier JM, Neimeyer RA. Predictors of grief following the death of one's child: the contribution of finding meaning. J Clin Psychol. 2008;64:1145–63.
17. Kemp C. Terminal illness: a guide to nursing care. New York: JB Lippincott; 1997.
18. Längle A. The method of personal existential analysis. Eur Psychother. 2003;4:59–75.
19. Lee V, Cohen SR, Edgar L, Laizner AM, Gagnon AJ. Clarifying "meaning" in the context of cancer research: a systematic literature review. Palliat Support Care. 2004;2:291–303.
20. Lee V, Cohen SR, Edgar L, Laizner AM, Gagnon AJ. Meaning-making intervention during breast or colorectal cancer treatment improves self-esteem, optimism, and self-efficacy. Soc Sci Med. 2006;62:3133–45.
21. Lewis CS. A grief observed. New York: Bantam Books; 1976.
22. Little M, Sayers EJ. While there's life … hope and experience of cancer. Soc Sci Med. 2004;59:1320–37.
23. Marris P. Attachment and society. In: Parker CM, Hinde JS, editors. The place of attachment in human behavior. New York: Basic Books; 1992.
24. Maslow A. Toward a psychology of being. Princeton, NJ: Van Nostrand; 1962.
25. McGrath P. Reflections on serious illness as spiritual journey by survivors of haematological malignancies. Eur J Cancer Care. 2004;13:227–37.
26. Nadeau JW. Families making sense of death. Thousand Oaks, CA: Sage; 1999.
27. Neimeyer RA. Constructivist psychotherapy. New York: Routledge; 2009.
28. Palmer RE. Hermeneutics. Evanston, IL: Northwestern University Press; 1969.
29. Pargament KI, Mahoney A. Spirituality, discovering and conserving the sacred. In: Snyder CR, Lopez SJ, editors. Handbook of positive psychology. London: Oxford University Press; 2002.
30. Park LC, Folkman S. Meaning in the context of stress and coping. Rev Gen Psychol. 1997;1:115–44.

31. Ricoeur P. History of truth (translated by CA Kelbley). Evanston, IL: Northwestern University Press; 1965.
32. Rose HJ. A handbook of Greek mythology. New York: Routledge; 2000.
33. Schlegel RJ, Hicks JA, Arndt J, King LA. Thine own self: true concept accessibility and meaning in life. J Pers Soc Psychol. 2009;96:473–90.
34. Tolstoy L. My confession, my religion, the gospel in brief. New York: Scribner; 1929.
35. Treadway DK. Home before dark. New York: Union Square; 2010.
36. True G, Phipps EJ, Braitman LE, Harralson T, Harris D, Tester W. Treatment preferences and advance care planning at end of life: the role of ethnicity and spiritual coping in cancer patients. Ann Behav Med. 2005;30:174–9.
37. Yalom ID. Existential psychotherapy, part IV. New York: Basic Books; 1980.
38. Folkman S, Greer S. Promoting psychological well-being in the face of serious illness. Psycho-oncology. 2000;9:11–9.

Chapter 11
The Patient's Personality as a Guide to Communication Strategy

Purvish M. Parikh, Kumar Prabhash, G.S. Bhattacharyya, and A.A. Ranade

Abstract Effective communication is a continuing challenge due to information overload, including easy access to unorganized information. The potential for miscommunication also depends on the patient's receptiveness. The process of imparting the message needs to be improved. Understanding the personality and "type" of the patient helps prepare the oncologist to overcome the challenge of communicating with clarity. A structured, stepwise approach ensures its success. Documentation of the entire process is part of due diligence and can prove useful in the future.

Keywords Patient preference • Communication strategy • Individualized • Oncology

Introduction

We are in an era of information overload. More is written in medical scientific journals every year than one can read in a lifetime. Couple this with the ease of access to information, via the Internet and using such devices as smart phones, tablets, and now near-field connectivity (NCF). No wonder we are faced with several new challenges in communicating with cancer patients and their families. The oncologist and other

P.M. Parikh (✉)
Indian Cooperative Oncology Network, 74 Jerbai Wadia Road,
Parel, Mumbai 400012, India
e-mail: purvish1@gmail.com

K. Prabhash
Tata Memorial Hospital, Mumbai, India

G.S. Bhattacharyya
AMRI, Kolkata, India

A.A. Ranade
Sahyadri Hospital, Pune, India

Table 11.1 Factors that need improvement during healthcare provider–patient communication (table taken from Kimberlin et al. [5])

Theme	Patients n (rank)	Caregivers n (rank)	Total n (rank)
Improve process of information exchange	186 (1)	129 (1)	315 (1)
Increase active participation of patient and caregiver in care process	105 (3)	92 (2)	197 (2)
Improve provider relationship-building skills	109 (2)	38 (3)	147 (3)
Overcome time barriers	34 (4)	29 (4)	63 (4)
Address fears regarding use of pain management medications	29 (5)	10 (6)	39 (5)
Foster appropriate involvement of family and caregivers	15 (6)	15 (5)	30 (6)
Improve coordination of care among providers	10 (7)	7 (7)	17 (7)

healthcare providers therefore need to be aware of and devise innovative strategies to make communication effective during (a) breaking the news to the patient about the diagnosis of cancer, (b) helping the patient navigate through therapy, (c) counseling the patient posttreatment, and (d) providing support for the terminally ill patient [1, 2].

Potential for Miscommunication

There is a potential for miscommunication during the process of information exchange between healthcare provider and patient. We know that the patient is usually under extreme duress, has a limited attention span, tends to cling to the positive aspects, and will remember only about 10% of what he or she is told [3–5]. The amount of useful information retained and understood depends on the active participation of both patient and caregiver, the relationship-building skills of the oncologist, the time devoted to the consultation, the patient's fear, and the level of coordination of care among the healthcare providers. According to a study done by Kimberlin et al. [5], both the patients and their caregivers indicated in focus group interviews that the process of information exchange needed to improve (Table 11.1). Other aspects that needed improvement included relationship-building skills and active participation of the patient and caregivers.

Patients also have a tendency to misquote. This is their "strategy" if they do not want to follow a particular line of therapy or advice given by their treating physician [6]. They often claim that another expert's recommendation was different. Such statements can lead to a soured relationship or miscommunication between healthcare professionals and should be guarded against. The best way to deal with it is to offer to talk directly to that colleague so that matters are crystal clear.

Communication Regarding the Unknown and the Frightening

It is important for healthcare providers to know that most human beings are not ready to face the diagnosis of a life-threatening illness such as cancer. This is because most of us think that we are invulnerable, that illnesses happen only to others. We tend to evaluate risk in two ways, voluntarily and involuntarily [7]. We can voluntarily decide to take a particular risk—for example, to learn to swim despite the risk of drowning. We think rationally and take measures to control the risk by having a coach who can rescue us from drowning. On the other hand, cancer falls in the realm of involuntary risk—risk that cannot easily be perceived. Patients are ill prepared for it and have very little time to respond when faced with such a diagnosis. Due to cancer's involuntary nature, patients tend to assume that the risk is high, and they panic [8]. Thus, the healthcare provider should remember that he or she has to don the mantle of the swimming coach and help the cancer patient navigate to safe shores.

Klein and Stefanek elegantly point out that people have different numerical abilities, and hence using heuristics can help explain the risk faced when a diagnosis of cancer is revealed for the first time [7]. People's motivational behavior, self-enhancement, tendency to appear rational, and ability to avoid regret are factors that influence their decision making. They prefer having control over their health outcomes, but do not understand enough about the disease. People tend to use their hearts rather than their minds. It is crucial that healthcare providers elicit perceptions of risk when helping their patients navigate through the process of decision making when faced with cancer. This is even more important when the patient is a child or an elderly person, dependent on someone else to make the right decision [9, 10].

Facing the Communication Challenge: Know Your Patient

The challenges we have (old and new) include dealing with the following types of patients:

(a) The "I-know-it-all" patient. This is typically a white collar, type A personality who has been at the helm in all important decision making his entire life. He is well qualified, part of senior management of a large organization, and used to processing tons of information provided by subordinates. He is used to being in the hot seat and feels that he can digest and understand the finer points of anything in seconds. He has downloaded terabytes of information from the Internet, tabulated and classified it, and comes for consultation already having selected what he thinks is the right line of treatment. It is an uphill task to explain to such a patient the difference between information, data, and insight. Just making him realize that there are a lot of unverified and often misleading (though usually well-meaning) opinions on the Internet that need to be distinguished from facts can take hours.

(b) The "It-can't-be-true" patient. This is the one who does not want to face reality. He will want second and third opinions, a rebiopsy or review of the biopsy by an "expert," and will move heaven and earth in the quest of someone who will say that the diagnosis of cancer is incorrect. Patience and assistance in setting up consultations is very helpful in such instances. Putting him in touch with other experts will hasten the process of going through this stressful time.

(c) The "I-don't-want-to-know" patient. This patient has poor coping abilities and will be the typical ostrich with his head in the sand. He will avoid any attempt to discuss the disease and its details and will want a "reliable" close relative to make decisions for him.

(d) The "I-am-going-to-die" patient. This is the typical "OMG" reaction—an expression so well known today. An eternal pessimist, he will expect the worse and has a tendency to go into depression and anxiety that needs pharmacological intervention. Such patients do poorly, and expert psychiatric help is often needed.

(e) The "Don't-tell-the-patient" family. This is common in Asian countries. The family (or at least its head) will be of the opinion that the patient is too frail to know the truth; that discussing cancer with him is likely to "kill" him; that he will not be able to bear the "shock"; hence, the diagnosis should be concealed from him. Here counseling the family is at least as important as communicating with the patient. Unless the family barrier is tackled, it will be difficult to have any meaningful dialogue with the patient. Takashi Hosaka et al. studied the results of disclosure or nondisclosure of the diagnosis of cancer in Japan, a community that prefers that patients not be told their diagnosis [11]. According to popular belief, nondisclosure protects the patient from anxiety, depression, and posttraumatic stress disorders (PTSD). Contrary to this belief, data showed that psychiatric disturbance was higher (48.9%) among patients who were *not* told their diagnosis as compared to patients who were (42.9%). Furthermore, patients not told their diagnosis often suspected what they were suffering from and even asked the interviewer about it. Such a situation is often the root of mistrust among cancer patients and disturbs the patient–family relationship. This study states that full disclosure with the help of communication sessions that involve medical, emotional, and practical conversations may lead to healthy patient–doctor relationships.

(f) The "Don't-tell-my-family" patient, on the other end of the spectrum, is the patient who wants to keep all the information to himself. This kind of patient is not unknown in Western culture. Such patients are worried about self-esteem, about what their peers will say, and even about losing their job or promotion. It is important to help them realize that they would be doing without an important pillar of support by excluding their immediate family. This can also lead to reversal of a disturbed family–patient relationship. Hence, it is vital to discuss coping skills with such patients.

Approach to Breaking Bad News

There is no good way of breaking bad news [12, 13]. The principle is to ensure that doing so causes the least amount of stress. This requires a strategy that matches the type of patient. Some benefit most from full disclosure in one session; some from gradual disclosure. Devising the right strategy needs close attention to several considerations; there is no rule of thumb that fits all.

Some of the steps necessary for an individualized approach to overcoming communication barriers include the following:

Step 1: Prepare the background: There are several insights that others in the healthcare team can provide the treating physician. Often these valuable allies are overlooked. Nurses, having more frequent and less formal interactions with the patient and the family, may attain a good understanding of the patient's psyche. By having a meeting with clinic and ward staff members, the primary physician will be better equipped to select the right approach for breaking bad news.

Step 2: Prepare adequate time and privacy: The patient and the family should know that this is an important consultation. This will ensure that the patient will be able to bring along his close confidant and primary caregiver. Physicians should provide a quiet, private room without interruptions to help with the process.

Step 3: Ensure adequate understanding: Convey the information in a simple, clear manner. Use a tone that has hope and compassion. Avoid technical jargon. Assuming that the patient has understood everything told to him is a potential pitfall that must be avoided. Asking counter-questions from time to time will verify the extent of the patient's perception and interpretation. Repeat the message several times until it is conveyed correctly. As an extra precaution, written information, including pamphlets, may be provided.

Step 4: Encourage patients to express feelings: Pause during the consultation to allow the patient to express his feelings. Nonverbal gestures and other clues are vital. Using touch to convey empathy, warmth, sympathy, encouragement, and reassurance is very helpful.

Step 5: Focus on the broad principle, not on the finer details: Convey whether the disease management approach is curative or palliative in intent, or is for symptom control. Treatment options should be introduced at this time. Discuss potential side effects only after the overall plan has been agreed upon. Avoid any statements that would indicate a sense of hopelessness, of abandonment, that nothing more can be done. Indicate that there is a definitive plan for follow-up and subsequent consultation.

Step 6: Offer assistance in telling others: If the patient does not belong to category F (vide supra), offer to help the patient talk to other family members and friends. Encourage them to discuss the matter among themselves and to write down points that remain unclear. That way their understanding can be improved to their satisfaction in the shortest possible time.

Step 7: *Documentation*: Giving the above information should be coupled with advice about other support services that can be of use to patients with advancing disease—such as cancer support groups, palliative care services, nutritional counseling. Document what has been conveyed to the patient, who will take on the role of primary caregiver, and the patient's reaction to the news. Include this information on the summary that goes to the referring doctor and other members of the healthcare team that will be involved in the patient's subsequent management.

Conclusion

Communication with the cancer patient is diverse and complex. Active listening is the key that is often forgotten [14]. Frustration can creep in when the interplay is complicated further by misunderstanding by other stakeholders, especially when family members (and sometimes patients themselves) believe that information from the Internet makes them experts. Great patience is required to tackle this delicate situation. That formal training in communication is not included in the training curriculum of physicians is an important gap that is only now being addressed. Using discussion groups and simulated case scenarios can be valuable in improving skills.

References

1. Girgis A, Sanson-Fisher RW. Breaking bad news: consensus guidelines for medical practitioners. J Clin Oncol. 1995;13(9):2449–56.
2. Step MM, Ray EB. Patient perceptions of oncologist-patient communication about prognosis: changes from initial diagnosis to cancer recurrence. Health Commun. 2011;26(1):48–58.
3. Stajduhar KI, Thorne SE, McGuinness L, Kim-Sing C. Patient perceptions of helpful communication in the context of advanced cancer. J Clin Nurs. 2010;19(13–14):2039–47.
4. Russell BJ, Ward AM. Deciding what information is necessary: do patients with advanced cancer want to know all the details? Cancer Manag Res. 2011;3:191–9.
5. Kimberlin C, Brushwood D, Allen W, Radson E, Wilson D. Cancer patient and caregiver experiences: communication and pain management issues. J Pain Symptom Manage. 2004;28(6): 566–78.
6. Parikh PM, et al. Communicating with the patient. Indian J Hematol Blood Transfus. 2001;19(3): 57–8.
7. Klein WM, Stefanek ME. Cancer risk elicitation and communication: lessons from the psychology of risk perception. CA Cancer J Clin. 2007;57(3):147–67.
8. Zikmund-Fisher BJ, Fagerlin A, Ubel PA. Risky feelings: why a 6% risk of cancer does not always feel like 6%. Patient Educ Couns. 2010;81(Suppl):S87–93.
9. Repetto L, Piselli P, Raffaele M, Locatelli C, GIOGer. Communicating cancer diagnosis and prognosis: when the target is the elderly patient-a GIOGer study. Eur J Cancer. 2009;45(3): 374–83.
10. Fletcher PC, Schneider MA, Harry RJ. How do I cope? Factors affecting mothers' abilities to cope with pediatric cancer. J Pediatr Oncol Nurs 2010;27:285–98.
11. Takashi Hosaka, Hisae Awazu, Isao Fukunishi, Toru Okuyama, James Wogan. General Hospital Psychiatry—May 1999 (Vol. 21, Issue 3, Pages 209–213).

12. Mack JW, Wolfe J, Cook EF, et al. Hope and prognostic disclosure. J Clin Oncol 2007; 25:5636–42.
13. Tomlinson D, Bartels U, Hendershot E, et al. Factors affecting treatment choices in pediatric palliative care: comparing parents and health care professionals. Eur J Cancer 2011; Jun 11. [Epub ahead of print].
14. Tomlinson D, Bartels U, Gammon J, Hinds PS, Volpe J, Bouffet E, Regier DA, Baruchel S, Greenberg M, Barrera M, Llewellyn-Thomas H, Sung L.: Chemotherapy versus supportive care alone in pediatric palliative care for cancer: comparing the preferences of parents and health care professionals. CMAJ. 2011 Oct 17. [Epub ahead of print].

Chapter 12
Challenges to the Disclosure of Bad News to Cancer Patients in the Middle East: Saudi Arabia as an Example

Ali Aljubran

Abstract Attitude towards disclosure of bad news to cancer patients in Saudi Arabia is still an unsettled issue. Recently, emerging data show clear contradiction between the public attitude, which is very conservative towards full disclosure, and the cancer patients' attitude. This chapter attempts to look into what governs the public attitude towards disclosure in Saudi Arabia as an example of what may affect attitudes in developing countries. It also brings some data from local surveys among physicians and patients as well as from public surveys with a comparative analysis of the Western literature in the past and at present to prove that attitude is dynamic and can be changed.

Keywords Attitude • Disclosure • Cancer • Communication • Psychosocial • Saud

Introduction

In a busy Tuesday morning clinic, I was about to see a new 67-year-old male patient who had been accepted by my clinic as a case of newly diagnosed metastatic colon cancer. After brief triaging, my nurse admitted the patient to the examination room. He was accompanied by his wife and son. While I was still in my office, the nurse informed me that the son wanted to talk to me before I went in to see his father. That was not an unusual request from a family member in the first clinic visit. In this area of the world, a close male relative, commonly the son or the husband, likes to give a briefing about the patient's recent health condition, but more importantly to say that the patient is not yet aware of the diagnosis and ask that he or she not be told.

A. Aljubran, MD (✉)
Medical Oncology, King Faisal Specialist Hospital and Research Center,
Riyadh, Saudi Arabia
e-mail: ajubran@kfshrc.edu.sa

The son was a 32-year-old school teacher. He was nervous and obviously overwhelmed by the new bad news that he decided to hide.

He started by saying that his father did not know about the diagnosis and that he would not be able to stand knowing the truth. I listened to his concerns about what he thought would be the negative impact of informing his father about the diagnosis and to his request that I not tell him. He thought that his mother, too, would not be able to cope with this situation, especially because she had recently had a heart attack; he asked that I not tell her as well.

It was a challenging situation, with two contradictory conceptions and attitudes: the socioculturally supported public attitude, which considers informing the patient about fatal or incurable conditions as merely adding to the patient's sufferings and thus wrong; and the ethically and scientifically supported attitude, which considers open discussion with the patient about the disease and available therapeutic options as a crucial step, not only because it is ethically required, but also because it is a necessary step in creating a healthy physician–patient relationship.

The son proposed to start the treatment, which in this case was noncurative chemotherapy, without even telling the father that it was chemotherapy, let alone discussing the side effects with him. He suggested that if his father were to ask about the intravenous therapy, he should be told that it is a plain intravenous fluid.

While the patient was waiting with his wife in the examination room, I showed my full understanding of the son's worries and told him that I truly believed that he was driven by a sincere wish to help his father at that difficult time. However, I stressed the ethical aspects of the matter and explained the great benefits to the patient of open discussion about the disease and therapy. I concluded the conversation by my usual statement that I am not in a position to hide any information from my patient; that I will follow the strategy of disclosing the diagnosis without going into details and outlining the proposed plan of therapy; then I will give more information at the patient's request. I offered the alternative that the son himself start breaking the news to his father at home, if he thought that would be more appropriate; then, when the patient returned to my office, I could reiterate the major points of information.

The son seemed confused and unable to make a decision. However, he decided at the end not to inform his father of the diagnosis and to decline therapy. In a final effort, I told him it would be unacceptable to make that decision on behalf of his father and it would have a negative impact on his father's health. He decided to leave the clinic along with his father and mother.

Two months later, the patient was brought to my clinic by his brother-in-law in very poor condition. He was on a wheelchair, cachectic, deeply jaundiced, and very weak. He was not able to talk much, but his brother-in-law told me that he had tried herbal medicine and went to Mecca, a sacred place in Islam, seeking cure. His condition had deteriorated with time, he had lost appetite and weight, and had become unable to walk. His condition appeared beyond any kind of therapy; only palliative care seemed appropriate. It was shocking to realize that he was still not aware of his diagnosis.

Two striking issues in this story need to be addressed: first, how far a male relative may go in taking over a patient's basic rights and responsibilities; and second, how much permission is given to him by the patient to do so. It was very obvious that the patient himself did not show any desire to intervene. He gave no sign that he would like to step in and take care of the whole situation. Was that because he was weak and affected physically and emotionally by his recent illness, so he trusted and authorized his very enthusiastic son to handle things? What made the son talk and make decisions on behalf of the father? And did the father really intend for him to run the complete show? These questions and more are addressed in an attempt to deeply understand the sociocultural background behind such attitudes.

Magnitude of the Challenge

Disclosing the diagnosis or prognosis to cancer patients in Saudi Arabia can be a serious challenge to the physician in his daily clinic practice. The public attitude towards full disclosure is still conservative. Physicians occasionally find themselves confronted with situations of clear contradiction between what they have learned as the correct ethics of medicine and what the public attitude dictates. In most of these situations, the family's request for nondisclosure of diagnosis and prognosis to the patient is the most contradictory and the most difficult to manage. The local sociocultural paradigm views the patient as an individual in an extended family, allowing or actually encouraging other family members to show their sympathy and support by sometimes taking over some or all of the patient's responsibilities and rights. Valuing the patient's autonomy and informed consent are not yet prominent or influential in Saudi society.

This chapter attempts to look into what governs the public attitude regarding disclosure of full information to the patient in Saudi Arabia, as an example of the issue in many developing countries; and into whether or not this attitude is amenable to various psychosocial, educational influences. At the end, there are some locally oriented and validated recommendations as to how to handle the patient's truth-telling issues.

Attitude is a hypothetical construct that represents an individual's degree of like or dislike of an item. Attitudes are generally positive, negative, or neutral views of an "object"—i.e., a person, behavior, or event [1]. Most attitudes in individuals are results of observational learning from their environment. The important question of whether attitudes change or not has been positively answered by many psychologists and sociologists. Unlike personality, attitudes are expected to change as a function of experience. They can be changed through the tools of persuasion or by social influence, such as social proof and authority [1].

Attitude Has Changed in the West

The general attitude among physicians in the West in the recent past was not in favor of fully discussing the diagnosis or prognosis with patients. In 1953, a questionnaire administered to 442 Philadelphia physicians regarding the issue of disclosure of diagnosis found that only 31% of the physicians surveyed stated that they always tell their patients the details of their diagnosis [2].

In 1960, a survey of 5,000 physicians found that only 16% stated that they always tell the patients their diagnosis [3]. Another survey 1 year later of 219 physicians in Chicago found that 90% stated that they generally do not inform patients of their diagnosis [4]. On the other hand, the public attitude was not so different.

In 1948, a public survey for the American Cancer Society covered many aspects of the public reaction to cancer. Information was collected by personal interviews of 1,244 adult persons. To monitor for changes in public opinions, two repeat surveys were conducted in 1955 and 1962. One relevant question was, "Supposing that a doctor finds out that a person has cancer, should the person be told?" Percentages of response with a clear yes were only 63, 64, and 60% in the years of 1948, 1955, and 1962, respectively [5].

Understanding Is the Key to Solutions

There was a combined medical and largely sociocultural background for such a conservative attitude towards disclosure. This background consists of many elements, including:

- The nature of the disease. Cancer was, and still is in many situations, viewed as a death sentence, and revealing the diagnosis to a patient was considered cruel and inhumane. Patients' relatives thought that disclosure of the diagnosis would lead to loss of hope and that the patient would become devastated and crippled and even die earlier.
- The extended family role in the face of less patient autonomy, in the past and to some extent in the present time, in many non-Western countries. A patient is primarily viewed as a member of a family rather than an autonomous person; and that therefore all decisions, including health-related decisions, should be made by family members. This assumption has been held in many societies and continues to be a major component in the sociocultural background of many non-Western countries.
- Paternalistic medicine and the principle of beneficence has helped physicians collude with patients' relatives in not explaining the status and prognosis of the disease to the patient in many settings.

The attitudes of both physicians and the public have undergone major changes in the West in the past 50 years. In a questionnaire that was administered to a group of physicians who attended the 1999 Annual Meeting of the American Society of Clinical Oncology, participants were asked about difficulties they had when approaching stressful discussions and communication strategies used in giving unfavorable information [6]. The questionnaire was completed by 167 oncologists. Sixty-four percent of them practiced in North America and Europe, and the remaining practiced in non-Western countries. In disclosing the cancer diagnosis and prognosis, physicians from Western countries were less likely to withhold unfavorable information from the patient at the family's request, avoid the discussion entirely, or use euphemisms. Another questionnaire given to both physicians and patients in the US and Japan confirmed this finding and revealed that both physicians and patients in the West are more inclined toward respecting patient autonomy and informed consent [7]. In that questionnaire sample, groups of Japanese physicians ($n=400$) and patients ($n=65$) as well as US physicians ($n=120$) and patients ($n=60$) were selected randomly. A majority of both US physicians and patients, but only a minority of Japanese physicians and patients, agreed that a patient should be informed of an incurable cancer diagnosis before the family is informed.

There is now a clear focus, both legally and ethically, on the issue of informed consent and patient autonomy. It is now an unshakable belief that telling the truth is a moral duty and that the patient has a need to know the truth in order to make decisions. The change in the attitude in the West over the 1950s and 1960s was multifactorial in etiology. Revelations by the post-World War II Nuremberg trials, which disclosed experimentation on humans without consent, showed the legal and ethical need for informed consent. The 1950s and 1960s was an era of social upheaval in the US, when movements promoting human rights were demanding rights for women, consumers, and finally patients, who began to demand that they be fully informed about their diagnosis, prognosis, and treatment options. Furthermore, advances in surgical and radiation oncology and the beginning of medical oncology gave more treatment options and increased survival in many cancers. These advances increased optimism about the cure of some cancers. These changes provided the momentum toward disclosing diagnoses to patients. On the physicians' side, there was greater recognition of communication as an effective means of enhancing patient understanding and compliance.

The Paradigm in Saudi Arabia

Attitudes are undergoing steady, albeit slow changes, in many non-Western nations, including Saudi Arabia. Public education, in addition to the increased cultural openness due to the communication revolution, and worldwide globalization are having some effect in changing a few aspects of the sociocultural atmosphere in Saudi Arabia. Because of the complicated political, social, and religious mix of values that govern Saudi society, changes, if allowed to happen, are slow and follow a cautious path. While the values of patient autonomy and informed consent are now rooted deep in the conscience of Western societies and control and shape the physician–patient relationship, these values are not yet prominent or influential in Saudi society. The patient is frequently thought of not only as an individual, but as part of a family; it is expected that family members will be intimately involved with decision-making.

Indeed, family members, and to a lesser extent friends, find themselves forced by their genuine cultural and mainly religious values to extend their help and support to their relatives or friends. They frequently find themselves allowed, and sometimes obliged, by the patient to come forward and take over some or all of the patient's responsibilities. This is the way they show sympathy and support to a sick relative or friend. It is commonly believed that patients (especially female patients) are very vulnerable and should not be left alone to handle the stress of knowing bad news or making decisions. This supportive attitude, unfortunately, can evolve into a dominating attitude that steals the patient's basic right to knowledge and decision-making.

Nevertheless, many patients (especially old women) accept this situation, where the dominating relatives (sons, most of the time) become the major players. These patients trust their dominating relatives and literally hand over some or all responsibilities.

Bedikian et al. conducted a survey of 100 adult patients and companions referred to the Department of Oncology at King Faisal Specialist Hospital, Riyadh in 1984 [8]. He found that only 16% of patients were told that they had "cancer," and 34% were told they had a "tumor." On the other hand, 69% of companions were told about the diagnosis of cancer. Another questionnaire was conducted almost 10 years later to assess physicians' attitudes toward sharing information and decision-making with patients in the setting of a serious illness [9]. Two hundred and forty-nine physicians from three different areas of the country participated in the study. Seventy-five percent of the physicians preferred to talk with close family members rather than patients. In the face of such an attitude, oncologists from King Faisal Specialist Hospital, Riyadh [10] tried to explain why physicians avoid telling their patients about their disease. They concluded that physicians may not know what to say or how to say it when they are about to break bad news. They may wish to avoid the difficulties of having to cope with a patient who is disturbed by the bad news: they may feel the patient simply will not be able to cope, or that it may take too much time and patience out of a busy work schedule. To further monitor any evolving change in attitudes, a recent study was conducted to assess physician and public views in Saudi Arabia towards involving the patient vs. the family in the process of diagnosis disclosure and decision-making. The study surveyed 321 physicians and 264 hospital attendees from six different regions [11]. In the case of a patient with incurable cancer, 67% of doctors and 51% of hospital attendees indicated that they would prefer to inform the patient of the diagnosis rather than the family ($P=0.001$). Assuming the family already knew, 56% of doctors and 49% of hospital attendees would tell the patient even if the family objected (difference not statistically significant). However, in the case of HIV infection, 59% of physicians and 81% of hospital attendees would inform the family about HIV status without the patient's consent ($P=0.001$). The authors concluded that there is a need for greater recognition of patient autonomy among physicians. These studies assessed only public and physician preferences and attitudes regarding disclosure, which are clearly conservative. At least one study has been conducted specifically to assess patient preferences towards disclosure of diagnosis and prognosis [12]. A small survey of 114 patients in a teaching hospital in the Eastern Province revealed that almost all (113 patients) wished to know all the information about their cancer, and only one patient preferred to know some information. All patients were against information being withheld. Almost all patients wanted to know the benefits and adverse effects of therapy (98 and 99%, respectively), and all wanted to know the prognosis of their disease. This study showed how the patient's preference is toward absolute disclosure, while the general public attitude is against full disclosure.

Locally Oriented Recommendations

Every healthcare provider involved in the care of cancer patients knows how difficult it can be to disclose the diagnosis to the patient. Disclosure of prognosis, especially after failure of therapy, is even more difficult. To overcome such difficulties, the following suggestions are provided:

1. Disclosure has to be a systematic process and has to follow guidelines for breaking bad news. These guidelines are set up to make the process of disclosure smooth and fruitful. They should be taught in medical school and be a part of postgraduate training.
2. Establishment of a support program for both patients and their families. There is no doubt that breaking bad news is a daily routine in the practice of oncology, putting a continuous psychological and emotional burden on physicians. Establishing a support program will definitely help physicians cope with the situation better and enable them to perform the task in an optimal way.
3. The argument for disclosure can be supported by many strong points, including the clear Islamic perspective to respect the patient and protect the patient's right to know and to freely make choices. It can also be supported by studies about patient preferences, which include evidence of benefit to the patient that is now undebatable [12]. These benefits include building a trustful relationship with the physician and the ability to make decisions, or at least share in decision-making, improving compliance, and last but not the least, planning the end of life.
4. More local research is needed to study all public, patient, and physician attitudes as well as signs of change and the underlying factors influencing change.
5. Finally, one of the most appropriate approaches, which fits patients in many developing countries, including Saudi Arabia, is what James Hallenbeck and Robert Arnold have described in an article titled "A Request for Nondisclosure: Don't Tell Mother" [13]. This model of negotiation with the family has been used and found to be very useful in the Saudi situation. This is a summary of the key points, with minor modifications to fit local clinical practice:

    - Unlike in many parts in the world, physicians in Saudi Arabia, as per the local sociocultural background, frequently need to establish a physician–family rapport in addition to a physician–patient rapport.
    - Respect the sociocultural background. Most of the time the family would like to know first. This can be acceptable provided that the patient is not denied the right to know.

- Try to understand the family's viewpoint and respond empathetically to their distress, keeping in mind that the aim is not to hide any information from the patient upon his or her request. Explain to them the benefits to the patient of disclosure and the practical difficulties associated with not telling the diagnosis.
- Explain the importance of truthfulness for you and negotiate how you will respond if the patient asks to be told the truth. Stress the point that "if he or she asks me to tell the truth, I must do so."
- Talk to the family about what the patient would want and explain that "you are fine with a family member being the decision-maker" if the patient concurs with the decision.

References

1. Attitude (psychology): From Wikipedia, the free encyclopedia. http://en.wikipedia.org/wiki/Attitude_(psychology). Accessed in December 2010.
2. Fitts WT, Ravdin IS. What Philadelphia physicians tell patients with cancer. JAMA. 1953;153:901–4.
3. Rennick D, editor. What should physicians tell cancer patients? N Med Materia. 1960;2:41–53.
4. Oken D. What to tell cancer patients: a study of medical attitudes. JAMA. 1961;175:1120–8.
5. Horn D, Waingow S. What changes are occurring in public opinion toward cancer: national public opinion survey. Am J Public Health Nations Health. 1964;54:431–40.
6. Baile WF, Lenzi R, Parker PA, et al. Oncologists' attitudes toward and practices in giving bad news: an exploratory study. J Clin Oncol. 2002;20:2189–96.
7. Ruhnke GW, Wilson SR, Akamatsu T, et al. Ethical decision making and patient autonomy: a comparison of physicians and patients in Japan and the United States. Chest. 2000;118:1172–82.
8. Bedikian AY, Saleh V, Ibrahim S. Saudi patient and companion attitudes toward cancer. King Faisal Spec Hosp Med J. 1985;5:17–25.
9. Mobeireek AF, Al-Kassimi FA, Al-Majid SA, Al-Shimemry A. Communication with the seriously ill: physicians' attitudes in Saudi Arabia. J Med Ethics. 1996;22:282–5.
10. Young D, Moreau P, Ezzat A, Gray A. Communicating with cancer patients in Saudi Arabia. Ann N Y Acad Sci. 1997;809:309–16.
11. Mobeireek AF, Al-Kassimi F, Al-Zahrani K, et al. Information disclosure and decision-making: the Middle East versus the Far East and the West. J Med Ethics. 2008;34:225.
12. Al-Amri AM. Cancer patient's desire for information: a study in a teaching hospital in Saudi Arabia. East Mediterr Health J. 2009;15:19–24.
13. Hallenbeck J, Arnold R. A request for nondisclosure: don't tell mother. J Clin Oncol. 2007;25:5030–4.

Chapter 13
Talking to a Child with Cancer: Learning from the Experience

Eulalia Lascar, María Angelica Alizade, and Blanca Diez

Abstract It is well known that communication with children who are suffering from a life-threatening condition is a big challenge and that, if it is open and honest, it can greatly lessen anxiety and fears. Besides, good communication improves the quality of life for kids and families, since it is a useful tool in order to promote the design and development of coping strategies during all the different moments of the illness through listening to their needs, expectations, fears, doubts, and feelings.

In this chapter, we want to highlight the actual situation in our country with the most relevant data on demographical, epidemiological, and cultural aspects and to outline the principal features of our style of communication, which has evolved over years of experience of work with children and families as one interdisciplinary team, the only way of accomplishing this difficult task.

The main aspects of communication and the way in which children express their thoughts, wishes, and feelings are presented in the drawings, pictures, and real stories that they shared with us.

We also want to add some brief observations about what happens to us professionals, because we strongly believe that this is the first step if we want to care for others.

Another important aspect is the contact with the siblings of the sick child; they are not usually considered when a strategy of communication is planned.

Finally, we mention some communicational aspects in the end of life stage.

Keywords Communication • Pediatric oncology • Pediatric palliative care

---

E. Lascar (✉)
Hospital de Niños Dr. Ricardo Gutierrez, Arce 441, 4th E, (1426) CABA,
Buenos Aires, Argentina
e-mail: eulalia.lascar@gmail.com

M.A. Alizade
Buenos Aires Psychologists Association (APBA), Buenos Aires, Argentina

B. Diez
Fleni, Neuro-Oncology, Buenos Aires, Argentina

With love, to the little ones, who teach us, every single day.

Introduction

Being able to communicate with children who are suffering from a life-threatening illness, as is cancer, is a big challenge in daily practice. We need to talk with children in many different situations. Sometimes we have to prepare and put the child at ease before a physical examination or an invasive procedure. This is a very common aspect of our work, and it is appreciated by the little patients and their families.

We know that timely explanations can greatly diminish stress and fears. Talking with children allows us to know whether there are any factors in the environment that can cause unexpected symptoms, and of course this knowledge helps us to manage such factors in advance and in the best way, paying attention to detail. Children need to know what is wrong and like to discuss diagnosis and treatment. As Dr. Roger Burne said, "there are no fixed rules for this situation; what matters is the professional's capacity to cope with the emotional and spiritual impact of what is said."

Communication is also an essential component of palliative care, which offers active and total care from the moment of diagnosis, during treatment, and relapse, also in the terminal stage when there is no possible cure, and even during the stage of mourning (see Fig. 13.1).

The Reality in Our Country

To explain how we communicate with the children with cancer and their families, we would like to describe some features of our country and its people that are quite different from those of most other countries in South America. Argentina is a very large country, with a continental area of 2,776,888 km^2. (France has an area of 543,988 km^2.) The total Argentine population is 40,091,359 (Census 2010), of which 25.6% are younger than 15 years old. The distribution of the population is very uneven. The average population density for the country as a whole is only 14.4 inhabitants/km^2. Remarkably, in the Federal District there are 13.647 inhabitants/km^2, while in the province of Santa Cruz there are barely 0.8 inhabitants/km^2. Most of the people live in cities (92%) (see Fig. 13.2). The ethnic predominance is Caucasian (mostly Spanish and Italian), with some mixture of aborigines and

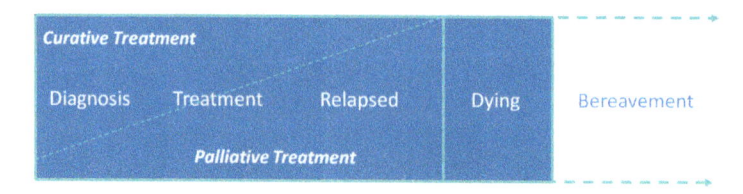

Fig. 13.1 Intervention time

Caucasians, and a minority of pure aborigines. It is, indeed, exceptional to find anyone of Black African descent.

We have reliable data about the general incidence of childhood cancer in Argentina since 2000 through ROHA (Registro Oncopediátrico Hospitalario Argentino). ROHA is a not-for profit institution committed to providing a resource for gathering and disseminating epidemiologic data on childhood cancer, describing its incidence and survival patterns, evaluating diagnosis and treatment, and raising awareness of the disease. ROHA gathers data from 91 sources, 12 regional registries, and 2 cooperative groups. Data are grouped by histological type and primary site, based on the International Classification of Childhood Cancer 1996 (ICCC) and the International Classification of Diseases for Oncology, third edition. Ninety-five percent of cancers are histologically confirmed. The percentage does vary by ICCC category from 86% for CNS (ICCC III+Xa) to 100% for leukemia (ICCC I) (see Fig. 13.3). Forty percent of the children, at some point in their treatment, migrate to hospitals located in other provinces that provide services of higher complexity (leukemias 30%, brain tumors 50%). Some of the patients and their families need to travel more than 2,500 km in order to receive medical treatment. The mother or a family member always stays in the hospital with the child.

In Argentina, pediatric oncology and palliative care treatments are included in the free medical program that is obligatory in the whole country. But its implementation is still deficient in most hospitals. It does not cover travel or lodging costs, with the consequent financial burden for the families. The majority of professionals do not yet understand the advantages of this modality of care, which includes the care and management of symptoms from the very beginning of the neoplastic disease, always in collaboration with the primary oncology team. During all these stages, it is necessary to offer effective support, which means helping each family to recognize its own needs, fears, doubts, hopes, expectations, and to be able to identify what this illness means to each family, which will differ according to its social level, beliefs, and cultural background and will also depend on its previous experience of the illness.

> Sabrina's parents didn't want to tell her that her hair would fall out due to the leukemia treatment. The twelve-year-old girl was proud of her long, straight hair. To this we should add that her aunt was resistant to telling her because it reminded her of the death of one of her family members, who had received chemotherapy with the subsequent loss of hair. She couldn't separate death from the loss of hair, and so was unable to focus on the curative treatment of her niece.

Oftentimes during the various stages of diagnosis and treatment when we perceive that communication between the members of the family is blocked and does not allow us to come to an agreement as to the management of information, we meet with the "extended family." We invite the parents and all family members, friends, and neighbors who are involved and, in some cases, a representative of their religion or ancestral tradition (native tribes). We organize meetings with siblings separately. We promote an open dialogue with whatever difficult issues there may be, adjusting our information to their way of thinking. From this meeting, we create a link with the child and the family and, on that basis, design strategies of management and support.

When dealing with babies, we have to take into account that they lack the necessary psychological mechanisms to help them fight pain OR fight against pain and that

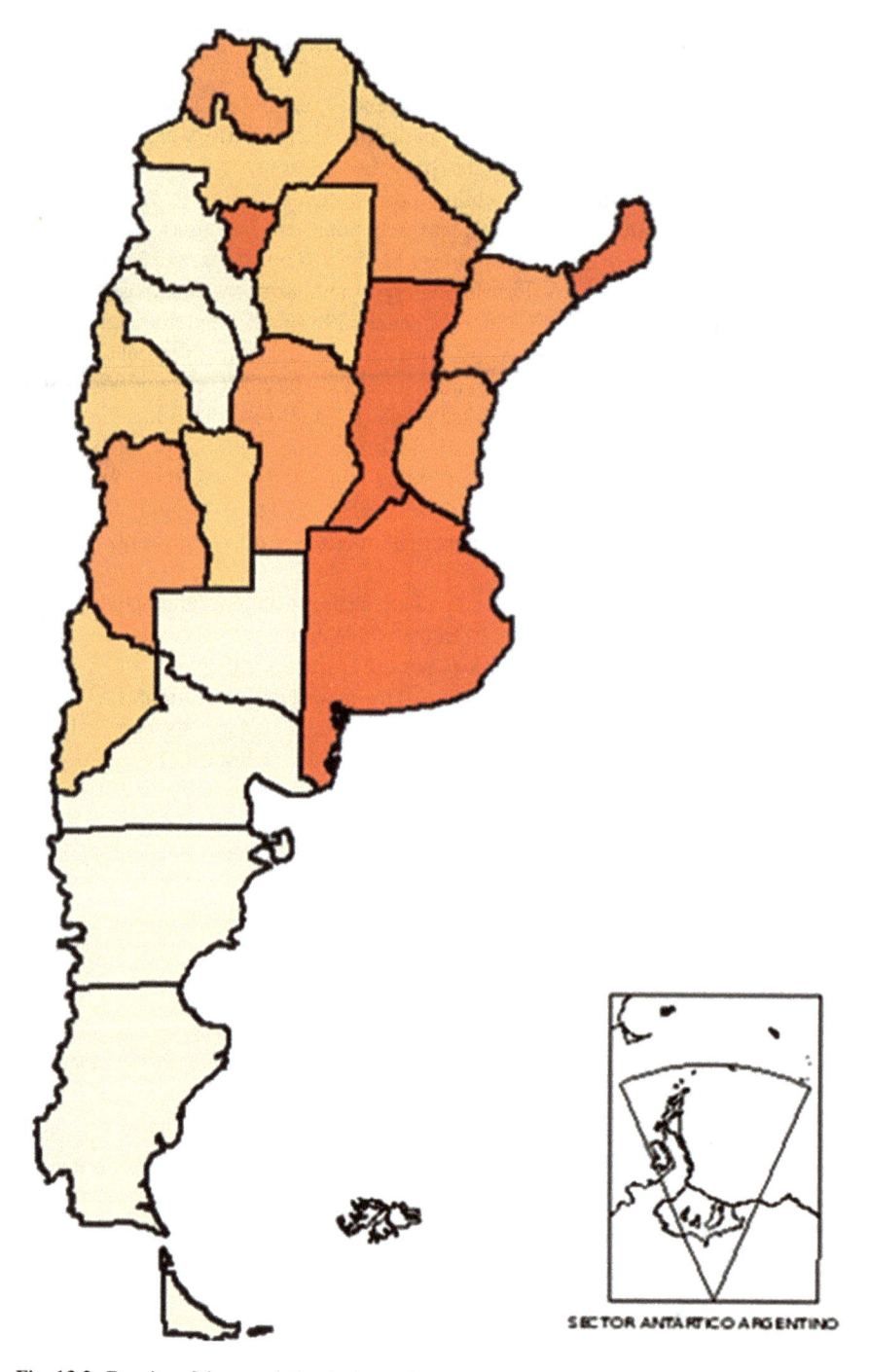

Fig. 13.2 Density of the population in Argentina

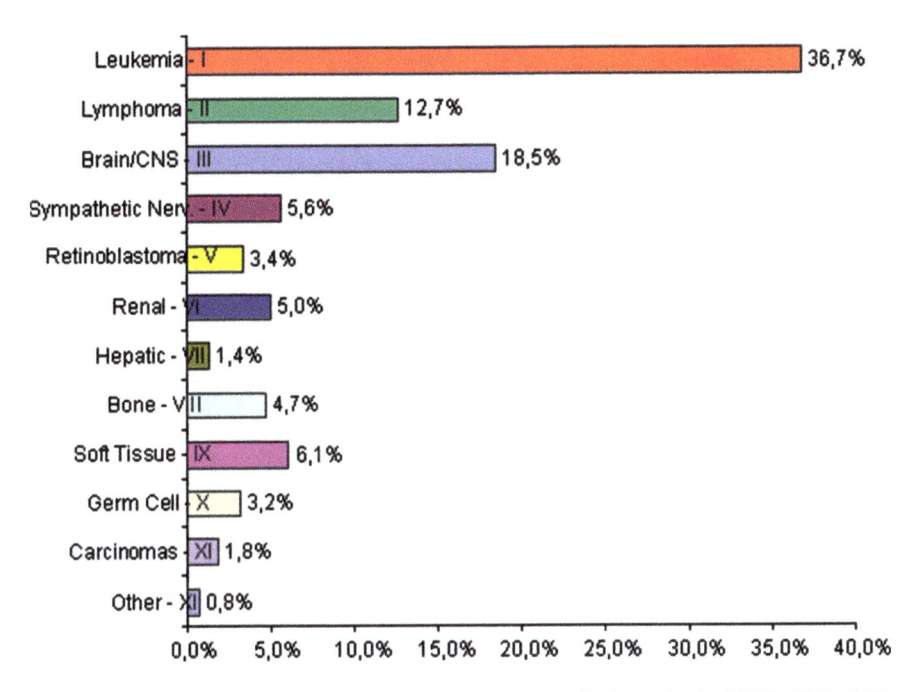

13 Talking to a Child with Cancer: Learning from the Experience

Type	Percentage
Leukemia - I	36.7%
Lymphoma - II	12.7%
Brain/CNS - III	18.5%
Sympathetic Nerv - IV	5.6%
Retinoblastoma - V	3.4%
Renal - VI	5.0%
Hepatic - VII	1.4%
Bone - VIII	4.7%
Soft Tissue - IX	6.1%
Germ Cell - X	3.2%
Carcinomas - XI	1.8%
Other - XII	0.8%

Fig. 13.3 ROHA (http://www.roha.org.ar). Childhood cancer in Argentina by ICCC, 2000–2008. Total number of cases: 11,445

their only means of communication is through their mothers. Both of them together create a wholeness of an illusion of self-sufficiency. Thanks to this bonding, the mother is usually able to provide adequate and efficient answers.

> We remember a 17-month-old girl who had been operated on for a CNS tumor and had to undergo a second surgery. Our team was called in due to the constant crying of the baby, whose sleepless and anguished mother hopelessly tried to calm down. The baby girl kept banging her head against the side of the cot and even against her mother's bosom. We suspected that she was suffering from headaches, so we indicated analgesia, which eventually soothed her. The crying also waned as soon as the mother felt the sympathy and support offered by the doctor and the team psychologist. This allowed the baby to change her outwardly aggressive behavior and cuddle up to her mother's breast.

At all ages, sick children can normally make a regression to that moment of symbiotic union with the mother they had at birth; it is a protective union and in this case necessary to help them cope with their suffering. That is why these mothers, who care tirelessly for their children day by day, merit all our admiration. So, they must be helped in order that they may gradually reestablish communication with the rest of the family, with the outside world and with themselves. This is one of the fundamental tasks of the health carers.

Within these strategies, we consider fundamental the creation of a space for communication in which we can include the whole family (siblings, parents, and extended family) as the unit of care, keeping the child in the principal role.

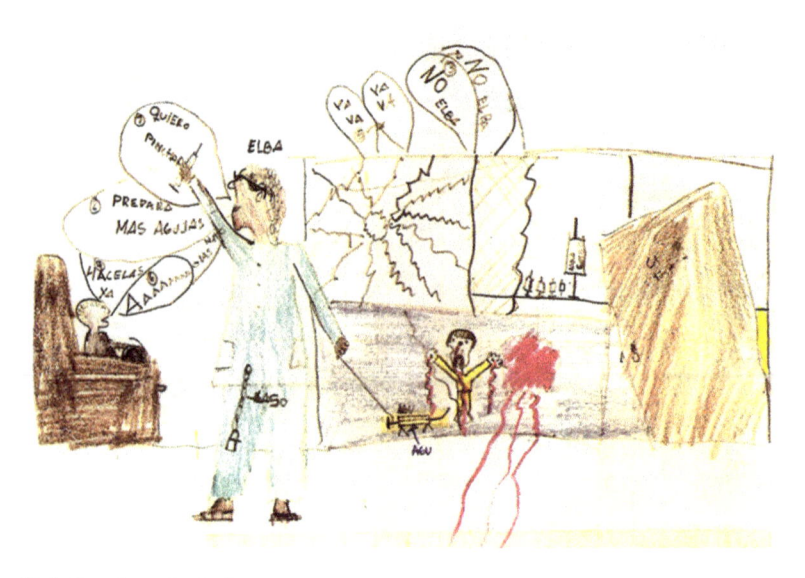

Fig. 13.4 Oncology day beds

An effective communication should be open. Open communication is defined as verbal and/or nonverbal free expression of positive and negative thoughts and feelings that may include the children's fears, questions, and concerns related to the illness, the treatment and prognosis, as well as the death and dying processes (see Fig. 13.4).

In our experience, an atmosphere of open communication helps children feel confident that they will receive an honest answer when questions are asked.

When we propose an open climate of communication from the beginning of the illness, this is reflected in how the child talks about death.

The first impression on the bond that we create with the family will determine its quality and will promote trust between team-patient-family.

When the team manages communication from the start, without lies, and informing step by step with the truth, a trusting bond with patient and family will result, which will become stronger with the passing of time.

The information should be tailored to the needs of the different stages that must be faced. It also must take into account the capability of the different family members to tolerate and work through certain information.

Talking with a child is always a two-way process and is not a one-time verbal conversation; it will include different expressions of feelings over a period of time, using different approaches, even by them.

The child knows what he needs, and sometimes he will set limits; it is a way for him to control his reality. It is important that the patient feels respected, in wishes and needs, by everyone around (see Fig. 13.5).

Fig. 13.5 "The entry of any doctor with bad news and nurses that come to prick me is prohibited. Thank you"

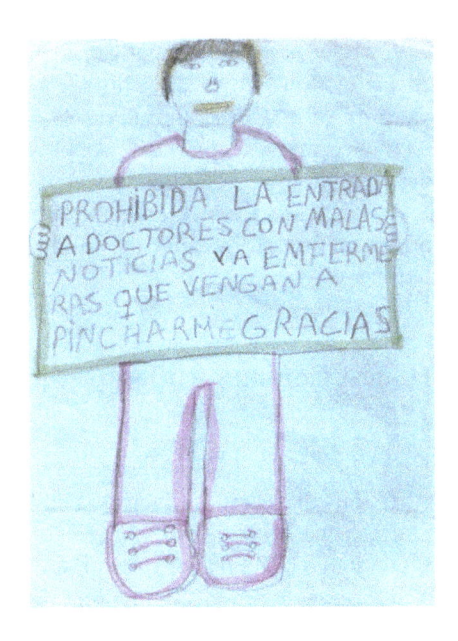

What Happens to Us Professionals

It seems that although many more professionals now value open and honest communication, this is still very difficult to put into practice. This is currently one of our educational goals.

Different distancing tactics (such as lies, jokes, answering with another question, speaking loudly, acting out) are still used regularly by doctors and are due to multiple factors: fear of being blamed, fear of handling the unknown, fear of unleashing a powerful reaction, fear of expressing their own emotions or unease to confront difficult issues.

> "If you listen carefully to your patients, they will speak not only of what is wrong with them, but also of what is wrong with you."
> Walker Percy (Love in the Ruins)

It will be necessary to adopt a new form of communication, which enables us to become involved with the patient and his parents, giving the latter full empowerment over what is, in the long run, their own job: to be "the principal carers"—always keeping a healthy distance that allows us to act in favor of the patient.

Within this frame of work, we can help the family to organize themselves and collaborate with the care of the sick child.

To listen is the key to care. We doubt that we could care for anyone if we don't know how to listen. This is essential. In our country, it is often very difficult to find privacy in the hospital setting; even the private ones are very noisy, and doctors in general do not consider privacy important. However, we always find a way to achieve this aim.

It will be necessary for active listening within a private space. Once the child has chosen with whom to share his feelings, the team will recognize that person as a valid spokesperson for the child.

In Argentina, feelings are usually expressed through physical contact, kisses, cuddles, hugs, with children as well as with adults.

In the case of a sick child, who has limited independence and freedom, it is important for us to perceive the desires for closeness and physical contact, to respect intimacy.

Honest Communication

We must have in mind:

- To only answer that which the child asks.
- To answer with the truth that is adequate to each moment.
- To not go beyond their questions.
- To follow the child's timing for awareness.
- To be able to recognize that which we don't know, being able to tell "I don't know, but I am trying to find out."

> F. Dolto says: "the child has the need to know the truth and has the right to it; often it will be painful to understand, but if another person mentions it, it will give the child an opportunity to integrate the truth and be aware of his humanity."

Talking with Children Is ...

- To listen carefully, that is, to be aware of the characteristic of their cognitive development and their previous experiences.
- To never lie.
- To use understandable terms, to not use euphemisms or empty phrases.
- Never to contradict and always to respect their beliefs and family customs.

> During a guided visualization, 3-year-old Javier, suffering from a neuroblastoma in its final stage, imagined traveling through space to a castle. When asked who was with him, he immediately answered: The Zorro! It was this film character that he choose to be his imaginary companion during his last days.

- To talk to the parents in the presence of the child, avoiding the famous conspiracy of silence.
- To always use the therapeutical triad in communication: empathy, honesty, and warmth.

The child may be very well aware of the fact that he or she is dying, but choose not to talk about it when there is no room to express it. It is we, as professionals, together with the parents, who are responsible for creating that space for communication.

If we fail to do this, the child will feel isolated and lonely and will not find with whom to share his doubts and anguish.

We should remember that the child usually expresses using symbolic language and metaphors. It's surprising to discover how some children protect their parents, as much as their parents protect them. It so happens that they can deny and cover up the existence of pain and other kind of discomfort so as not to distress their parents.

> A 16 year old teenager said: "I have been putting up a struggle for a long time. If I go on fighting it is only for my mum's sake; if it were up to me I would give up."

Key Aspects for Effective Communication with Children

- Their mental level of development and the different concepts about illness and death that they may have.
- A child of 5 years of age doesn't have the capacity to understand death as a permanent fact, it will be more like an absence. The absentee can come back at any moment, which is why it is not recommendable to tell children "he's gone on a trip;" this will only increase the belief in an absent life. They must be helped in their own terms to process a situation that is nonreversible, making it clear that the loved one (the person he or she loves) is no longer there and will not come back.
- Children often repeat the same questions and we must be tolerant with this, always giving the adequate answer. If told that the deceased is in the cemetery, the child may ask: "who will take him food?" We must explain patiently that the person is dead, and that means that the deceased one does not eat any more, does not breathe, does not walk, or do any of the activities that the child does.
- The existing communication system within the family. We have learned that each family has its own existing communication system and we must respect it. To pretend to change it would be arrogant and can be damaging for the child, since a fissure in the relationship of the team with the parents will thus become apparent and may cause the child to lose confidence in the caring team. The majority of our families find it very difficult to talk about illness and death.

> Maria, a teenage girl, with a tumor in her lower maxillary bone, complained about having nightmares with threatening contents. Her parents had asked the team not to tell her what the diagnosis was. The parents referred to the illness as a "little ball" that had to be removed. As the nightmares persisted and produced much anguish, a meeting was organized with both parents. The team's psychologist explained to them that the nightmares were reflecting the fear generated by that which was hidden from her. "That which is not said" took on dimensions more terrifying than reality, appearing in her dreams in the shape of monsters and ghosts. The parents understood this interpretation perfectly and the suffering of the daughter. Finally they were able to confess their own difficulties to tell Maria face to face that she had cancer. The sole idea of telling her the truth overwhelmed them with despair. They blamed themselves for not having been able to protect her from this illness; they felt they had failed her as parents.
>
> We respected their decision of not telling her the truth, but agreed that they should be the ones to tell her, once they felt ready to do so. During the sessions with the psychologist

Fig. 13.6 Patricia

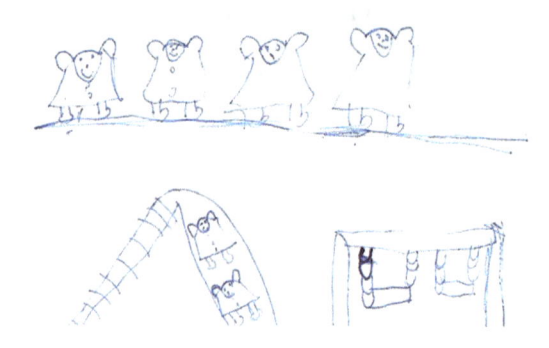

she inquired, without naming the disease, what information Maria had of it. It turned out that she had quite a lot of information. She had seen films on TV about bald children with cancer, and she also knew that the mother of one of her classmates had had cancer, etc.

So, gradually, as we brought this theme into our psychotherapeutic sessions, mentioning the different types of cancer and the different types of treatment for it, her nightmares began to diminish. Eventually, when her parents were able to put the facts of the diagnosis simply to her, they all felt greatly relieved.

- An attitude of mutual pretence is often employed when parents act that they are not concerned in order not to worry their children, and children pretend they are not worried because they do not want to upset their parents. We can confront the parents openly with the suggestion that they may be using this attitude and they often agree that they are. As they reach an understanding of what is happening with the child, they can offer him/her an open space to express their feelings. Sometimes they need more time to be prepared to cope with this.
- Another approach is to offer opportunities for children to communicate obliquely. In this case, teachers and psychologists can have a particular role in applying other types of communication. In order for communication with children to be possible, one must be knowledgeable of the normal evolutionary development of children and adolescents and must integrate the cognitive-emotional and social dynamic aspects in the therapeutic approach.
- The child expresses through play and symbolic language. The illness, and the discomfort that it can produce, can sometimes be represented in drawings, or in role-playing, as the "bad guys" that attack, and where the strength of their defenses will be evidenced by the result of the final battle.

Patricia, 8 years old, suffering from a Sarcoma localized in the cervicolateral area, which caused her severe pain, never drew the necks in her series of drawings of little girls, which she was very fond of doing, as is shown in figure (see Fig. 13.6).

The fantasies concerning the medication and injections can be depicted as monsters and caricatures (see Fig. 13.7).

- School age children are eager to know, they want answers to the myriad of questions that may arise in their minds, be they explicit or not. To encourage their

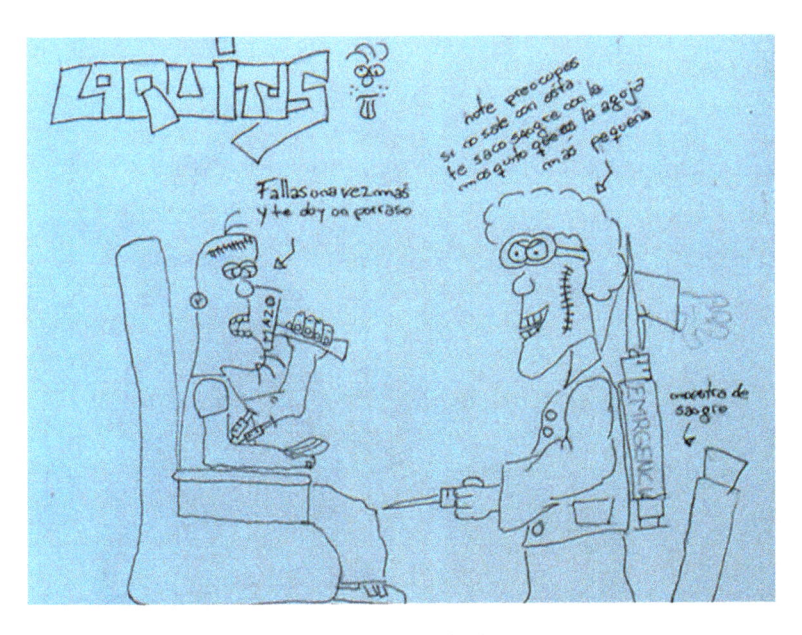

Fig. 13.7 Fantasies concerning the medication and injections

- curiosity and give them information of their illness, operations and medical procedures, will help the child to lower anxiety, and at the same time will enrich his life through these experiences.
- Children find it very easy to incorporate medical terms; they are very attentive and can reproduce with great precision certain medical and nursing procedures that they must go through. They transform that which they must suffer passively into an active game. Making active that which is passive is a valuable psychotherapeutic technique for psychological processing and produces cathartic results.
- In Pediatric Oncology, where treatments are aggressive and continually threaten the child's emotional balance and stability, the use of toy animals in games allows the child to distance from reality and enter the symbolic realm easily. The toy, be it a bear, cat, dog etc., will take on the function of symbolic starters. In psychodramatic theory, this object will function as a bridge between his inner world and the recognition of the outside world; it acts as a means of communication between the psychotherapist and the child. It can be made to say or act that which has not yet been able to be expressed in words. Winnicott writes the transitional object and other transitionary phenomena, often a blanket or soft piece, toy, enable the child to move from the concrete to the symbolic, to enter the world of imaginative play.
- The families who practice systems of denial and avoidance present the hardest problem of all. In these cases, we always bring to mind the stages described by E. Khubler Ross, where hope is always present. Even when the reasons for denial are understandable, this attitude is very stressful for professionals.

Fig. 13.8 Communication through pictures

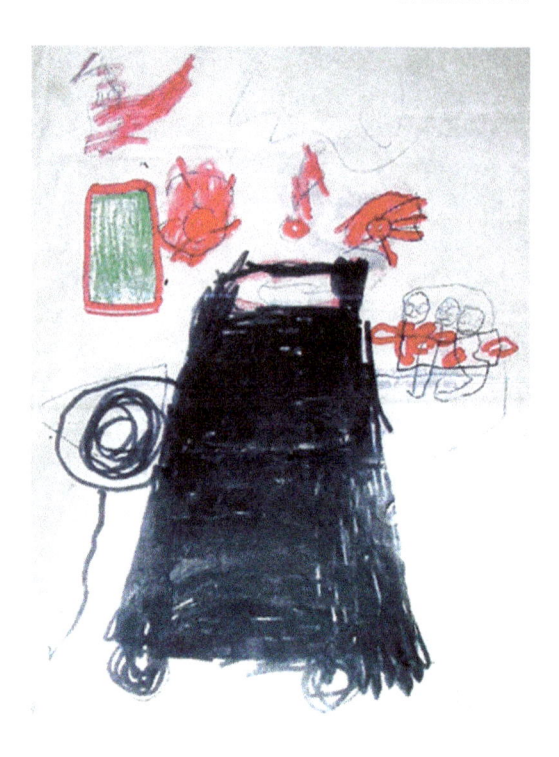

- Children may choose their own method for communication, either through drawings or paintings. Both are easily accessible to most and provide opportunities to express themselves. As in play, children can communicate specific messages.

    When Alejandra, 5 years old, was undergoing treatment for leukemia she did the drawing pasted below; the members of the team became worried by its contents, we feared that she might be suffering a relapse. Then we found out that there was another 15 yr old girl in the same room with her, who was in the terminal stages of an ocular Rabdomiosarcoma, with an important protrusion of her eye. We decided to move Alejandra to another room, and her next drawing was rampant with colorful flowers and butterflies (see Fig. 13.8).

Communicating with the Siblings of the Sick Child

Siblings are often ignored and hurt by adults. It is as important to listen and to talk with them as with their sick brother or sister. They can feel very confused and scared by the sadness of their parents and by their incapacity to comfort them.

They can also be angry with their parents, feeling that they have let their brother or sister become sick, worried by their own fantasies, in regard to death and to their own health. Very often, siblings refer to various physical symptoms: headache, stomachache, dizziness, etc.; in our experience, we often observe that siblings will ask to see their pediatricians. Changes also occur in their school performance, such as depression and anxiety, as they can be jealous of the time their parents spend with the sick child. These are all real needs that deserve to be taken into account and be alleviated. A feeling of guilt is often present, as well as is the fantasy that they can become infected with the same disease. That is why we consider it very important to foster the participation of siblings in the care of the sick child. Making them feel helpful, like getting involved during the whole process, will act as a preventive measure for both their physical and mental health.

When Death Approaches: Talking to a Child with Cancer That Is No Longer Curable

> A little girl aged 9, two days before dying of leukemia, gave her hospital pediatrician the picture that is shown below. She began by drawing the figures above, and then afterwards, she drew a line and completed the picture at the bottom, with what looks like a black box (see Fig. 13.9).

When the time of death is closer, our goal is to accompany the process, in order to reduce anxiety and fear as much as possible. Another important goal is to facilitate communication between the family members and with the health carers.

Little children do not understand what death is; for them everything is either absence or presence. Their only need is to feel accompanied and to know that they will never been abandoned. They need to feel the protection offered by their family and the health carers.

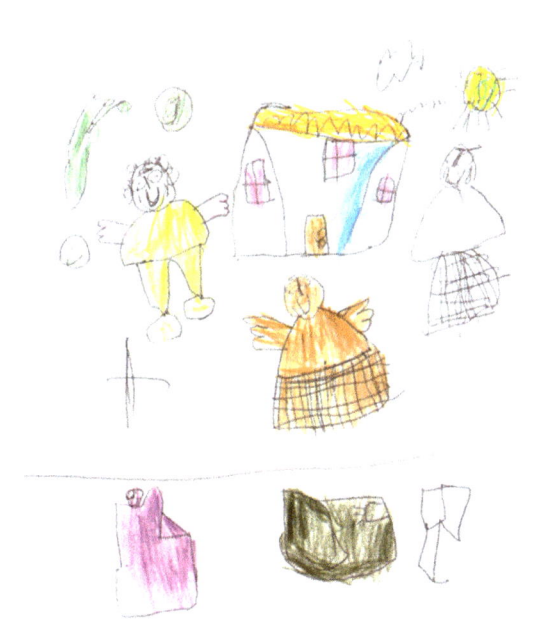

Fig. 13.9 Picture from a little girl, 2 days before dying of leukemia

Nearing adolescence, the appearance of fear and anger can be prevalent. In such cases, it will be important to offer them other opportunities to express their feelings.

"A cancer diagnosis is likely to have a devastating effect when it occurs, but it is possibly especially problematic during adolescence. The many challenges faced by adolescents have led to a concern for their psychosocial well-being. The review of the literature has identified that amongst the psychological challenges; there is uncertainty and fear around the status and progression of the cancer [1]." The bitterness of a young adolescent who is dying can probably cause more problems to the family and the medical staff than any other reactions experienced by other age groups of patients in the terminal phase.

When confronted with a relapse or the deterioration of health, it is important that the patients, who have received adequate and complete information about their illness, continue to receive this modality of communication from the team. Sometimes we see that when curative treatment fails, it results in the interruption of the communication between the sick child, his parents and doctors, which, of course, will cause a subsequent increase of anguish, and the appearance of symptoms like insomnia, irritability, lack of interest, nightmares, anger, etc.

The quality of the questions put forward by adolescents will give us an idea as to how much they will be able to tolerate the answers given. Some teenagers need more information than others, such as details of the disease and the treatment. For this type of patient, all the information given will be reassuring, as this will secure for them an intellectual control over the situation, which is known as one of the defensive mechanisms typical in adolescence.

It is during this stage when many children and teenagers find a way of carrying out a plan so as to say good-bye to their parents, siblings, friends, and doctors.

We can remember some cases in which little children gave away their toys, their favorite clothes, etc. to their siblings or friends. In some cases, they can also leave messages as a farewell.

> Diana, a teenage girl aged 14, who clearly knew she was close to death, but that had never wanted to talk about it, left her mother a message in the letter-box of her mobile phone. She had been hospitalized some days before her condition worsened. When her mum went home after her death, she felt deeply moved on retrieving the phone messages when she heard her daughter's: "Hello mommy, I hope that you are well, don't cry. I love you a lot!"

> Geronimo, aged 5, in the terminal phase of a neuroblastoma, organized a barbecue for all the family, including the extended family. He himself phoned each of them. When everybody was there, he got the camera and took a photograph of the whole group, saying at the same time: "I want to take you all along with me." He died peacefully three days later.

When talking with the parents during the bereavement stage, we can observe the effects of a good farewell from their child or, on the contrary, the guilt or regret at not having said the truth in time.

If we used all the possible tools at our disposal, in the communication with sick children, and we allowed them, at the same time, to establish a fluid communication with us, it would help a normal development of the bereavement process, adjusted to the particular characteristics of each family who has lost a child.

"A man who works with his hands and his head is a technician, but a man who works with his hands, his head and his heart is an artist."

–St François d' Assise. (Olivier Messiaen's Opera Saint Francois D'Assise)

Acknowledgment We do wish to acknowledge, with gratitude, the very much we have learned from talking with children, our patients, and their families.

To our friends and colleagues, Prof. Jorge Roca, Prof. Sonia Steed, and Estela Goldschläguer MD., for their help in translation and, most importantly, for sharing our thoughts and feelings.

"Talking to a child with cancer. Learning from the experience" © 2011 E. Lascar, M. A. Alizade, B. Diez

Reference

1. Singh K., Hodgson D. Journal of Radiotherapy in Practice Vol. 10, © 2011 Cambridge University Press.

Chapter 14
Effective Communication with Older Cancer Patients

Lodovico Balducci and Martine Extermann

Abstract This chapter reviews the special issues related to communication with older cancer patients. The first part of the chapter is a brief review of the current knowledge related to the treatment of cancer in the older-aged person, the second concerns the content of the message and its delivery.

The content of the message is derived from the current knowledge of the subject and may be so summarized:

- The treatment of cancer may be beneficial to subjects of all ages and chronologic age is not a contraindication to cancer treatment
- Given the diversity of the older population it is important to sort out patients who are more likely to benefit from cancer treatment and those who are not. A comprehensive geriatric assessment is the only validated instrument that does estimate the risk of mortality of older individuals and the risk of surgical and medical complications
- Long-term complications of cancer treatment in older individuals, including the risk of functional dependence and cognitive decline, are still largely unknown

The delivery of the message needs to account for common perceptive changes of aging. As the tactile sensations are the best preserved in older individuals, touching the patient while talking to him/her may improve the effectiveness of the message. Likewise, the use of simple words and the delivery of written information are beneficial for patients with attention and memory disorders. The presence of a caregiver may facilitate the delivery of the message as long as the practitioner keeps the patient as the center of the interview.

Keywords Communication • Cancer • Aging elderly • Toxicity • Clinical research

L. Balducci, MD (✉) • M. Extermann, MD, PhD
Senior Adult Oncology Program, Moffitt Cancer Center, Tampa, FL, USA
e-mail: lodovico.balducci@moffitt.org

Cancer in the older person is the most common form of cancer, but the information about the treatment of cancer in individuals 70 and older is limited [1]. With the exception of large-cell lymphoma [2–4], older patients have been largely excluded from clinical trials of cancer chemotherapy [5, 6]. Even in the case of lymphoma, the elderly population enrolled in trials was highly selected in terms of function and comorbidity [2–4].

The diversity of the older population is the main obstacle to clinical trials in the elderly. Other obstacles include comprehension of the trial, as clinical research is a relatively young discipline; practical difficulties of access to care; and so-called ageism [7], the prejudice toward aging that may affect practitioners, the family, and the patient himself/herself.

The discussion of treatment options in the elderly is thus marred by the following problems:

- Inadequate information
- Individual assessment of risks and benefits
- Access to care issues
- Comprehension of treatment plans and of clinical trial principles
- Clear definition of treatment goals

In this chapter, we will review the information we already have related to the management of cancer and aging, the information we need to obtain, and how we can communicate this information to the patient. We assume that effective communication is essential to provide the most effective treatment and to conduct meaningful research.

What We Do Know

Aging involves progressive loss of the functional reserve of multiple organ systems, increased prevalence of chronic diseases (comorbidity), increased use of medication (polypharmacy), and the appearance of the so-called geriatric syndromes, conditions that are typical of, albeit not unique to, aging. Altogether, these changes conspire to reduce a person's life expectancy, susceptibility to stress, and ability of independent living [8]. Aging is universal, but it occurs at different rates in different individuals; thus it is poorly reflected in chronological age. At most chronological age is a landmark, beyond which an individual assessment of physiological age is advisable. That landmark is commonly placed at age 70.

The basic questions related to the treatment of the older cancer patient include the patient's life expectancy, tolerance of treatment, and the risk of long-term complications [8].

Several models based on a comprehensive geriatric assessment may be used to estimate a person's risk of mortality. As an example, the investigators of the San Francisco Veterans Hospital have been able to predict the mortality risk of individuals of different ages based on function and comorbidity [9, 10].

The geriatric assessment has also been used to predict therapeutic complications in older cancer patients [11]. The Preoperative Assessment of Cancer in the Elderly (PACE) estimates the surgical risk of individuals 70 and over, while the Chemotherapy Risk Assessment Score in High-Age Patients (CRASH) predicts the risk of acute hematological and nonhematological complications [12]. Both instruments are evolving with the inclusion of more variables and of more treatment conditions (such as multimodality treatment). At present, they provide an accurate estimate of the risk of treatment in individual patients.

Even in healthy elderly individuals, age is a risk factor for some acute complications of chemotherapy, including chemotherapy-induced myelosuppression, mucositis, and peripheral neuropathy [8]. The risk of neutropenia and neutropenic infections may be ameliorated with the prophylactic use of filgrastim and pegfilgrastim in patients receiving moderately toxic chemotherapy [13], and the risk of mucositis with the prophylactic use of keratinocyte growth factor (seldom used due to cost) [14] or of supersaturated solutions of calcium phosphate [15].

Long-term complications of cancer chemotherapy are known only in part. Age is a risk factor for anthracycline-induced acute myelogenous leukemia [16, 17] and congestive heart failure [18, 19]. It is debated whether age is a risk factor for "chemo brain" [20, 21].

What We Need to Know

Current information allows the practitioner to make evidence-based treatment-related decisions. This information still needs to be refined and updated.

Missing information. The PACE and the CRASH scores have demonstrated that a comprehensive geriatric assessment is useful to predict death risk and therapeutic complications. It is not clear, however, how many additional elements of the geriatric assessments should be included in these models. For example, studies conducted at our institution as well as by other investigators showed that polypharmacy is associated with an increased risk of chemotherapy-related toxicity [22]. In particular, the number of drugs a patient was assuming as well as the risk of adverse interactions among these drugs were associated with increased incidence of chemotherapy-related toxicity. These findings beg the question whether polypharmacy is an independent risk factor for the PACE or the CRASH scores. Other elements that may fine-tune these scores include anemia, serum albumin levels, concentration of inflammatory cytokines, leucocyte telomerase length, frailty index, and allostatic load [23–28]. The more insight we gain in the biology of aging, the more precise we can become in predicting mortality and therapeutic complications. Anemia has been associated with increased risk of chemotherapy-related toxicity in patients of all ages [29]. In the older person, it may reflect a condition of progressive functional decline and increased susceptibility to stress [29]. The prevalence of sarcopenia increases with age. This condition has been associated with a number of therapeutic complications [30]. Aging has been defined as a progressive inflammation, and the concentration of inflammatory cytokines in the circulation has been associated with reduced life expectancy, functional dependence, dementia, osteoporosis, and other geriatric syndromes [25]. In individuals of the same age, the length of leucocyte telomeres has been associated with reduced life expectancy and increased incidence of cancer and geriatric syndromes [23, 24]. Aging has also been defined as loss of homeostasis, and the degree of this loss is reflected in the so-called "allostatic load" that assesses the loss of self-regulation of a number of physiologic functions [27]. Frailty is an important construct in geriatrics. It indicates a critical reduction of functional reserve so that a minimal stress may precipitate functional dependence [28]. The relationship of frailty and cancer treatment is unknown.

In addition, the influence of social issues on survival and tolerance of treatment is unknown. Common sense suggests that a home caregiver is essential to the administration of effective treatment. A home caregiver should be able to take the patient to regular clinic visits and to the hospital in case of emergencies, to support the patient's emotional needs, and to assist the patient in daily activities. Thus, the education and support of the caregiver should be part of the treatment equation. In the case of other diseases, such as Alzheimer's disease and stroke, caregiving is associated with decreased life expectancy and serious medical and emotional complications [31].

As mentioned, some of the long-term complications of cytotoxic chemotherapy in the aged have been recognized. These include acute myeloid leukemia/ myelodysplasia and cardiac dysfunction [16–18]. Little is known about three other potential complications that may be devastating for older individuals: cognitive decline, functional dependence, and frailty. It is controversial whether cancer chemotherapy is associated with increased incidence of dementia [20, 21]. Of more interest, however, is whether cancer chemotherapy may lead to decreased cognition that impairs daily function even if it does not reach the level of impairment that one calls dementia.

Functional dependence is arguably the most destructive and costly complication of aging. It is reasonable to assume that strenuous medical treatment may accelerate the development of functional dependence, but this assumption is unproved as yet. The relationship of cancer and frailty is completely unknown. The main question is whether frailty may represent a long-term complication both of cancer and its treatment.

In addition to cure, prolongation of survival, and symptom relief, the main goal of cancer management in the elderly is prolongation of "active life expectancy." This is the period of time during which the patient is able to keep living independently. What interventions, if any, may help preserving functional independence during and after cancer treatment is unknown.

Clinical research in elderly cancer patients. It is clear that individuals 65 or 70 and older are recruitable in clinical studies, as demonstrated in the recent CRASH study [26], in the many trials exploring the need of growth factor support after chemotherapy in the elderly [32–36], and in a recent trial of adjuvant treatment of breast cancer in women 65 and older [37]. What is less clear is the design of clinical studies answering the questions that are specific to age.

Randomized clinical trials are essential to demonstrate that cancer treatment is beneficial irrespective of age. They have proved that women over 64 do benefit from adjuvant breast cancer therapy [37], that individuals over 69 benefit from adjuvant fluorouracil for colorectal cancer [38], and that filgrastin and pegfilgrastin reduce the risk of neutropenic infection in patients over 64 receiving chemotherapy [32–36]. However, randomized clinical trials are conducted with selected patients and cannot account for the diversity of the older population lest they accrue an unrealistically high number of individuals.

Pharmacological studies are also important to establish the effectiveness and safety of new medications in older individuals. With aging, there is a decline in glomerular filtration rate, liver mass, splanchnic circulation, and gastrointestinal absorption, in addition to a reduced functional reserve of virtually all organ systems, that need to be accounted for in the development of new drugs [10].

Only well-planned community-based prospective studies in which all the relevant information related to aging is collected (function, comorbidity, social support, laboratory parameters) may embrace the diversity of the older population and identify patient profiles for whom a determined type of treatment is indicated or contraindicated. Despite some logistic difficulties, the CRASH study showed that this type of investigation is feasible and may include community practitioners.

Communication

After a review of what we know, what we don't know, what we need to know, and how to get the information we need, we are able to discuss concretely how we can communicate with the older cancer patient. We will explore separately the message we should deliver and the communication techniques to deliver it.

The message. The centerpiece of the message is that cancer treatment may be beneficial irrespective of age [2–4, 10]. Dispelling ageism is essential to deliver effective cancer treatment to patients who are skeptical themselves, may be accompanied by skeptical family members, and may have been referred by skeptical practitioners. This optimistic message should be modulated according to the disease under consideration. It is imperative for older individuals to understand that chemotherapy may cure large-cell lymphoma and multimodality treatment may cure rectal cancer with sphincter preservation. Meanwhile, it should be emphasized that the treatment of acute myelogenous leukemia seldom leads to cure and might accelerate death [39], and that the benefits of adjuvant chemotherapy for most forms of breast cancer are marginal. The message also should be modulated to individual patient characteristics. For example, it is unreasonable to offer any form of adjuvant chemotherapy to patients with less than 5 years to live or to those whose comorbidity makes chemotherapy prohibitively toxic.

The balance of risk and benefit should be adjusted to the patient's personal values or desires. Meanwhile, it needs to be emphasized that we still don't know some critical information, such as the effects of cancer and cancer treatment on functional dependence, and that our models to predict life expectancy and tolerance of treatment are not watertight.

It is also essential to identify the patient's primary caregiver, to insist on the designation of a primary caregiver, and to instruct both patient and caregiver of the potential problems arising during treatment, including the risk of neutropenic infections and other emergencies that may require immediate medical attention and substantial investment of the caregiver's time. It may be helpful to explore proactively with the caregiver coping techniques that may sooth the emotional burden of caregiving [31, 40]. These may include respite time, as well as instructions about the management of common problems that may occur.

Last, but not least, it is important to emphasize the need of clinical research to obtain the information necessary to provide safer and more effective treatment, encourage patients to enroll in open trials, and allow practitioners to include personal information in a large database of older individuals, from which prognostic and predictive variables may eventually be derived.

The delivery of the message. Some general principles may help in delivering this complex, multifaceted message.

The most important principle is to respect the patient's autonomy, an endowed characteristic that cannot be diminished by disease or by any form of cognitive impairment. In the name of this autonomy, the patient must feel to be the center of attention and under no circumstances should feel neglected. This is important even when the patient's comprehension is clearly compromised by cognitive decline or hearing or visual impairment [41]. As tactile sensations are the best preserved with aging [41], hand-holding is a very effective way to make the patient feel included in any discussion occurring in his/her presence. Frequent smiles and eye contact also go a long way in fostering this feeling. One should make every effort to avoid overlooking the patient and communicating exclusively with the caregiver and other family members. Even individuals who have been described as severely demented maintain some ability to make decisions about their management, and this autonomy should be respected. Nobody is so demented that he/she cannot decide whether to have meat or fish for dinner!

Respect for the patient's autonomy also requires that the practitioner get to know the patient, including his/her personal values or desires. On the initial visit, after greeting the patient, I thank him/her for trusting his/her life to me, and I make sure that no factors, such as my Italian accent or the patient's poor hearing, interfere with our communication. I also try to acknowledge the patient's profession: I will refer to the patient as doctor if he/she holds a doctoral degree, as reverend if he/she is a minister, or with his/her rank if he/she is a retired military person. In addition to underlining respect for the patient's autonomy, this approach allows me to get the patient's confidence, to identify potential home caregivers, and to recognize the patient's values, including what he/she expects from the treatment. For some individuals, the prolongation of life is paramount, especially if they have some landmark to meet, such as a birth, wedding, graduation, or anniversary. For others, the most important thing is to remain independent to the end. For most, the goals of treatment become defined during a number of conversations with the practitioner.

Many older individuals nowadays are highly sophisticated and know how to navigate the Internet and ask proper questions. Yet some medical concepts, such as adjuvant chemotherapy, prolongation of survival in the absence of a cure, and mainly treatment choice and clinical trials, may be novel for them. It is important then to take all the time necessary to explain that the role of the practitioner is to help explore all treatment alternatives, but eventually the treatment decisions need to be negotiated with the patients; that virtually most forms of treatment are gambles, with the odds stacked in favor of the patients.

While the design of modern clinical trials may be difficult for the noninitiated to understand, it is important not to underestimate the ability of older individuals to comprehend the rationale of clinical research. A number of studies have demonstrated that individuals 65 and older were as willing as younger ones to participate in clinical trials, if they were offered to them [42].

Finally, while compassion is always paramount, it is important to present a realistic picture of the potential outcomes. In addition to showing respect for the patient's autonomy, this approach will gain and maintain the patient's confidence.

Conclusions

Effective communication is the key to effective treatment. Practitioners discussing cancer treatment as well as cancer research with older individuals need first of all to be convinced that cancer treatment may be worthwhile. Second, they need to be familiar with the assessment of physiological age so that the treatment can be modulated according to the patient's individual characteristics and desires. Third, the home caregiver should be included and empowered in any communication, as he or she is an integral part of the treatment team.

Any discussion should recognize and preserve the patient's autonomy, even when the cognitive capacities are reduced. Use of touch and other nonverbal forms of communication may be particularly effective in patients with cognitive or sensorial impairments.

References

1. Balducci L, Ershler WB. Cancer and ageing: a nexus at several levels. Nat Rev Cancer. 2005;5:655–62.
2. Lee KW, Kim DY, Yun T, et al. Doxorubicin-based chemotherapy for diffuse large B-cell lymphoma in elderly patients: comparison of treatment outcomes between young and elderly patients and the significance of doxorubicin dosage. Cancer. 2003;98(12):2651–6.
3. Coiffier B, Lepage E, Briere J, et al. CHOP chemotherapy plus rituximab compared with CHOP alone in elderly patients with diffuse large-B-cell lymphoma. N Engl J Med. 2002;346(4):235–42.
4. Pfreundschuh M. How I treat elderly patients with diffuse large cell B cell lymphoma. Blood. 2010;116(24):5103–10.

5. Talarico L, Chen G, Pazdur R. Enrollment of elderly patients in clinical trials for cancer drug registration: a 7-year experience by the US Food and Drug Administration. J Clin Oncol. 2004;22:4626–31.
6. Unger JM, Coltman Jr CA, Crowley JJ, et al. Impact of the year 2000 Medicare policy change on older patient enrollment to cancer clinical trials. J Clin Oncol. 2006;24(1):141–4.
7. Lewis JH, Kilgore ML, Goldman DP, et al. Participation of patients 65 year of age and older in cancer clinical trials. J Clin Oncol. 2003;21(7):1383–9.
8. Balducci L, Colloca G, Cesari M, et al. Assessment and treatment of elderly patients with cancer. Surg Oncol. 2010;19(3):117–23.
9. Lee SJ, Lindquist K, Segal MR, et al. Development and validation of a prognostic index for 4-year mortality in older adults. JAMA. 2006;295(7):801–8.
10. Carey EC, Covinsky KE, Lui LY, et al. Prediction of mortality in community-living frail elderly people with long-term care needs. J Am Geriatr Soc. 2008;56(1):68–75.
11. Pope D, Ramesh H, Gennari R, et al. Preoperative assessment of cancer in the elderly (PACE): a comprehensive assessment of underlying characteristics of elderly cancer patients prior to elective surgery. Surg Oncol. 2006;15(4):189–97.
12. Extermann M, Boler I, Reich R, et al. The CRASH score (chemotherapy risk assessment scale for high-age patients): design and validation. Am Soc Clin Oncol Proc. 2010:Abstract 9000.
13. Smith TJ, Katcheressian J, Lyman GH, et al. 2006 update of recommendations for the use of white blood cell growth factors: an evidence-based clinical practice guideline. J Clin Oncol. 2006;2006(24):3187–205.
14. Rosen LS, Abdi E, Davis ID, et al. Palifermin reduces the incidence of oral mucositis in patients with metastatic colorectal cancer treated with fluorouracil-based chemotherapy. J Clin Oncol. 2006;24(33):5194–200.
15. Sonis ST. Pathobiology of oral mucositis: novel insights and opportunities. J Support Oncol. 2007;5(9 Suppl 4):3–11.
16. Lyman GH, Dale DC, Wolff DA, et al. Acute myeloid leukemia or myelodysplastic syndrome in randomized controlled clinical trials of cancer chemotherapy with granulocyte colony-stimulating factor: a systematic review. J Clin Oncol. 2010;28(17):2914–24.
17. Gruschkus SK, Lairson D, Dunn JK, et al. Use of white blood cell growth factors and risk of acute myeloid leukemia or myelodysplastic syndrome among elderly patients with non-Hodgkin lymphoma. Cancer. 2010;116(22):5279–89.
18. Pinder M, Duan Z, Goodwin JS, et al. Congestive heart failure in older women treated with adjuvant anthracycline chemotherapy for breast cancer. J Clin Oncol. 2007;25(25):3808–15.
19. Herhman DL, McBride RB, Eisenberger R, et al. Doxorubicin, cardiac risk factors and cardiac toxicity in elderly patients with diffuse B cell non Hodgkin's lymphoma. J Clin Oncol. 2008;26: 3159–65.
20. Heck JE, Albert SM, Franco R, Gorin SS. Pattern of dementia diagnosis in surveillance, epidemiology and end results breast cancer survivors who use chemotherapy. J Am Geriatr Soc. 2008;56(9):1687–92.
21. Baxter NN, Durham SB, Phillips KA, et al. Risk of dementia in older breast cancer survivors: a population-based cohort study of the association with adjuvant chemotherapy. J Am Geriatr Soc. 2009;57(3):403–11.
22. Extermann M, Popa MA, Druta M, Wallace K, Brunello A, Balducci L. Drug interactions assessed with drug interaction facts are associated with increased risk of chemotoxicity in older cancer patients receiving chemotherapy. In: The 100th Annual Meeting of the American Association for Cancer Research, Denver, CO, April 2009, Abstract 5450.
23. Willeit P, Willeit J, Mayr A, et al. Telomere length and risk of incident cancer and cancer mortality. JAMA. 2010;304(1):69–75.
24. Houben JM, Giltay EJ, Rius-Ottenheim N, et al. Telomere length and mortality in elderly men: the Zutphen elderly study. J Gerontol A Biol Sci Med Sci. 2010;66(1):38–44.
25. Ferrucci L, Corsi A, Lauretani F, Bandinelli S, Bartali B, Taub DD, et al. The origin of Age-related pro-inflammatory state. Blood. 2005;105:2294–9.

26. Maggio M, Guralnik JM, Longo DL, Ferrucci L. Interleukin-6 in aging and chronic disease: a magnificent pathway. J Gerontol A Biol Sci Med Sci. 2006;61(6):575–84.
27. Yang Y, Kozloski M. Sex differences in age trajectories of physiological dysregulation: inflammation, metabolic syndrome, and allostatic load. J Gerontol A Biol Sci Med Sci. 2011;66(5):493–500.
28. Walston J, Hadley EC, Ferrucci L, et al. Research agenda for frailty in older adults: toward a better understanding of physiology and etiology: summary from the American Geriatrics Society/National Institute on Aging Research Conference on Frailty in Older Adults. J Am Geriatr Soc. 2006;54(6):991–1001.
29. Ferrucci L, Balducci L. Anemia of aging: the role of chronic inflammation and cancer. Semin Hematol. 2008;45:242–9.
30. Glass D, Roubenoff R. Recent advances in the biology and therapy of muscle wasting. Ann NY Acad Sci. 2010;1211:25–36.
31. Belle SH, Burgio L, Burns R, et al. Resources for Enhancing Alzheimer's Caregiver Health (REACH) II Investigators. Enhancing the quality of life of dementia caregivers from different ethnic or racial groups: a randomized, controlled trial. Ann Intern Med. 2006;145(10):727–38.
32. Zinzani PG, Storti S, Zaccaria A, et al. Elderly aggressive histology non-Hodgkin's lymphoma: first line VNCOP-B regimen: experience on 350 patients. Blood. 1999;94:33–8.
33. Sonneveld P, de Ridder M, van der Lelie H, et al. Comparison of doxorubicin and mitoxantrone in the treatment of elderly patients with advanced diffuse non-Hodgkin's lymphoma using CHOP vs CNOP chemotherapy. J Clin Oncol. 1995;13:2530–9.
34. Osby E, Hagberg H, Kvaloy S, et al. CHOP is superior to CNOP in elderly patients with aggressive lymphoma while outcome is unaffected by filgrastim treatment: results of a Nordic Lymphoma Group randomized trial. Blood. 2003;101:3840–8.
35. Doorduijn JK, van derr Holt B, van der Hem KG, et al. Randomized trials of granulocyte-colony stimulating factor (G-CSF) added to CHOP in elderly patients with aggressive non-Hodgkin's lymphoma. Blood. 2000;96(11):133a.
36. Balducci L, Al-Halawani H, Charu V, et al. Elderly patients receiving chemotherapy benefit from first cycle pegfilgrastim. Oncologist. 2007;12(12):1416–24.
37. Muss HB, Berry DA, Cirrincione CT, et al. Adjuvant chemotherapy in older women with early stage breast cancer. N Engl J Med. 2009;360:2055–65.
38. Sargent DJ, Goldberg RM, Jacobson SC, et al. A polled analysis of resected colon cancer in elderly patients. N Engl J Med. 2001;345:1091–7.
39. Dombret H, Raffoux E, Gardin C. New Insights in the management of elderly patients with acute myeloid leukemia. Curr Opin Oncol. 2009;21(6):589–93.
40. Haley WE. Family caregivers of elderly patients with cancer. Understanding and minimizing the burden of care. J Support Oncol. 2003;1(4 Suppl 2):25–9.
41. McGilton KS, Boscart V, Fox M, et al. A systematic review of the effectiveness of communication interventions for health care providers caring for patients in residential care settings. Worldviews Evid Based Nurs. 2009;6(3):149–59.
42. Kemeny MM, Peterson BL, Komblith AB, et al. Barriers to clinical trials participation of older women with breast cancer. J Clin Oncol. 2003;21:2268–75.

Chapter 15
"I Never Died Before...": End-of-Life Communication with Elderly Cancer Patients

Stein B. Husebø and Bettina S. Husebø

Abstract The frail elderly are more vulnerable than others. They will increasingly develop chronic or incurable diseases followed by physical and psychosocial limitations. Old age is often connected with cognitive failure and pain. There is a high need for resources, competence, teaching, and research focusing on long-term and palliative care for these individuals. A large violation of human dignity is that the frail elderly in their last month and days are left alone dying, that communication on, and relief of, the developing suffering is ignored. The greatest violation of human dignity we can imagine is that dying patients are transferred between home, hospitals, or nursing institutions shortly before death. They often die in transport or shortly after arrival. The highlight of life is ignored: that a unique human being is dying. Planning communication and palliative care can provide the needed safety and quality of care for cancer patients and the frail elderly in their last months of life. This advanced planning will also enable more patients to die at home or in nursing facilities, preventing unnecessary emergency transferals of the dying to hospitals. How a person dies remains in the memory of his or her family: disturbing, hindering, and destroying the process of grief, or relieving it, as a highlight of dignity and caring farewell.

Keywords Cancer • Dementia • Communication • Dying • End-of-life care • Frailty • Old age • Ethics • Palliative care • Dignity

---

S.B. Husebø, MD (✉)
Dignity Centre, Red Cross Nursing Home,
Ellerhusensvei 35, 5035 Bergen, Norway
e-mail: sthusebo@c2i.net

B.S. Husebø
Department of Public Health and Primary Health Care,
University of Bergen, 5035 Bergen, Norway
e-mail: Bettina.husebo@isf.uib.no

Oddvar: The Other Side

A phone rang late one Sunday evening. The nurse on the phone said, "Oddvar's wife is here. She says he must have pneumonia." Oddvar was 84 years old. He had been in the nursing home for the last 3 years. He suffered from prostatic cancer, pain, and dementia, with increasing cognitive failure. The last 2 months he was bedridden, in the end stage of dementia. Communication was no longer possible. His wife still saw him every day and cared marvelously for him.

In our nursing home, our physicians are on call 24 h a day. I drove to the nursing home and examined Oddvar. Then we sat down in the ward room: his wife, the nurse, and I. His wife looked at me and said, "He has pneumonia, right?" "Yes," I replied. "You are a good doctor." "Then we should give him penicillin, Doctor Husebø, shouldn't we?" "To give penicillin is one side…" I replied. "I have an important question for you. You know Oddvar better than anyone else. What would he have wanted in this situation?" After some seconds she replied: "He was a very proud man… He would have wanted to be dead years ago."

"That is the other side," I said. "But doesn't it mean a lot of suffering to die from pneumonia?" "Earlier we said pneumonia is the friend of old people," I answered. "And we can relieve his suffering sufficiently if problems develop." "Doctor Husebø, then we should not give him penicillin. But you must know, I love him very deeply."

Oddvar received palliative care and not penicillin. He died peaceful 4 days later, with his wife at his side.

My question, "What would he have wanted?" means "What is the presumed consent?" Oddvar's wife openly stated that he would have seen death as a relief. On the other side she loves him and is not quite ready to let him go. To ask her, "What do *you* want us to do?" probably would lead to therapeutic intervention and penicillin. He might have lived longer, for some more days or weeks.

Nina: "I Never Died Before"

Three weeks earlier, Nina, 67 years old, was referred from hospital to the palliative care ward in our nursing home. Her breast cancer had been diagnosed 6 years ago. Now she had extended skeletal and brain metastases and was receiving maximal doses of cortisone to relieve the symptoms of high brain pressure. During the last years Nina had gone through a vast list of therapy interventions, including radiation, surgery, hormones, and several chemotherapies. She received chemotherapy in hospital until the day of admission to our nursing home.

Following her recent medical condition and the rapid development of complications, Nina's prognosis was poor. According to our experience, she would become unconscious in the following weeks, probably days, and would die within a month.

That is my knowledge and understanding. What about hers?

15 "I Never Died Before…": End-of-Life Communication with Elderly Cancer Patients

Nina was a special person. She cheered and cared for all, her family, the nursing staff, her physician. Despite rapid deterioration of her condition, she kept on fighting for survival time. Her and her family's behavior remained exclusively optimistic. They never addressed the end of life coming close.

Should I tell her? What should I tell her?

I was convinced she knew she was dying. She also knew that the time left runs out. As Leo Tolstoy wrote in his outstanding novel *The Death of Ivan Ilych* 130 years ago [1], Ivan and Nina, and almost all dying persons, have reflections, phantasies, and fears about dying and death. They increasingly experience loneliness and isolation as a burden if they are left alone with their concerns.

My task in these situations is not to tell, but to listen: to sit down with open ears and heart [2]. To give her the signal that I am ready when she is. That she can share whatever she needs to share. That she can ask whatever she has in her mind, also regarding what there is of "unfinished business."

I sat down and listened. She listened to my silence. Then she looked at me and said, "Well, Dr. Husebø, we both know, don't we? Soon I will be dead. Nobody talks about it. We are all brave and optimistic. In hospital, the physicians totally avoided the question of death and dying. But it is there, all the time, in my head. I am not afraid of death. When I am dead, I will be relieved. But, I am afraid of dying…"

Then, with a brave smile in her face: "I never died before. How is it going to be? Can you help me to be prepared? Will I suffer?"

We openly discussed her situation, present and future challenges, also the limited time left. I explained that probably in the next weeks due to her brain metastasis she would become unconscious, despite maximal dosage of cortisone. "If we then prolong the cortisone, we prolong the time of the dying process," I said. "If we stop cortisone then, you will die within the next days…." "Please, Doctor Husebø, when I become unconscious, stop the cortisone and let me die in peace," she said.

"There is another obstacle, Doctor Husebø. You have met my daughters and the three grandchildren. As I said, I am ready to go. But my feeling is that they are not. Behind our optimistic approach and behavior there is a wall, a lot of grief, and fear of addressing it. Could you help us, to find a way, to open the door?"

"Interesting," I thought. Shortly after Nina arrived in the nursing home, one of her daughters phoned me and said, "Our mother is a marvelous person. She always fought her illness with rare courage and optimism. Please don't destroy her hope by frank truth. Leave her innocent. Let her die happily as she is…"

Two days after my conversation with Nina we all met in her room: the two daughters, the sons-in-law, the grandchildren, a nurse, and I.

"I have asked Doctor Husebø to join us, allowing us to talk openly about my illness and future," Nina opened.

Surprisingly, further communication was interrupted by the youngest participant, her 5-year-old granddaughter. She jumped into Nina's bed and asked, "Grandmother, will you soon be dead?"

In the following minutes we witnessed a conversation between the dying grandmother and her grandchild that none of us will forget, because of the innocent attitude, questions, and openness of the child. We shared concerns, hope, grief, tears, and laughter. They all knew that Nina's death was coming closer. But locked doors prevented them from talking together. The locked doors were opened by a 5-year-old child. The door remained open until Nina peacefully died with the family present 3 weeks later.

Liv: "Thank You for Your Openness. I Will Go Home and Die Where I Have Lived"

As the responsible anesthetist, I met Liv, 74 years old, for preoperative preparation. Eight months before, she had been operated on for colon cancer. She developed multiple bowel metastases. Now she had fistula from the bowels, followed by thin feces delivery from the vagina and urinary tract. Surgery was planned for the next day.

Her general condition was extremely poor. I rapidly developed doubt for the success of this intervention and found the surgeon responsible for the operation.

"Will she survive the operation?" I asked. "Well," he answered, "she will die soon, but my hope is that we can provide some relief… We have no choice." "And postoperative complications?" "You are the intensive care specialist," he answered. "What do you think?" "She probably will develop postoperative infections and die on a respirator," I responded. "But we have no choice," he said. Then we discussed the interesting question: Who has choice?

Together we went to Liv, sat down, and discussed her situation, as openly as we had discussed it together. She listened. Then she asked some questions, before saying, "You tell me that I have a choice between an operation followed by high risk of complications, or going home. Regardless how I choose, I will die in the following weeks, perhaps a month or two. Did I get you right?" "Yes." "Thank you for your openness," she said. "I will go home and die where I have lived."

Maria: "You Killed My Wife"

Maria, age 79 fell at home and fractured her right hip. She was admitted to the hospital for orthopedic surgery. After 5 days in the hospital she was referred for rehabilitation. Three weeks later, with poor benefit of rehabilitation, she was transferred to our nursing home as a long-term patient.

Her general condition at admission was extremely poor: weight 44 kg, hardly any food and fluid intake. Mobilization from bed was not possible. Communication was only fragmentary, due to severe cognitive failure.

In the previous 3 years she had been admitted to hospital five times, seeing nine different specialists. The result from these referrals was seven diagnoses. By the time of referral to our nursing home she had received 13 drugs. Among the diagnoses were Parkinson's disease, cervical cancer, heart failure, and dementia. Consistent from all the specialists was the diagnosis of dementia. Her dementia was never properly focused on or assessed and was poorly communicated to her family.

The caregiving staff experienced Maria's husband as difficult and demanding. He hardly ever came to see her. He accused us, saying that we were killing his wife. He threatened us with lawyers and the police.

Four weeks after her admission, she rapidly developed severe heart failure. The situation worsened. Despite maximal therapeutic efforts, including intravenous penicillin due to pneumonia, she fell unconscious.

At a meeting with her husband and son the next day, the husband demanded that we restore Maria's health and weight to the situation before she fell. He also demanded transfer to the hospital. He totally ignored our statement that severe dementia was the main problem, and that Maria was close to death. His threats of lawyer and police were dominant.

After passionate, but totally fruitless, searching for bridges of communication, we again concluded that there was no indication for hospital admission. During the next 2 days Maria's health further deteriorated. All death-prolonging interventions were stopped. The focus was changed towards optimal palliative care. Two days later she died peacefully in the nursing home. The family was not present.

Four days later her husband accused us to the police of being responsible for Maria's death: we had killed his wife.

Communication with Elderly Patients at End of Life

Oddvar, Maria, Liv, and Nina represent some of the central communication and ethical challenges in end-of-life care of the frail elderly [3]. These patients suffered from a variety of chronic and incurable diseases. Cancer, pain, and dementia are common. Many need care day and night. Due to advancing cognitive failure they often loose the ability to understand their choices or to make competent decisions [4].

With high levels of precision we knew that Oddvar, Maria, Liv, and Nina would die within the next days or weeks. Most doctors, with their clinical experience, competence, and attitude, have the background to know when the time left becomes limited to days, weeks, or months. When we know, our focus should be on preparatory communication with patient, family, and staff, also on planning optimal palliative care (http://advancecareplanning.org.uk).

In Liv and Nina's situations informed consent was the central challenge for communication and ethics [5]. Informed consent is first of all based on information. Without open information, informed consent cannot be established [4]. All of us have difficulty in the dark finding the road home. When the map and the information provided are misleading and we don't know our position, we are lost.

In Liv's situation we could ask: Why is she going to the hospital? Why is she accepting surgery? The answer is clear: she is brave. She has a family who needs here. She fights for survival as long as it and quality of life are within reach. She knows that the end of her life is coming closer. When the surgeon suggests an operation, she accepts, trusting his advice, expecting gain of time and quality of life. When we openly discuss costs, side effects, and benefits of interventions compared with no interventions, this gives her the needed information and strength to choose to go home and die there, cared for by her family. Without this openness, informed consent would not have been established [6, 7].

Nina also knows. But she needs someone she trusts to support her in talking about her "unfinished business," allowing her and her family to say farewell before it is too late.

Oddvar and Maria represent more challenging patients. For them informed consent is out of reach. Presumed consent and advanced directive become the central targets for communication and ethics.

Oddvar's wife was prepared. She had over years seen and experienced the development of Oddvar's dementia. She knew and trusted the caregiving staff and nursing home physician and vice versa. There had been several open, preparatory meetings, discussing the challenges for Oddvar and his relatives in the present and future. She loved him. She cared for him. It was difficult for her to let him go. But with support she accepted this as the best solution. That evening we easily reached a consensus, also regarding Oddvar's presumed consent.

Maria's husband was not prepared. Several hospital admissions and specialist assessments kept the focus on a large variety of diagnoses and therapeutic interventions. The multiple options that were offered established expectations in him: "There is a solution somewhere, a radical therapy withheld or yet not discovered, that will cure my wife, bring her back to good health for more good years together."

The healthcare system did not establish the needed preparatory communication. A variety of therapy options were provided. Focus and communication on the central challenges were absent.

In Maria's situation, despite efforts and competence, we did not succeed. It was not possible to establish the needed trust and consensus in the short time left before Maria died. The husband denied. He fought, not accepting her death. He kept on fighting after her death. It is understandable that he needed enemies. We became his favorite targets. The name of this denial and fight is *grief*. Grief is the strongest expression of love. Denial can develop into a severe burden upon the grieving process.

The husband and we strongly disagreed on the basic ethical questions. For Maria's husband lack of appropriate medical assessment and interventions was the problem. He fought for the unrealistic goal of rehabilitation, to restore her health to what it was years ago. For us, as the caregiving team, the key problem was irreversible—severe dementia, followed by rapidly developing life-threatening complications.

Although it was difficult and challenging, we decided to protect Maria's dignity. We took charge and responsibility, refused to admit her to the hospital, and focused on palliative care. The autopsy of Maria showed severe Alzheimer disease, without doubt the central reason for her health problems and deterioration over the last years. The legal authorities supported our judgments.

In most developed countries, Maria would have been admitted to the hospital in the last days before death. In a majority of hospitals artificial nutrition, PEG-tube, pharmacological and technical measures would have been provided until she finally died. In many countries a lawyer or the court would intervene for life-prolonging measures. Through these interventions she might have lived some more days, but at what costs, with what life, of what quality, with what dignity?

The Life Perspective

Some of us are born into privileged societies. For many the life project is strongly limited, often to the question of food, housing, and daily life survival. In most developed countries, we face a growing tendency toward the more or less realistic expectation: society will take care of us when we get old and dependent upon others for care.

In Norway, the number of persons over the age of 67 will double by 2050, and those over 80 years old will increase by more than 100% by 2050 [8]. Every year, 44,000 inhabitants die, 40% in hospitals and 40% in nursing homes (NHs) (http://www.ssb.no). Seventy thousand people in Norway have dementia, 34,000 of whom live in a NH, with about 14 months' mean length of stay before death [9]. Almost 80% of the dying NH patients have diagnoses of dementia and heart failure, and 14–27% have cancer [4]. They have complex mental health problems, such as agitation and aggression, disabilities and social needs, compounded by widespread prescription of potentially harmful psychotropic drugs [10].

In our older years we are more or less healthy and develop more or less dependency on others. Most of us develop incurable diseases: cancer, heart failure, stroke, dementia, or cognitive failure. Few of us die healthy, "with our boots on." The majority of us will in the last weeks, months, or years before we die need care day and night.

What makes the challenges for good communication and ethics in caring for the frail elderly so special?

The frail elderly are more vulnerable than others. They increasingly develop chronic or incurable diseases followed by physical and psychosocial disabilities. Old age is often connected with cognitive failure. Their frailty and illnesses make them dependent on care and the healthcare system. The healthcare system focuses more on old people's diseases than on long-term care, quality of life, and dignity in their final years and days. The dying elderly are admitted to hospitals and kept alive with lack of respect for informed or presumed consent. There is a high need of resources, competence, teaching, and research focusing on long-term and palliative care for the frail elderly. Dying and death for the frail elderly rapidly comes closer every day. For the dying frail elderly, death can mean relief and no longer represents the final enemy to fight.

All of us contribute to this situation, in daily life, in society, and in our families: frailty, dependency, dying, and death continue to be denied, poorly communicated, and hidden.

The reality for the frail and dying elderly, soon to be ourselves, is often cruel. Societies are overwhelmed by the costs of long-term care [11]. Instead, the healthcare systems have well-established strategies for economic gain, offering and carrying out therapy with poor or no benefit to health for the frail elderly.

The key question in ethics is: *What is a good life*? When caring for frail elderly patients, a second question arises: *What is a good decision to enable and support a good life for our patient*?

Following these two basic ethical questions a variety of new central questions arises, such as: *Has the patient received and understood appropriate information regarding his or her health, options for medical or caring interventions? Also regarding benefits, costs, side effects, and consequences of these interventions? Are we withholding and hiding necessary information? Why? Is it in some end-of-life situations ethically acceptable not to tell the patient the truth? Is it morally acceptable to give information to the relatives while excluding the patient?*

The Roles of the Key Persons

The frail elderly patient is the key person. To support and give strength to his or her maximal autonomy and dignity must be the central goal for communication and ethics. That means that communication about the condition, situation, options for therapy and care, and prognosis for the patient should never take place without the patient present.

There are a few, but important, exceptions to this basic rule, such as: patients with severe dementia and cognitive impairment, the unconscious or psychotic patient, and the dying patient in his or her final days and hours. On the average 60% of dying patients will be unconscious at the end of their life [12, 13].

What is important is not only the information *to* the patient, but, even more, the information *from* the patient, such as: *What information was received previously?* (Patients will not tell what the information was, but what they understood it to be.) *What are the patient's expectations and goals? What is the patient's life project? Who are the important relatives and caregivers?*

Elderly patients live in or are connected to a family system, where spouse, children, and other relatives have more or less close roles for the care and important decision-making [14]. From the beginning, with the patient present, important relatives should be invited to and included in the communication process, also contributing with information, communication, and questions of importance for the patient's and family's well-being.

The caregiving staff, in home care and institutions—nurses, assistant nurses, physical therapists, occupational therapists, and others—often have a major, but underappreciated, role [15]. Often they care for frail elderly patients over a long period. Often they have unique information, observations, competence, and experience regarding the patient and his or her situation. They know the actual large and small questions to be faced. They often can, better than anyone else, review the physical, psychosocial, and spiritual challenges and the patient's life project. Often they realize that the patient is dying long before the physician does. They should be included and participate in all communication processes and decision-makings regarding frail elderly patients [16].

Frail elderly patients need proper medical and interdisciplinary assessment. On the average each patient in our nursing homes has seven chronic and/or severe diseases [17]. On the average, each nursing home patient daily receives up to 13 different drugs [18–20]. Together with the focus on care and psychosocial integration, strategic communication, and ethical challenges, we must establish a map of the patient's health and illnesses, of good and recommended medical interventions, restoring or contributing to health [21]. The physician must also make up his or her mind what interventions or treatments should *not* be recommended, especially when the expected outcome is poor and the expected negative side effects are dominant.

The care of frail elderly patients with multiple diseases and dying elderly patients can be burdensome. Some physicians' strategies towards these patients may be to avoid them, to overlook that they are dying, to withhold important information, to support unrealistic hopes, to offer meaningless interventions, or to unnecessarily admit them to hospitals [22].

The good physician is a caring, humble, skilled, and compassionate communication partner and advisor, who also addresses the patient's impending death. The good physician will openly bargain with patients, supporting them to find their optimal solution.

Truth hurts. But deceit hurts more. To focus solely on hope of survival will leave the patient without hope when survival is out of reach [23].

As Victor Frankl has written, to know establishes power and hope; not to know is followed by hopelessness and powerlessness [24].

From his years in prison Vaclav Havel wrote: "Hope is not optimism, not the expectation that everything will end well, but the expectation that something will give meaning, regardless of how it ends" [25].

Communication: Patients with Cognitive Failure

As in the situation of Oddvar and Maria, a large number of frail elderly persons lack the ability to understand and choose, especially the rapid increasing number of patients with dementia and cognitive failure. How do we communicate and choose with them? And in these situations what are the basic principles respecting their dignity?

Some patients with severe cognitive failure still have their autonomy. But their autonomy now becomes increasingly vulnerable and dependent on proxies, which can create strain. The main characteristic of these proxies is that they are close relatives or caregivers. Their knowledge and closeness to the patients can support us with vital information like: *What is the life story and life project of the patient? What were the central values? Are there formal or informal advanced end-of-life directives? What is the presumed consent?*

With severe cognitive failure autonomy is severely reduced. There still will be many small or large autonomy challenges, like: *Get out of bed? Shower or bath? Tooth brush? Company? Physical and psychosocial activity? A walk? Wheelchair? What to eat, and when? When go back to bed? What kind of music do I like? Can I sing? Can I care for someone or something, like a neighbor patient, a pet, or a flower?*

Also, large and basic ethical questions develop: *Home, nursing home, or hospital? Drugs: benefit or side effects?* There will be challenging problems due to cognitive failure and behavioral disturbances: *Locked doors, sedation, or skilled environment therapy? Access to competent caring staff and doctors? Artificial nutrition? Prolonging of the death process? Pain assessment and symptom relief? Establish palliative care?*

Communication now grows more complicated. The proxies are needed partners in the discussion of ethical questions. They should speak for the patient, and protect the patient's autonomy and dignity. Additionally, proxies must contribute to skilled assessment and relief of pain and other symptoms [26]. Although elderly persons tend to have more painful diseases, they have been found to report less pain. They receive fewer analgesic drugs than their younger counterparts. With impaired cognition, patients' ability to report pain and other symptoms decreases, leading to the interpretation by staff members that elderly persons with dementia have less pain than mentally healthy controls [27]. Thus, when elderly adults in pain also have severe dementia and reduced communicative abilities, they are at high risk to develop behavioral disturbances like agitation and aggression [28]. Recently, it was demonstrated that individual pain treatment reduced agitation in nursing home patients with moderate and severe dementia.

Preparatory, inclusive communication provides the solution. The patient (if possible), close relatives, a representative of the caregiving staff, and the doctor meet several times. Challenges now and until the patient dies are reviewed and discussed. A consensus, a preparatory palliative plan for action is established.

How the physicians and caregiving staff play their roles as communicators can enable or prevent a good communication process. Improvement is needed in the competence and attitude in ethics, communication, and palliative care for the frail elderly, also in teaching and research. Long-term care usually means low budget, low status, lack of adequate competence, and severe discrimination against the frail and dying elderly.

The Dying Frail Elderly: The Palliative Plan

The largest violation of human dignity is that frail elderly people in their last hours and days are left alone with their dying, that communication on, and relief of, the developing suffering is ignored.

The greatest violation of human dignity we can imagine is that dying patients are transferred between home, hospitals, or nursing institutions shortly before death. They often die in transport or shortly after admission. The highlight of life is ignored, that a unique human being is dying.

Preparatory communication, skilled assessment of pain and other symptoms, and planning can provide the needed safety and quality of care for cancer patients and the frail elderly in their last months of life. Advanced planning will also enable more patients to die at home or in nursing facilities, preventing unnecessary emergency transfers of the dying to hospitals [29].

The plan must provide the needed information regarding communication and ethics, and also a concrete plan for palliative symptom control of expected developing symptoms, such as pain, dyspnea, nausea, death rattle, delirium, anxiety, agitation, or panic [17]. The potentially needed drugs should be available at the bed site. The professional carers must have competence and support for using them when appropriate.

A cell phone number for contact with the responsible physician in emergencies will provide the needed security for patient, family, and professional caregivers. The plan should be signed by the responsible physician and nurse, and a copy left at the bedside in case unexpected complications develop.

How a person dies remains in the memory of his or her family—disturbing, hindering, and destroying the process of grief; or relieving it, as a highlight of dignity and a caring farewell.

References

1. Tolstoy L. The death of Ivan Ilych. Melville House, NY, 2008. ISBN 9781933633541.
2. Doust J, Del Mar C. Why do doctors use treatments that do not work? For many reasons—including their inability to stand idle and do nothing. BMJ. 2004;328(7438):474–5.
3. Husebo BS, Husebo SB, Hysing Dahl B. Old and given up for dying? Palliative care units in nursing homes. Illn Crisis Loss. 2004;12(1):75–89.
4. Detering KM, Hancock AD, Reade MC, et al. The impact of advance care planning on end of life care in elderly patients: randomised controlled trial. BMJ. 2010;340:c1345.
5. Nishimura A, Mueller PS, Evenson LK, et al. Patients who complete advance directives and what they prefer. Mayo Clin Proc. 2007;82(12):1480–6.
6. Young AJ, Rodriguez KL. The role of narrative in discussing end-of-life care: eliciting values and goals from text, context, and subtext. Health Commun. 2006;19(1):49–59.
7. Rodriguez KL, Young AJ. Perceptions of patients on the utility or futility of end-of-life treatment. J Med Ethics. 2006;32(8):444–9.
8. Engedal K, Haugen PK. Demens. 4th ed. Tønsberg: Aldring og Helse; 2006.
9. Sintef Unimed. Pasientkartlegging ved Bergen Røde Kors Sykehjem. Oslo: Sintef Unimed, 2003; STF78A034507.
10. Selbaek G, Kirkevold O, Engedal K. The prevalence of psychiatric symptoms and behavioural disturbances and the use of psychotropic drugs in Norwegian nursing homes. Int J Geriatr Psychiatry. 2007;22(9):843–9.
11. Batavia AI. Disability versus futility in rationing health care services: defining medical futility based on permanent unconsciousness—PVS coma, and anencephaly. Behav Sci Law. 2002;20(3):219–33.

12. Brandt HE, Ooms ME, Deliens L, et al. The last two days of life of nursing home patients—a nationwide study on causes of death and burdensome symptoms in The Netherlands. Palliat Med. 2006;20(5):533–40.
13. Brandt HE, Deliens L, Ooms ME, et al. Symptoms, signs, problems, and diseases of terminally ill nursing home patients: a nationwide observational study in The Netherlands. Arch Intern Med. 2005;165(3):314–20.
14. Williams SW, Williams CS, Zimmerman S, et al. Emotional and physical health of informal caregivers of residents at the end of life: the role of social support. J Gerontol B Psychol Sci Soc Sci. 2008;63(3):S171–83.
15. Oliver DP, Porock D, Oliver DB. Managing the secrets of dying backstage: the voices of nursing home staff. Omega J Death Dying. 2006;53(3):193–207.
16. Bottrell MM, O'Sullivan JF, Robbins MA, et al. Transferring dying nursing home residents to the hospital: DON perspectives on the nurse's role in transfer decisions. Geriatr Nurs. 2001;22(6):313–7.
17. Husebo BS, Husebo S. [Nursing homes as arenas of terminal care–how do we do in practice?]. Tidsskr Nor Laegeforen. 2005;125(10):1352–4.
18. Brulhart MI, Wermeille JP. Multidisciplinary medication review: evaluation of a pharmaceutical care model for nursing homes. Int J Clin Pharm. 2011;33(3):549–57.
19. Tjia J, Rothman MR, Kiely DK, et al. Daily medication use in nursing home residents with advanced dementia. J Am Geriatr Soc. 2010;58(5):880–8.
20. Dwyer LL, Han B, Woodwell DA, et al. Polypharmacy in nursing home residents in the United States: results of the 2004 National Nursing Home Survey. Am J Geriatr Pharmacother. 2010;8(1):63–72.
21. Gjerberg E, Forde R, Bjorndal A. Staff and family relationships in end-of-life nursing home care. Nurs Ethics. 2011;18(1):42–53.
22. Husebo SB. Communication, autonomy, and hope. How can we treat seriously ill patients with respect? Communication with the cancer patient: information and truth. Ann N Y Acad Sci. 1997;809:440–59.
23. Husebo SB. Is there hope, doctor? J Palliat Care. 1998;14(1):43–8.
24. Frankl V. Man`s search for meaning. New York: Washington Square Press; 1984. ISBN 0451523806.
25. Havel V. Letters to Olga. New York: Henry Holt and Company; 1989. ISBN 0805009736.
26. Husebo BS, Strand LI, Moe-Nilssen R, et al. Pain in older persons with severe dementia. Psychometric properties of the Mobilization-Observation-Behaviour-Intensity-Dementia (MOBID-2) Pain Scale in a clinical setting. Scand J Caring Sci. 2010;24:380–91.
27. Husebo BS, Strand LI, Moe-Nilssen R, et al. Who suffers most? Dementia and pain in nursing home patients: a cross-sectional study. J Am Med Dir Assoc. 2008;9(6):427–33.
28. Husebo BS, Ballard C, Sandvik K, et al. Efficacy of treating pain to reduce behavioural disturbances in residents of nursing homes with dementia: cluster randomized clinical trial. BMJ. 2011;343:1–10.
29. Husebo BS, Husebo SB. [Ethical end-of-life decision making in nursing homes]. Tidsskr Nor Laegeforen. 2004;124(22):2926–7.

Chapter 16
Communication with Cancer Patients about Palliative and End-of-Life Care

Guido Biasco, Matteo Moroni, and Ludovica De Panfilis

Abstract Communication with a cancer patient and his/her family takes place in a dynamic way. Steps of communication concern the seriousness of the illness and the chances of cure, the ineffectiveness of treatment, the opportunity to start a palliative care program, and end-of-life decisions. The moment when palliative care should be offered depends on the attitude of the team that is in charge of the patient. In general, palliative care is offered when cancer-directed therapy is no longer effective. Nevertheless, there is an increasing trend to suggest palliative care earlier, at the diagnosis of cancer, not at the end of the treatment, thus encouraging synergy between palliative care providers and oncologists. This attitude can both increase the quality of life of the patient and limit the risks of a discontinuity of clinical management. The decision about the start of palliative care should be based on candid communication between physicians and patients, so as to allow the latter to make well-grounded decisions concerning treatment and the time necessary for each possible intervention to be carried out. Physicians should know the case history and the possibilities offered by palliative care as well as have cross-cultural competence to understand and speak in relation to the culture, expectations, and real needs of the patient and his/her family at each stage of illness.

Keywords Communication • Palliative care • Cancer • Language

G. Biasco, MD (✉) • M. Moroni MD, PhD
Academy of the Sciences of Palliative Medicine, Via Aldo Moro, 16/3,
40010 Bentivoglio, Italy

"Giorgio Prodi" Center for Cancer Research,
University Alma Mater Studiorum, Bologna, Italy
e-mail: guido.biasco@unibo.it; matteodoc1974@libero.it

L. De Panfilis
Academy of the Sciences of Palliative Medicine, Via Aldo Moro, 16/3,
40010 Bentivoglio, Italy
e-mail: Ludovica.depanfilis@hotmail.it

Introduction

Palliative care and hospices have developed rapidly in the last 50 years [1]. Together with this development, a growing number of studies on state-of-the-art palliative and end-of-life care in oncology, along with new practical guidelines, advocate for clear and compassionate approaches to helping cancer patients and their families make choices about delicate matters such as pain control, advanced directives, and place of death [2–4].

When and how should one talk to a cancer patient about palliative and end-of-life care? This question is at the root of an endless series of observations, remarks, and researches but still lacks a specific answer. The stereotype of telling the truth in any case is consistent with the need to properly inform patients and their families about the seriousness, hopes, and prognosis of a life-threatening illness. In this way ethics is respected, however it may be applied. There is no simple formula to guide one in this matter, but there are some general principles that are applicable. Understanding them will enable and enhance communication about palliative programs to achieve the best quality of life for dying cancer patients. These principles, bearing on *cancer*, *communication*, *palliative care*, and *end-of-life care*, will be analyzed in this chapter. The language and meaning of each word are basic for the systematic analysis both of the information to be given to the patient and his/her family and for discussion within the scientific community. This is the starting point, to identify when and how to begin a conversation on palliative care, being aware that the conclusion will be a analytic picture rather than a final statement.

Cancer. Palliative care originates and develops mainly for facing the needs of cancer patients. However, the word *cancer* is often used in a not-very-accurate way in this context. Too often we generically refer to a patient with a bad prognosis as a cancer patient. When referring to palliative care, we should limit the discussion to patients with late-advanced cancer, who represent a large, but not the only, group of cancer patients. Also, the group of patients suffering from late-advanced cancer is not homogeneous. The type of cancer, the staging, the possibilities of treatment are different, implying that the evolution of the prognosis is also different.

Some types of cancer, such as exocrine pancreas or lung cancer, have a poor, short-term prognosis; others, such as breast or neuroendocrine cancer, have a long-term prognosis, lasting even for years. The distinction between short and long prognosis is not a marginal question when considering palliative care, since the prognosis can influence the modalities of intervention, and, more importantly, can determine when to start palliative care. Depending on the evolution of a variety of cancer processes, how and when to start palliative care is inevitably variable.

Palliative care. A recent analysis carried out on a group of students at the University of Bologna Faculty of Medicine confirms the common opinion that language and the meaning of words in palliative medicine are extremely confused [5]. Hence the question, how shall we communicate clearly if we do not use correct and commonly shared terms? In particular, what do we mean by palliative and end-of-life care? Palliative care, palliative medicine, end-of-life care, supportive care are often referred to as if they were synonymous but often do not signify the real situations [6–11].

Expressions that have recently come into use include "end-of-life support" and "dying trajectory"; these terms construct a different reality around death so as to counter the "wrongness" of death and promote its "normalization," the rightness of a clinical course that focuses on "dying" [12]. Often a patient is referred to a palliative care team following "treatment interruption" or because "there is no further treatment." Thus palliative care becomes "no treatment," but care or "management" services; whereas, in fact, patients may receive palliative care *during* treatment, including radiation and/or chemotherapy. "Symptom management" can mean "symptom management only," implying a less effective course of action or a second-rate decision [13]. Such language denies palliative care its speciality, its role in providing qualified care during illness, with the consequence that such services are sometimes considered merely as "hand-holding." Inaccurate language is the reason for the recent definition of palliative care as "room for confusion" [14].

Communication. This word is used by sociologists, anthropologists, philosophers, and linguists to describe the specific nature of human relationships as they are or may be, relationships of mutual participation and understanding. The term is basically synonymous with life with others, coexistence, and indicates how this coexistence happens. Communication is an on-going process, needing time, environment, cultural background, and social setting. These factors enrich communication and mark it as subjective, evolutionary, empathic, not schematic.

Communication in oncology is a delicate issue. Sensible communication between patient and physician is necessary for the patient and for the positive outcome of treatment. Words can support therapy and are an integral part of it [15]. There are basic communication skills required throughout the different steps of the disease: being able to ask the right questions at the right time, to listen, to keep to the main topic; to be aware of the patient's implicit questions; to distinguish the cognitive from the emotional; to speak empathically; to deal with difficult moments [16].

Truth is one of the important concepts in the semantic area of communication. The communicative action claims the truth, and sharing is its objective. Truth and information clearly sum up the substance of communication, implying a complete linguistic structure and an ideal speaker [17].

Within the medical field, truth has objective, subjective, and relational aspects and evolves in time under the influence of several factors—the peculiarities of physician, patient, and the patient's family, as well as the social and cultural setting and the environment. The importance of truth-telling in conversations between physicians, professional caregivers, and patients must be understood [18]. There is a particularly heated discussion on how and when to tell the truth; many issues must be considered, including the seriousness of the illness, the presence of physical and psychological suffering, the impact of prejudice and social stigmatization, the effect of certain treatments [19]. Especially when dealing with incurable disease, the main problem is *how* to tell the truth; it is necessary to create a proper moment to tell, to understand what is said, to help the patient think and show his/her emotions. All this goes beyond the simple obligation to inform [20].

Instead of the Latin and Anglo-Saxon models usually referred to when discussing communication in medicine, which have opposite structures and methods, the best approach for communication seems to be a patient-centered one that takes into account his/her beliefs and values without forgetting that the individual is unique. This kind of communication is inherent in the treatment known as "tailored palliative care," which involves the rediscovery of human value, caregiving, and the sharing of the patient's pain and personal situation [21].

When to Start Palliative Care: Is Earlier Better?

A milestone article by Dr. Temel and coworkers, recently published in the *New England Journal of Medicine*, suggests that the intervention of a palliative care team earlier than usual with cancer patients shows good outcomes [22]. The research was carried out on metastatic non-small-cell lung cancer patients at diagnosis. Patients were randomized in two groups: the first one received standard oncological care, with palliative care services given when the treatment was no longer effective, as usually happens. The second group received palliative care services early, at their diagnosis; the palliative care team collaborated with the oncologists.

The results of this study show for the first time in a very pragmatic way that cancer patients who received palliative care early, at their diagnosis, had a better quality of life and longer survival compared to patients who received oncological care in the more usual manner. However, the excellent outcomes obtained in the study should be given careful consideration, particularly regarding the generalizability of the results—always a delicate issue when trying to reach an evidence-based method of palliative care [11].

First of all the typology of patients should be considered. The study included patients with short life expectations, 70% of whom died in the course of the study, the median survival time being 5.7 months. These data show that results cannot be automatically transposed to patients having a longer course of illness. Under these circumstances a palliative care team intervention should be considered in relation to the stage of the illness. In other words, it is necessary to determine if the intervention by a specific palliative care team, as the article suggests, is useful early, at the diagnosis, independently of cancer staging; or whether it is advisable to set standard criteria to indicate the optimum moment for the start of palliative care.

In Italy there is growing attention being paid to the integration of palliative care in oncology somewhat earlier than the end-of-life stage [23]. However, too-early intervention could lead to three problems. First, the issue of expertise: Perhaps a palliative care team is not necessary at the early stage of illness, when treatment is still possible for a patient with still-good performance status. During this stage, the patient and his family need mainly good communication and possibly psychological support, both of which can be provided by the oncology team. At this point palliative care is part of the treatment, and it should be considered as supportive care, improving the efficiency of the anticancer therapy.

As previously mentioned, the need to outline a comprehensive and common language is relevant in palliative care. If we mean palliative care as "caring" and not "curing," not a "supportive treatment," then we will only reinforce the semantic and operative confusion underlying this specialty [7, 12, 24–27].

Second, the criteria to standardize the stage at which it is advisable to start palliative care have not been well defined. This impedes the generalization of research in palliative care. The homogeneity of study groups is always under discussion. Data concerning the demographic aspects of patients, the type of cancer, its staging, patients' performance status are not enough. Homogeneity criteria of study groups in different trials have not yet been established, with consequences related to the transposition of data.

Lately there has been a growing interest in the massive analysis of the whole human genome [28]. This process may find its application also in research on the end of life and incurable chronic diseases. Perhaps a standard molecular basis is the most solid future we can hope for, but at present we must seek for pathological and clinical markers that are not yet generally recognized.

The third problem that the earlier-than-necessary intervention of a palliative care team could involve is the matter of cost. A palliative care team has its own cost. Temel's article depicts a saving in therapeutic and diagnostic aggression, as well as in frequency of hospitalization. During the early stage of a cancer illness, cost excesses and the savings that may result from excess reduction are quite rare. At that stage the palliative care team cost could exceed what is saved by appropriate tests.

Temel's work does not describe the relationship between oncologists and the palliative care team. Even though the details provided on the roles played by both teams are accurate, there is no evidence of how they cooperated. This aspect is relevant to pragmatic research: since it was an open survey, it was necessary to exclude the possibility that the presence of a palliative care team might have influenced the behavior of the oncologists. Furthermore, the professionals forming the palliative care team are also significant: palliative care teams are not all homogeneous; their composition often depends on the immediate circumstances. Consequently, the assumption that a generic palliative care team operating early in the cure of cancer patients may be useful to patients and their families must be critically assessed. Finally, the willingness of patients and their families must be taken into consideration. The intervention of a team in addition to that the patient usually deals with must be carefully considered. Here communication, language, and the sensitivity to understand the needs and expectations of a patient who is diagnosed with cancer are important. Cross-cultural considerations, social status, cultural level, heterogeneity of perspective in approaching cancer, as well as end-of-life matters, are hot topics in palliative care; they cannot be overlooked when making organizational choices.

Is There a Better Way to Tell Patients about Palliative Care?

The way we select words to identify and describe values, ideas, methods, and disciplines is never neutral. This selection of words often reflects relative power and social dynamics. Language is, indeed, product and producer when used with respect to the surrounding reality.

Palliative medicine is typical of a specific historical and cultural background, which can be defined as the Western setting, with its own peculiarities that make it differ from other cultures. Also, the meaning of certain concepts, such as health and illness, pain and death, varies a lot on the basis of the historical, geographical, and anthropological backgrounds of reference. As far as the concept of pain is involved, for instance, our culture has removed any ground of discussion. Pain is not to be talked about, not to be proved; it symbolizes weakness, precariousness. Pain is removed from daily experience, from personal conscience, and from the theoretical system at the basis of scientific and social disciplines [29]. Likewise, the concept of death: it is first of all a natural, biological event. It is perceived as the outcome of wrong therapy; it questions the physician's "infallibility." Death is incomprehensible because it is part of a system of beliefs that makes it look like something that has to be hidden, forgotten, and changed into a private, upsetting event. This is a cognitive mismatch with death that is morally wrong, however biologically inevitable [12].

The progress of science has made it possible to replace the paternalistic Hippocratic paradigm with the so-called bioethical paradigm, which is founded on morality in evolution. This morality is built upon individuals' quality of life and self-fulfillment. It is also founded on a peer-to-peer relationship between doctor and patience, linked together by the therapeutic alliance [30]. Within the field of medicine, one of the developments of this bioethical setup is palliative medicine, the philosophy of which can be summarized by the expression "taking care" of the entire patient. Palliative medicine is meant to be a sort of counterculture born in a context of infallibility and within a mentality built upon the power of curing. It is intended to use words, methods of curing, approaches, and values appropriate to a concept of health as a set of physical, social, existential, and psychological conditions that all together represent indicators of the quality of life, rather than a mere clinical approach. The ideal model is designed around the patient's needs and is centered on the individual and his/her background. This focus, together with a clear communication approach, effectively allows and promotes improvement of the patient's quality of life [31].

According to what has been illustrated so far, communication is very important from several points of view; it has to be analyzed beginning from the concept of individualized treatment and, above all, from the new paradigm of palliative care. This means much more than the simple communication in palliative care; we are actually referring to the patient's perception of change when a shift to palliative care occurs. This perception of change implies certain issues on the level of communication. How and when shall we inform the patient about it? Is there an ideal way and time to do this?

First of all it is important to go back to the perception of terms. The semantic ambiguity of the words in palliative medicine ends up disorienting the community and showing the inner confusion of the discipline regarding its aims—that is, the concept of active and global cure linked with the concept of care and assistance, also definable with the expression "system of support" [12]. The term "palliative" evokes negative emotions; it has always been associated with desperate situations, in which nothing more can be done. Palliative care hence has a negative connotation; its founding philosophy, summed up by the expression "the patient is incurable but not unable to be taken care of," is never emphasized.

The term "palliative," within the frame of an individualized approach to global care, can have a much wider meaning and can differ from the term "end-of-life care." To have a palliative care team working together with an oncological team not only implies positive outcomes for the oncological team, but is beneficial to the patient, in terms of both quality of life and effective communication [22, 32]. Talking about palliative care from the beginning would actually avoid the clash that might arise when a patient is told to start this path following a negative prognosis. Because the shift to palliative care is connected to the idea of a desperate situation, it is perceived by the patient and his/her relatives as a surrender of the physicians to the disease. The palliative aspects of pain relief and quality of life improvement are completely ignored when compared to the tragedy of an upcoming death [33].

The cultural background implies also a different perception of the meaning of *truth*. In Western culture the individual is seen as autonomous, independent, self-determined, and rational. It is for this reason that interpersonal relations generally involve open verbal communication. However, this is a culturally univocal perspective; it has to be replaced by culturally based, culturally informed communication that allows gradual negotiations between physician, patient, and the patient's family regarding not only the best treatments, but also the best kind of dialogue [34]. It is only by knowing the individual's cultural background and by being aware of his/her needs, that appropriate communication and, hence, effective treatment are possible. This is the reason why the only feasible answer to the question whether there is a universally suitable way to talk about palliative care to the patient is that there is no method that always works, that is effective for all cases. What *is* certain is the importance of acknowledging the patient's inherent value because of his/her status and background. To discuss this kind of care in advance is definitely the right way to improve the perception of the term "palliative."

This complete, individualized communicational approach, which is typical of palliative medicine, has to be considered as part of an intermediate ethic between two contrasting classical models—one based upon the principle of autonomy, the other one based upon the sanctity of life. Autonomy cannot be reduced to total freedom of choice; but in the field of palliative medicine, it is a source of the physician's duty to inform and to test the deep understanding of the information given. Furthermore, it can also imply the physician's ability to listen to and comprehend the patient's requests, under the perspective of "controlled autonomy." We can define palliative medicine by borrowing a theory from Carol Gilligan, "ethics of the cure" [35]: the necessity of regarding the moral life as recognizing the contextual character of our decisions, which, in turn, are influenced by innumerable factors; and the necessity of having an attitude of care and responsibility towards others.

The Multifaceted, Dynamic Process of Communication

In the course of its work with a cancer patient the care team can interact with the patient alone; the patient along with family members or friends, who might be involved in decision-making; and the patient, family members, and professional caregivers, who would probably not be involved in decision-making but could be involved in other ways. It is in these settings that the distinctive features of the course of the illness occur. At the early stage of illness there is a substantial period in which the patient's response to treatment is constant. This is followed by a period of decline of general conditions due to relapse or being off therapy. Finally, there is a rapid decline to death, when the seriousness of the illness can lead from palliative to end-of-life care.

Communication with cancer patients in the periods of palliative and end-of-life care has, therefore, a very dynamic background, starting with a more-or-less stable relationship between physician and patient, with communicative skills and coping strategies changing in relation to the stage of the illness. The physician must be prepared and properly trained to change both the subject and the form of communication, but we should not forget that the patient is not passive; it follows that listening also must be dynamic [36]. Moreover, there should not be misunderstandings, such as misinformation about the diagnosis (at the early stage) and prognosis (at the active post-treatment and later stages).

In this dynamic process of communication the relationship between the physician and the patient is asymmetric. A professional with a technical and cultural background cares for and addresses a person with a specific problem but usually without the same knowledge. There is asymmetry in communication even when the patient is a physician, because of possible subconscious defense mechanisms and the need to rely on a colleague with specific expertise. These preliminary remarks are useful in underlining that communication between physician and patient is by its nature a shared process. It follows the following scheme: person has a problem → person consults an expert → expert evaluates problem → expert suggests solution → person makes decision about solution → person and expert prepare to face together the steps of the decision. This procedure is integral to informed consent.

From a communication, relational point of view, cancer developing through its different stages can be considered a "matter of a couple," in which physician and patient are somehow forced to seek new energies, emotions, and skills that usually are outside the average relationship as it moves through diagnosis and treatment. A remarkable variable related to the contribution that each member can give to these conversations is the extreme heterogeneity of point of view between physician

16 Communication with Cancer Patients about Palliative and End-of-Life Care

Table 16.1 Questions and problems in a clear and dynamic conversation

Actor
Question
Background
Physician
When do I communicate the bad news/prognosis? How shall I tell it?
Whom shall I tell it to? What kind of options can I offer?
Little time to tell bad news that need appropriate and dedicated time
Communication skills are not included in training programs of the medical schools yet
To the patient? To the patient and caregivers?
Which option shall I offer the patient, considering that traditional treatments could give him/her hope while palliative care could discourage him/her?
Patient
What's happening now? What is my physician going to tell me? Do I really trust my physician?
What am I going to do with the news he/she will tell me?
Changing of the overall view: from recovery to cure
Will the subject of the conversation be fully understood? The relationship between physician and patient is obviously based on confidence: is the expert I choose and who has been caring for me so far giving me a real assessment of my situation?
Can the view/imagination of the consequences of the news that the patient is receiving dramatically change his or her coping strategies?
Decision about my life, my family, my desires to express and to realize, DNR statements, more days or better days?

(often not only an oncologist) and patient [37]. In conversations communication should be appropriate, proactive, and responsible; both parties should face their problems (Table 16.1) [38, 39]. Questions may remain the same throughout the course of illness, but as happens in married life, the setting of the discourse changes. In this complex setting the role of "empathic opportunities" may be seen—those moments when the patient starts a more human and relational dialogue with his/her physician to outline, within a professional relationship, a really shared treatment process, based on the patient's real needs and expectations of appropriate clinical management by the physician. The physician must at this point also take into account outcomes not strictly biomedical. This is real and deep empathy, which requires that physicians have a double skill: to catch the empathic opportunities and to manage them without escaping for fear of being or feeling inadequate to manage them [40, 52]. Considering that communication as a dynamic, empathic, bidirectional process, the best way to gain the necessary skills is by a gradual approach. Such an approach also has the benefit of respecting the patient during his/her process of gaining awareness. Communication improves a lot when empathy and the ability to dialogue merge together with consciousness of the cultural and personal needs of the individual involved [41]. This needs time to be achieved.

The division of time into two essential stages with different subjects can facilitate dynamic communication, enabling a more delicate and aware approach to palliative care (Table 16.2). Hope, not illusion, is the basis for the communication process; it

Table 16.2 Division of time-illness in two essential stages having different subjects as a help for dynamic communication

Stage	Subject
I	Diagnosis and treatment to cure illness
	No symptoms or few symptoms
	The physician has a lot to say/the patient has a lot to know and decide upon
	Many issues that physician and patient need to talk about
II	Advanced cancer
	Many symptoms
	Nothing more to do
	Great need for care
	Last decisions to take for both physician and patient

can create realistic dynamic discourse and enhance the development of clear communication between physician and patient, allowing such communication to:

1. Create realistic hope based on the realistic clinical situation of the patient (the right step at the right moment or, in case of an unaware or not fully aware patient, a process of truth-telling in small doses appropriate to the psychocognitive skills of the patient and his or her family).
2. Create the proper opportunity to face emotions such as anger and frustration (an "emotional corner" dedicated to the resolution of "what is not still"). The achievement of realistic communication can optimize the time available by using the meetings between physician and patient to exchange views not only about treatment possibilities but also on their impact on the patient.
3. Create an individualized care plan, including control of symptoms, the setting of care (e.g., hospice, home) and of death, and any aggressive therapy.

Improving Cross-Cultural Palliative and End-of-Life Care

In discussing palliative care, the cultural diversity between health professionals and patients may result in a clash of point of views, beliefs, or ethical standards [43]. Differences can also arise in communication styles as well as in the language spoken by different cultures [44]. Palliative and end-of-life care do not have universal rules; hence the need to strike a balance between different cultures and beliefs [27, 45]. This is a delicate issue if we consider that ethics and law in Europe and the Western world are based on the view that the individual is autonomous and self-assertive. Eurocentric beliefs and values are often assumed to be universal; but in more community-centered cultures the family, not the individual, is "the ethical unit of care." When physician and patient are of different cultures, misunderstandings of the opportunities offered by palliative care can arise [46].

Expectations with regard to palliative care are different in different cultures. For instance, in the US African Americans wish to prolong life more than non-Hispanic whites [47]. This attitude of *vitalism* illustrates the multifaceted nature of culture where religious, social, and historical factors are inextricably linked [48]. International studies show that terminally ill patients who consider religion very important are less likely to acknowledge their impending death and more likely to ask for life-prolonging care than those to whom religion is less important. Fear of dying far away from the family leads to strong preferences for palliative home care. In the US, African Americans, Hispanics/Latinos, and Asian Americans have been shown to have significant mistrust of their physicians for general medical care [49]. Professional caregivers trained for multicultural conversations are prepared to answer properly the many ways that patients express their distress and fears [50, 51]. It follows that professional caregivers should be well trained in cultural competence so as to establish a proper relationship with patients and their families and reduce the likelihood of miscommunication and open conflicts during the course of illness [26, 42].

Truth-telling is a more delicate issue. A culturally appropriate response to cancer patients who may wish not to know avoids blunt disclosure, while families are helped to see the positive value of patients' involvement in treatment decisions [53]. African American family members and non-Hispanic white family members have different communication expectations as far as end-of-life care is concerned [26, 54]. Non-Hispanic white participants wanted more factual information about medical options, prognosis, quality of life, and cost implications; while African American participants tended to value the protection of life at all costs and requested spiritually focused information about suffering and spiritual guidance to support them in the decision-making process. Notably, non-Hispanic white participants tended to exclude family participants in end-of-life discussions, while African American participants preferred to include more family, friends, and spiritual leaders.

Conclusion

Informing cancer patients and their families about the possibilities of palliative and end-of-life care may imply communicating to them a poor prognosis. Therefore, this kind of communication needs to be carefully measured and based on what patients know or wish to know, as well as on treatment options and the stage of illness when a palliative care program can be started.

Since there are no standardized rules to respect these needs, to be appropriate, communication must follow personalized modalities. Each patient has a unique identity, which depends in part on his/her social, economic, and cultural background as well as his/her own culture and education. This is the reason why a great part of the discourse on palliative care must originate from a basic element, the physician's training and awareness. The American Society of Clinical Oncology identifies candid conversation with cancer patients and their families, including the communication of treatment options and goals, as a basic issue [21]. This cannot be a single conversation, but needs to be regularly modified and updated throughout the course of each cancer patient's illness. An early discussion on palliative care would enhance a humanized and individualized communication approach; palliative care deals with individual suffering at any phase of the disease. Working in advance on communication regarding feasible recourse to palliative care would also allow the gradual introduction of news to the patient on the basis of his/her own sensibility and needs. Therefore, communication concerning palliative care cannot happen in a single moment; rather, it must be dynamic, depicting the situation that the cancer patient is going through.

Communicating means being understood, and this implies having a common, shared language as well as the ability to understand the expectations of patients and their families, their cultural identity. Language is still somewhat confused, and a preliminary conversation is necessary to identify a vocabulary that the patient can understand. This interaction requires that physicians be trained so as to gain flexibility as well as the ability to listen to and be understood by patients, with full respect for their autonomy. The education and training provided by medical and specialty schools in most countries is doing very little to prepare oncology professionals to discuss terminating or not starting futile care, and to join with the patients and families in the transition from active to palliative and end-of-life care [54, 55].

The ability to understand and be understood should be connected with expert knowledge of palliative care, knowing what it can offer and how it can be delivered during the course of the illness. Divergent social and cultural assessments, not only economic resources, result in different methods of providing palliative care and require that local policy makers identify palliative care models adaptable to the specific needs of the people. The example of Italy supports this concept. Home care in the southern part of the country is linked to a social structure that allows for the development of such a model. In contrast, in northern Italy, in which the socioeconomic and cultural assessments are characterized by a dynamic lifestyle and a projection toward Continental and Anglo-Saxon social models, the development of a modern palliative care organization, with residential and at-home care, is well accepted and developed [5]. In Italy, as in other Western countries, the interplay of several factors influences the organization and delivery of palliative care.

In conclusion, physicians should not only be well trained in cancer treatment, but also aware of palliative care options. When and how to start talking about palliative care cannot depend on the occasions that may be offered by the clinical setting. These tasks demand even greater sensitivity and preparation when clinical encounters occur with patients and families from diverse socioeconomic, ethnic, and cultural backgrounds. Cross-cultural competence is a key requirement for individualized, candid communication about treatment and also about care for the cancer patient and his/her family (Fig. 16.1).

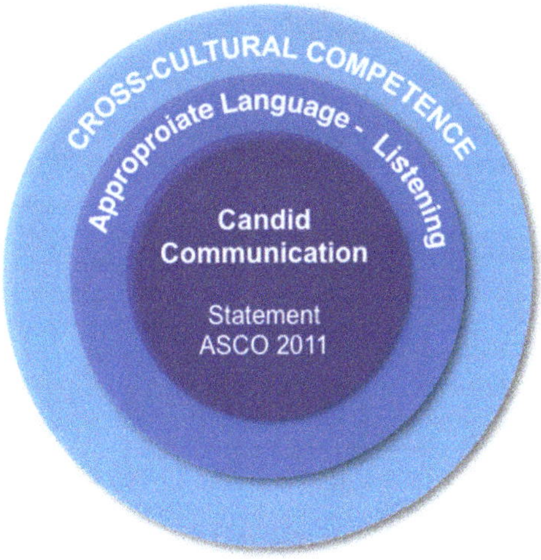

Fig. 16.1 Cross-cultural competence is a key requirement for individualized candid communication about treatment and care for the cancer patient and his/her family (Guido Biasco, MD, Bologna, 30 July 2011)

Acknowledgments The authors are grateful to Mrs. Cristina Musiani for her support in the translation and revision of the manuscript.

References

1. Clark D. From margins to centre: a review of the history of palliative care in cancer. Lancet Oncol. 2007;8:430–8.
2. Breivik H, Cherny N, Collett B, et al. Cancer-related pain: a pan-European survey of prevalence, treatment, and patient attitudes. Ann Oncol. 2009;20:1420–33.
3. Ferris FD, Bruera E, Cherny N, et al. Palliative cancer care a decade later: accomplishments, the needs, next steps-from the American Society of Clinical Oncology. J Clin Oncol. 2009;27:3052–8.
4. Teno JM, Condor SR. Referring a patient and family to high-quality palliative care at the close of life: "We met a new personality… with this level of compassion and empathy". JAMA. 2009;301:651–9.
5. Biasco G, Baider L. Cultural, social and political factors in providing palliative care. In: Ramaswamy G, editor. American Society of Clinical Oncology Educational Book. 47th Annual Meeting Spring; 2011. p. 107–10.
6. Pastrana T, Junger S. A matter of definition—key elements identified in a discourse analysis of definitions of palliative care. Palliat Med. 2008;22:222–32.
7. Portenoy RK. Palliative medicine: from paradigm to best practice. J Palliat Med. 2008; 11:1092–3.
8. O'Connor M, Payne S. Discourse analysis: examining the potential for research in palliative care. Palliat Med. 2006;20:829–34.
9. Hanks GW. The mainstreaming of palliative care. J Palliat Med. 2008;11:1063–4.
10. Fadul N, Elsayem A, Palmer JL, et al. Supportive versus palliative care: what's in a name? Cancer. 2009;115:2013–21.
11. Currow DC, Wheeler JL, Glare P, et al. A framework for generalizability in palliative care. J Pain Symptom Manage. 2009;37:373–86.

12. O'Connor M, Mellar PD, Abernethy A. Language, discourse and meaning in palliative medicine. Prog Palliat Care. 2010;18:66–71.
13. Zikmund-Fisher BJ, Lacey HP, Fagerlin A. The potential impact of decision role and patient age on end-of-life treatment decision making. J Med Ethics. 2008;34:327–33.
14. Fallon M, Smith J. Terminology: the historical perspective, evolution and current usage— room for confusion? Eur J Cancer. 2008;44:1069–71.
15. Costantino Cipolla, Giuseppe Remuzzi. Introduzione in Dire, fare, curare. Parole tra medici e malati, a cura di Costantino Cipolla e Giuseppe Remuzzi, Franco Angeli, Milano; 2008. p. 7–12.
16. Back AL, Arnold RM, Baile WF, Tulsky JA, Kelly Fryer-Edwards K. Approaching difficult communication tasks in oncology. CA Cancer J Clin. 2005;55:164–77.
17. Habermas J. Theory of communicative action, Vols. 1 and 2. Boston: Beacon Press; 1984.
18. Fallowfield L, Jenkins WA, Beveridge HA. Truth may hurt but deceit hurts more: communication in palliative care. Palliat Med. 2002;16:4297–303.
19. Surbone A. Truth telling and ethical issues: an overview, UICC World Cancer Congress, Bridging the gap. Transforming knowledge into action. July 8–12, 2006, Washington, DC.
20. Baider L, Surbone A. Cancer and the family: the silent words of truth. J Clin Oncol. 2010;28:1269–72.
21. Peppercorn JM, Smith TJ, Helft PR, et al. American society of clinical oncology statement: towards individualized care for patients with advanced cancer. J Clin Oncol. 2011;29:755–60.
22. Temel JS, Greer GA, Muzikanskj A, et al. Early palliative care for patients with metastatic non-small-cell lung cancer. N Engl J Med. 2010;363:733–42.
23. Casadio M, Biasco G, Abernethy AP, Bonazzi V, Pannuti R, Pannuti F. The National Tumor Association Foundation (ANT): a 30 year model of home palliative care. BMC Palliat Care. 2010;9:12.
24. Biasco G, Surbone A. Cultural challenges in caring for our patients with advanced cancer. Letter. J Clin Oncol. 2008;26:1–2.
25. Ashley EA, Butte AJ, Wheeler MT, et al. Clinical assessment incorporating a personal genome. Lancet. 2010;375:1525–35.
26. Kagawa-Singer M, Valdez A, Yu MC, Surbone A. Cancer, culture and health disparities: time to chart a new course? CA Cancer J Clin. 2010;60:12–39.
27. Surbone A. Cultural competence in oncology: where do we stand? Ann Oncol. 2010;21:3–5.
28. Astolfi AL, Biasco G, Bruera E, Surbone A. Progress in genomic technology: a new challenge for the palliative medicine? J Pain Symptom Manage. 2010;40:7–9.
29. Gaines AD, Juengst ET. Origin myths in bioethics: constructing sources, motives and reason in bioethics. Cult Med Psychiatry. 2008;32:303–27.
30. Bruera E, Hui D. Integrating supportive and palliative care in the trajectory of cancer: establishing goals and model of care. J Clin Oncol. 2010;28:4013–7.
31. Bradley CT, Brasel KJ. Core competencies in palliative care for surgeons: interpersonal and communication skills. Am J Hosp Palliat Care. 2007;24:499–507.
32. Feeg VD, Elebiary H. Exploratory study on end-of-life issues: barriers to palliative care and advance directives. Am J Hosp Palliat Care. 2005;22:119–24.
33. Kagawa Singer M, Blackhall LJ. Negotiating cross-cultural issues at the end of life. JAMA. 2001;286:2993–3001.
34. Gilligan C. In a different voice: psychological theory and women's development. Kingle edition; 1993.
35. Goldzweig G, Meirowitz A, Hubert A, et al. Meeting expectations of patients with cancer: relationship between patient satisfaction, depression and coping. J Clin Oncol. 2010;28:1560–5.
36. Keating NL. Physician factors associated with discussion about end-of-life care. Cancer. 2010;116:998–1006.
37. Seno VL. Being-with dying: authenticity in end-of-life encounters. Am J Hosp Palliat Med. 2010;27:377–86.
38. Mack JW, Weeks JC, Wright AA, Block SD, Prigerson HG. End-of-life discussions, goal attainment and distress at the end-of-life: predictors and outcomes of receipt of care consistent with preferences. J Clin Oncol. 2010;28:1203–8.

39. Pollak KI, Arnold RM, Jeffreys AS, et al. Oncologist communication about emotion during visits with patients with advanced cancer. J Clin Oncol. 2007;25:5748–52.
40. Surbone A. Cultural aspects of communication in cancer care. Support Care Cancer. 2007;14:789–91.
41. Stubenrauch JM. Study: few physicians discussing end-of-life options with advanced-stage patients. Oncology. 2010;25:26–8.
42. Fadiman A. The spirit catches you and you fall down: a Hmong child, her American doctors, and the collision of two cultures. New York: Farrar Straus & Giroux; 1997.
43. Barnato AE, Chang CH, Saynina O, et al. Influence of race on in-patient treatment intensity at the end of life. J Gen Intern Med. 2007;22:338–45.
44. Kagawa-Singer M, Chung RC-Y. Towards a new paradigm: a cultural systems approach. In: Kurasaki KS, Okazaki S, Sue S, editors. Asian American mental health: assessments, theories and methods. New York: Kluwer; 2002.
45. Haas JS, Earle CC, Orav JE, et al. Lower use of hospice by cancer patients who live in minority versus white areas. J Gen Intern Med. 2007;22:396–9.
46. Born W, Greiner K, Sylvia E, et al. Knowledge, attitudes, and beliefs about end-of-life care among inner-city African Americans and Latinos. J Palliat Med. 2004;7:247–56.
47. Loggers ET, Maciejewski PK, Paulk E, et al. Racial differences in predictors of intensive end-of-life care in patients with advanced cancer. J Clin Oncol. 2009;27:5559–64.
48. Collins KS, Hughes DL, Doty MM, et al. Diverse communities, common concerns: assessing health care quality for minority Americans. New York: The Commonwealth Fund; 2002.
49. Rhodes R, Teno JM. What's race got to do with it? J Clin Oncol. 2009;27:5496–8.
50. Brawley OW, Smith DE, Kirch RA. Taking action to ease suffering: advancing cancer pain control as a health care priority. CA Cancer J Clin. 2009;59:285–9.
51. Kagawa Singer M, Valdez Dadia A, Yu M, et al. Cancer, culture and health disparities: time to chart a new course? CA Cancer J Clin. 2010;60:12–39.
52. Bruera E, Palmer JL, Pace E, et al. A randomized, controlled trial of physician postures when breaking bad news to cancer patients. Palliat Med. 2007;21:501–5.
53. Shrank WH, Kutner JS, Richardson T, et al. Focus group findings about the influence of culture on communication preferences in end-of-life care. J Gen Intern Med. 2005;20:703–9.
54. Evans WG, Tulsky JA, Back AL, et al. Communication at times of transitions: how to help patients cope with loss and re-define hope. Cancer J. 2006;12:417–24.
55. Back AL, Arnold RM, Baile WF, et al. Faculty development to change the paradigm of communication skills teaching in oncology. J Clin Oncol. 2009;27:1137–41.

Chapter 17
Communication with Patients with Hereditary Cancer: Practical Considerations Focusing on Women's Cancers

Karen Carapetyan, Julia Smith, and Franco Muggia

Abstract Advances in our understanding of genetic pathways associated with hereditary cancers carry with them a responsibility to provide patients and their families with up-to-date concepts of cancer screening and prevention. In addition, cancers arising in carriers of BRCA mutations may be more responsive to new treatments (such as with the so-called poly-(ADP-ribose) polymerase [PARP] inhibitors) that seemingly have greater efficacy against these hereditary tumors. Access to appropriate educational materials for both patients and families coupled with dialogue between biomedical specialists is a necessary ingredient for providing optimal guidance when facing BRCA and other known genetically related cancers. Much can also be learned by emerging literature by patients and their families. Through examples, we emphasize the special needs of these patients in ongoing communications with their physician and related health advisors.

A diagnosis of cancer has an impact not only on patients but also on their families. Beyond prescribing therapeutic interventions for a particular patient at diagnosis, physicians must take into account preceding illnesses in the family. When there is a known familial predisposition to a particular cancer, a cancer diagnosis carries additional emotional impact and may determine subsequent decision-making,

K. Carapetyan
Department of Medicine, New York University School of Medicine,
462 1st Avenue, NB 7N24, New York, NY 10016, USA
e-mail: karen.carapetyan@nyumc.org

J. Smith (✉)
Department of Medical Oncology, New York University Medical Center,
160 East 34th Street, New York, NY 10016, USA
e-mail: Julia.Smith@nyumc.org

F. Muggia
Department of Medicine, New York University Langone Medical Center,
New York University Medical Institute, 550 1st Avenue, New York, NY 10016, USA
e-mail: Franco.muggia@nyumc.org

not only on the part of the afflicted woman, but also of other family members. Therefore, guiding a patient through the implications of a positive genetic test or a compelling family history requires an awareness of family dynamics beyond what may have been addressed by a genetic counselor. We describe here issues pertaining specifically to (1) women who have been diagnosed with ovarian cancer and are subsequently found to carry BRCA mutations, (2) women diagnosed with breast cancer and are screened for BRCA mutations, Lynch Syndrome, or other hereditary conditions. Finally, we emphasize the development of educational materials for women at risk as a useful tool in such communication, based on experiences at various institutions, including the Lynne Cohen Program for Women at High Risk of Cancer at Bellevue Hospital Center and New York University Clinical Cancer Center [1].

Keywords Breast • Ovarian • BRCA genes • Risk reducing surgery

Patients with Ovarian Cancer and BRCA Mutations

It is tragic when a woman (and family member of a patient) develops advanced ovarian cancer because preventive measures were not or could not be instituted. However, even with diagnostic advances, women are most often discovered to have stages III and IV ovarian cancers. Nevertheless, treatment even in these late presentations may be associated with long-term survival. Such women face issues about their risks for developing breast and other cancers, and a number of other challenges. For example, we previously reported [2] on unusual clinical features in patients with BRCA mutations who over the years developed both breast and ovarian cancers. Among these features were unusual metastatic sites for ovarian cancer (such as brain and bone) coupled with ambiguity in the epithelial markers that reflected disease with a primary either in the breast or the ovary.

A diagnosis of ovarian cancer in a woman who carries a deleterious mutation of BRCA1 or -2 casts a shadow on all other decisions. The reason behind such a statement is that after such a presentation of the ovarian cancer, even if complete remission is achieved with chemotherapy, there is a lifetime risk of relapse. The possibility of relapse should be taken into account in all subsequent decisions. Often, when well patients are seen by breast cancer specialists as breast cancer risks begin to be addressed, recommendations for bilateral mastectomies and reconstructions are not unusual. However, should such recommendations not be given in close communication with the gynecologic oncology team? It is not uncommon to find a lack of communication among various specialists as they interact with the patient, as illustrated by this clinical vignette.

Clinical Vignette 1

A 36-year-old woman, the mother of two teenage children, with a positive family history of breast cancer at age 55 in her mother, underwent gynecologic surgery following a short history of pelvic pain and discovery of bilateral adnexal masses.

After total abdominal hysterectomy and bilateral salpingo-oophorectomy, omentectomy, and lymph node dissection, she was diagnosed with a high-grade serous carcinoma, stage IIC, and an intraperitoneal (IP) catheter was inserted. At cycle 1, IP cisplatin caused severe emesis, and IP paclitaxel a week later was associated with abdominal pain. Cycle 2, at a reduced dose of cisplatin tolerance, was better; but when the second IP paclitaxel was given, the pain intensified, suggesting catheter complications, requiring emergency surgery with removal of the catheter. She subsequently completed her chemotherapy with intravenous carboplatin and paclitaxel. In addition to being very symptomatic, she became distraught at learning that she was a BRCA1 mutation carrier (testing being encouraged in all women diagnosed with high-grade ovarian cancers because of emerging therapeutic implications). One year after diagnosis, she was beginning to regain her well-being and emotional balance. Upon "friendly" advice, she consulted a "high-risk" clinic; the recommendation from the consultant was that she should undergo risk-reducing bilateral mastectomies. Such advice exacerbated her feelings of helplessness. We pointed out that risk-reducing surgery may be the preferred option under many circumstances for women with deleterious BRCA mutations with no further childbearing expectations; in her instance, breast magnetic resonance imaging (MRI) surveillance (which had already been instituted) was suitable to her medical circumstances [3]. Two years later, she is continuing with such surveillance. Better communication at the time of her breast cancer clinic consultation could have prevented much emotional distress.

Rarely, ovarian cancer is discovered incidentally or at risk-reducing surgery in stage I, where the probability of prolonged (>5 year) disease-free survival exceeds 75%. In this setting, surgical intervention to reduce the risk of breast cancer might be more strongly contemplated by physicians and patients alike. Again, advice should be provided by a team of specialists, rather than unilaterally making recommendations even if they are considered standard for the prevention of breast cancer.

The decision of surveillance vs. risk-reducing surgery in women with a diagnosis of ovarian cancer is surfacing with increasing frequency. Recent studies have clearly shown that ovarian cancer patients with BRCA mutations have a significantly better outlook than those with a sporadic background [4] and that they respond better to up-front and subsequent chemotherapies [5]. With the possibility that agents with little toxicity such as PARP inhibitors [6] can be used for maintenance to delay recurrences, one should give consideration to clinical trials addressing issues of secondary prevention, including the risk of breast cancer. In the meantime, the main focus in managing this challenging group of patients should be in enhancing communication with the patients regarding issues of risk-vs.-benefit ratio in surveillance (usually ongoing in any woman carrying a diagnosis of ovarian cancer) vs. additional surgical interventions.

Much remains to be learned about special features of BRCA-mutated ovarian cancer. We do know that these are usually of the high-grade serous subtype with prominent peritoneal spread of disease; also, as noted above, their responsiveness to chemotherapy leads to a better outcome, stage for stage, as compared to the sporadic variety [4]. We also have learned from risk-reducing surgery that the fimbria of the Fallopian tubes are a common site of origin, and that often such origins are accompanied by "p53 signatures" in the epithelium—that is, there are areas of positive immunohistochemistry to p53, pointing to mutations in this tumor suppressor as an early event [7]. As noted earlier, we have reported on unusual distributions of disease and coexistence of abnormalities in CA125 and CA27.29 in patients with a history of both breast cancer and ovarian cancer, leading to confusing clinical findings [2]. Also, perhaps because of their better outcome, patients with ovarian cancer and BRCA mutation may be on treatment longer than other women with this disease. This may account for the occasional development of other malignancies not usually associated with BRCA mutations, such as squamous carcinomas of head and neck origin, and with high incidence of renal complications and hypertension in up to 25% of patients on continuous treatment for more than 4 years [8]. This type of information may be relevant in addressing preventive issues for women with ovarian cancer and BRCA mutations.

Patients with Breast Cancer and BRCA Mutations

Breast cancer is much more amenable to surveillance than ovarian cancer, beginning with the expanded use of yearly mammography during the past 40 years. Mammographic screening in high-risk populations has begun before the age of 40, but its sensitivity has been hampered by the accompanying high mammographic density. To improve the sensitivity in the surveillance of high-risk population of women, attention has turned during the past decade to MRI. This imaging modality has aided in detecting cancer in premenopausal women and in the recognition of frequent multicentric disease within the breast. Studies have established the power of yearly MRI in avoiding the occurrence of interval cancers as a sensitive, specific tool for surveillance for both patients already carrying a diagnosis of breast cancer and their at-risk family members [3]. Its effectiveness in early detection has enhanced both the awareness and the detection of breast cancer problems in the population at large, more so in women diagnosed with these cancers at an early age and their families. Close communication between oncologists, genetic counselors, and other practitioners is needed to provide the best possible guidance to these women, and we elaborate on what has been learned by others.

Clinical Vignette 2

A powerful story has been told by one of two daughters of a woman who developed breast cancer in her 40s and, after navigating through the physical and emotional consequences of difficult surgery and adjuvant chemotherapy, went on to experience an intra-abdominal malignancy that would take her life within a decade. After witnessing the cruel illness that would take her mother's life, likely because of the then yet-to-be defined BRCA mutation–related breast-ovarian cancers, the daughter,

Jessica Queller, went on to tell how her mother's illness affected her decisions when she was to test positive for a BRCA mutation—decisions that she took very much on her own. This is described in her moving website: http://www.jessicaqueller.com/. Jessica's initial actions in obtaining genetic testing provided the very basis for the issues of doctor–patient communication in this setting and underscore the importance of effective communication that reaches out beyond the scientific issues.

The impact of genetic cancer risk assessment on communication of cancer risk information within families is not fully known but is emerging in part through such autobiographical descriptions. There is little research, however, in examining patient and family member responses to genetic information. Existing research on hereditary cancer syndromes can yield information on three major issues: (1) how patients understand their risk of disease following genetic counseling and testing; (2) their emotional responses to the information; and (3) their adoption of recommended risk-reducing strategies. Prior research suggests that genetic counseling and testing may improve patient understanding, but patients might still not fully understand the meaning of their results for disease risk. The exchange of information is at the core of cancer genetic counseling. Preferably, such exchange supports a "caring, professional relationship that offers guidance, but allows individuals and families to come to their own decisions," as put forward by the Proposed International Guidelines on Ethical Issues in Medical Genetics and Genetic Services (1998) [9].

Women with inherited BRCA1 or BRCA2 gene mutation have 56–83% risk of breast cancer by age 70, with substantial risk beginning at age 30. Subjects at high risk of inheriting a cancer may process risk information differently than the general population, likely because of their prior family experiences. However, little is known about clinical, demographic, or psychosocial predictors that impact risk perception in these groups. Many of these women will develop breast cancer at a young age, and oncologists need to be aware of the more pronounced issues in this age group, such as fear of death, loss of fertility, premature menopause, relationship stress, disruption of medical insurance coverage, and financial loss [10]. The American Society of Clinical Oncology (ASCO) has recommended that oncologists discuss fertility issues with young breast cancer patients who have not completed their families as soon as the possibility of a need for systematic adjuvant therapy becomes apparent [11, 12]. Unfortunately, many patients are not made aware of the fact that their treatment may compromise their fertility until treatment is completed. Today, there are several effective fertility preservation options available for patients. Embryo cryopreservation after in vitro fertilization is the most established method with live birth [11].

Breast cancer in pregnancy is expected to be more frequent among women with BRCA mutations. Management of pregnancy associated with breast cancer requires a multidisciplinary approach. Mammography, ultrasound, and breast surgery are safe in all trimesters. Breast feeding should be avoided if chemotherapy or tamoxifen are to be administered post partum. For young women diagnosed with breast cancer, the diagnosis is devastating. It may be difficult for them to share their concerns with their husbands and relatives. It is hard for them to take time off for surgery and accompanying systemic treatment when they are working, studying, trying to keep their business afloat, or looking after their young children.

Patients with Lynch Syndrome and Other High-Risk Situations

Increasingly, one is able to identify families carrying cancer-predisposing genes. Because cancers associated with Lynch syndrome lead to an array of cancers in both men and women, recognition is more difficult than those associated with deleterious BRCA mutations. Communication about cancer risks to both patients and their families is also more complex. Increasingly, however, awareness of susceptibility to colon cancers in both men and women, and of susceptibility to endometrial and, to a lesser extent, ovarian and breast cancers in women, is leading to screening recommendations. Since women carriers of mutations in one of the mismatch repair genes associated with Lynch syndrome have lifetime risks of 40–60% of developing endometrial cancer, it is important that gynecologists be involved in providing appropriate guidance and surveillance measures to these families. Henry Lynch's contributions to the science of uncovering these hereditary genes and to the families that have benefited from these efforts are being recognized at the two Joint Meetings on Hereditary Breast and Ovarian Cancers, which were organized by the Bari Cancer Institute Giovanni Paolo XXIII and New York University (co-chairs Angelo Paradiso and Franco Muggia, in 2009 and 2011).

Rarer genetic syndromes conferring enhanced lifetime risks towards a wide range of cancers pose many challenges to effective communication between physicians and patients or their families. These include Li-Fraumeni, Cowden, and Peutz-Jeghers syndromes, among others. As more is learned about pathogenetic mechanisms leading to improved treatments, educational measures will undoubtedly improve. Examples of using educational materials to enhance communication between groups at high-risk of cancer and health providers are described in the next section.

Educational Material for Women at Risk

In 2001, the Lynne Cohen High Risk Clinic opened a high-risk clinic at Bellevue Hospital Center, including New York University (NYU) School of Medicine faculty, as a service for underserved minority women at high risk for breast and ovarian cancer [1]. This program from the outset was free of charge, because it was initially conceived to couple service with research. At the time, it was the first in the New York tristate area (including New Jersey and Connecticut) to offer outreach, screening, and education to high-risk women. Women who feared that they were at high risk met a bilingual nurse who explained the sequence of the visit and assisted them in filling out a comprehensive clinical and research questionnaire. Visits were then arranged with a physician (often a medical oncologist or a gynecologist oncologist) and, if they were deemed possibly at high risk, with a genetic counselor. Because of the success at Bellevue, the Lynne Cohen Foundation for Ovarian Cancer Research decided in 2003 to fund the same program in the NYU Cancer Institute for insured women. In this program, the women are offered genetic testing when appropriate, surveillance, clinical trial opportunities, and support groups.

Finally, a consortium was formed under the Foundation's aegis to include three other institutions (University of Alabama, University of Southern California, and MD Anderson Cancer Center). This group, as well as NYU, collaborates in sharing assessment tools, educational goals, and maintenance of a registry for research purposes. As shown on the website of the Lynne Cohen Foundation for Ovarian Cancer Research, the three daughters of Lynne Cohen are at the helm of this organization, which is devoted to supporting research on screening and prevention of this disease: http://www.lynnecohenfoundation.org/.

The NYU Cancer Center has also been involved with the Memorial Sloan Kettering Cancer Center in Project Hope, an education and predictive/preventive program for women at risk of development of ovarian cancer. The mission is to reduce the incidence of ovarian cancer and improve outcomes for women treated for it as a result of research and education (www.projecthopeforovariancancer.com). An outgrowth of this collaboration has been the development of educational materials to enhance the awareness of the community-at-large toward ovarian cancer. It uses a graded approach in suggesting assessment tools tailored to the risk of individual women.

Similarly, in 2005 the Hollings Cancer Center received funding from the Wachovia Foundation to fund a 5-year breast cancer initiative to identify and provide clinical services for women at high risk for breast cancer. These funds support a nurse practitioner, educational materials, a genetic counselor, and other educational initiatives important to the success of the program. The aims of this service are to: (1) Provide education to women about risk factors, risk reduction, breast self-examination, and surveillance procedures in clinical and outreach interventions; (2) Provide genetic counseling and screening for women at high risk; (3) Devise and evaluate protocols for managing women at high risk; (4) Identify and evaluate women at high risk for developing breast cancer; (5) Provide emotional support to women and their family members who are at high risk; (6) Facilitate participation in research related to prevention, early diagnosis, and treatment. This group has been successful in launching major research initiatives in the pathology, epidemiology, and treatment of breast cancer.

In conclusion, as our recognition of hereditary risks for cancer continues to increase, it is important that health organizations keep pace in their communications with patients and their families about issues beyond cancer treatment, to prevention and surveillance. Educational materials reaching out to lay people and health practitioners will become an important vehicle for future communication.

References

1. Smith J, Baer L, Blank S, Dilawari A, Carapetyan K, Alvear M, et al. A screening and prevention program serving an ethically diverse population of women at high risk of developing breast and/or ovarian cancer. Ecancermedicalscience. 2009;3:123.
2. Dilawari A, Cangiarella J, Smith J, Huang A, Downey A, Muggia F. Co-existence of breast and ovarian cancers in BRCA germ-line mutation carriers. Ecancermedicalscience; 2009.
3. Warner E. Impact of MRI surveillance and breast cancer detection in young women with BRCA mutation. Ann Oncol. 2011;22 Suppl 1:144–9.

4. Tan DSP, Rothermundt C, Thomas K, Bancroft E, Eeles R, Shanley S, et al. "BRCAness" syndrome in ovarian cancer: a case–control study describing the clinical features and outcome of patients with epithelial ovarian cancer associated with *BRCA1* and *BRCA2* mutations. J Clin Oncol. 2008;26:5530–6.
5. Safra T, Borgato L, Nicoletto MO, Rolnitzky L, Avraham SP, Geva R, et al. BRCA mutation status and determinant of outcome in women with recurrent epithelial ovarian cancer treated with pegylated liposomal doxorubicin. In: American Society of Clinical Oncology-National Cancer Institute-European Organisation for research and treatment of cancer annual meeting on molecular markers in cancer. Hollywood, FL, 18–20 Oct 2010.
6. Calvert AH, Azzariti A. The clinical development of inhibitors of poly(ADP-ribose)polymerase (PARP). Ann Oncol. 2011;22 Suppl 1:i53–9.
7. Muggia F, Safra T, Dubeau L. Review: BRCA genes: lessons from experimental and clinical cancer. Ann Oncol. 2011;22 Suppl 1:i7–10.
8. Muggia F, Cannon T, Safra T, Curtin J. Delayed neoplastic and renal complications in women receiving long-term chemotherapy for recurrent ovarian cancer. J Natl Cancer Inst. 2011;103(2):160–1.
9. McBride CM, Kaphingst KA. Patient responses to genetic information: studies of patients with hereditary cancer syndromes identify issues for use of genetic testing in nephrology practice. Investigator Social and Behavioral Research Branch, National Human Genome Research Institute, Bethesda, MD. Semin Nephrol. 2010;30(2):203–14.
10. Ford D, Easton DF, Stratton M, et al. Genetic heterogeneity and penetrance analysis of the BRCA1 and BRCA2 genes in breast cancer families. Breast Cancer Linkage Consortium. Am J Hum Genet. 1998;62:676–89.
11. Lee SJ, Schover LR, Patridge AH, et al. American society of clinical oncology recommendations of fertility preservation in cancer patients. J Clin Oncol. 2006;24:2917–31.
12. Pieterse AH, van Dulmen AM, Ausems MGEM, Beemer FA, Bensing JM. Communication in cancer genetic counselling: does it reflect counselees' previsit needs and preferences? Br J Cancer. 2005;92:1671–8.

Part III
The Physician

Chapter 18
Physicians' Emotions in the Cancer Setting: A Basic Guide to Improving Well-Being and Doctor–Patient Communication

Maria Die Trill

Abstract It is common knowledge that confronting death is quite anxiety-provoking. Continued exposure to suffering, physical and mental deterioration, disfigurement, loss and pain elicits significant emotions in medical staff working in the oncology setting. In addition, disease chronicity, which facilitates the development of intense doctor–patient relationships, complex medical decision-making, and unconscious attitudes towards helping interact with clinical pressure and other factors and may result in tiredness, emotional confusion, helplessness, and lack of empathy, all of which may interfere in the staff's general sense of well-being as well as in their relationship with patients. Identifying and elaborating one's feelings adequately in this context, taking into account personality traits, personal history, and intrapsychic variables, is of primary importance for oncology staff members in order to develop efficient communication skills with patients and their families.

The purpose of this chapter is to provide some insight into the importance and the need of a basic "self-analysis" that can lead to an increased sense of well-being, enhanced skills in dealing with cancer, and improved doctor–patient communication in the cancer setting. Suggestions are provided as to what staff members can ask themselves in order to identify deep emotions that stem from the interaction of their daily work and their personal lives. Guidelines and suggestions as to how to manage certain personal and patient issues are provided as well. The need to focus on the satisfactions derived from working in oncology is emphasized.

Keywords Oncology staff • Staff emotions • Communication • Staff well-being • Burnout • Staff helplessness

M.Die Trill, PhD (✉)
Department of Oncology, Psycho-Oncology Unit, Hospital General Universitario
Gregorio Marañón, Calle Maiquez, 7, 28007 Madrid, Spain
e-mail: mdietrill@gmail.com

The practice of medicine is an art, not a trade;
A calling, not a business;
A calling in which your heart will be exercised equally with your head.

Sir William Osler

Introduction

Medical staff working in oncology are usually confronted with emotionally complex tasks on a daily basis. These experiences start early on, when medical students are put through a grueling course and exposed to death, pain, sickness, and what William Osler called the perplexity of the soul, at younger ages than most of their nonmedical peers. During the years that follow, doctors are encouraged to tackle difficult problems with inadequate support, having to pretend that they have more powers than they actually do [1]. Walking next to those suffering pain, physical and mental deterioration, losses, and death adds to the burden of difficult medical decision-making and ethical issues that staff is usually expected to deal with in a professional and efficient manner. It also turns communication with patients into situations that elicit complex feelings that are frequently difficult to handle.

Cancer has become a long, chronic disease in the past few years. Staff usually share intense, complex and at times, emotionally chaotic moments with patients and their families all along the oncological process, throughout continued and palliative care. The result of this sharing and accompanying is the development of relationships with deep levels of intimacy and bonding between health professionals, patients, and family members.

Stress, sadness, hopelessness, anger, and feelings of impotence occur, undeniably, in the oncology staff. Questions about their own professional skills, unconscious attitudes towards helping, and other issues involved in patient care play a significant role in how professionals deal with the difficulties related to working in oncology. In addition, the lack of time to grieve patient loss is very limited or even worse, nonexistent, for many oncology professionals. Due to an increased clinical pressure, among other things, doctors hardly have time to acknowledge and become aware of the feelings they develop that are associated with disease progression and with patients' deaths and losses.

The price for continued exposure to suffering, loss, and death; difficulties in identifying and elaborating one's own feelings adequately; and specific personality traits and intrapsychic variables is usually stress, tiredness, burnout, lack of empathy, and deteriorated communication skills with patients. The purpose of this chapter is to provide some insight into the importance and the need of a basic "self-analysis" that can lead to an increased sense of well-being, enhanced skills in dealing with cancer, and improvement in communication skills in the oncology setting. What are the most difficult issues for each physician in patient care and why are they more difficult for some workers than for their colleagues? Why do some suffer burnout, extreme helplessness, feelings of despair or sadness if they supposedly have voluntarily and freely chosen a caregiving profession? Why is it easier to help some patients or families than others? These and other relevant questions will be raised throughout the chapter. Guidelines and suggestions as to how to manage certain personal and patient issues are provided as well.

Despite this chapter referring to physicians working in oncology, most professionals involved in cancer care experience all or some of the feelings described below: mental health professionals, nurses, etc. Most of what is described here could be applied to all. However, physicians must deal with several tasks that ordinarily only they undertake. For example, the author believes that probably one of the most difficult tasks doctors are confronted with is the personal relationship and communication with the patient, because it entails a significant emotional load that is frequently difficult to deal with and for which physicians, as other professionals, have not been provided with the necessary skills. Deciding what treatment protocol a patient should receive is the result of a rational decision-making process based on scientific evidence and usually supported by a medical team. Telling a patient he has developed new metastatic disease implies confronting one's own feelings and simultaneously dealing with those of the patient in a one-to-one situation. It is the responsibility of the doctor to inform of a cancer diagnosis, of disease progression, of treatment failure, and of the need to initiate palliative care while caring medically for the patient and dealing with his own and the patients' feelings. Not an easy task to perform.

Professionals' Feelings in Cancer Care

Can any doctor honestly say that he has never felt bored or irritated, attracted or interested in certain patients? Do we not, at times, resent the demands of people for whom the disease seems to have become a way of life? [2]. In addition to such feelings that are common in the medical environment, intense relationships with cancer patients and their families usually develop within brief periods of time in the oncology setting. It is quite difficult to walk through the complex cancer experience without feeling at least part of the sadness, despair, and anguish that patients experience and that characterizes the disease process, irrespective of its prognosis. Moving from one loss to another, from one death to another exposes physicians to suffering and frequently, death, in a continued manner. Oncology professionals, however, tend to not give themselves the necessary time and "permission" to identify and deal with their own emotions, let alone grief. They usually do not have the skills to develop new insights as to what their feelings are in specific situations with patients and their families, and therefore are limited in their ability to elaborate these emotions. Unresolved emotional tension may tend to accumulate.

Personality traits and intrapsychic variables are important sources of physician distress as well. For example, the need to attend to everyone's needs but their own will adversely impact on medical staff. Frequently, such an attitude is generalized and maintained throughout nonprofessional relationships. It is not infrequent for staff to become the reference for friends and family when these encounter difficulties.

Generally, professionals expect much more of themselves than they would ask of others around them. As a consequence, they not only care for their patients in their work environment, but tend to behave as caretakers in their daily personal lives.

Caring for the severely ill and dying may elicit significant distress in the physician who has not resolved his unconscious feelings of omnipotence [3]. Spikes and Holland [4] describe the ways in which the omnipotent healer reacts to the seriously ill and dying patient. These feelings of omnipotence may find expression in the physician's image as the powerful healer, as indestructible, and/or as a destructive force. And each of these attitudes may, in turn, have adverse effects on his ability to provide optimal care for the patient. For example, a physician who experiences death anxiety without being aware of it may respond with false reassurance or with avoidance to patients' questions about prognosis, especially when it is poor. Other physicians may respond with a definite answer to the question when actually it is impossible to predict the temporal outcome of the patient's disease. The physician in this case gives little consideration to what the particular question may mean to that specific patient. However, by responding in these inappropriate ways, he wards off his disappointment with his professional fallibility and preserves his image as a "powerful almighty healer." On the long run, the physician will tend to experience feelings of personal failure, frustration, hopelessness and helplessness, and anger. This tends to occur when a physician feels he has nothing left to offer a patient with advanced illness who he believes "will die despite anything that I do." It will not be until the doctor becomes aware of the numerous things that he has already done and can still do for the patient that he will become more conscious of his feelings of despair that resulted from his need to succeed by saving the patient from dying. The doctor in this case has not evaluated his caretaking abilities in a realistic manner and was, therefore, unaware of his limitations as a professional. Too often healthcare professionals have high demands on themselves and great difficulty respecting their own limits. The duty in the healthcare domain is to cure patients when possible, and to care for those that cannot be cured [5].

Being exposed to advanced and terminal illness in a continued manner may elicit death wishes in the professional who views himself as a powerful healer. The physician may even feel angry towards patients who refuse further treatment and express their wish to be left alone to die. In this case, anger follows his feelings of guilt and self-reproach. Such death wishes stem from the fact that the physician views the patient as a constant reminder of his inadequacy [4]. Other times and in places where the doctor–patient relationship responds to a more hierarchical model, the physician may respond inappropriately when confronted with obsessive-type patients who make "too many questions" about their disease. The doctor here may feel that his medical knowledge or more so, his medical skills, are being questioned.

Confronting death is quite anxiety-provoking. Empathizing with the dying exacerbates such anxiety and confronts the physician with his own death. This is particularly the case with physicians caring for patients with whom they share certain characteristics and/or identity (i.e., age, profession, social status, cultural background, etc.). Anger or, on the other hand, excessive compassion and false reassurance may result from this process.

The physician's image of himself as so powerful that he can cure is related to his image of himself as a destructive force: if he can cure, he can also harm. A conscious derivative of his attitude are his worries that he may harm the patient, especially when treating him with potent pharmacologic agents or a complex surgical procedure or treatment [3]. These fears may also become evident in the communication process with the patient, where the physician may fear hurting the patient with negative medical information such as a poor prognosis, advancing disease, or by responding with honesty to questions such as "How soon will I die?" in the context of a poor prognosis.

Different authors have tried to explain why some people develop traits that lead them to choose caretaking professions. For example, human behavior tends to repeat itself in situations in which there are unresolved unconscious conflicts. Salvation fantasies have been described among professional caretakers as a product of psychological adaptation to an early childhood trauma, which can be a loss, a deception, etc., in the context of object relations in infancy [6, 7]. Such relations are positive and intense and their disruption is experienced as profound and permanent (for example, the birth of a new sibling that displaces attention from parents or primary caretakers). The result of this complex psychological process is a series of personality traits that include profound sympathy towards suffering together with an obligation to rescue and alleviate, and egocentric traits. Among the "negative" aspects of this process Atwood [7] has described difficulty in developing emotional intimacy: the person learns to give but has difficulty receiving. Dependent personalities are therefore common among caretakers, although dependency is not consciously experienced. Eliott and Guy [8] reported that parentified children internalize a caretaking role and later fulfill, by means of their profession, their need of closeness and intimacy that were not met in childhood. In another study, Paris and Frank [9] reported that medical students were more likely to have experienced medical illness in their family and concluded that traumas of childhood are "repaired" by giving to others in adulthood what they would have wanted to give or be given as a child. Unresolved issues related to one's own trajectory may also catch the clinician in an "impossible mission" according to Stiefel [5], which can exhaust him unless acknowledged, worked through, and integrated.

Oncology staff have also been described as significantly resilient as well [10]. Resiliency is an innate energy or motivating life force present to varying degrees in every individual, exemplified by the presence of particular traits or characteristics that, through application of dynamic processes, enables an individual to cope with, recover from, and grow as a result of stress or adversity. The avoidance of suffering observed in those not working in healthcare professions may lead us to believe that oncology staff have an impressive ability to tolerate suffering, more so than the general population.

It is therefore not surprising to find up to 30% of medical oncologists suffering from psychiatric morbidity, twice as much prevalence as identified in the general population, and up to one third of clinicians reporting high levels of emotional exhaustion, lack of motivation, and low levels of personal achievement [11].

Some Relevant Questions: Proposal of an Introductory Guide to Self-Analysis

Training health professionals with communication skills training programs is a promising approach to changing negative attitudes and improving doctor–patient communication skills in the cancer setting [12]. However, the author believes that communication skills training needs to necessarily be accompanied by a basic exercise of introspection in which the professional ought to find honest responses to some basic questions and issues that he needs to confront. Taking time to respond to the following may throw some light into many inner feelings. Their identification will facilitate the understanding of physicians' reactions to various patients and situations that are encountered in the work situation. It will also potentiate the development of optimal management of one's own emotions in the complex oncology setting, the result being enhanced relationships with patients, families, and an increased sense of personal and professional well-being. This does not intend to be an exhaustive guide to self-questioning. The purpose is rather to provide the reader with some basic initial questions and issues that may give place to more thorough and elaborate psychotherapeutic work, guided by a professional.

- *Questions about one's personal career choice*: One should initially raise questions that will allow him to understand why he has chosen a caretaking profession. This will enable the caretaker to identify his original motivations. The influence of early development and life trajectory on career choice has already been illustrated [5, 8, 9]. It may well be that health caretakers have chosen their particular work for reasons such as resolving past losses, relieving feelings of guilt, trying to give new meaning to their lives, assuming a sense of special calling, or proving that they can care for the seriously ill better than others cared for their own ill relatives. A sense of disillusionment with previous jobs or professions or a need to prove to oneself or others that one is competent has also been identified as a motivating factor [13].

    – Identify the factors that you believe led you to choose your profession. What comes to your mind when you ask yourself: "Why did I choose this profession initially?"
    – Have family expectations or variables influenced your decision? In what manner?
    – Did any early experience with illness or death influence your career choice? In what way?
    – Have you ever felt guilty about having/not having behaved in a specific manner, for example? Can that have influenced your career choice? Does "saving" or helping people relieve your guilt feelings?

- *Expectations and awareness of professional limitations*: Too often healthcare professionals have high demands on themselves and a great difficulty in respecting their own limits as to what they can do [5]. Identifying one's expectations in the workplace can facilitate acknowledging one's own limitations.

- Think of the time in your life when you first decided to become a caretaker. What were your aims, hopes, and expectations?
- Is the work you perform similar to what you imagined it would be before starting to work? How is it different from your initial expectations?
- What were your expectations of yourself in the care of the severely ill or dying patients when you started working as a professional caretaker?
- Which are the most difficult aspects of your job? Why do you think they are difficult for you? How do you confront such difficulties?
- Had you anticipated encountering such difficulties before starting your job?
- How would you define success in your job? Do you consider yourself a successful professional? Why? Do you consider you have fulfilled your initial expectations regarding your performance?
- What are your limitations in the workplace? How do you feel when you think about them?
- Can you identify a patient or situation that made you feel limited professionally? How did you manage the situation and your own personal feelings?

- *Grief-related issues*: Identifying what we feel in the context of continued exposure to loss and death is an important issue. Sooner or later, those who avoid conscious grief collapse, usually with some form of depression [14]. Grieving is a necessary psychological process if we want to avoid dragging the pain throughout a lifetime. Avoidance of grief together with feelings of helplessness that easily tend to develop in oncology is usually a setup for burnout and disillusionment in the workplace. Past losses, especially if unresolved, can lead to difficulty when individuals are constantly confronted with death. There is some evidence, for example, that early parental death may predispose individuals to become depressed when exposed to later loss situations [15]. In addition, unresolved grief can precipitate a delayed grief reaction, which can be triggered quite unexpectedly, particularly in circumstances similar to the first loss. However, it should be mentioned that persons who have never suffered any losses or who have seldom had to test their capacity to cope under adverse conditions may experience great distress when confronted with numerous deaths [13]. Becoming aware of the meaning of each patient loss is therefore of utmost importance.

  - Is there anything that you do after a patient with whom you had a long or intense relationship dies or is referred to a different professional or medical team? In other words, how do you grieve patient loss? Why?
  - Does the above help you give some closure or grieve efficiently? Is there anything that could help you deal with the loss in a more effective way?
  - Can you identify what specific patient losses have meant to you? Can you understand why they have affected you in the way they have?
  - Does confrontation with death and loss in the workplace elicit feelings related to previous losses in your life?
  - What previous experiences have you had with death in your personal life? How have they affected you? How have they influenced your attitude towards death in the cancer setting? Do they affect the care you provide dying patients? In what ways?

- *Transference and countertransference*: Transference is a psychoanalytic concept that refers to the unconscious feelings the patient experiences towards his analyst during psychotherapy. Transference is experienced by patients towards their physician in the medical setting. That is the case of patients who "fall in love" with their doctors. Such feelings are the echo of reactions that the patient experienced during his childhood towards a significant person. Transference can be positive (e.g., love, affection, admiration, etc.) or negative (e.g., anger, frustration). Countertransference refers to the feelings that the therapist inadequately projects onto the patient and that are also "remains" of past relationships. One difference between countertransference and identification with a patient is that the former is the result of an unconscious process, while the latter is conscious. Keep in mind that transference and countertransference are only two of the many variables that affect relationships to patients. However, some questions one may want to ask himself in an effort to identify what may (or may not) be the result of countertransference are as follows [16]:

    - Did I ever feel depressed or angry during or after an interaction with a patient?
    - Have I ever felt the need to impress a patient or be considered "special" by him/her?
    - Have I ever felt that nobody can care for a specific patient better than I can?
    - Have I ever found myself repeatedly arguing with the same patient? Why?
    - Have I ever experienced feelings of significant affection or anger repeatedly towards a specific patient?
    - If the response to any of the above is affirmative, you may want to ask yourself why you think you responded in such ways to patients. Can you identify why you experienced such feelings and reactions?
    - Have you experienced such feelings/reactions in the past, with a significant person in your life? Can you define who the patient represented for you or who he/she reminded you of?
    - Can you define a relationship between your reactions in the past and those occurring later on in the workplace?
    - Can you identify any personal, unsatisfied needs that you may unconsciously have expected to satisfy through your interaction with a patient?
    - Have you or any of your patients suffered because of countertransference issues?

- *Issues related to helplessness*: Feeling helpless is a common reaction to cancer and its treatments. Helplessness is not always consciously experienced since it may confront us with our personal and professional limitations. However, it may adversely affect optimal patient care as well as the physician's sense of well-being and professional achievement.

    - Have you ever experienced feelings of helplessness while carrying out your work?
    - When do you recall feeling helpless for the first time in your work with cancer patients? Describe the patient or situation.

- How did you deal with such feelings of helplessness? Did you share them with anyone? With whom? How did this person react?
 - Which of the following generate or increase your feelings of helplessness: (a) Any specific type of tumor or disease process? Specify which one. (b) A particular type of patient or family (e.g., unadapted families; patients or family members with specific personality traits, physical appearance, age, etc.)? (c) Patients or family members belonging to any specific social, cultural, or ethnic group? Specify which. (d) Patients or family members that behave in a certain manner, e.g., the hostile patient, the quiet patient, etc.
 - How do you recognize feelings of helplessness in yourself when working with cancer patients? In other words, what are the first manifestations of such feelings?
 - What measures, if any, do you adopt to prevent the development of feelings of helplessness and to avoid the interference of such feelings with optimal patient care?
 - If you cannot identify a situation where you experienced feelings of helplessness in the oncology setting, how have you avoided them?

Discovering patterns in our responses to specific patients, families, or situations in the medical setting may well be a major first step in identifying significant insights. For example, one may realize that he tends to respond with anger repeatedly when confronted with the serious illness or impending death of older female patients. One may then question what woman/women in his life has suffered a serious illness or died, and what feelings and behavior this situation elicited in him. Did the individual feel helpless, impotent, and frustrated for not being able to alleviate the suffering of this significant woman in his past life? Is the current response to dying females in the cancer setting related in some way, to the previous life experience? The answer is most likely, affirmative. Identifying such patterns of behavior will help us respond in more appropriate ways to patients and their families, and will enhance self-understanding.

Where Does One Go from Here? Some Basic Suggestions

Communication skills training is a basic first step in finding effective ways of communicating with cancer patients, feeling more effective in doing so, and reducing feelings of helplessness throughout the communication process. However and as previously mentioned, in addition to participating in such training programs where skills and knowledge of specific communication techniques are acquired, additional steps are necessary in order to handle emotions efficiently.

Identification of and working through intrapsychic stressors can considerably reduce psychological distress in the professional and thus provide effective, long-lasting support of the oncology clinician. The more we are aware of our emotions, the less we are emotion-driven and able to perceive a given situation adequately [5].

Dealing with our feelings however is not an easy task, especially if these are considered unwanted or undesirable. After identifying specific emotions that tend to arise in specific patient encounters, we may not know how to behave or how to deal with such uncovered feelings. Where we go from here will depend on multiple variables. Some may choose to block such feelings, ward them off once again, fearing that they will experience an emotional overload that they will be unable to control. These professionals will not move forward in their approach to patients and difficult situations. Others, on the other hand, may decide to elaborate the newly identified emotions, work through them in ways that will enhance their relationship to patients, and facilitate the communication process with them. If the doctor understands how he feels in situations that are uncomfortable for him and why he feels that way, he will be able to control such unpleasant feelings and focus more effectively on the patient and on the task he is to perform.

Some may choose to consult a mental health professional in order to give some meaning to their new "emotional discoveries." Others may want to deal with them on their own. Yet others may find great support when sharing their work-related emotions with colleagues at the workplace. Consultation with a mental health professional may take place on an individual or group format. For example, weekly staff meetings with a psycho-oncologist may foster supportive relationships among staff members that make it easier for them to deal with their feelings. According to Spikes and Holland [4] the psycho-oncologist may:

(a) Encourage the staff to ventilate their feelings towards specific patients under their care and attempt to foster awareness of the origins of these attitudes
(b) Employ reality testing with the staff to help to convince them that their feelings of worthlessness and despair have an irrational basis; to reduce their feelings of guilt, and to enable them to function more effectively
(c) Encourage open expression of grief about the impending or actual loss of particular patients
(d) Emphasize the use of a team approach in the medical setting such that the staff can support the professional responsible for the care of a specific patient
(e) Encourage doctors to find their own level of tolerance for dealing with difficult patients and the feelings they evoke

Following the Socratic dictum "Know thyself," it remains clear that recognition and analysis of personal feelings is therefore imperative in the cancer setting. Access to feelings and fantasies and abilities to communicate needs must however be in balance with an ability to maintain adequate defenses against stresses evoked by the disease, hospitalization, and death.

Learning to share the responsibility of care with coworkers is essential and will decrease the possibility of a staff member feeling overburdened. It also implies that one is aware of his own limitations as a professional specialized in cancer care. Setting limits may be difficult for some professionals, especially in work environments that demand meeting the total physical, psychological, and spiritual needs of patients and families. Defining why one has difficulties in setting such limits (e.g., need for recognition and approval, etc.) may be an excellent starting point. Recognizing that one cannot cope with a specific patient or situation is not a sign of weakness but rather, of maturity, and enables the medical professional to withdraw before reaching the saturation point and/or to define more effective ways of handling the situation and his own feelings. As Holmes [2] illustrates, the search for the good doctor is an illusion. Psychoanalyst Winnicott [17] reassured mothers that to be "good enough" was preferable to striving to be ideal. Mothers who are good enough provide children with the opportunity to learn to cope effectively with disappointment and failure in the context of love. Similarly, if the physician can, without complacency, bring his good and bad parts together to become a good enough doctor, he should be content, as his patients will be, despite sometimes feeling let down by him.

Providing continuity of care is another task at times difficult to carry out: overspecialization of oncology professionals places the patient in a position in which he is referred from one specialist to another throughout the cancer process, and places the physician in a position in which he cannot provide care at all times throughout the disease. Depending on his attitude towards death, for example, it may either be alleviating or distressing for a medical oncologist to be unable to care for a terminally ill patient that he has become attached to during the treatment phase because he is to be followed by a palliative care professional at the end of his life. Occasionally visiting the patient or making brief telephone calls during the palliative treatment, despite not treating him medically, may facilitate closure and mourning and may reduce the physician's sense of abandoning the patient or not caring for him at a difficult time.

Finding strategies for coping with grief is also imperative in the cancer setting in order to avoid accumulation of unresolved losses as well as the development of chronic sorrow. The first step towards this sometimes difficult process is to acknowledge the loss and explore its meaning and the feelings associated with it. Going through the feelings that the loss entails, as difficult as this may be, is necessary to give some closure. Identifying how past losses affect the present ones as well as defining rituals to acknowledge the loss also help. Coming to grips with one's concept of life and death should precede this psychological work.

Increasing the physician's perception of control is essential. Cancer is a disease that reduces this perception. Setting up realistic treatment goals, becoming aware of one's own limitations in controlling the disease as described above, and identifying the things that one does to cure the patient or improve his quality of life are of fundamental importance.

Identifying what have been described as "great moments in helping" can often reveal one's purpose in helping. Thinking of helping situations that have touched the professional most profoundly reminds him of his mission as a helper [18].

Satisfaction Derived from Working in Oncology

In order to balance our feelings in the workplace, professionals must not overlook the satisfaction derived from working in the cancer setting. As important as identifying one's own fears, frustrations, and pain is to become aware of what keeps professionals going, what the sources of job satisfaction are in working with those that suffer and sometimes die. Among these sources of satisfaction medical staff should remember:

- It is a privilege to share intense and private moments with patients and their families.
- Professionals have an opportunity to play an important role during critical moments of patients' and families' lives, and are in a unique position to help them navigate throughout the cancer process.
- Working in the cancer setting places professionals in a highly valued social group.
- Not everyone can tolerate exposure to suffering as much as the medical staff nor can dedicate their professional life to cancer. This enables the development of a feeling of being special in some way.
- Confronting life and death issues helps prioritize and value important aspects of life in addition to accelerating a process of emotional maturity.
- One may repress the frustration that emerges at times in the cancer setting, or may choose to feel sufficiently strong to be generous.
- One may feel emotional numbness in the face of suffering, but may also choose to tolerate the human condition.
- One may run away from emotionally charged patient encounters, but may also feel privileged to share extraordinary moments.
- One may experience guilt feelings or may decide to experience a special gratitude and a refined appreciation of life.
- One may feel intellectually overwhelmed or may choose to feel intellectually challenged in their daily tasks.

References

1. Smith R. All doctors are problem doctors. BMJ. 1997;314:841.
2. Holmes J. Good doctor, bad doctor—a psychodynamic approach. BMJ. 2002;325:722–3.
3. Friedman HJ. Physician management of dying patients: an exploration. Psychiatry Med. 1970;1:295–305.
4. Spikes J, Holland J. The physician's response to the dying patient. 2011. http://internationalpsychoanalysis.net/wp-content/uploads/2011/04/StrainPowerpoint11. Accessed 15 Apr 2011.
5. Stiefel F. Support of the supporters. Support Care Cancer. 2008;16(2):123–6.
6. Stolorow RD, Atwood GE. Messianic projects and early object relations. Am J Psychoanal. 1973;33(2):213–5.
7. Atwood GE. On the origins and dynamics of messianic salvation fantasies. Int Rev Psycho Anal. 1978;5:85–96.
8. Eliott DM, Guy JD. Mental health professionals versus non-mental health professionals: childhood trauma and adult functioning. Prof Psychol Res Pract. 1993;24:83–90.
9. Paris J, Frank H. Psychological determinants of a medical career. Can J Psychiatry. 1983;28:354–7.
10. Grafton E, Gillespie B, Henderson S. Resilience: the power within. Oncol Nurs Forum. 2010;37(6):698–705.
11. Ramirez AJ, Graham J, Richards MA, Cull A, Gregory WM. Mental health of hospital consultants: the effects of stress and satisfaction at work. Lancet. 1996;347:724–8.

12. Barthe J, Lannen P. Efficacy of communication skills training courses in oncology: a systematic review and meta analysis. Ann Oncol. 2011;22(5):1030–40.
13. Vachon M. Staff stress in hospice care. In: Davidson GW, editor. The hospice: development and administration (chapter 6). Washington, DC: Hemisphere Publishing Company; 1985. p. 111–27.
14. Bowlby J. Attachment and loss. Loss, sadness and depression, vol. 3. London: The Hogarth Press and the Institute of Psychoanalysis; 1980.
15. Brown G, Harris TJ, Copeland JR. Depression and loss. Br J Psychiatry. 1977;130:1–18.
16. Relling-Garskof K. Transferring the past to the present. Am J Nurs. 1987;87:477–8.
17. Winnicott D. Transitional objects and transitional phenomena. London: Tavistock; 1951.
18. Larson D. The helper's journey. Working with people facing grief, loss and life-threatening illness. Brunsville, NV: Research Press; 1993.

Chapter 19
The Setting, the Truth, and the Dimensions of Communication with Cancer Patients

Ursula Klocker-Kaiser and Johann Klocker

Abstract The basis of any human coexistence is communication. Communication is also the basis of every therapeutic action. The more severe and threatening the illness is, the more important the communicative interaction between the affected persons (the patient and his family) and the medical professional or team. According to Watzlawick it is not possible not to communicate; therefore, it is wise to concede special significance to the communication between patient and medical professional and thus to support the therapeutic action. At the centre of communication between patient and medical professional is talk about information, in the so-called pretreatment interview, which is never easy. This presents both the bearer as well as the recipient of bad, life-threatening news with a heavy emotional burden.

Keywords Communication • Family members • Relevant truth • Holistic approach

The Setting: Several Short Conversations Including Family and Nursing Staff

The pretreatment interview should be carried out by the attending physician with the patient. Experience shows that it is very beneficial when information is transmitted in several short talks rather than in a single, usually long one. Because of the subject matter and emotional weight of what is being said, the patient often cannot grasp the information in an initial conversation. This is probably a self-defence mechanism of humans (life-threatening news does not register because of the emotional overload). This makes further conversations and opportunities to ask questions necessary.

U. Klocker-Kaiser, MD • J. Klocker, MD, Ph.D (✉)
Klinikum Klagenfurt am Wörthersee, St. Veiterstrasse 47, Klagenfurt 9020, Austria
e-mail: u.klocker@kabeg.at; j.klocker@kabeg.at

With the patient's consent it is advisable to include nursing staff (nurses, carers) and family members in further talks.

The advantages of including nursing staff are as follows:

- The implicit permission to ask the nursing staff questions
- The possibility for the nursing staff to pass on information to patients because the information status is known
- In this way a team is presented (doctor-nurse/carer)

Including family members has these advantages:

- The information is given to the family, and the content can be discussed with the patient within the family.
- The information is thus consolidated within the family, and there is greater understanding about what has been said.
- The support of the family can thus be encouraged and accordingly strengthened.

In principle, conversations with family members should always be carried out in the presence of the patient. One-to-one talks with family members should be the exception. Even if the patient and family members receive the same information in separate conversations, there is a different understanding of what has been said because of differences in perception and suppression. This situation can easily lead to speechlessness within the family (differently understood information separates). The family wants to spare the patient, and the patient wants to spare the family. However, if the patient and family members talked together, a clear basis for discussion within the family is created.

The Truth

Without a doubt, the patient should encounter openness and honesty. It would be arrogant to believe that in such a difficult situation—as contact with the ill is—it would be possible to "lie mercifully". Since not only words but the whole person communicates, deviating from the truth constitutes a fundamental imbalance and is not suitable as a means of communicating with the ill.

It is therefore not a question of whether the seriously ill should or should not be informed of the truth; it is a matter of introducing the truth at the right time and in the right measure when talking to the patient. This requires a high degree of sensitivity and readiness to reflect.

Three principles can be defined for dealing with the truth:

Assessment of the Patient's Capacity to Comprehend

One can inform a patient of a truth only if he/she is capable of comprehending it. To avoid giving either too much or too little, the main focus of the pretreatment interview should be toward determining, how much truth can be given to this patient at this moment? "It can also be inhuman to, as it were, force knowledge about a person's death on him and thus to put him in a state of hopelessness" [2].

Focus on the Relevant Truth

A widely held philosophical position nowadays views truth as relative. This concept seems dubious to us when dealing with the ill. We find the concept of *relevant truth* more suitable. The dialogue with the patient should be guided toward those aspects that are relevant for his/her recovery and also for his/her future lifestyle and plans. These aspects can be recognised only in a detailed discussion with the patient or the patient and his/her family. Relevant truth is a dynamic concept.

Holistic Approach

Limiting treatment to the physical aspects of disease can only be reductionist. This results in curing for the sake of the cure. In the process the search for meaning is all too easily excluded. Being committed to the truth, the attending physician must also be prepared to deal with its emotional, intellectual, and spiritual aspects if the patient so wishes. In principle, the patient should not be left alone with his/her questions.

The Three Dimensions of Communication

The dimensions of dialogue in a conversation between medical or nursing staff and patients and their family members as defined by Meerwein in 1985—*emotional warmth, patient centredness, information content*—remain a helpful framework (Fig. 19.1).

This means that the information, the cognitive-verbal part of a conversation, is only one component of the communication; there are other important components of

Fig. 19.1 The three dimensions of a doctor (or nursing staff)—patient conversation (I, W, P) according to Meerwein (1985)

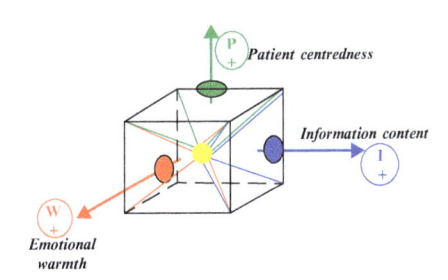

the communication in the emotional-nonverbal domain. This also means that if the cognitive-verbal and the emotional-nonverbal messages are not consistent with one another, the message does not register, because more importance is attached to the nonverbal-emotional aspect of the information. It also means that every communication has a factual and a relationship aspect, and the relationship aspect in turn determines how the content is received. Thus information can be taken in only when *attention to the patient* and *emotional warmth* form the basis of its communication.

When doctor and patient are first getting to know one another, the nonverbal dimensions of their dialogue dominate, while the informational content remains largely in the background. As already mentioned, particularly in the case of emotionally draining news, the information does not register. For this reason alone it makes sense to have several short conversations (step-by-step information). In the initial conversations the dimensions *emotional warmth* and *patient centredness* should be emphasised, thus preparing the way for the dimension of *informational content*. In further conversations it is possible to have an informational talk based on a well-prepared interactive basis.

Seven thoughts on communication between medical professionals and people affected by cancer are:

- Clarification and information are—if presented thoughtfully with appropriate emotional warmth and regard for the individual—stress reducing. As a result the patient feels accepted and valued.
- Hope can and should be communicated by focusing on the best possible progress.
- Natural compassion (not pity) should be the basis for the communicative interaction.
- Acknowledging the momentary situation and setting positive, even if small, goals are the central focus.
- Caring inquiries (e.g., What does this mean for you?) are appropriate. Breaks in the conversation give the patient emotional space.
- Offer further support.
- Good communication saves time.

References

1. Bräutigam W, Meerwein F. Das therapeutische Gespräch mit Krebskranken. Bern: Fortschritte der Psychoonkologie Hans Huber; 1995.
2. Frankl VE. Anthropologische Grundlagen der Psychotherapie. Bern: Hans Huber; 1975.
3. Holland JC. The human side of cancer. New York: HarperCollins; 2001.
4. Klocker JG, Klocker-Kaiser U, Schwaninger M. Truth in the relationship between cancer patient and physician. Ann N Y Acad Sci. 1997;809:56–65.
5. Schulz KH, Schulz H. Krebspatienten und ihre Familien. Stuttgart: Schattauer; 1998.
6. Senn HJ. Wahrhaftigkeit am Krankenbett bei Tumorpatienten. Thieme, Stuttgart: Onkologie für Krankenpflegeberufe; 1992.
7. Watzlawick P, Beavin JH. The pragmatics of human communication. New York: Norton; 1967.

Chapter 20
Improving Communication Effectiveness in Oncology: The Role of Emotions

Maria Antonietta Annunziata and Barbara Muzzatti

Abstract Through communication, physicians disclose to their interlocutors (who become *patients*) the course of their disease (with the diagnosis), and again through communication doctors announce the recovery from disease, or its progression, or the helplessness of medicine in coping with it. Communication in medicine has, then, very strong ethical and personal implications that inevitably include personal interpretations of life and suffering, as well as the establishment of a genuine doctor–patient relationship and listening to and recognizing the patients' and one's own emotions. Emotions represent an important aspect of the communicative task of physicians. In the present chapter (1) we will introduce the doctor–patient relationship as an element intrinsic to communication and its emotional aspects; (2) we will describe the principal emotions of patients along the disease course, as this is marked by various medical communications; (3) we will then focus on the subject of physicians' emotions, and (4) list the principal strategies and resources that emotions (both doctors' and patients') will or should stimulate in physicians themselves. Increasing communication efficacy, improving the doctor–patient relationship, and adherence to therapy, as well as reaching greater well-being both in patients and in healthcare providers are the principal reasons that should encourage physicians to focus on this communicative-relational element and to look for occasions for specific training.

Keywords Cancer • Communication • Emotion • Professional relationship • Oncology
• Bad news

M.A. Annunziata (✉) • B. Muzzatti
Centro Di Riferimento Oncologico Aviano, National Cancer Institute,
Unit of Oncological Phsychology, Aviano, PN, Italy
e-mail: annunziata@cro.it

Introduction

It has been estimated that an oncologist will give on average 35 pieces of bad news a month, thus achieving the remarkable number of 20,000 during the course of a career [1, 2]. Communication is a medical action, comparable to a technical and technical-specialist practice, even if it is often taken for granted as being peculiar to Man and should therefore be a "natural" skill. Through communication, physicians disclose to their interlocutors (who become patients) the course of their disease (with a diagnosis), and again through communication doctors announce the recovery or the progression of disease or even the helplessness of medicine in coping with it.

Communication in medicine has, then, very strong ethical and personal implications that inevitably include personal interpretations of life and suffering, the establishment of a genuine patient–physician relationship, and the ability of recognizing and listening to patients' and one's own emotions. Healthcare providers seem to be increasingly aware of the difficulties in this task. They point out the necessity of specific training on this issue [1, 3] by reporting as particularly difficult the discussion of topics of strong emotional impact, such as the high cost of drugs for patients they know cannot afford them and topics relating to treatment failure [2]. During medical visits, these difficulties may be observed in the little importance given to the emotional and psychosocial content of discussions compared to their biomedical and organizational content [4], even though the literature is unanimous (e.g., [5]) in showing that patients elicit, appreciate, and pursue the possibility of venting their own experiences and emotions in their care process. The attention paid to emotional issues, as opposed to cognitive and informative issues, seems to correlate with satisfaction and trust in patients and with requests for further information, adherence to therapy, and better quality of life [6–9]. For example, literature data show that patient-focused communication is associated with more important and significant health results [10]. A communicative style focused on patients includes empathy, reassurance, and active listening [11] and can improve the psychological adaptation of patients [12–15], their capacity for making decisions, adherence to therapy, and satisfaction with treatment [16]. Patients who have been given the opportunity to discuss their emotions with a caring staff member have been shown to have less distress than those not given this opportunity [17]. They also seem to have a better understanding of their disease and show improvement in remembering information [18–20].

Emotions, then, represent an important aspect of the physicians' communication task. In the following sections, we will introduce the doctor–patient relationship as an intrinsic element of communication and its emotional aspects; we will then describe the principal emotions of patients along the disease course, the steps of which are marked by various medical communications; we will subsequently focus on the subject of the physicians' emotions and will finally list the principal strategies and resources that emotions (doctors' and patients') should stimulate in physicians themselves.

Even though we tend to differentiate emotions, mood states, and feelings according to the length and degree of reactivity to a circumscribed and recognizable event (see, for instance, [21]), on these pages we will employ the term "emotion" in its broader sense, meaning all that belongs to the affective-emotional sphere of individuals in contraposition with rationality. Talking about emotions means focusing on the physiological, cognitive, and behavioral activation that follows a stressful event; on behavioral styles (cf. the construct of emotion-focused coping); on what involves any life experience and consequently the course of disease as well. In oncology, the disease path is marked by several phases, each validated by a medical communication. To make this communication effective and to assure the recipient's, as well as the sender's, well-being, the physician must take into consideration the emotions that the content of the communication itself may elicit. In oncology, we define as "bad news" those communications in which the adjective "bad" defines the emotional impact of the communication content.

The Emotions in the Physician–Patient Relationship

A relationship is a situation of mutual influence between two individuals that involves their emotions, expectations, motivations, and values—that is, with all that pertains to their own subjectivity. A good relationship—where the evocation of life experiences and events and transferring one's experiences (the unveiling of intimate life experiences) to the interlocutor are possible—can be achieved through communication that starts from the recognition of the Other as a human being and then accepts everything the Other brings along, emotions included.

The relationship is "real" and produces mutual personal evolution (Balint). After the relationship, in fact, the interlocutors are different: they each share something about the other person on the subject of their communication.

The relationship is the fundamental element in all specialties of medicine and in all environments, but it is more difficult where the space and time given to the relationship are narrower and more constraining (e.g., the hospital) and in serious pathologies like cancer.

The physician–patient relationship has the disease as a starting point. This involves both interlocutors in a radically different way than in most relationships: the physician is an expert on disease (objective knowledge), while the patient is an expert on illness (subjective knowledge and experiences).

Disease puts patients in an emotionally difficult situation; the more serious the disease, the more complex the situation. This feeds the patient's need for being taken care of, especially when his/her physical status causes fear and preoccupation. In oncology more than in other fields, sick persons need medicines for their bodies, but also for their souls.

The physician–patient relationship is founded on care. Taking care of others motivates the physicians' encounter with patients from the start and allows the ethical fulfillment of the technical action. Thanks only to a caring attitude, the objectifying moments of diagnosis and therapy acquire profound and authentic humanity.

In oncology, the cure must include taking care of the sick person. Caring fills a need for warmth, closeness, and trust and has a fundamental role for the human being from early childhood, as numerous scientists have demonstrated with their research (e.g., Harlow's, 1959 research on the Rhesus monkey; Spitz's study of orphanages and children deprived of maternal care).

Starting from the technical-scientific development in the latter half of the last century, physicians have increasingly identified themselves with the curing, the technical, and the specialistic aspects of medicine. Relational competences, summarized in the human dimension of the "medical action," were put in the background and considered unnecessary. Even emotions—a fundamental component of any relationship—have always been considered disturbing and have therefore been set aside from the medical scene, even through detachment education (which is different from therapeutic distance).

Today, medicine and physicians find themselves involved in profound transformations. The advances in learning, scientific knowledge, and technology have had ample repercussions on clinical practice and have opened new issues on an ethical level that can be solved only with awareness and with the involvement and participation of patients.

Dealing with collaborative patients who fully understand the situation they are in and want to become protagonists of their disease implies taking care of their soul and welcoming their emotions; this is the only way to eliminate their confusion and restore them to reason, which is a fundamental step for their understanding and choice. Nowadays, recognizing and respecting patients' subjectivity is crucial, as is focusing on their expressivity and decisions and harmonizing technical and relational competences. The communication of the diagnosis in oncology is an example of how these aspects of the medical action interact.

The role of the physician, then, becomes more complex and articulated and requires new skills and competences. *The physician is expected to recover from the past the attention to the human dimension of suffering that inevitably marks every encounter with disease and pain.*

Today, physicians can find themselves facing situations that require "less technique" and are "more relationship focused"; the acquisition of communicative-relational competences is thus fundamental. The physician–patient relationship depends on many factors, including biographies and emotional and clinical experiences; it certainly is a relationship in which both partners are involved with all their emotions.

Patients' Emotions

Human beings feel the greatest need for caring in hard times, when they lack health and certainty in the future, when they are scared, confused, and unable to take care of themselves. Especially when life-threatening, disease induces in patients strong emotions, preoccupations, and the need for being taken care of, help, and trust. Patients often tend to put themselves in a condition of emotional inferiority to physicians; this needs to be corrected, because their emotions represent an important element of the cure (understanding and retaining information) and also of caring (acceptance, comfort, nonjudgment, openness, trust). The possibility of patients participating in their own course of therapy is increased by having their confused and intense emotions acknowledged.

In oncology, two multidisciplinary constructs capture the relevance of emotions in the disease and cure processes: emotional distress and cancer-related fatigue. Emotional distress, especially in the presence of anxious and/or depressive states, affects a high percentage of oncological patients [22]. To emotional distress, we must add cancer-related fatigue, which, being a multifactorial syndrome, involves fatigue and emotional as well as physical-behavioral indolence [23]. These two aspects can interfere with medical communications (reducing the reception, comprehension, and recollection of information); they can also be an explicit object of communication, as they are the possible outcomes of treatments and could elicit the request for specific supporting interventions.

The Diagnostic Phase

Obtaining the diagnosis of a serious disease establishes certainty on a pathological state. But paradoxically, this gives way to a sequence of uncertainties about prognosis, life expectation, efficacy of treatment, and collateral effects. Obtaining an oncological diagnosis is rarely a distinct event; more frequently, it is the outcome of a process that can be articulated in several (more or less invasive) medical examinations and in various evaluations with different specialists. In this phase, the certainty of the diagnosis can be preceded by uncertainties, caused by the examinations in progress and by the inevitably cautious communications of healthcare providers. Typical communications in this phase concern the symptoms: their evaluation starts the medical consultation, the reports (often incomplete), the diagnosis itself (naming the disease), the therapeutic options with their respective pros and cons, and the prognosis (not necessarily given by physicians, more often presumed by patients themselves). The emotional range of fear (tension, fear, anxiety, terror, panic) is associated with the unknown—in particular, with what could menace integrity and safety; it is, then, understandable that fear accompanies the subject in this phase, which ends exactly with the acceptance of the role of "patient" by the subject him/herself. Other common emotional experiences in this phase are the sense of guilt (e.g., for having overlooked symptoms or screening guidelines or for not having adopted prevention behaviors), embarrassment or shame (induced by medical procedures or by the possibility of being sick), and rage and blame (self-directed, not directed towards care providers or any scapegoat or transcendent entity). Moreover, sadness and depressive states, being associated with real or imagined loss, are related to a sense of loss of autonomy, independence, social and working status, and to the reduction or procrastination of one's own life objectives, all associated with the experience of cancer.

The Phase of Treatments

Undergoing cancer treatment means confronting uncertainty once again: uncertainty of the efficacy of the treatment itself and of its extent (whether full recovery or temporary remission of symptoms).

Cancer treatments have immediate, long-term, or late side effects, tolerance of which varies from patient to patient. Not infrequently, treatments need adjustment during therapy; these modifications may affect their administration, length, or effects. In this phase, it may also be necessary to take into consideration possible permanent side effects (infertility or disability are among the most severe examples) that could considerably reduce future quality of life. The subjective significance given by patients to side effects, to the limitations imposed by treatment, or to late or long-term effects helps in understanding the emotional experiences of patients in this phase. Further manifestations of anxiety and depression are isolation experiences and the fear of abandonment, first by care providers then by relatives and friends.

Follow-Ups, Remission, and Long-Term Cancer Survival

Although physicians may welcome the therapy results as "satisfactory" (with a reduction of tumoral mass, for example), patients often cannot fully understand the importance of therapeutic outcomes; this is due to the presence of side effects (that limit their quality of life and well-being), to the preoccupations that these side effects engender, and to the possibility of a relapse. The periods preceding or following follow-ups can be particularly anxiety-inducing for patients. In this phase, they may show preoccupation and fear for the eventuality that their descendant (whether potential or real) also might get cancer.

Nevertheless, patients tend not to tell doctors about their emotional turmoil, as if assuming that this is the "natural" price to pay for recovering; it is the physician's task to investigate and legitimate this uneasiness.

Furthermore, emotional uneasiness, depressive and anxious experiences, and preoccupations can extend for a very long time (they might also appear later), thus also characterizing long-term cancer survival. In this stage, it is particularly important for patients to adhere to screening and follow-up programs, for both oncological and other potential diseases; anxiety, preoccupation, and unrealistic optimism can interfere with the understanding of these practices and with adherence to therapy.

Finally, once the diagnostic step is over and treatments have been finished, from an emotional point of view patients can develop aspects of posttraumatic growth: they report experiencing serenity, peacefulness, trust, and gratitude [24].

Relapse

From an emotional point of view, communicating a relapse is in general harder than communicating a diagnosis: relapse elicits further emotions and mood states, such as impotence, defeat, abandonment, ambivalence, and the impossibility of trusting again. These are normal reactions when facing failure (and relapse is perceived as such), and it is therefore normal that patients live and express them. It is also equally important for the therapist not to combat them ineffectively, through false expectations and unrealistically optimistic behaviors.

From Active to Palliative Care

Communicating the inefficiency of the treatments available and that medicine can succeed only in controlling symptoms may lead patients to experience defeat, depression, loss, impotence, and abandonment. Many reasons (discretion, shame, fear of bothering caregivers or of preventing further therapeutic attempts and the self-perceived burden to caregivers) can hinder patients in expressing their own emotional world; it must not be forgotten that in this phase patients value quality of life more than prolonged survival [9]. Hope, then, is a state of mind that is essential to well-being; nevertheless, it must not be based on groundless elements or fed by colluding caretakers' and relatives' attitudes.

Finally, it must not be forgotten that the patient's emotional state fluctuates frequently between positive and negative emotions; and that pain, soporific, or confusional states—often effects of palliative treatments—can affect the emotional sphere.

Genetic Counseling

A genetic test for those tumoral forms of cancer for which a familiar/genetic predisposition is known, involving in the screening ascendant and descendant relatives, can provide only probabilistic data. These risk percentages are not certain data, from which a unique prophylactic therapy can follow [25]. Beside the cognitive difficulties engendered from such test results, patients are challenged from an emotional point of view; they may become preoccupied about their own health status and that of their descendants, with anxiety and ambivalence about taking prophylactic or, more simply, secondary prevention measures. A sense of shame is not uncommon, especially regarding one's partner or relatives. When patients have already had children, they often develop a sense of guilt and of "suspension" for the possibility of having transmitted to them their genetic "weakness." But if they have not yet had children and decide on the basis of genetic tests not to have children, besides a sense of guilt towards their partner, they could also experience emotions of bereavement and loss.

The Physician's Emotions

For a long time, it was believed that emotional-affective dynamics, projections, and defenses were restricted to the psychoanalyst's office. Today, we know that transference and countertransference occur in all relationships, especially in meaningful, need-motivated, and asymmetrical relationships. Balint highlighted the importance of countertransference, of the feelings and emotions felt by physicians for patients in a care relationship. Certainly, pain, fear, impotence, and confronting death are very powerful activators in the physicians' unconscious.

In general, physicians tend to undervalue the influence of their mood state and emotions on their actions in relation to patients. Their education made them believe that professional behavior and therapeutic distance require emotional detachment, the absence of affective involvement, and the denial of those feelings that the encounter with a suffering Other inevitably triggers in themselves.

In general, it is correct to speak about "therapeutic distance" (as a reflexive component in the relationship), and attention must be paid to the process of identification with patients. Nevertheless, this does not mean that experiencing emotions and feelings is not allowed, but rather that physicians have to learn to identify and listen to them, in order to not be overwhelmed and to recognize what patients experience. Feelings, emotions, mood states are indispensable for understanding the context in which doctors operate; they allow for empathy. Understanding and accepting the Other in an empathic way require the recognition of one's own emotions and feelings.

When doctors tell patients a bad prognosis by referring only to technical data and formal procedures, they achieve detachment as the outcome of defensive behavior, finalized in distancing the distress and suffering that patients can bring. Then the physicians' behavior is determined by the emotions, and thus often lacks the necessary awareness that would allow transforming a difficulty into experience, personal growth, and help for patients.

Especially in oncology, where daily encounters with suffering and death are inevitable, unheard and unrecognized emotions compromise the communication and the relationship between physician and patient.

Communicating bad news in oncology is a medical action; like all other medical actions, it has to be prepared through self-listening, by focusing on one's fears and motivations, and listening to the Other: "How could he/she react?" and "How will I react to his/her responses?"

Listening to emotions gives consistency and coherence to actions. It is not merely a matter of controlling emotions, but also of knowing how to listen and recognize them. Listening and recognizing one's own emotions are necessary for both self-care and care for the Other; this is what medical advances have allowed one to forget. Even though physicians may not be aware of it, their communication with patients is strongly influenced by their own emotional experiences. Emotions, if recognized and managed, besides helping clinicians in understanding the context in which they work, can therapeutically benefit the relationship, rather than being a hindrance, as they often seem to be.

Recognizing how emotions organize experience and behavior and influence actions, thoughts, and choices is fundamental for physicians to avoid behaving exclusively emotionally. It is possible to learn from experience, to grow, and be of help only by recognizing one's own emotions, even when they are confused and imprecise.

Entering a relationship with the Other requires beginning a path of research and undertaking that, starting from oneself, could help in opening one to the patient's suffering. Education in self-care and encountering one's own emotions allow one to create the climate for the development of relational skills, so that they become more conscious acts. This means that these skills can be learned and developed and that their development can, in turn, contribute to making both the patients and the world of their relationships mature.

Emotional Challenges in the Physician–Patient Relationship

The fundamental prerequisite for creating a welcoming context that allows patients to feel sufficiently at ease to tell their stories and express their experience of the disease, the treatments, and their consequences is focusing on emotions. This certainly is the most delicate task for physicians, along with the informative and communicative duties pertaining to their role.

In communicating, physicians should focus on the emotional prominence of what they say, on the specific meaning that the communication has for patients in relation to the phase of life the patients are in, their aspirations, values, and projects. Doctors should practice empathic listening to connect them with their own emotions and their patients'. Then they should validate the patients' emotions engendered by the disease, its consequences and evolution. Physicians should encourage patients to express emotions and to take care of them, as they are an inseparable component of the body–mind unit and of the multidimensional biological, psycho-social experience that the disease is. Finally, doctors should always allow patients to keep hope alive; for this purpose, both trust and emotional impact are essential.

Today, there is growing agreement that communicative skills can be taught in educational training sessions [26] that give physicians more confidence in their competence and improve their objective performance, with special attention to patients and their needs [27–30]. A 3-day intensive training program produces significant subjective and objective changes [31]; continual education is necessary to reinforce and consolidate the acquired skills [26, 29, 32].

Nevertheless, it is reductive to think about the physician–patient relationship only in terms of technical protocol or as an acquisition of communication skills. Although the teaching and learning of technical knowledge can be planned and programmed, how to facilitate affective growth and activate the process of emotional growth in caring contexts is not yet clear.

Scientific and technological learning demands more and more space and commitment; this inevitably subtracts attention from the soul. Education for self-care teaches the physician how to transform external events into profound internal experiences, how to feel better with oneself and one's patients, and how to make patients feel better. Learning communicative skills in specific training can be positively encouraged by the ability of clinicians to draw on profound and less explicit "knowledge" derived from experience, from critical self-listening, from doubting, and most of all, from the memory of past difficulties.

More and more educational training on communication skills is being organized (e.g., [33, 34]). To realize personal development and relational skills, it is nevertheless necessary to learn how to sustain one's own experience, by listening to what happens inside and by expressing it. For this aim, to allow the understanding of the experience, it can be useful to share it. This involves creating an opportunity of encounter and reflection that, through self-narration and representation, permits one to recognize feelings and emotions unconditionally; this is the fundamental step of a personal process of development.

Conclusions

Today medicine and physicians are undergoing profound transformations. Advances in learning, scientific knowledge, and technology have had significant repercussions on clinical practice, opening new issues on an ethical level. Even the doctor–patient relationship has achieved new meanings, and the language itself evidences this evolution: *clinical encounter, care relationship,* and the medical profession as a *helping profession* are now commonly used expressions.

Through communication, the physician introduces patients to the path of their disease and accompanies them along it, which is a difficult and painful experience. Emotions are an integral part of this experience, and clinicians have to take them into account; they influence the global well-being of patients, their quality of life, their therapeutic choices. Welcoming and taking charge of emotions represent an important burden for doctors: it connects them with their own emotions and destroys the shield of detachment and paternalism that in the past they had built for self-defense and protection. But at the same time, it adds important elements to their clinical practice, which are necessary to establish a therapeutic plan that matches the biological–psychosocial needs of patients, so that patients will be more and more involved and informed.

The asymmetry of the paternalistic role of the past thus gives way to an asymmetry founded on the recognition and recovery of patients' subjectivity, encouraging their expressive and decision-making possibilities.

It is increasingly evident today that technical and relational competences have to harmonize reciprocally; communicating bad news is an example of how these two aspects of medical action integrate. To reach a correct diagnosis, doctors obviously have to master the technical competences, but the phases of the "path" by which a diagnosis is communicated require the ability to build a relationship and to realize an encounter.

The role of physicians becomes, then, more complex and articulated and requires deeper and more refined skills. Doctors are asked to recover a competence that in reality they already had: the attention to the suffering human dimension that marks, inevitably, all encounters with disease and pain, both patients' and doctors'. Today, there is a new awareness of how these aspects can work together to enhance the technical-specialistic aspects at every step of the disease course.

Managing patients' emotions is achieved through the ability to recognize and listen to one's own emotions—in a personal growth path—and through the learning of communication skills in specific educational training, which makes possible greater well-being for both patients and physicians.

References

1. Paul CL, Clinton-McHarg T, Sanson-Fisher RW, Douglas H, Webb G. Are we there yet? The state of the evidence base for guidelines on breaking bad news to cancer patients. Eur J Cancer. 2009;45(17):2960–6.
2. Dimoska A, Girgis A, Hansen V, Butow PN, Tattersall MH. Perceived difficulties in consulting with patients and families: a survey of Australian cancer specialists. Med J Aust. 2008;189(11–12):612–5.
3. Daugherty CK, Hlubocky FJ. What are terminally ill cancer patients told about their expected deaths? A study of cancer physicians' self-reports of prognosis disclosure. J Clin Oncol. 2008;26(36):5988–93.
4. Hack TF, Pickles T, Ruether JD, Weir L, Bultz BD, Degner LF. Behind closed doors: systematic analysis of breast cancer consultation communication and predictors of satisfaction with communication. Psychooncology. 2010;19(6):626–36.
5. Fujimori M, Uchitomi Y. Preferences of cancer patients regarding communication of bad news: a systematic literature review. Jpn J Clin Oncol. 2009;39(4):201–16.
6. Arora NK, Gustafson DH. Perceived helpfulness of physicians' communication behavior and breast cancer patients' level of trust over time. J Gen Intern Med. 2009;24(2):252–5.
7. Seetharamu N, Iqbal U, Weiner JS. Determinants of trust in the patient-oncologist relationship. Palliat Support Care. 2007;5(4):405–9.
8. Neumann M, Wirtz M, Bollschweiler E, Mercer SW, Warm M, Wolf J, et al. Determinants and patient-reported long-term outcomes of physician empathy in oncology: a structural equation modelling approach. Patient Educ Couns. 2007;69(1–3):63–75.
9. Epstein RM, Street Jr RL. Patient-centered communication in cancer care: promoting healing and reducing suffering. Bethesda, MD: National Cancer Institute, NIH Publication No. 07–6225; 2007.
10. Stewart MA. Effective physician-patient communication and health outcomes: a review. Can Med Assoc J. 1996;152:1423–33.
11. Dowsett SM, Saul JL, Butow PN, Dunn SM, Boyer MJ, Findlow R, et al. Communication style in the cancer consultation: preferences for a patient-centred approach. Psychooncology. 2000;9:147–56.
12. Roberts CS, Cox CE, Reintgen DS, Baile WF, Libertini M. Influence of physician communication on newly diagnosed breast patients' psychologic adjustment and decision-making. Cancer. 1994;74:336–41.
13. Sardell AN, Trierweiler SJ. Disclosing the cancer diagnosis: procedures that influence patient hopefulness. Cancer. 1993;72:3355–65.
14. Fogarty LA, Curbow BA, Wingard JR, McDonnel K, Somerfields MR. Can 40 seconds of compassion reduce anxiety? J Clin Oncol. 1999;17:371–9.

15. Schofield PE, Butow PN, Thompson JF, Tattersall MHN, Beeney LJ, Dunn SM. Psychological responses of patients receiving a diagnosis of cancer. Ann Oncol. 2003;14:48–56.
16. Fallowfield LJ, Jenkins V. Effective communication skills are the key to good cancer care. Eur J Cancer. 1999;35(11):1592–7.
17. Devine EC, Westlake SK. The effects of psychoeducational care provided to adults with cancer: meta-analysis of 116 studies. Oncol Nurs Forum. 1995;22:1369–81.
18. Maguire P, Tait A, Brooke M, Thomas C, Sellwood R. Effect on counselling on the psychiatric morbidity associated with mastectomy. BMJ. 1980;281:1454–6.
19. McArdle JM, George WD, McArdle CS, Smith DC, Moodie AR, Hughson AV, et al. Psychological support for patients undergoing breast cancer surgery: a randomised study. BMJ. 1996;31:813–6.
20. Maguire P, Brooke M, Tait A, Thomas C, Sellwood R. The effect of counselling on physical disability and social recovery after mastectomy. Clin Oncol. 1983;9:319–24.
21. Oatley K. Emotion: a brief history. Oxford, UK: Wiley-Blackwell; 2004.
22. Winn RJ, McClure JS. Clinical information & publications, distress management: clinical practice guidelines. In: NCCN clinical practice guidelines in oncology. Guidelines for supportive care, version 1. National Comprehensive Cancer Network. 2008. http://www.nccn.org/professionals/physician_gls/f_guidelines.asp. Accessed Apr 2009.
23. National Cancer Control Network. Clinical practice guidelines in oncology cancer-related fatigue. 2009. http://www.nccn.org/professionals/physician_gls/PDF/fatigue.pdf.
24. Calhoun LG, Tedeschi RG. Handbook of post-traumatic growth. Mahwah, NJ: Erlbaum; 2006.
25. NCCN clinical practice guidelines in oncology. Genetic familial high-risk assessment: breast and ovarian. 2008. http://www.nccn.org/professionals/physician_gls/f_guidelines.asp4.
26. Maguire P. Can communication skills be taught? Br J Hosp Med. 1990;43:215–6.
27. Fallowfield L, Lipkin M, Hall A. Teaching senior oncologists communication skills: results from phase I of a comprehensive longitudinal program in the United Kingdom. J Clin Oncol. 1998;16(5):1961–8.
28. Razavi D, Delvaux N, Marchal S, Bredart A, Farvacques C, Paesmans M. The effects of a 24 hr psychological training program on attitudes, communication skills and occupational stress in oncology: a randomised study. Eur J Cancer. 1993;29A:1858–63.
29. Bird J, Hall A, Maguire P, Heavy A. Workshops for consultant on the teaching of clinical communication skills. Med Educ. 1993;27:181–5.
30. Baile WF, Lenzi R, Kudelka AP, Maguire P, Novack D, Goldstein M, et al. Improving physician-patient communication in cancer care: outcome of a workshop for oncologists. J Cancer Educ. 1997;12:166–73.
31. Fallowfield L, Jenkins V, Farewell V, Saul J, Duffy A, Rebecca E. Efficacy of a cancer research UK communication skills training model for oncologists: a randomised controlled trial. Lancet. 2002;359:650–6.
32. Delvaux N, Merckaert I, Marchal S, Libert Y, Conradt S, Boniver J, et al. Physicians' communication with a cancer patient and relative. A randomized study assessing the efficacy of consolidation workshops. Cancer. 2005;103(11):2397–411.
33. Caminiti C, Annunziata MA, De Falco F, Diodati F, Fagnani D, Isa L, et al. HUCARE project: humanization of cancer care in Italy: results after the first year of implementation. Ann Oncol. 2009;(Suppl 8–B15).
34. Passalacqua R, Caminiti C, Annunziata MA, Borreani C, Diodati F, Fagnani D, et al. Psychosocial care of Italian adult cancer patients: a large collaborative, hospital-based quality improvement project (HUCARE). In: 35th European Society for Medical Oncology (ESMO) congress, Milan, Italy, 2010.

Chapter 21
Binary Thinking, Hope, and Realistic Expectations in Communication with Cancer Patients

Jerome Lowenstein

Abstract Sitting for many years on the ethics committee of our medical center, I have come to recognize that when the details of a complex ethical issue are reviewed, examined from different perspectives, and discussed—i.e., "slowed down"—the analog appearance of the process often breaks down to reveal the digital, yes/no nature of our judgments.

Keywords Hope and realistic expectations • Binary logic and medical ethics • The whole truth

Binary thinking, seeing the universe as either A or B, is pervasive and is not limited to obvious polarities such as right/left, up/down, in/out. Qualitative descriptions such as larger/smaller, warmer/colder are essentially binary distinctions, albeit modified by a quantitative component. These things we take for granted—we are born with these binary distinctions. I have come to recognize the much more pervasive effects of binary thinking. If I were writing this essay 20 or 25 years ago, I would be using a typewriter whose 30 or 40 keys would each control a single printer's striker representing a unique letter, number, or symbol. The only binary feature of the typewriter would be the "shift key" used to print capital letters, numbers, and some symbols; and, sometimes, a key to shift from the black to the red ribbon.

Today, though keyboards are still an important component of computers, cell phones, iPhones, and all manner of electronic devices, there are no strikers; behind every keyboard lurks a binary logic system. Typewriters have been replaced by word processors. What happened to the "writer" of typewriter?

Word processors operate on a binary system in which different combinations of "on" and "off" represent each letter of the alphabet and punctuation symbols in a

---

J. Lowenstein (✉)
Department of Medicine, NYU Langone Medical Center, 530 1st Avenue,
New York, NY 10016, USA
e-mail: Jerome.Lowenstein@nyumc.org

language not dissimilar from the Morse code. With another on/off signal, the word processor can generate an almost limitless series of different fonts, symbols, and alphabets.

Binary systems are not limited to word processors. The continuous stream of news clips that runs around the NY Times building and all of the flashing, brightly colored images that surround Times Square are generated by lights going on or off. Television images are composed of pixels, small lights that either "on" or "off". The higher the definition, the more pixels. It is as simple as that. The binary nature of digitized images is not apparent when the density of pixels is great; but when the image is enlarged, the "graininess" reveals the digital nature of the image. Sometimes this digitized effect is desirable. That would appear to be the case for pointillist paintings or portraits by Chuck Close. For me, portraits by Chuck Close have the grainy quality of a greatly magnified image—perhaps that is their attraction.

But this is not the only way in which our universe is becoming binary. I say "becoming" because it was not always this way. Sound, whether it is the voice, music, or the many musical and musical sounds around us, represents vibrations of varying wavelengths and amplitudes. A continuous spectrum of these frequencies and amplitudes characterizes spoken language, instrumental music, and song. Some musical instruments divide the spectrum of wavelengths into discrete "tones." The piano, harpsichord, banjo, guitar, lute, and mandolin all have frets, raised bands that allow the instrument to produce discrete notes that represent a portion of the spectrum. Other instruments—violin, viola, cello—permit the full spectrum of tones, including the quarter-tones and glissandos used in many kinds of music. Surely there are no "stops" or frets in the human voice.

From the earliest recordings made in the laboratory of Thomas Edison, voices and music retained the full range of tones. Analog recordings capture not only the primary tones, but also many of the overtones. With digital sound recording, which has come, increasingly, to replace analog recording, tones are reduced (or transformed) into discrete groups; this division is somewhat arbitrary. These digitized sounds are represented by various combinations of binary signals that are able to closely approximate the sound perceived when a voice transmits a melody to the human ear—closely, but not exactly, since overtones and other features of analog sound are lost. For all the convenience that comes from having music stored, free of surface noise, on a thin compact disc (CD) or an iPOD, or transmitted electronically to a variety of multicolored hand-held devices, the sound is not the same; many people can readily distinguish digitized music from the richer analog music. Most of us recognize the "machine" quality of the voice that directs us when we seek to find a train schedule, buy a movie ticket by telephone, or follow the route guided by a GPS system in our car.

What accounts for the dramatic inroads that binary logic has made in our language, music, and visual perceptions over a very short period of time? Technology has made it possible to digitize images and sounds, but I suspect that there is another factor that made binary thinking take hold so quickly. Julian Jaynes argued in his 1976 classic, *The Origin of Consciousness in the Breakdown of the Bicameral Mind* [1] that our understanding of things is aided by metaphor, particularly metaphors

Fig. 21.1 Binary Vision

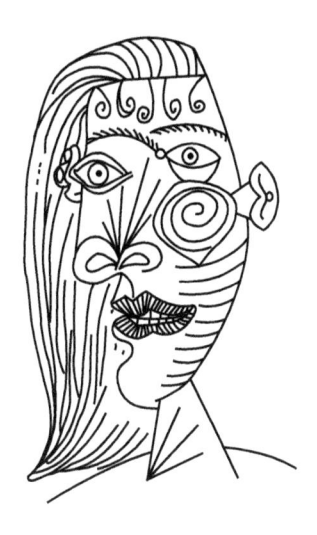

that relate to our bodies. The propensity to judge things as "one the one hand, and on the other" is hard to separate from our anatomy. Remy Charlip, a wonderful children's book artist, wrote of two octopi who married and went down the aisle "arm in arm in arm in arm...."

It should not be unexpected to learn that binary systems have been modeled on biological systems. Nerve conduction and brain function can be seen as based on binary systems. Light strikes the retina, a specialized extension of the brain where receptors (rods and cones) respond in an all-or-none manner to generate an electrical signal, which travels along the optic nerves to specific areas of the visual cortex, where a "quantum" of neurotransmitter chemical is released, again in an all-or-none phenomenon, and evokes a response in the brain cells. The intensity, color, apparent depth, and other qualities of the image are the result of the number and pattern of the stimulated "on" receptors. Is this different from the image on my TV screen or the overwhelming array of "images" that occupy every building face on Times Square?

While much of our biology may be binary and intuitive, this paradigm often breaks down just when we need it most. Those who understand particle physics assert that energy exists at the same time as a wave and as a particle; I find that I cannot hold these two different images side by side in my mind. Even more striking is my inability to "picture" states beyond the three-dimensional modes that I've grown up with. It must yield an exciting view of the nature of the universe for physicists who can imagine the curvature of space and time or understand string theory. I envy that capacity. If the problems posed by physics seem too abstract, contemplate this line drawing by Picasso, which presents the viewer with a woman's face seen from two angles at the same time...but Picasso was a genius (Fig 21.1).

Why am I so interested in binary thinking? I confess that I am not certain that I can discern the difference between analog and digital sound recordings, and I am not troubled by the impact of binary thinking in most aspects of my life—most, but not all. There are two areas, very important to me, where the all-or-none model represents a serious problem for me. Just as fine music requires analog sound to preserve its subtle variations and a fine watercolor needs the blurred edges created by the brush rather than the sharp edge created by collage, the analysis of ethical issues and the balance of truth telling and reassurance in medicine require the equivalent of analog thinking. As a first approximation, each of these would appear to be based on finely graded "analog" thinking, but I do not find this to be the case. Like digitized visual images, composed of blinking lights or pixels, that break down into their faceless on/off signals when slowed down or magnified, I find that when these issues are examined closely—i.e., slowed down—their binary composition becomes very apparent.

Sitting for many years on the ethics committee of our medical center, I have come to recognize that when the details of a complex ethical issue are reviewed, examined from different perspectives, and discussed, the analog appearance of the process often breaks down to reveal the digital, yes/no nature of our judgments. Countless times I have listened to a member of our committee give a very insightful, nuanced description of the issue at hand and propose a clear, reasonable solution only to hear a second, third, and fourth equally carefully nuanced analysis of the ethical issue. Each aspect of the issue, seen from a different perspective, generates its own response, all-or-none; and like Humpty Dumpty, we, the group, find it hard to put the pieces back together in a satisfactory way. This is seen very clearly in the area of truth telling.

The following, from *The Midnight Meal and Essays about Doctors, Patients, and Medicine* [2] summarizes some of my thoughts about truth telling;

> Attitudes and expectations of patients and physicians with regard to revealing the truth have undergone dramatic changes over the past 25 years. When I was a medical student, house officer and during the early years of my medical practice, the prevailing dictum (or so I believed) was that the truth should be used judiciously, as with any treatment administered by the physician. Patients rarely questioned the actions of their physicians. The word "cancer" was rarely spoken and patients usually were told that radiation treatments, hormones or chemotherapeutic drugs were given to "prevent problems." The prevailing notion today is very different. *Paternalism* has been rejected in favor of *patient autonomy* and the view that "full disclosure" is a requisite for good medical practice. Greatly increased patient awareness of sophisticated issues regarding diagnostic and treatment aspects of many illnesses is in part responsible for the dramatic change in the role of truth in the physician-patient relationship. In no small degree this shift can also be traced to the climate of fear of malpractice actions in medicine today.
>
> Reflecting on my own life and medical encounters of members of my family, I am not sure that I am ready to reject a measure of paternalism. Our society cannot and should not return to the time, not very long ago, when patients were told very little and were expected to listen to the advice of a physician "who knew best." I do, however, think something important has been lost when a physician feels that every doubt and concern, however remote, unlikely, or frightening, must be shared with the patient. This form of presenting the "whole truth" to the patient bears a striking resemblance to the manner in which the *Physicians Desk Reference* lists all the potential side effects of each drug. While it may be appropriate for the PDR, and I have some doubts about this, I surely do not feel that the physician should "reveal all" in the same way as a package insert. "Truth" and "facts" are not discrete, defined entities, like so many colored marbles, to be handed to the patient to accept or reject. The words physicians speak to patients often linger in their mind and in their memories. They are repeated, examined and reexamined, as patients seek reassurance, guidance or solace. We have all heard our own words or the words of other physicians

repeated, by patients, years after they were spoken. I am quite sure that there are times when what has been said has had greater consequences for the patient's well being than the medications or treatments prescribed. It seems to me that what is said to a patient or a patient's family should reflect the physician's fullest understanding of the needs of the patient in the same way as the choice of a medication or advice regarding surgery. For some patients this will require "full disclosure," by which I mean an effort to fully educate the patient, recalling that the linguistic root of the word doctor is *dichter* meaning, "to teach." For other patients, or under other circumstances, it may be more appropriate to use the truth judiciously. The decision is not a simple one and, I submit, cannot be made according to a uniform rule or universal principle. The issue has been made very much more difficult by the fact that less than full disclosure has been judged, at times, as malpractice. The decisions of how much truth is called for or is appropriate, like the question of how much treatment is appropriate, should reflect the physician's fullest understanding of the patient's life rather than society's current attitudes about paternalism and truth telling.

Having devoted my career to the care of patients, in the role of primary physician or specialist, I frequently find myself in a quandary trying to reconcile my dual roles as providing reassurance and support on the one hand, and providing information about the likelihood of success of a treatment or the prognosis of an illness on the other. I find myself returning to thoughts that I expressed almost 15 years ago [3].

It is often much more difficult to give reassurance than advice, guidance, and counsel. It is easy when the diagnosis is clear cut, the condition benign, self-limited or curable, and the prognosis excellent. This makes the day for the physician. Often, however, it is apparent to both the physician and the patient that the outcome cannot be predicted or that the prognosis is, in fact, very poor. This is painful for both the physician and the patient. A colleague recently confided that he felt acutely uncomfortable with a patient who had cancer and her husband because, "they hung so much on every word, looking for reassurance." He explained, "I just try to keep it light with them....at least it seems to help me." How can the physician give reassurance or be reassuring when the patient has AIDS, advanced cancer, or Alzheimer's disease? When we know that the need for reassurance is great, how are we to respond? In many situations it is apparent to the patient, as it is to the physician, that the outcome cannot be predicted or that the prognosis is, in fact, very poor.

Having struggled with some of these issues for almost 30 years, I have learned that the need for reassurance under these circumstances calls for the physician to use his or her relationship with the patient, rather than a measured, guarded assessment, to provide support. The more uncertain the future and the more bleak the prognosis, the greater is the need of patients for the support that can come from knowing that an educated caring physician is fully committed to seeing them through their illness, in a word, "being there." This is reassurance. The patient's call for reassurance is not a call for magic, miracles, or omniscience. It is a cry for a "human connection." Reassurances that pain will be controlled, dignity will be preserved, that the patient's wishes will be respected, and that the patient will not be left to face death alone require a significant commitment from a caring physician, and do not require a "warning label".

I fully recognize the difference between *hope* and *realistic expectations*. Hope is not a statistical issue; it is a state of mind. No matter how solid the database on which a prognosis is based, I am aware that we all—physicians and patients alike—respond as though the issue is binary. I can hear you say, "Yes, but life or death is a binary issue." But is it? Death is all-or-none (binary), but dying is not a binary process—it is an analog process with an almost endless series of gradual transitions. I feel that in many things—dealing with illness, facing end-of-life decisions—the outcome is not binary but rather is a question of quality—quality of life; and this, despite efforts at quantification by questionnaire, is basically an analog function.

I am left with the question, How do I hold onto hope, which is never dependent on reality; and uncertainty, which is always present?" Are there individuals who share the physicist Richard Feynman's gift of being able to hold such opposing views in their minds at once? Who can honestly be both optimistic and realistic? Optimism relates to the future; hope is a thing of the present. To hold these views simultaneously is to collapse time, to be in the moment. Are those individuals who achieve this recognized as healers?

References

1. Jaynes J. The origin of consciousness in the breakdown of the bicameral mind. NY: Houghton, Mifflin Company; 1976.
2. "The Whole Truth…?" from J. Lowenstein. The midnight meal and other essays about doctors, patients, and medicine. London: Yale University Press; 1997. pp. 76–80.
3. "Reassurance and the warning on the label" from J. Lowenstein. The midnight meal and other essays about doctors, patients, and medicine. London: Yale University Press; 1997, pp. 35–39.

Chapter 22
A Physician's Personal Experiences as a Cancer-of-the-Neck Patient: Communication of Medical Errors to Cancer Patients and Their Families

Itzhak Brook[*]

Abstract This chapter presents my personal experiences as a physician who underwent laryngectomy for hypopharyngeal squamous cell carcinoma. I describe the numerous medical and surgical errors that occurred during my hospitalizations at three medical institutions. They were made by physicians, nurses, and other medical providers. Medical errors should be prevented as much as humanly possible. Ignoring them can only lead to their repetition. Disclosure practice can be improved by strengthening policy and supporting healthcare professionals in disclosing adverse events. Increased openness and honesty following adverse events can improve provider–patient relationships. There are important preventive steps that can be implemented by each institution and medical offices. Educating the patient and their caregivers about the patient condition and planned treatment is of outmost importance. These individuals can safeguard and prevent mistakes when they see deviations from the planned therapy.

Keywords Cancer • Hypopharynx • Surgery • Errors

Medical and surgical errors are very common in the hospital setting [1]. Recent studies had shown that errors occur in up to 40% of patients hospitalized for surgery, and up to 18% of them suffer from complications because of these errors [2]. These mistakes encourage medical malpractice lawsuits and increase the cost of medical care, the length patients' hospital stays, and their morbidity and mortality [3].

---

[*]Dr. Brook is the author of the book: *My Voice: A Physician's Personal Experience with Throat Cancer*. The book can be read at http://dribrook.blogspot.com/. Printed copy of the book can be obtained at https://www.createspace.com/900004368.

I. Brook, MD MSc (✉)
Department of Pediatrics, Georgetown University School of Medicine,
4431 Albemarle Street, NW, Washington, DC 20016, USA
e-mail: ib6@georgetown.edu

The recent development of a mandatory bedside checklist is a simple, cost-effective method to prevent many of these errors [4].

As an infectious diseases specialist for 40 years, I was not aware how common these errors are until I became a patient myself after being diagnosed with hypopharyngeal carcinoma; until I had to deal with these errors as a patient, not a physician.

Despite the fact that the small cancer (T1, N0, M0) was surgically removed and I received local radiation, after 20 months a local recurrence at a different location (pyriform sinus) was discovered (T2, N0, M0). Unfortunately, my surgeons were unable completely to remove the tumor by laser after three attempts. At that point, I elected to undergo complete pharynolaryngectomy with flap reconstruction at a different medical center, which had more experience with this type of cancer. The tumor was completely removed and no local or systemic spread was noted.

Although the care I received at all institutions was overall very good, I realized that mistakes were being made at all levels of my care. Despite these experiences, I feel great gratitude to the physicians, nurses, and other healthcare providers who supported and cared for me through my difficult and challenging hospitalizations.

This chapter describes the medical errors I encountered in my care during my hospitalizations at three medical centers and how the medical staff responded to them. What made it difficult for me to abort many of these mistakes was my inability to speak after I underwent laryngectomy. Fortunately, I was able to abort many of these errors, but not all. In each instance, I will discuss the optimal approach toward handling communication of these errors with the patient.

Failure to Diagnose Cancer Recurrence

My surgeons failed to diagnose the recurrence of my cancer in a timely fashion, although they examined me using an endoscope on a monthly basis after my initial surgery. I had been complaining of sharp and persistent pain in the right side of my throat for 7 months. They kept reassuring me that since there were no cancerlike findings, the pain was most likely due to irritation of the irradiated airway mucosa by reflux of stomach acid. Even after they increased the acid-reducing medication I was taking, the pain did not subside.

The recurrence was finally observed by an astute resident, who was the first physician who, while performing an endoscopic examination, asked me to do a valsalva maneuver (exhale while closing my mouth). This maneuver allows visualization of the pyriform sinus, where the tumor was located. I was wondering why my experienced head and neck surgeons failed to perform such a basic procedure before. Had they done it earlier, my tumor (which was 4×2 cm) would most likely have been observed and removed at an earlier stage.

I was also examined by a radiation oncologist just 3 weeks earlier, who had seen no abnormality when he performed an endoscopic examination of my upper airway. This specialist confessed to me later that he actually did not look down into the area where the new cancer was found because his instrument broke down during his examination. Although I was angry at his failure to do the test appropriately, which delayed the diagnosis of the malignancy, his honesty and willingness to admit that his examination was incomplete made it easier for me to forgive him. I also had deep appreciation for his kindness, care, and compassion and kept returning to him for my care. I also did not realize that radiation oncologists are less experienced than otolaryngologists in performing endoscopic examinations.

Failure to Remove the Recurrent Cancer Using Laser

The first error during my hospitalization was that my surgeons, using laser, mistakenly removed scar tissue instead of the cancerous lesion. The cancerous lesion was farther down in the pyriform sinus. It was a week before the error was discovered by pathological studies. This error could have been avoided if frozen sections of the lesion, not just of the margins, had been analyzed. This error meant that I had to undergo an additional laser surgical procedure 10 days later to remove the tumor.

The circumstances that led to notifying me about the error were very upsetting for me. Following the initial surgery, my surgeons informed me they were able to remove the cancer in its entirety by using the laser, and all the margins of the removed area were clear of cancer. I was therefore spared from more extensive surgery, which would have included removal of tissues in the right side of my neck, requiring their replacement by tissues transplanted from my thighs or shoulder areas. However, as was planned, the entire lymph gland system in the right side of my neck was excised and was going to be studied for the presence of metastasis within a few days. I felt great relief when I heard the news and felt very fortunate. Even though there was still uncertainty about the final pathological results, the alternative was much worse.

The day of my discharge finally arrived a week after my surgery, and I was expecting to hear from my surgeons about the final pathological report before going home. The last day was dragging on and on, and my discharge orders were not in yet. Finally, at about 4:30 p.m. the chief otolaryngology resident, accompanied by a junior resident, walked into my room and asked me to follow them to the Otolaryngology Clinic. I was a little surprised, because all I expected to receive from them were my discharge papers. They explained to me that they wanted to reexamine my upper airways one more time using endoscopy. This made sense and seemed reasonable to me; I assumed that they wanted to perform a final examination prior to my discharge. I expected this would take only a few minutes and I would finally be allowed to go home.

In the clinic, they directed me to an examination room. I sat on the examination chair, and the senior resident numbed my upper airway and inserted the endoscope downward through my nose. He seemed to concentrate on one area and asked the junior resident to also observe it. They mumbled something to each other and nodded their heads in agreement. I asked them if everything was okay, but they did not respond. After completing their examination, they left the room without saying a word and closed the door. It felt strange to sit on the examination chair waiting for their return, but no one came back for a long time.

After 30 min, I left the examination room and searched the clinic to no avail, finding no one. The long wait was very unnerving and did not make any sense to me. However, I had no suspicion that there was anything wrong.

After about 50 min, the two residents, accompanied by the two senior surgeons who performed my surgery, walked into the examining room and delivered to me the most distressing and upsetting news.

The chief surgeon began, "I would like to discuss with you the results of the pathological examinations. I have some good and some bad news. The good news is that there are no signs of cancer spreading into the lymph glands on the right side of the neck. The bad news is that the tumor is still in your hypopharynx. We have not yet removed it. The endoscopic examination done today confirmed that it is still where it was before."

Words cannot express my feelings when I heard this. I was stunned. My first response was utter surprise and disbelief. Anger and loss of trust came later. Accepting my situation and making decisions for the best course of action came last.

The surgeon proceeded to explain that the tissue they removed with the endoscope was not the tumor, but rather scar tissue that looked abnormal. That abnormal area was only half an inch away from the cancer, but was higher up in my airway, so that when they inserted the endoscope, they observed it right away. Because that area looked very suspicious, they assumed that it was the tumor. They removed it and sent it to the pathological laboratory without confirming that what they took out was indeed cancerous. They then proceeded to take biopsies around the resected area. These biopsies were immediately frozen and inspected in the operating room and were found to be cancer-free. When the pathology laboratory read the resected tissue suspected to be cancerous several days later, to the surprise of everyone, there were no cancer cells to be seen, and the tissue contained only scar tissue. To my question why they did not analyze frozen sections of the tissue suspected to be cancerous in the operating room, the surgeon responded "We were convinced that what he had removed was the cancer."

Obviously, the surgeons erroneously assumed that they had removed the cancer. However, if they would have requested that the pathologist who was present in the operating room confirm this by looking at the frozen sections of the suspected cancerous lesion, the error would have been discovered right away and they would have proceeded to search and ultimately remove the cancer, which was so close by.

The surgeons discovered their mistake only when the pathological report came back and showed only scar tissue in the specimen. What was left now to do was to go back and attempt to remove the actual tumor. The surgeons informed me that they were planning to do just that in 2 days.

I was puzzled and upset by the incompetence of the surgeons. I had so many disturbing questions for them: "Why is it not the standard of care to immediately study by frozen section the removed tumor right in the operating room? This could have prevented me from needing another surgical procedure. Furthermore, this failure has delayed the removal of the cancer for 9 additional days. How could you have missed finding the tumor you observed several times before?"

What was even more upsetting was that a few days prior to the surgery, my surgeon reassured me that he was going to take biopsies of the cancer before removing it and confirm the presence of cancer at the site. His email just prior to my surgery said, "We will take multiple mapping biopsies, from both your new primary site and the old site."

Later, I learned from the otolaryngologist that another adverse consequence of the failure to remove the cancer on the first surgery was that each surgery induces extensive local swelling and inflammation, rendering immediate new surgery in the affected area more difficult. This was especially significant in my case because my tumor was located at a very narrow area that is difficult to access and visualize. In other words, the best chance for successful removal of the cancer by laser had been in the first surgery. After the initial surgery, the narrow passage where the tumor was situated became inflamed, irritated, and swollen, and its diameter was therefore reduced. This made any follow-up interventions more difficult because insertion of an endoscope and visualization of the area were harder.

It was very difficult for me to contain my feelings of extreme anger and my loss of trust; but I knew it was inappropriate for me to express these emotions freely as I wished I could. I was very vulnerable and depended on these surgeons, who were still taking care of me. I had had close professional relationships with many of them for over 27 years and liked them very much as individuals. I only wished I could tell them how angry I was and walk away to get treatment elsewhere. I regretted not having had the laser surgery done by surgeons who had more experience with this procedure.

I realized then that experience is very important in this kind of surgery. Since throat cancer frequency is diminishing in this country, there are fewer patients with this type of cancer and surgeons consequently have less experience removing it. With so few throat cancer patients, it is no surprise that expertise in its removal and care is concentrated in just a few places. Obviously, my surgeons had very little experience using laser to remove my type of cancer. I was wondering why the department head, the one that used the laser, stated that if he felt that he could not remove my cancer with laser, he would have told me so. I sympathized with his honest self-confidence, because even though I am not a surgeon, I had probably manifested similar self-assurance whenever I talked with patients and their family members. However, as I became older and more experienced, I often admitted my shortcomings and deferred decisions to physicians who were more experienced in areas I was not. Since I liked my surgeons very much, I ignored consideration of their competence in this procedure when I made my decision to let them operate on me.

Although the error made by my surgeons was very regrettable, their honest admission and acceptance of responsibility made it easier for me to endure it. Even though the surgeons suggested that I could seek care in another center, I decided to give them a second chance to remove the cancer.

Failure to Respond to Breathing Difficulties in the Surgical Intensive Care Unit

I have experienced hazardous situations because of nursing errors. On one occasion, one day after my major surgery while I was still in the Surgical Intensive Care Unit (SICU), I experienced an obstruction of my airway and reached for the call button. It was not to be found, as it had fallen to the floor. I tried to call the attention of the staff, and even though I was a few feet away from the nursing station, I was ignored until my wife happened to arrive about 10 min later. I was helpless in asking for assistance without a voice and was desperately in need of air while medical personal passed me by.

When my wife went to the nurses' station to complain about what happened, she was rudely rebuffed by the SICU attending physician, who told her not to interfere with his medical rounds. I insisted that the incident be reported to the nurse supervisor, but even when she showed up a few hours later, she did not seemed to be concerned and explained that my nurse was busy caring for other patients. I was too sick to pursue the matter any further.

When I brought this incident to the attention of the head surgeon, he just shrugged his shoulders and told me that he had little influence on what happened in the SICU, but he assured me that things would be much better for me when I was moved to the otolaryngology floor, where he ran things. He told me that the staff there was more familiar with patients with my kind of operation, so the care there would be much better and more customized to my needs.

The unwillingness of my surgeon to act upon my complaint was very disappointing and upsetting to me. Instead of dealing with the problem in the SICU that cares for his patients when they are critically ill, he comforted me by promising better care when I will be less in need of it.

Failure to Respond to Breathing Difficulties in the Otolaryngology Ward

A similar incident took place on the otolaryngology floor a week later, when the nurse did not respond to my call to suction my airways. I felt difficulty in breathing, as mucus that had built up in my trachea was obstructing my airway. I pressed the call button in my room, but no one came to my assistance. I was able to get the attention of a nurse assistant, who told me that my nurse was on a break. Since the nurse assistant was not trained in suctioning airways, she promised to look for a nurse who could help me. The nurse finally came to assist me 15 min later. I learned that she was on the phone ordering supplies during all that time.

This was a very distressing event, as I was agitated and struggling to breathe in the middle of the otolaryngology ward. There were two residents and several nurse assistants on the floor, yet no one helped me for what felt like a very long time. It is obvious that even on a ward dedicated to people with breathing difficulties and breathing issues, there were many distractions that prevented physicians and nurses from paying attention to their patient's immediate needs.

I brought the incident to the attention of the nurse supervisor and the head surgeon but never received any feedback from them about what was to be done to prevent such incidents in the future. The lack of response by these medical providers was inappropriate and contributed to my frustration and anxiety.

Premature Oral Feeding

The most serious error in my hospital care was feeding me by mouth with soft food a week too early. Early feeding by mouth after laryngectomy with free flap reconstruction can lead to failure of the flap to integrate and lead to its failure. This premature feeding continued for 16 h. Only my persistent questioning brought this to the attention of a senior surgeon, who discontinued it. I wondered what would have happened had I not continued to question the feeding and when (or if) the error would have been eventually discovered.

Even though I repeatedly requested an explanation from my physician of how this error occurred, I received no response. I learned later by looking in my medical records that this occurred because the order to start oral feeding was intended for another patient and was erroneously transcribed into my chart.

This was another example of the complete lack of communication by the physician to explain and apologize for the mistake. Accepting responsibility for the error and explaining what steps were being taken to prevent such a mistake in the future would have been the appropriate way of handling the situation.

Nursing Errors

Some of the errors by nursing and other staff included the following (Table 22.1): not cleaning or washing their hands and not using gloves when indicated, taking an oral temperature without placing the thermometer in a plastic sheath, using an inappropriately sized blood pressure cuff (thus getting alarming readings), attempting to administer medications by mouth that were intended to be given by nasogastric tube, dissolving pills in hot water and feeding them through the feeding tube (which caused burning in the esophagus), delivering an incorrect dose of a medication, connecting a suction machine directly to the suction port in the wall without a bottle of water, forgetting to rinse away the hydrogen peroxide used for cleaning the tracheal breathing tube (thus causing severe irritation), forgetting to connect the call button when I was bedridden and unable to speak, and forgetting to write down verbal orders.

Table 22.1 Medical errors experienced by the author

Physicians' errors
Failure to detect cancer recurrence
Early feeding
Removal of scar tissue instead of the tumor
Forgetting to write down orders
Nurses' errors
Not responding to calls
Forgetting to connect the call button when the patient is bedridden and unable to speak
Not cleaning or washing hands or using gloves when indicated
Taking oral temperature without placing the thermometer in a plastic sheath
Using an inappropriately sized blood pressure cuff (thus getting wrong readings)
Attempting to administer medications orally intended for nasogastric tube
Delivering an incorrect dose of medication
Administering medication through the nasogastric tube that were dissolved in hot water (thus causing esophageal burning)
Connecting a suction machine directly to the suction port without a bottle of water
Forgetting to rinse the hydrogen peroxide after cleaning the tracheal breathing tube (thus causing severe irritation)

Even though I always notified the nurse supervisors and in many cases the resident and/or attending physicians about the errors, I was never informed what action was taken to prevent similar mistakes in the future.

Conclusions

All of the errors in my care made me wonder what happens to patients without medical education, who cannot recognize and prevent an error. Fortunately, despite these errors, I did not suffer any long-term consequences. However, I had to be constantly on guard and stay vigilant, which was very exhausting, especially during the difficult recovery process.

I realized that the help of a dedicated patient advocate, such as a family member or friend, is very much needed for all hospitalized patients. Although my family members are not in the medical profession, they were instrumental in preventing many errors.

My experiences taught me that it is very important that medical staff members openly discuss with their patients the errors that were made in their care. The occurrence of errors weakens patients trust in their caregivers. Admission and acceptance of responsibility by the caregivers can bridge the gap between them and the patient and reestablish the lost confidence. When such a dialogue takes place, more details about the circumstances leading to the mistake can be learned and preventing similar mistakes in the future is more likely. Open discussion can assure patients that their caregivers are taking the matter seriously and that steps are taken to make their hospital stay safer.

Not discussing the mistakes with patients and their family members increases their anxiety, frustration, and anger, which can interfere with the patients' recovery. Furthermore, such anger may also lead to malpractice law suits.

Obviously, medical errors should be prevented as much as humanly possible. Ignoring them can lead only to their repetition. I am sharing my experiences in the hope that they will encourage better medical training, contribute to greater diligence in care, and increase supervision and communication between caregivers. It is my hope that my presentation will contribute to the reduction of such errors and lead to a safer environment in the hospital setting. It is also my hope that medical care providers will openly discuss mistakes with their patients.

References

1. Tezak B, Anderson C, Down A, Gibson H, Lynn B, McKinney S, et al. Looking ahead: the use of prospective analysis to improve the quality and safety of care. Healthc Q. 2009;12:80–4.
2. Griffen FD, Turnage RH. Reviews of liability claims against surgeons: what have they revealed? Adv Surg. 2009;43:199–209.
3. Studdert DM, Mello MM, Gawande AA, Gandhi TK, Kachalia A, Yoon C, et al. Claims, errors, and compensation payments in medical malpractice litigation. N Engl J Med. 2006;354:2024–33.
4. Byrnes MC, Schuerer DJ, Schallom ME, Sona CS, Mazuski JE, Taylor BE, et al. Implementation of a mandatory checklist of protocols and objectives improves compliance with a wide range of evidence-based intensive care unit practices. Crit Care Med. 2009;37:2775–81.

Chapter 23
Communication with Cancer Patients in Family Medicine

Mustafa Fevzi Dikici, Fusun Yaris, and Fusun Aysin Artiran Igde

Abstract Family medicine is the point of first medical contact within the healthcare system. Patient perspective and patient-centered communication are very important in family medicine. Family physicians assess the illnesses and complaints presented to them, dealing personally with most, serve as the patients' advocate, explaining the causes and implications of illness to the patients and their families, serve as an adviser and confidant to the family. BATHE (background, affect, trouble, handling, empathy) is a method for communication in family medicine while practicing bio-psychosocial medicine. The communication process with cancer patients in the daily practice of family physicians will be evaluated in this chapter.

Keywords Communication • Cancer patient • Patient-centered care • Family medicine • Primary care • General practice • Continuity of care

Cancer Epidemiology for Family Physicians

Family medicine/general practice is the point of first medical contact within the healthcare system [1, 2]. In a family practice of 2,000 people, approximately eight patients are diagnosed with cancer each year and four patients die of the disease. Large increases are predicted in the incidence and prevalence of cancer. People with cancer visit their family physicians (FPs) about twice as often as other patients, and most say they turn to their FPs first rather than a cancer center if their symptoms worsen [3]. Because 45% of cancer patients die usually within 5 years, the average family doctor will have three to four patients die of cancer yearly. If a FP practices 40 years, he/she will have had 160 cancer patients who died [4].

M.F. Dikici, MD (✉) • F. Yaris, MD, Ph.D. • F.A. Artiran Igde, MD
Department of Family Medicine, Ondokuzmayis University School
of Medicine, Samsun, Turkey
e-mail: mdikici@omu.edu.tr

In 2006, crude cancer incidence was 261.6 for men and 175.9 for women per 100,000 in Turkey [5]. A family physician with a patient panel of 3,000 patients would have approximately 1,500 women and 1,500 men. That means that the family physician would have approximately four (3.92) new male cancer patients and three (2.64) new female cancer patients each year.

The Family Physician's Role in Cancer Care

The diagnosis of cancer may be made in FP's office; however, the diagnosis is only suspected by the FP. The patient then needs to be examined by one or more other physicians, who are usually strangers, to confirm the terrifying suspicion of cancer. The FP's role is in some ways even more crucial once he/she has turned the diagnostic work over to specialists. The FP must be able to explain what will happen. He/she needs to be completely clear with the specialists as to what the patient is expecting, what the patient has been told, by whom, and under which circumstances the diagnosis of cancer will be told to the patient and family. The patient should learn the cancer diagnosis from the family physician if possible. The patient and family will be more likely to understand this bad news and to accept the empathy and compassion they need when the diagnosis is conveyed by the FP, who has had a long relationship with the patient. The patient and family need to know that the FP is intimately involved in the patient's care, and he/she will not delegate such an important duty of giving bad news to another physician. In addition, the FP needs to let the patient and family know that he/she will continue to play an important role in the patient's care [4].

The cancers of the patients of the FP will originate in different organs, with several types. To understand an individual patient's disease, the treatment options, risks, side effects of treatment, and prognosis seems impossible. The FP knows the patient and family best, and the FP is obliged to be the patient's and family's advocate. The FP needs to have the ability to reveal and share the sources of information about the disease and communicate this clearly to the patient and all specialists involved in the care [4].

The FP must remember that the oncologist sees the patient in the context of the stress of serious illness, while the FP has a much broader frame of reference. Whether the patient is cured of cancer or experiences progressive disease, the patient and family will return to the care of the FP. The FP must realize that the diagnosis of cancer does not eliminate the need for care for other medical problems. The FP must be willing to share uncertainty with the patient. The ability of the FP to confront uncertainty may provide important relief to the patient and family, especially if things do not go as predicted [4].

The FP needs to know how to deal with difficult issues at the end of life. The patient's family experiences many problems in caring for their loved one—anxiety, depression, guilt, helplessness, isolation, income loss, etc. The most important information for the caregivers is that they will not be abandoned by the FP. This situation permits calling for help when the family is overwhelmed [4].

One of the foremost skills of the family physician is the ability to use effectively the knowledge of interpersonal relations in the management of patients. This powerful element of clinical medicine is the specialty's most useful tool [6].

Communication needs special attention in cancer patients. Family doctors should have capabilities of breaking bad news to the patients and relatives, longitudinal care of the patient, palliative care, and dying patients' care. Care of a cancer patient in primary care requires highly developed communication skills. Cancer may involve progressive loss in the patient's functional capacity, and the patient needs medical, psychological, and social support. The family and caregiver of the patient with cancer may also need support [6].

Breaking Bad News

Breaking bad news is difficult. Training doctors in this is beneficial [7]. Here is a summary of suggestions for breaking bad news [8]:

1. *Preparing the environment*: The physician prepares a peaceful atmosphere before giving the bad news.
2. *Understanding what the patient knows, wants to learn*: Almost all patients want to hear the truth, but there is a limit to how much patients can bear at a single encounter.
3. *Giving information*: Breaking bad news is a painful experience for the physician as well as the patient. The FP blends reassurance and encouragement with the bad news and chooses the words carefully. The way of giving bad news is important in the encounter.
4. *Developing empathetic behavior*: The physician explains that he/she understands her/his patient's feeling. The physician remains flexible on the comments and suggestions after the patient's response. By attending to the patients' reactions, the physician learns about the fears and concerns of the patient.
5. *Closing the interview appropriately*: The patient needs time to digest the news. The family may be involved in the discussion and ask questions. Appropriate time is necessary for the interview. A second interview can be recommended to clarify everything better [7, 8].

Family Physician–Oncologist Collaboration

We need primary care doctor–specialist collaboration in the care of a cancer patient. This collaboration also needs special communication skills [9]. Cancer survivors in general have multiple care needs after the primary treatment of their cancer, including management of symptoms resulting from disease or treatment, monitoring for late effects of treatment, follow-up tests to monitor for recurrence, and promotion of health [10]. As the complexity of treatment for cancer increases, the need for coordination of care and sharing of knowledge increases. Multidisciplinary cancer care has been shown to improve survival and adherence to evidence-based guidelines. That is a standard feature of high-quality cancer care [11]. Potential implications of optimized shared care include more informed patient-centered decision-making, better adherence to treatment, closer match between patient goals and treatments, and more appropriate care in a common care plan [12]. Many studies reinforce the importance of good communication and collaboration between family physicians and the oncology team in order to keep the former involved at all phases of the cancer and to promote shared care in cancer follow-up [13].

What Cancer Patients Want

Studies suggest that the majority of patients want prognostic information and shared decision-making. When discussing prognosis, patients' communication preferences include, but are not limited to, the following: realistic, complete information, an opportunity to ask questions, to be treated as an individual, to trust the competence of the physician, reassurance of sufficient pain control, and to maintain hope. Despite this, there also is evidence for relative independence between the patient's desire for information and his/her preference for participation in decision-making. Patient satisfaction, emotional health, and regret may be related to congruence between preferred and actual participation; however, physicians often have difficulty determining what patients want [14].

The patient's perspective has a critical role in the process of a consultation with the family physician [15]. The following are aspects of the patient's perspective [16]:

- The patient's thoughts about the nature and cause of the problem
- The patient's feelings and fears about the problem
- The patient's expectations of the physician and health care
- The effect of the problem on the patient's life
- Prior experiences
- Therapeutic responses

Patient-Centered Care

Patient-centered care is being respectful and responsive to individual patient preferences and personal values [17]. Patient-centered care is the ability to adopt a person-centered approach in dealing with patients and problems, to develop and apply the general practice consultation to bring about an effective doctor–patient relationship, and to provide longitudinal continuity of care as determined by the needs of the patient [1].

Research has shown that the components of the patient-centered approach have positive relationships with a variety of worthy outcomes, such as patient recovery, emotional health, physical function, and physiological outcomes [18, 19]. Other advantages are patient satisfaction and adherence, physician satisfaction, fewer malpractice suits, and saved time [19]. Programs that encourage patients and physicians to communicate in a more patient-centered way have resulted in improved outcomes. This method can be taught during medical education [20].

The patient-centered model is a reasonable representation of the realities of medical practice; the model guides physicians in their complex work of patient care. Because the method grew out of medical practice, rather than being borrowed from other disciplines, it has immediate applicability for both the novice as well as the experienced physician [19]. The model applies to the majority of patient–doctor interactions. It describes what physicians do when they are functioning well with the patients, providing a conceptual framework for the physician [19].

Patient-Centered Communication

Family physicians assess the illnesses and complaints presented to them, dealing personally with most and arranging special assistance for a few. The FP explains the causes and implications of illness to the patients and their families and serves as an adviser and confidant to the family. The FP receives intellectual satisfaction from this practice, but the greatest reward arises from the depth of human understanding and personal satisfaction inherent in family practice. Patients have adjusted somewhat to a more impersonal form of healthcare delivery and frequently look to institutions rather than to individuals for their health care; however, their need for personalized concern and compassion remains. Patients consider a good physician to be one who shows genuine interest in them; who thoroughly evaluates their problem; who demonstrates compassion, understanding, and warmth; and who provides clear insight into what is wrong and what must be done to correct it [6].

For clinicians who want to inform patients and undertake shared decision-making, the goal of effective communication presents a number of challenges. To begin with, the probabilities to be discussed are small. For each screening test done, the chance of finding and effectively treating an early cancer is quite low. Likewise, the chance of causing harm, such as a false-positive screen followed by an invasive test resulting in complications, is also very unlikely, though possible. Using accurate terms that patients can understand is only the first step, however; the decision-making process should take into account the patient's perceptions, values, and preferences [21]. Physician behaviors indicating interpersonal competence and genuine concern, such as listening and caring, providing information, answering questions, and patience promote trust [22].

Discussion of the Prognosis

While guidelines exist for discussing prognosis with patients, there is no firm evidence supporting any one approach. Researchers have found that patients prefer a realistic and hopeful style when disclosing prognosis. Hope is conveyed partly by discussing all the treatment options. Cancer patients in Western cultures report a preference for knowing their diagnostic findings, prognosis, and probability of successfully treating their disease. Not all cultures endorse such a preference; physicians from non-Western cultures may be more reluctant to disclose prognostic information than Western physicians. Others have described the practical difficulties of determining if a specific cancer patient really wants to know his/her prognosis. It is common for patients not to understand their prognosis, which may hinder decision-making and treatment. Both the patient and the physician affect the discussion of prognosis. This discussion may be hampered by the different focuses of the patient and the physician. Patients are focused on the impact of cancer on their lives and their discomfort and pain. Physicians, by contrast, are focused on the illness, particularly on its progression and treatment. Eliciting and validating patient concerns and an attentive tone of voice promote a satisfactory discussion of the cancer patient's prognosis [23].

Practicing Biopsychosocial Medicine

The physician's awareness of the impact of stress on the overall problems presented by patients is critical for determining the appropriate course of treatment. Many physicians are unaware of their considerable capability to influence the thinking and behavior of their patients. Therapeutic talk is direct conversation that focuses patients on their strengths and choices. It makes patients feel better, more competent to deal with the circumstances of their lives, and connected, through a positive relationship with their physician. It changes the story that patients are "inadequate" and that "no one cares" [6].

BATHEing the patient gets to the core of psychosocial problems and often elicits evidence of anxiety or depression. Depression can be treated effectively after the diagnosis, using brief sessions and therapeutic talk, with or without medication [6] (Table 23.1).

BATHE (background, affect, trouble, handling, empathy) is not the only technique a clinician can employ, but it also tends to bring order out of what is frequently a chaotic and open-ended approach to psychosocial assessment. In the process, it helps bridge the gap between the biomedical and the psychosocial in a way that is meaningful for contemporarily trained physicians. By asking pointed, focused questions, which lend themselves to brief but reasonably comprehensive answers, the physician is able to incorporate this very necessary form of assessment into a format that can enable one to deal with large numbers of patients. Family physicians have a responsibility to each patient to provide comprehensive health care, but they also have a responsibility to the community to care for a number of patients. The proper blending of these two responsibilities can be facilitated by this technique [6].

Table 23.1 BATHE

Item	Question
B: Background	A simple question can elicit the context of the patient's visit: What is going on in your life?
A: Affect	Some questions allow the patient to report her/his current feeling state: How do you feel about that? What is your mood?
T: Trouble	A question can help the physician and the patient focus on the situation's subjective meaning: What about the situation troubles you most?
H: Handling	An assessment of functioning can be elicited by a question: How are you handling that?
E: Empathy	Some statements can legitimize the patient's reaction: That must be very difficult for you

Ownership

The physician's inquiry into the patient's psychosocial status is designed to produce enhanced comprehension on the part of the physician of the overall dimensions of a patient's presenting problem. It is not designed to enable the physician to assume responsibility for the patient's particular situation, but rather to assess the patient's situation so that therapeutic suggestions can be made, enabling the patient to deal with his or her problem more effectively. The patient continues to own his or her problem, but the family physician is better able to help the patient in the resolution of the problem because the physician has a comprehensive understanding of the derivation of the problem. This is true whether the problem is predominantly biomedical or psychosocial, because each invariably has a component of the other ingrained in the patient's overall situation. Ownership of the problem remains with the patient, but what emanates from the doctor–patient relationship is the understanding on the part of the patient that the physician is there to help. The physician's skills and abilities to help are enhanced by assessing and understanding the array of influences working on a given patient [6].

Forms of Therapeutic Talk

Giving Advice

Although patients ask for advice, getting them to focus on their own resources with some guidance for developing alternatives is always more effective. When the physician gives advice or directly solves a problem, it does not empower the patient. It is better to make patients aware of their own strengths and their abilities to assess and exercise their own options. However, there are certain suggestions that the physician can make that focus primarily on the process of dealing with problems. Patients should be instructed to focus on the "here and now," to look at their options and to apply the tincture of time. Along with the physician's support and the opportunity to return to discuss the situation further, this is often enough to diminish a patient's stress level and trigger a significant positive change in the patient's affective response. Using the BATHE technique to structure subsequent visits is highly effective [6].

Distinguishing among Thoughts, Feelings, and Behavior

There are other brief interventions that the family physician can employ [6]. Patients must learn to differentiate among thoughts, feelings, and behavior. Thoughts are related to our beliefs and the stories that we tell ourselves about the world, other people, and ourselves. Everyone makes these judgments, expectations, and generalizations. Physicians must acknowledge the patients' views before being able to challenge them [6].

Feelings are emotional responses to a situation based on thoughts and judgments. Feelings must be expressed and accepted. In this process, feelings change. Feelings also change when irrational thoughts and unrealistic expectations are altered [5].

Behavior consists of the actions we take. Our behavior is the only thing in this life that we can control. Helping patients focus on their behavior and make positive adjustments in their lifestyle is probably the most important intervention a physician can make. Even a depressed patient should be encouraged to express thoughts and feelings related to being defeated and discouraged, but the patient also should be given instructions to take daily walks, regardless of whether the activity holds any enjoyment [6].

Assuming There Are Options

When patients are overwhelmed, they lose sight of the fact that they still have choices. The physician's suggestion that there are always options and that the patient needs to explore them cues the patient in a positive direction. It is not the physician's task to generate these options, it is the patient's responsibility. The physician communicates the expectation that the patient can do this and will return to report the results. This therapeutic intervention helps patients be more open to possibilities; to look at their world, including themselves, in a new way; and to become aware of having choices [6].

Changing the Story

Encouraging patients to reinterpret their situations is useful. Every trying circumstance can be seen as an opportunity to learn a necessary lesson. This approach is called reframing. Physicians can point out that there are four healthy options for handling a bad situation [6]:

1. Leaving it alone dictates exploring the best and worst possible outcomes that may result and planning for an appropriate time to make a move.
2. Changing it requires an investigation of what is possible and what additional resources can be brought to bear.
3. Accepting it requires recognizing that if things could be different they would be different.
4. Reframing it means finding a way to interpret the situation as a positive or necessary learning experience [6].

Listening Well

During communication, an attentive tone of voice invites conversations about difficult topics. An attentive tone of voice also indicates physician mindfulness, characterized by purposeful attention to one's own thoughts and feelings in a nonjudgmental fashion [22].

A good physician must be a good listener. Of all the communication skills essential to rapport, the ability to listen well is probably the most important. All the information in the world about body language, vocal messages, and nonverbal cues is of limited value unless it helps the physician be a better listener. In the short time available to take a history, the aim is to obtain, in addition to essential facts, insight into the human being. This seems easy, but listening is the most complex and difficult of all the tools in a doctor's repertory. One must be an active listener to hear an unspoken problem. The appearance of readiness to listen is aided by bending forward and maintaining eye contact. The physician can discourage a patient from talking by looking away or writing in the medical record. Well-chosen questions can be rendered useless by inappropriate nonverbal behavior. For many people the opposite of talking is not listening; it is waiting to talk. Effective listening requires focusing on what is being said and on the tone of voice, facial expression, and body movements. Hearing what someone says and truly listening to what they are saying are quite different [6]. Analyses of doctor–patient interviews reveal that, on average, the doctor rather than the patient does most of the talking; although the physicians, when questioned, usually imagine the reverse [8].

How Family Physician–Patient Communication Influences Patient Health Behavior

The literature points to two pathways through which physician communication might lead to behavior change in the patient. First, if physicians explicitly prescribe a specific behavioral change, patients are more likely to change that behavior than in the absence of a personal recommendation. Second, if physicians communicate with appropriate personal rapport, such as warmth, openness, and interest, patients will be more likely to attempt the prescribed behavior change. In an earlier study of the effects of physician–patient communication on breast cancer screening among women aged 50 and over, the biggest predictor of mammography use, conditional on physician recommendation, was found to be patient-perceived physician enthusiasm for the test [24].

There are large variations across countries in physicians' intentions of informing patients and relatives about prognosis. In most countries, there is potential for improvement in these intentions. There is a positive association of training in palliative care and younger age of the physician with a more proactive approach to prognosis discussion [25]. When patients are informed and involved in decision-making, they are more compliant with medical recommendations. Joint decision-making requires patients to be fully informed about alternatives and potential risks of treatment and to have trust in their physician [26].

Primary Palliative Care

FPs deliver the majority of palliative care to their cancer patients, generally in an effective way, especially when they have specialist support [27]. Improved communication is necessary throughout treatment and care [28] (Table 23.2).

Web-based tools also may be useful for improving communication between the family physicians and palliative care patients, caregivers, and proactive patient management [29].

Table 23.2 A practical model for primary palliative care—identify, assess, plan care

Identify palliative care patients	Communicate information within the team
	Record and communicate about the patients
	Identify caregivers and their needs
Assess and respond to patient and caregiver need (patient-centered care responding to needs)	Physical problems, holistic/psychosocial needs
	Discuss the needs with patients and caregivers according to their agenda
	Plan regular response to need
	Support, symptom control
	Refer
	Communicate better with patients, caregivers, and staff
Plan care	Nominate specific coordinator in practice
	Communicate with team members and others
	Caregiver support anticipated, education, empowerment
	Discuss preferred place of care
	Drugs, equipment needed
	Out of hours crisis care
	Terminal phase planned according to protocol
	Staff support
	Plan of proactive support, further contacts

Conclusion

In the light of the core competences, family doctors have the responsibility in the care of cancer patients in their population from the beginning to the end of the cancer period. Characteristics of the family medicine specialty interface with the cancer patients' needs for the continuity of patient-centered and comprehensive care.

References

1. Evans P. (Ed.) The European Society of General Practice/Family Medicine. The European definition of general practice/family medicine, Wonca Europe 2002. Barcelona: WHO Europe Office; 2002.
2. Dikici MF, Kartal M, Alptekin S, Cubukcu M, Ayanoğlu SHA, Yaris F. Concepts, task in family medicine and history of the discipline. Turk Clin J Med Sci. 2007;27(3):412–8.
3. Sisler JJ, Brown JB, Stewart M. Family physicians' roles in cancer care. Survey of patients on a provincial cancer. Can Fam Physician. 2004;50:889–96.
4. Walsh E. Cancer care. In: Saultz JW, editor. Textbook of family medicine. New York: McGraw-Hill; 2000. p. 585–602.
5. Cancer Control Department of the Ministry of Health of Turkey. http://www.kanser.gov.tr/index_en.php. Accessed 17 Apr 2011.
6. Rakel RE. The family physician. In: Rakel RE, editor. Textbook of family medicine. 7th ed. Philadelphia: Saunders Elsevier; 2007. p. 3–14.
7. Dikici MF, Yaris F, Cubukcu M. Teaching medical students how to break bad news: a Turkish experience. J Cancer Educ. 2009;24(4):246–8.
8. Silverman J, Kurtz S, Draper J. (Eds.) Relating specific issues to core communication skills. In: Skills for communicating with patients. 2nd ed. Oxon: Radcliffe Medical Press; 2005.
9. Foy R, Hempel S, Rubenstein L, Suttorp M, Seelig M, Shanman R, et al. Meta-analysis: effect of interactive communication between collaborating primary care physicians and specialists. Ann Intern Med. 2010;152(4):247–58.
10. Haggstrom DA, Arora NK, Helft P, Clayman ML, Oakley-Girvan I. Follow-up care delivery among colorectal cancer survivors most often seen by primary and subspecialty care physicians. J Gen Intern Med. 2009;24 Suppl 2:S472–9.
11. Davit B, Philip J, McLachlan SA. Team dynamics, decision making, and attitudes toward multidisciplinary cancer meetings: health professionals' perspective. J Oncol Pract. 2010;6(6):e17–20.
12. O'Toole E, Step MM, Engelhardt K, Lewis S, Rose JH. The role of primary care physicians in advanced cancer care: perspectives of older patients and their oncologists. J Am Geriatr Soc. 2009;57 Suppl 2:S265–8.
13. Aubin M, Vézina L, Verreault R, Fillion L, Hudon E, Lehmann F, et al. Family physician involvement in cancer care follow-up: the experience of a cohort of patients with lung cancer. Ann Fam Med. 2010;8(6):526–32.
14. Trice ED, Pierson HG. Communication in end-stage cancer: review of the literature and future research. J Health Commun. 2009;14 Suppl 1:95–108.
15. WcWhinney IR. Illness, suffering and healing, doctor-patient communication. In: WcWhinney IR, editor. A textbook of family medicine. New York: Oxford University Press; 1997. p. 83–128.
16. Naumberg EH. Interviewing and the health history. In: Bickley LS, Szilagyi PG, editors. Bates' guide to physical examination and history taking. 8th ed. Philadelphia: Lippincott Williams and Wilkins; 2003. p. 21–57.

17. Miada V, Peck J, Enis M, Brar N, Miada AR. Preferences for active and aggressive intervention among patients with advanced cancer. BMC Cancer. 2010;10:592.
18. Stewart M, Brown JB, Donner A, McWhinney IR, Oates J, Weston WW, et al. The impact of patient-centered care on outcomes. Fam Pract. 2000;49(9):796–804.
19. Brown JB, Stewart M, Weston WW. (Eds.) Why is practicing patient-centered medicine important? And breaking bad news. In: Challenges and solutions in patient centered care. Oxon: Radcliffe Medical Press; 2002. Introduction.
20. Dikici MF, Yaris F. Standardized and simulated patient program in Ondokuz Mayis University School of Medicine. Turk Clin J Med Sci. 2007;27(5):738–43.
21. Barrett B, McKenna P. Communicating benefits and risks of screening for prostate, colon, and breast cancer. Fam Med. 2011;43(4):248–53.
22. Hillen MA, de Haes HC, Smets EM. Cancer patients' trust in their physician—a review. Psychooncology. 2011;20(3):227–41.
23. Shields CG, Coker CJ, Poulsen SS, Doyle JM, Fiscella K, Epstein RM, et al. Patient-centered communication and prognosis discussions with cancer patients. Patient Educ Couns. 2009;77(3):437–42.
24. Fox SA, Heritage J, Stockdale SE, Asch SM, Duan N, Reise SP. Cancer screening adherence: does physician–patient communication matter? Patient Educ Couns. 2009;75(2):178–84.
25. Voorhees J, Rietjens J, Onwuteaka-Philipsen B, Deliens L, Cartwright C, Faisst K, et al. Discussing prognosis with terminally ill cancer patients and relatives: a survey of physicians' intentions in seven countries. Patient Educ Couns. 2009;77(3):430–6.
26. Beck RS, Daughtridge R, Sloane PD. Physician-patient communication in the primary care office: a systematic review. J Am Board Fam Pract. 2002;15(1):25–38.
27. Mitchell GK. How well do general practitioners deliver palliative care? A systematic review. Palliat Med. 2002;16:457–64.
28. Thomas K. (Ed.) Introduction. In: Caring for the dying at home: companions on the journey. Oxon: Radcliffe Publishing; 2005. p. 3–ßß13.
29. Dy SM, Roy J, Ott GE, McHale M, Kennedy C, Kutner JS, et al. Tell us™: a web-based tool for improving communication among patients, families, and providers in hospice and palliative care through systematic data specification, collection, and use. J Pain Symptom Manage. 2011;42(4):526–34.

Chapter 24
How to Train Teachers of Communication Skills: The Oncotalk Teach Model

Walter F. Baile

Abstract Just as communication is a skill that must be learned, teaching communication skills requires a methodology based upon known educational principles. "Positive psychology," which emphasizes skills needed to produce results; adult learning theory, which emphasizes the "activation" and motivation of learners; and social learning theory, which promotes the importance of practice in learning skills; all inform the implementation of specific techniques to promote learning. These techniques include providing realistic examples of teaching scenarios; ensuring a relevance to common challenges faced by learners; a respect for individual learners' skill level; providing cognitive "road maps" that guide the learner as "how to do it" in communicating effectively; respect for the self-generated goals of the learner; and an opportunity for learners to practice in a safe environment. An efficient way of teaching communication skills is to apply these principles in a small group setting where learners can support and learn from one another. This chapter describes a teaching format based upon these concepts applied to a course for teaching communication skills to medical oncology fellows. It illustrates how the process of teaching oncology attending physicians from major cancer centers to teach communication skills was implemented using a "retreat" model with distance learning. It identifies skills necessary to be a teacher of communication skills by describing not only the skills targeted for development in the fellows but in a parallel fashion the skills applied by the faculty themselves in promoting the development of the learners.

W.F. Baile (✉)
Departments of Behavioral Science and Faculty Development, Program on Interpersonal Communication and Relationship Enhancement (I*CARE), The University of Texas MD Anderson Cancer Center, P.O. Box 301402, Unit 1426, Houston, TX 77030, USA
e-mail: wbaile@mdanderson.org

Introduction

It has been said that communication skills are the cornerstone of comprehensive oncology care [1]. However, it is also clear that the core competencies of giving bad news, explaining clinical trials, discussing end-of-life decisions, and holding family meetings to decide issues such as removing patients from ventilators are extremely challenging and stressful for oncology practitioners [2]. Yet only now are these topics being introduced into training programs in oncology, but often in an ineffective way that does not result in the acquisition of meaningful skills [3, 4]. In fact, medicine almost seems still wedded to the concept that the above-mentioned communication skills can be acquired through careful observation of senior clinicians or are merely extensions of "bedside manners." The counterpoint to this is the demonstration in clinical trials and in longitudinal studies that extensive training is, indeed, required to learn these skills; and that even senior clinicians do not necessarily improve in these skills during the course of a long career [5–7].

The notion that communication is a skill is central to the discussion of how we teach and prepare learners to teach these skills. Fundamentally, communication is a set of defined verbal and nonverbal behaviors that can be observed, recorded, coded, measured, and taught [8–10]. Take, for example, the simple behavior of asking a patient about their understanding of their medical situation before giving them bad news. We and others have observed [11, 12] that this question is commonly left out of bad news discussions, although it is recommended by guidelines on breaking bad news [13, 14]. However, this behavior can be easily learned by clinicians once the usefulness of having the information is pointed out, the impact on patient satisfaction is explained, and the clinicians find the correct way of asking and make a conscious effort to practice it. With enough practice, the behavior can become part of a clinician's interviewing armamentarium. The same is true for some of the complex behaviors noted above, such as giving bad news or responding to emotions. We have shown in Oncotalk a residential workshop to assist medical oncology fellows in improving their communication skills [10], that these behaviors can be acquired through a combination of didactic education and skills practice in a coaching environment [11, 15]. Specifically, over a period of 5 years our group has trained approximately 150 medical oncology fellows to learn skills of breaking bad news, discussing transition to palliative care, and discussing end-of-life issues, using actors who portrayed the part of patients and learners who agreed to dedicate 3 days in a retreat setting to focus on learning these skills. In this paradigm experienced faculty coached the learners in a model based upon Lipkin's small-group learning [16].

Fellows who were trained worked together in small groups and received feedback about their performance from both colleagues and faculty that encouraged them to continue to practice their communication strengths and also to work on their "learning edges"—the skills they were less confident in.

Educational Principles

Oncotalk and Oncotalk Teach (which is the subject of this chapter) are anchored in theories about the doctor–patient relationship and also in educational principles [17–20] that explain how adults learn new information. First among these is that communication is a skill that can be observed, described, learned, and taught. Communication behaviors can be conceptualized as a hierarchy of skills. At the base are fundamental, less complex skills, such as that involved in asking patients about their perception of their illness. On the top rest more complex skills, such as responding to a patient's emotions or monitoring one's own emotional reactions to a patient's emotions. Learners gain confidence in communication skills by acquiring more simple skills first. These can be built upon to acquire more complex skills through coaching and practice [21]. Second, the functions of communication go well beyond conveying information, serving other important functions for the patient and family, such as establishing rapport, listening to concerns, dealing with emotions, and reassuring the patient. In this regard communication may be said to be "therapeutic," in that patients perceive these communication strategies as being helpful in supporting them through the various crises of cancer, such as diagnosis, recurrence, intractable side effects, failure of treatment, and end of life [22].

Educational theory provides an answer to the question: What makes communication skills work? Experts agree that the essential elements that enhance the effectiveness of communication skills training include the following [23, 24].

The training must be realistic. The communication challenges that learners encounter must be constructed in such a way that they are medically accurate. Otherwise, learners will be distracted by the need to clarify details that to them may not seem to conform to practice. For example, if one wants to challenge the learner to talk to a patient about transition to palliative care, you must be sure that the patient is scripted to have tried most treatments particular to his or her disease. Otherwise, you could end up in a discussion about whether the discussion is relevant to the patient at this point in the course of his/her illness. The facilitators and course organizers who conduct the training must be knowledgeable about the relevant medical details. In both Oncotalk and Oncotalk Teach the investigators went to great lengths to script cases that represented evidence-based treatments of common oncological diseases.

The training must be based on situations that the learner finds relevant. Constructing learning challenges that the learner will rarely encounter will not usually engage or motivate the learner. Attempting to teach geriatricians about talking to the mother of a newborn with a birth defect will seem irrelevant to them.

The tasks should be challenging enough to engage the learner. For example, most learners will find that dealing with strong emotions in a patient will challenge them more than making eye contact.

Teaching should respect the learner's skill level. Making the communication challenge too easy will bore the learners; making it too difficult will make them frustrated or anxious.

Teaching should focus on the goals and needs of the learner. When learners identify their challenges and then set their own goals for learning, they are more likely to be fully engaged.

Learners learn best when they are told and shown what to do and then have a chance to practice it in a safe environment. Lectures or explanations provide the rationale for any approach and a cognitive framework for understanding the "how to do it." Demonstrations of the technique then make it "come alive," while practice imprints the learning into the learner's skill repertoire.

The fundamental educational theories that drive the above concepts are *positive psychology*, which states that learning should focus on skills and techniques that are needed to produce a result and deemphasizes "errors" of the past; *adult learning theory*, which posits that learner activation is necessary for skill development and behavior change; and *social learning theory*, which states that teaching skills require that learners engage in simulated encounters. It also explains how small-group learning through the contributions of others in the group can accelerate the learning process [25]. Other educational principles acknowledge the importance of *reflective practice* in helping learners be aware of their skills and correct them [26]. In challenging learners to reflect on where they "got stuck" in an interview with a standardized patient (SP), they can not only learn the powers of self-observation, but be empowered to come up with new solutions to try and to attain confidence in their own ability to improve their communication skills.

This background was essential to a second communication skills teaching effort [27] we initiated to create a cadre of teachers in medical oncology who could transmit communication skills to fellows while mentoring them during clinical interactions in the everyday setting of the oncology clinic or inpatient hospital service. We chose this format because it seemed more practical for everyday teaching and because the skills required to conduct small-group teaching, as in Oncotalk [11], were beyond the reach of most novice teachers in communication skills. Thus the teaching model that evolved for Oncotalk Teach consisted of three skill sets. First, helping the learners you are mentoring or supervising set realistic communication goals for a clinical encounter before entering the room with the patient. Second, determining whether to intervene in the encounter you are observing between fellow and his/her patient and/or family. Third, debriefing the fellow about the encounter with the patient/family and the goals for the encounter by giving effective feedback. These skill sets were conceptualized as the beginning, middle, and end of an encounter with each fellow (see Table 24.1 for skills). In order clearly to identify all of the different persons taking part in the learning process, the physicians who designed the course and served as small-group facilitators were called "investigators"; the medical oncology faculty who were the primary learners were called "faculty"; and the palliative care physicians who took on the role of medical oncology fellows were called "fellows."

24 How to Train Teachers of Communication Skills: The Oncotalk Teach Model   279

Table 24.1 Master learning road map for Oncotalk Teach

The key teaching skills in the master cognitive map	What the teacher does to optimize learning	How the teacher knows he/she did it right
Beginning: faculty identifies learner goals (goals should be specific, learner generated, relevant to the conversation, challenging enough but not beyond the learner's competency)	Creates a plan to observe a substantive conversation Negotiates a specific goal with the fellow	Fellow names the goal Goal has observable endpoint
Middle: faculty sets up some type of skill practice and observes learner	Collects primary observational data about skill practice Intervenes if learner gets "stuck"	Fellow attempts to use skill in conversation with patient
End: faculty gives feedback and closes with one really good take-home point	Asks learner for self-assessment specific to goal Links feedback observation to their learner goal Builds on learner strengths in feedback Asks for "the most important" take-home point	Learner evaluates self using descriptive endpoints previously negotiated Learner accepts feedback as clearly relevant to own learning goal Learner feels like he/she can do better next time, practices the task Learner names a take-home point that is one of the key points from this encounter

Source: Back AL, Oncotalk Teach, University of Washington, Fred Hutchinson Cancer Research Center-

Components of Oncotalk Teach

In the following paragraphs the format for teaching is presented in detail. A description of the teaching plan may be found at http://depts.washington.edu/oncotalk/faculty_tch.html.

Investigators

The investigators served as workshop organizers and facilitators for the small groups. The workshop itself was funded by a 5-year grant from the National Cancer Institute (USA) as an educational intervention. The planning for the grant was led by Anthony Back, MD, of the University of Washington, Seattle and the Fred Hutchinson Cancer Center, a medical oncologist, who served as lead investigator. Coinvestigators were James Tulsky, MD, from Duke University Medical School, and Robert Arnold, MD, from the University of Pittsburgh, both well-known palliative care physicians. The author of this chapter, a psychiatrist, served as the fourth investigator; and Kelly Edwards, PhD, a medical ethicist and expert at small-group facilitation was the fifth member of the team. The planning for the grant took about 8 months, and the first year of the grant was devoted to the actual nuts and bolts of the workshop design.

Since the project involved a totally new approach to training faculty in teaching communication skills, the first year was a pilot year for the project. In year 2 the project was tweaked, when it was realized that some of the faculty needed a refresher in their own communication skills before they could jump into the role of teachers. For this reason a half-day Oncotalk-like communication skills training was added at the beginning of the retreat.

The investigators all had experience in small-group facilitation. However, it was necessary to have biweekly conference calls to work out a manual to provide the program of the retreat. For each retreat the investigators met for a full day prior to the initiation of the actual work with the learners to go over the plan and rehearse the standardized fellow and actors. Very few details were left to chance. The retreat also benefited from two coordinators hired under the grant who handled its extensive administrative aspects. A shared knowledge of facilitation and the basic approach to the learners are outlined in the paper "ABC of Learning and Teaching in Medicine: Teaching Small Groups" [18]. In Oncotalk Teach the investigators relied on core facilitation skills [28] to accomplish their learning objective, to create a cadre of teachers of communication skills in medical oncology.

Facilitating a group of experienced learners such as faculty had both its advantages and challenges. It is a great advantage when learners already have some experience in teaching, as many of our faculty already had. It was also a significant advantage that the learners came into the course motivated and voluntarily giving up their time to engage in a new educational endeavor. This, to a large degree, is what made the course successful. Teaching experienced learners is not without its challenges, and at times we encountered learners who were not open to changing their attitudes about teaching or who overestimated their own skills. However, this was rare. The investigators had learned a considerable amount about the faculty beforehand, since all faculty members completed an application that requested not only basic data about their academic areas of interest and their teaching experience but also a statement explaining their motivation for enrolling in the workshop. The investigators were careful to select applicants who demonstrated a commitment to teaching as a central part of their career. For these reasons there were few significant problems in engaging the learners in the group activity.

Facilitation skills require knowledge of both group process (see Fig. 24.1) and of how learners learn (see Fig. 24.2). There was a shared understanding among the investigators that the core facilitation skills needed to make the workshop successful included the following:

- Learners begin an experience at different levels of ability, and one task of the investigator is to help the learners assess their current skills and be guided toward building new ones
- Learners work best when they have clear goals and are challenged to meet those goals

24 How to Train Teachers of Communication Skills: The Oncotalk Teach Model

The Life of the Group

Forming

Storming

Norming

Performing

Adjourning

Participation
Giving + Feedback
Support and Encouragement
Showing Enthusiasm
Asking Questions

Fig. 24.1 Life of the group (adapted from Tuckman). Groups move through stages of development from forming (getting to know each other; dealing with anxiety about the task) to storming (struggling to understand the task; dealing with the realities of working together) to norming (group begins collaborative effort to resolve problems) to performing (functioning together smoothly to accomplish tasks through their participation, encouragement to the interviewer, and giving feedback), and adjourning (completing learning task, articulating take-home message)

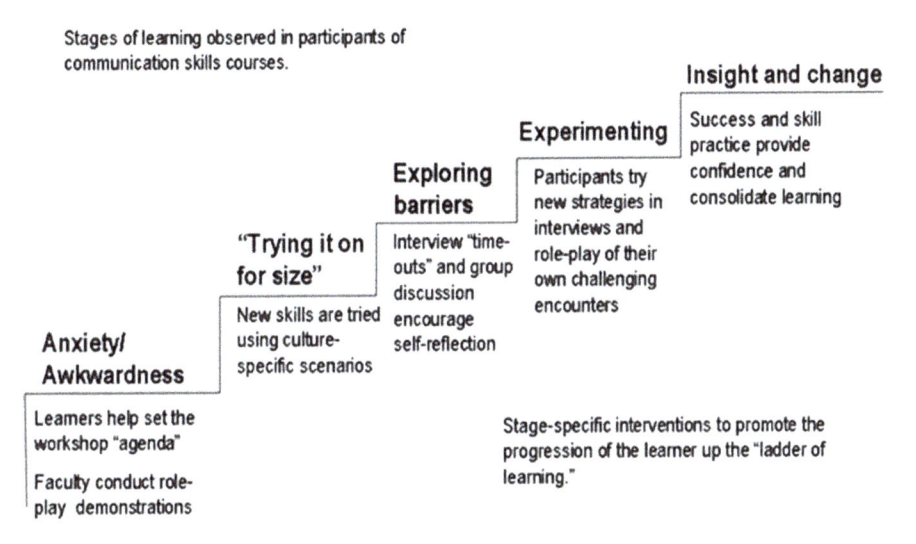

Stages of learning observed in participants of communication skills courses.

Insight and change
Success and skill practice provide confidence and consolidate learning

Experimenting
Participants try new strategies in interviews and role-play of their own challenging encounters

Exploring barriers
Interview "time-outs" and group discussion encourage self-reflection

"Trying it on for size"
New skills are tried using culture-specific scenarios

Anxiety/ Awkwardness
Learners help set the workshop "agenda"
Faculty conduct role-play demonstrations

Stage-specific interventions to promote the progression of the learner up the "ladder of learning."

Fig. 24.2 Life of the learner. Specific facilitator strategies such as clearly articulating goals, being transparent in thinking, and tolerating dissent can move the group smoothly to performing [38]

- Respecting the learners' efforts and praising their accomplishments are core elements in moving learners forward
- Trusting the group to make observations and participate in the learning of fellow group members enhances group performance
- Understanding how to give learners feedback about their performance is an essential skill, but understanding how to encourage learners to assess themselves is even more important

- Facilitators must provide group leadership, keeping the group on time, staying on task, being flexible in meeting learners' needs, and being responsible for guiding the learners toward their goals while keeping the group engaged and giving feedback about group performance
- Creating an open and positive environment that allows discussion, experimentation, and dissent
- Sharing the responsibility for achieving the goals of the learners with the group
- Setting ground rules, such as being on time, and employing effective listening to provide structure for the group
- Being able to manage the process (e.g., factors such as anxiety of a learner or boredom in a group that may impair the learning task)

Faculty Learners

The learners, who were called "faculty," were recruited from medical oncology teaching programs around the country. All submitted a CV and a statement as to what their current role in teaching was and why they were interested in the course. Faculty had various degrees of experience in teaching, but all expressed a commitment to pursue teaching as part of their academic careers. Each cohort consisted of 20 faculty who had varying degrees of academic rank. Several of the faculty were medical oncology program directors at their institutions.

Fellows

In order to create an educational environment in which the skills outlined may be learned and practiced, we recruited palliative care doctors from around the United States to take the role of standardized fellows so the faculty could practice in real time the skills associated with the beginning, middle, and end. That is, we constructed personae for our palliative care doctors to immerse themselves in when interacting as fellows with the faculty. Each fellow was given a persona that reflected a common challenge easily encountered in supervising fellows. Thus Dr. A was a fellow not so secure in his/her skills, Dr. B was a fellow who was almost totally focused on technical skills, etc. Each fellow was set up to present a patient to the faculty in a small group-learning setting. The patients were played by actors from Aspen, Colorado and had been part of our previous Oncotalk teaching program. Each actor had a patient role and a character challenge. For example, patient A was a highly emotional 45-year-old mother of a 5-year-old child who had metastatic melanoma. Other cases included lymphoma, prostate cancer, lung cancer, and breast cancer.

Teaching Format

The task for each faculty member was first to interact with the fellow about goal setting, then to interact with the patient and fellow in the actual clinical visit, and finally to debrief the fellow after the visit. Faculty was guided by a "cognitive road map" in the form of a lecture, which preceded each practice session. The modules for a retreat held over two sessions were as follows:

- Breaking bad news
- How to set goals for the learner
- Giving feedback to learners
- Take-home messages

Faculty worked in groups of five, with an investigator facilitator. Each faculty cohort consisted of 20 learners who came to Aspen twice over a 1-year period. Each learning session lasted 2 days and was separated from the next session by approximately 8 months. Distance learning via online cases provided faculty with continuity of skill development between learning sessions. Both faculty and investigators could comment on the cases and contribute to an online discussion. Each learning session had different goals. For each cohort, session one consisted of a 1-day communication skills course on giving bad news, followed by an introduction to mentoring fellows in real-time encounters with standardized fellows who had to give bad news to simulated cancer patients. In session two this skill was reinforced and an added skill was introduced—mentoring fellows through difficult patient encounters. In this exercise, fellows presented themselves to faculty asking them if they could discuss a difficult case. The case was an extension of the encounter with the same standardized patients whom they had seen earlier in the session. However, a psychosocial dimension was added: in one case the patient had hinted at suicide; another had booked a flight to Mexico in order to obtain alternative treatment. The purpose of the exercise was to help coach the fellow through the difficult encounter. Each of these challenges was preceded by a didactic presentation lasting 30 min that included breaking bad news, how to set goals for a fellow, and how to give feedback and mentor a distressed fellow with a difficult case. After each lecture, several of the investigators performed a role-play that illustrated the skills to be practiced in the subsequent encounters with standardized patients. A sample schedule is presented in Tables 24.2 and 24.3. After faculty divided into groups of five, each guided by an investigator, the faculty worked primarily with their small groups for the rest of the workshop, coming together as a large group mainly for didactic sessions and spending the rest of the time practicing with the standardized patients. Because this work was necessarily intense and often draining, the faculty was given various amounts of time off for recreation, attending to needs at home, and reflection. Thus, one entire afternoon after lunch was left to the faculty to decide what to do. In order to maintain a sense of the group, however, almost all meals were taken together. This provided an opportunity to build group cohesiveness and to enhance the relaxed atmosphere that we believed would contribute to learning.

Table 24.2 Example of use of cognitive map in practice session

Master cognitive map	An outpatient "learner talks" example	An inpatient "teacher talks" example
Beginning: faculty ask fellows for their learning goals; and help fellows identify strategies that will enhance likelihood of success in the encounter	You (a faculty member) ask the fellow at the beginning of an afternoon clinic session to identify a communication skill that the fellow wants to work on that day. The fellow says he has to give bad news to a patient and is pretty sure he/she will get upset. He is not sure how to respond. You spend a minute discussing how he might acknowledge the patient's emotion and give him/her space to emote. You and the fellow agree that he will try making an empathic response if the patient gets upset. You offer to intervene if he gets "stuck"	Before a family conference, you (a faculty member) ask the fellow what he/she would like to learn about doing a family conference. The fellow would like to watch to learn "how to do it better" and doesn't feel that he/she really knows how. You suggest that an important first step is to ask about what the patient and family understand, and to observe how you do that
Middle: the faculty observes the skill, then gives feedback	You watch the fellow tell the patient that his/her CT shows that the colon cancer has progressed. When the patient seems sad, the fellow successfully remains silent and says, "I know it's tough for you to hear that." The patient responds, "Well, what's next?" After the visit, during feedback, the fellow's self-assessment is that he/she thought it went pretty well. The faculty points out that the fellow did a great job in giving the patient space and being empathic. You point out that sometimes it takes more than one empathic response to lower emotions	You conduct the family conference. Afterwards, you spend 2 min asking the fellow what he/she observed about eliciting patient/family understanding. (The skill practice is observation in this case.) The fellow is able to remember your exact question and expresses some surprise that the question was so simple but useful
End: the teacher closes with one really good take-home point	You ask the fellow about his/her take-home learning point. The fellow says that it is really hard to be quiet; he/she had to resist wanting to jump right into the treatment plan	You ask the fellow about his/her take-home learning point. The fellow cites the question to elicit the family's perception. You agree and suggest that the fellow conduct that part of the next family conference

Source: Back AL, Oncotalk Teach, University of Washington, Fred Hutchinson Cancer Research Center

As mentioned previously, small-group learning was the key educational experience for the faculty. Day 1 of the retreat was given to honing their own communication skills, day 2 of the first retreat and days 1 and 2 of the second retreat were given to practicing coaching the fellows through challenging encounters. During 2 of these 3 days investigators would meet with a group of five faculty, and each would take a

Table 24.3 A sample Oncotalk Teach retreat day

7:30–8:00 Breakfast
8–8:30 Didactic presentation with faculty demonstration
8:00–12:00 Skills practice with SPs and SFs (25 min per learner) with one 15-min break
12–1 PM Lunch
1:00–1:30 Didactic presentation with faculty demonstration
1:30–4:00 Skills practice (in Oncotalk Teach 2 skills practice involved meeting with fellows alone to discuss "A Difficult Case")
4–6:30 Free time
6:30–7:30 Dinner
7:30–8:30 Small-group reflective exercise
8:30 Faculty debriefing

Note: The schedule varied slightly with each retreat, but the core elements of the didactic presentations and skills practice remained the same. While the faculty and the investigators had dinner together, the standardized fellows met with an educational specialist over dinner to debrief them on the encounters. One faculty member debriefed the standardized patients after each group of practice sessions. On day 2 the last didactic session involved a discussion of take-home messages and planning for implementation of teaching at each faculty home institution. On day 1 of the first retreat and day 2 of the second retreat learners met with SPs other than those used in the skills practice for an audio recorded evaluation session

turn coaching a fellow through an encounter with a patient. The work of the faculty with the fellow was seen as being divided into three parts. In the first part the faculty meets with the fellow to go over their goals for the encounter. The goals varied with the type of challenges scripted for the standardized patients and were laid out in a didactic session before the encounter. For example, if the goal of the encounter was to give bad news to a patient about poor results from chemotherapy, then the goal of the faculty was to discuss with the fellow how he or she might go about doing that. Prior to this encounter the approach of the faculty was also discussed with the investigator to review his/her plan on how to approach the fellow—that is, to help frame the approach to helping the fellows set goals, review their knowledge about giving bad news, and set up a situation in which the faculty might have to intervene in the encounter with the patient. This represents five stages for each encounter: investigator briefs faculty; faculty briefs fellow; fellow and faculty encounter patient; faculty debriefs fellow; investigator debriefs faculty.

The role of the investigator is complex: to act as both a coach for the faculty and the group and to keep the action and involvement of the group moving. It was especially important to keep the group engaged and to encourage them to give feedback to the faculty about their performance. In keeping with the idea that feedback is best received when it is specific, constructive, and in keeping with the goals of the learner, the investigator often asked the faculty what skills they would like the group to watch for as they engaged with the fellows. Thus, each faculty who was observing and not interviewing during a particular encounter was assigned a skill to watch for. In order to make the feedback more relevant and specific, they were asked to write down their observations and the actual phrases the faculty-interviewer used. This assignment served to underscore the faculty's responsibility to fellow group members. It tended to encourage group members who might otherwise be more passive and reluctant to participate in giving feedback. The investigators borrowed extensively from the previously mentioned models of learning and group dynamics in constructing the learning experience. In addition, they understood that learners progress through a series of stages, as illustrated in Fig. 24.1. In this model the faculty skills evolved through a series of stages, beginning with experimenting with an approach, assessing and reflecting on barriers to executing the skill, modifying the approach with feedback, and finally reaching some level of success in enhanced communication competence. Likewise, a model of group functioning was used to guide facilitators in the work of the group. It was based upon a model of group learning first articulated by Tuckman [29], who advocated a conceptual framework of group evolution through a series of stages (see Fig. 24.2). The work of the facilitator in this context is to move the group quickly to "performing," in which they are functioning at a high level of learning.

Faculty presented with various levels of skills, so it was necessary for facilitators to respect the "starting point" for each faculty. Finding the "learning edge" for individual faculty members respected the facts that on the one hand the investigators did not want to set unrealistic goals for less advanced learners, but on the other hand they wanted to construct appropriate communication challenges for learners who were more advanced.

Didactic Anchors

Didactic presentations formed the "roadmap" for faculty to follow. They are the "what-to-do" component of the teaching process. Didactic presentations are basically the curriculum of the communication skills course; they guided the faculty through the skills practice. They are the skills to be learned such as breaking bad news, disclosing a medical error, or talking to patients about end-of-life issues. In Oncotalk workshops each skills practice was preceded by a 30-min didactic presentation in which the skills were presented. For example, in discussing how to break bad news the SPIKES protocol was taught [13]. In a workshop lasting 3 days there might be as many as four didactic presentations, each followed by a practice session. In a workshop on discussing end-of-life issues with patients, didactic presentations might include basic communication skills such as establishing rapport, then breaking bad news, then transition to palliative care, then end-of-life discussions. It is important that the skills build upon one another and progressively challenge the learner.

Faculty Demonstrations

At the end of each didactic presentation investigators often chose to demonstrate the skills in question through a brief (10 min) role-play, in which one investigator member plays the doctor and another the patient. By "seeing" what the skills looks like, faculty is better prepared to practice it. We have also found that faculty favorably perceive the willingness of the investigators to engage in the same activity (role-playing in front of the group) that they are asking the learners to do.

Other Strategies That Promote Learning

Recreation. "Time off" for faculty provided a break from the intensity of the learning process. In a 3-day workshop, giving one afternoon off and not finishing later than 5 PM will provide time for recharging batteries and reflecting on the learning process.

Reflective exercises [26]. Helping learners be reflective and aware of their communication is an essential part of the workshops we conduct. Several exercises in which the small groups come together to reflect on a question, such as "think about a time when you recognized that you were a healer in an interaction with a patient and family," writing responses to this question, and sharing it with the group can serve to support the idea that communication is often a metacognitive skill in which awareness of the impact of our communication with others and the impact of their communication on us can guide us toward the intentionality needed to be effective communicators.

Parallel process. This concept describes a strategy for the facilitator in guiding the faculty to use the skills he or she may see in the interaction with the facilitator or group in coaching their interaction with the patient. For example, when facilitators praise learners, listen to them, are empathic toward their struggles, and urge them to reflect, they are demonstrating how these skills can be used in the interaction with the patient. The investigator-faculty interaction mimics that of the faculty–patient.

Open role-play. This gave faculty the opportunity to bring their own most challenging cases for consideration. In this format a faculty chose to show the group what a difficult communication looks like (e.g., dealing with a fellow who felt communication was too "toucy-feely"). The faculty, assisted by the investigator can step into the role of their patient. This is accomplished when the investigator interviews the faculty in the role of the fellow by asking questions such as, what year fellow are you, what are your interests. The investigator also "sets the scene" by asking the role-playing faculty to "set the scene" of the encounter (e.g., clinic visit) and to describe as the fellow what his resistance about. By immersing the faculty in the role of their fellow the group then see the communication challenges and surmise the underlying feelings and attitude of the fellow. A second phase of the encounter begins when one of the group members volunteers to conduct the interview. The faculty "in the shoes" of the fellow can then experience the encounter as if he/she were their fellow and empathically understand what the fellow needs from the faculty. A third phase begins when the faculty in the role of the fellow then switches back into the role of himself/herself to try out the most effective communication strategy, knowing what that was in the role of the fellow. Using this strategy requires that the investigator be confident in the use of role-reversal and in setting up the situation by interviewing the learner in the role of the patient.

Investigator debriefing. It is helpful for the investigators to get feedback on their own skills and to be able to brainstorm about challenges that come up during the course of the workshops. We accomplish this by having a trained observer periodically sit in our sessions and use a checklist of investigator skills to provide us with feedback. Debriefing of the sessions is another way to promote investigator development and support. Facilitation can be challenging and even stressful, as when you have learners who are struggling or resistant. Debriefing the learning sessions in a group with other investigators allowed us to brainstorm difficulties, celebrate successes, and get feedback on managing challenges.

Evaluation

Assessing the efficacy of workshops such as Oncotalk Teach can be done in a number of ways [30–32]. Feedback from learners regarding aspects of the workshop, such as skills of the facilitators, realism of the standardized fellows, the group experience, the milieu, can provide important quantitative information. Qualitative information that describes the experience of the group members and their take-home points also can be collected [33]. More quantifiable information can be obtained on knowledge gained by quizzing the participants on the key teaching points of the didactic sessions. Finally, standardization of interview scoring can allow the investigators to expose learners to interviews before and after the session to compare improvement in interviewing with standardized patients who were not part of the workshop [34]. Encounters about giving bad news, for example, are recorded before and after the workshop, scored, and compared to scores after the workshop [14]. For our workshop we chose to use standardized fellows and standardized patients to evaluate the faculty's ability to coach fellows in a clinic setting both before and after the workshop. In this format faculty have 20 min to meet with the fellow, sit in on an interview with the fellow, and debrief the fellow. These encounters are all audiotaped and then coded for skills taught in the workshop. Before- and after-the-workshop comparisons are then made. This data for Oncotalk Teach is currently being analyzed.

Faculty development focusing on teaching in the clinic or at the bedside is only one way that oncology faculty can be prepared to teach communication skills. Approaches other than small-group learning have been used to enhance the communication skills of practitioners. Faculty can be trained to use videotapes of interviews with discussion, can encourage presentation of cases with discussion, and can engage in modeling and demonstrations using role-playing [34–37].

In conclusion, teaching faculty in communication skills can be extremely rewarding. Considering the number of potential learners whom faculty can reach in teaching these skills over the course of a career, the time spent at residential retreats seems modest. One of the main barriers cited in the literature as an obstacle to teaching communication skills is the absence of qualified teachers. Oncotalk Teach is one model for accomplishing this. However, it takes time, motivation, and skill to master both the principles of effective teaching and the wherewithal to implement them. To accomplish these, institutions must be aware that demands on faculty to generate clinical income and research may be incompatible with the goal of creating excellent teachers in communication. Effective teachers are made, not born.

Acknowledgments The author would like to Acknowledge the Principle Investigator of Oncotalk Teach Dr. Anthony Back whose vision, inspiration and organizational skills were responsible for the design and implementation of Oncotalk Teach. Co-investigators Bob Arnold, Kelly Edwards and James Tulsky were awesome in their roles as facilitators for the faculty participants.

References

1. Fallowfield L, Jenkins V. Effective communication skills are the key to good cancer care. Eur J Cancer. 1999;35:1592–7.
2. Back A, Arnold RM, Tulsky JA. Mastering communication with seriously ill patients: balancing honesty with empathy and hope. New York: Cambridge University Press; 2009.
3. Hoffman M, Ferri J, Sison C, Roter D, Schapira L, Baile W. Teaching communication skills: an AACE survey of oncology training programs. J Cancer Educ. 2004;19(4):220–4.
4. Hebert HD, Butera JN, Castillo J, Mega AE. Are we training our fellows adequately in delivering bad news to patients? A survey of hematology/oncology program directors. J Palliat Med. 2009;12(12):1119–24.
5. Fallowfield L, Jenkins V, Farewell V, Solis-Trapala I. Enduring impact of communication skills training: results of a 12-month follow-up. Br J Cancer. 2003;89(8):1445–9.
6. Fukui S, Ogawa K, Ohtsuka M, Fukui N. Effect of communication skills training on nurses' detection of patients' distress and related factors after cancer diagnosis: a randomized study. Psychooncology. 2009;18(11):1156–64.
7. Butow P, Cockburn J, Girgis A, Bowman D, Schofield P, D'Este C, Stojanovski E. Tattersall MH; CUES Team Increasing oncologists' skills in eliciting and responding to emotional cues: evaluation of a communication skills training program. Psychooncology. 2008;17(3):209–18.
8. Delvaux N, Merckaert I, Marchal S, Libert Y, Conradt S, Boniver J, Etienne AM, Fontaine O, Janne P, Klastersky J, Mélot C, Reynaert C, Scalliet P, Slachmuylder JL, Razavi D. Physicians' communication with a cancer patient and a relative: a randomized study assessing the efficacy of consolidation workshops. Cancer. 2005;103(11):2397–411.
9. Butler L, Degner L, Baile W, Landry M; SCRN Communication Team. Developing communication competency in the context of cancer: a critical interpretive analysis of provider training programs. Psychooncology. 2005;14(10):861–72; discussion 873–4.
10. Kissane D, Bultz B, Butow PM, Findlay LG. A core curriculum for training communication skills training in oncology and palliative care. In: Kissane DW, Bultz B, Butow P, Finlay IG, editors. Handbook of communication in oncology and palliative care. Oxford, England: Oxford Press; 2010. p. 101–231.
11. Back AL, Arnold RM, Tulsky JA, Baile WF, Fryer-Edwards KA. Teaching communication skills to medical oncology fellows. J Clin Oncol. 2003;21(12):2433–6.
12. Costantini A, Baile WF, Lenzi R, Costantini M, Ziparo V, Marchetti P, Grassi L. Overcoming cultural barriers to giving bad news: feasibility of training to promote truth telling to cancer patients. J Cancer Educ. 2009;24(3):180–5.
13. Baile WF, Buckman R, Lenzi R, Glober G, Beale EA, Kudelka AP. SPIKES—a six-step protocol for delivering bad news: application to the patient with cancer. Oncologist. 2000;5(4):302–11.
14. Girgis A, Sanson-Fisher RW. Breaking bad news: 1. Current best advice for clinicians. Behav Med. 1998;24(2):53–9.
15. Back AL, Arnold RM, Baile WF, et al. Efficacy of communication skills training for giving bad news and discussing transitions to palliative care. Arch Intern Med. 2007;167(5):453–60.
16. Lipkin M, Caplan C, Clark W, et al. Teaching medical interviewing. The Lipkin model. In: Lipkin M, Putnam S, Lazare A, editors. The medical interview. Clinical care, education and research. New York: Springer; 1995.
17. Cranton P. Understanding and promoting transformative learning: a guide for educators of adults. New York: Jossey-Bass; 1994.

18. Jaques D. ABC of learning and teaching in medicine: teaching small groups. BMJ. 2003;326:492–4.
19. Silva DH. A competency based communication skills workshop series for pediatric residents. Bol Asoc Med P R. 2008;100(2):8–12.
20. Epstein RM, Street RL. A Framework for patient centered communication in cancer care. In: Epstein RM, Street RL, editors. Patient centered communication in cancer care. Bethesda: US Department of Health and Human Services, National Institutes of Health, National Cancer Institute, NIH Publication No. 07-6225. 2007. p. 17–38.
21. Epner D, Baile WF. Wooden's pyramid: building a hierarchy of skills for successful communication. Med Teach. 2011;33(1):39–43.
22. Parker PA, Baile WF, de Moor C, Lenzi R, Kudelka AP, Cohen L. Breaking bad news about cancer: patients' preferences for communication. J Clin Oncol. 2001;19(7):2049–56.
23. Kurtz S, Cook LJ. Learner centered communication training. In: Kissane DW, Bultz B, Butow P, Finlay IG, editors. Handbook of communication in oncology and palliative care. Oxford, England: Oxford Press; 2010. p. 583–95.
24. Fallowfield L, Jenkins V. Current concepts of communication skills training in oncology. Recent Results Cancer Res. 2006;168:105–12.
25. Shein EH, Bennis WG. Personal and organizational change through group methods; the laboratory approach. New York: Wiley; 1965.
26. Fryer-Edwards K, Arnold RM, Baile W, Tulsky JA, Petracca F, Back A. Reflective teaching practices: an approach to teaching communication skills in a small-group setting. Acad Med. 2006;81(7):638–44.
27. Back AL, Arnold RM, Baile WF, Tulsky JA, Barley GE, Pea RD, Fryer-Edwards KA. Faculty development to change the paradigm of communication skills teaching in oncology. Clin Oncol. 2009;27(7):1137–41.
28. Bens I. Facilitating with ease. 2nd ed. San Francisco: Jossey-Bass; 2005.
29. Tuckman B. Developmental sequence in small groups. Psychol Bull. 1965;63(6):389–99.
30. Konopasek L, Rosenbaum M, Encandela J, Cole-Kelly K. Evaluating communication skills training courses. In: Kissane DW, Bultz B, Butow P, Finlay IG, editors. Handbook of communication in oncology and palliative care. Oxford, England: Oxford Press; 2010. p. 683–705.
31. Duffy FD, Whelan G, Cole-Kelly K, Frankel R, et al. Assessing competence in communication and interpersonal skills: the Kalamazoo II report. Acad Med. 2004;79(6):495–507.
32. Geeta MG, Krishnakumar P, Rajasree KC, et al. Effectiveness of communication skills training on perceptions and practice of pediatric residents. Indian J Pediatr. 2011;78(8):979–82.
33. Nikendei C, Bosse HM, Hoffman K, Moltner A, Hancke R, et al. Outcome of parent physician communication skills training for pediatric residents. Patient Educ Couns. 2011;82(1):94–9.
34. Back Al, Arnold RM, Baile WF, Tulsky J, Oncotalk Teach video series. 2011. http://depts.washington.edu/oncotalk/videos/. 2012, March 15.
35. Pinsky LE, Wipf JE. A picture is worth a thousand words practical use of videotape in teaching. J Gen Intern Med. 2000;15:805–10.
36. Spagnoletti CL, et al. Implementation and evaluation of a web-based communication skills learning tool for training internal medicine interns in patient-doctor communication. J Commun Healthcare. 2009;2(2):159–72.
37. I *CARE. Interpersonal communication and relationship enhancement. www.mdanderson.org/icare. 2012, March 15.
38. Baile WF, Fryer-Edwards K, Back A, Tulsky J, Arnold R. Teaching communication skills to oncology fellows: the ABCs of using psychodynamic principles. Psychooncology. 2005;14 Suppl 12:IV-1.

Chapter 25
Communication Skills Training of Physicians in Portugal

Luzia Travado

Abstract Communication skills training for oncologists and cancer physicians in Portugal has received little attention in the past. Only more recently the interest for the skills of communication and the possibility of its training has raised attention in the medical community. GPs have shown more interest in this area and have included it in their residency activities. Some initiatives on Doctor–Patient Communication and Relationship skills targeting medical students and medical professionals have been conducted at the university level for undergraduate and postgraduate level as well as by professional societies in cancer care. The Pilot Program on Communication Skills Training for cancer physicians under the umbrella of the National Coordination for Oncological Diseases is presented. The need for including CST in educational programs for medical doctors and clinical professions is discussed, as well as opportunities for change.

Keywords Communications skills training in Portugal • Doctor–patient communication and relationship skills • Communications skills in clinical oncology

Communication skills training for oncologists and cancer physicians in Portugal has received little attention in the past [1]. Traditionally, medical education, although it promoted a humanistic practice, did not include, in its undergraduate and postgraduate curricula, regular learning and training activities in communication skills [2, 3]. Also as recertification of physicians' skills or knowledge is not required [4], there is no demand for communication skills training (CST) or credits given to it. As such, its value as a core-component in a doctor–patient relationship and for physician's lifelong learning process has been much undervalued [3], leaving it only to personal motivation and initiative. Specifically doctors working with cancer patients, namely

L. Travado (✉)
Clinical Psychology Unit, Central Lisbon Hospital Centre, Hospital de S. José,
Rua José António Serrano, 1150-199, Lisboa, Portugal
e-mail: luzia.travado@chlc.min-saude.pt

surgeons, oncologists, radiotherapists, and others, are not required to practice nor taught specific and useful communication skills to help them deal with the difficult moments throughout the disease process of communicating bad news to patients and families, which left this area much unattended [1].

The clinical practice of medicine in Portugal, as in other countries, has been criticized as being too biomedical and centered in its technology and on the doctor's agenda, which has become detrimental of the humanistic aspects of the doctor–patient relationship and good communication that characterize a more patient-centered approach [5–7]. Only more recently the interest for the skills of communication and the possibility of its training has raised attention in the medical community. The scientific evidence that a good doctor–patient communication may improve patients' clinical outcomes [1, 8] and also their satisfaction with care [9–11], along with CST having shown to be efficient in improving the skills and in reducing physicians burnout [12–17], appearing in papers published in medical journals and in congress presentations internationally and nationally, has brought some attention to this area along with some recognition for the need to include it in medical education and training [18, 19].

CST at University Level and for GP's

Some examples of change can be given. The Department of Medical Psychology of the School of Medicine, University of Oporto, has initiated in 2001 a communication skills program as a practice class included in the Doctor–patient relationship topic of the Medical Psychology course for undergraduate students of medicine [20]. More recently, this department has developed a program called Clinical Communication Skills at postgraduate level addressing the need for advanced education in this area for professional practitioners in clinical settings [21]. The program is 1 year long with a total of 270 h comprising theoretical presentations, role-modeling, role-playing, and small groups exercises, addressing basic and advanced communication skills and communication in special situations, including issues of self-awareness and self-help (ibidem). Its contents and methodology as well as its preliminary results from the 2008 program have been presented showing beneficial effects on participants' communication skills as in their self-confidence. The participants in the study were a group of 25 health professionals, including physicians, nurses, clinical psychologists, and physiotherapists (ibidem).

Other initiatives at the University level in Medicine Schools have been conducted, namely at the School of Medical Sciences of the New University of Lisbon, which offers a postgraduate course of 50 h on *Doctor–Patient Communication and Relationship* targeting medical professionals [22]. Also, the Students Association of the Institute of Medical Sciences Abel Salazar in University of Oporto has recently advertised a *Doctor–Patient Communication* program with basic and advanced modules with an emphasis on practicing the skills with simulated cases and role-playing, including managing difficult communication situations, such as dealing with emotions, breaking bad news (BBN), and how to deal with a difficult patient, for their associated students [23].

The residency training for a General Practionner (GP) or as in Portugal we call it—Family Doctor—has long recognized the importance of the doctor–patient relationship and communication and its added value in the consultation and in the outcome of the clinical encounter [3, 10, 11, 24]. The *Portuguese Journal of General Practice* [Revista Portuguesa de Clinica Geral] has devoted almost an entire issue discussing the topic of the *Doctor–patient communication and relationship* and its relevance for the clinicians' daily practice [19]. It recalls the initial Balint groups developed in the 80s as a way to debrief, discuss, and improve the difficulties in the doctor–patient encounter that were adopted in some training locations of GPs in the North of Portugal [25, 26]. It mentions the "portfolio of critical incidents" in the consultation as an important reflexive tool for self-learning and improvement of communication skills and a valuable tool for tutorial assistance at postgraduate or residency level [27]. Also a recent book was published by José Nunes, a Portuguese GP, on *Communication in Clinical Context* [18] to inform and assist clinicians in this area and in the training provided for the residency of GPs under the Primary Care module of which he is one of the main leaders in the country.

Nevertheless, it is widely recognized that communication skills encompass not only understanding the techniques that are essential to develop the skills, but also envisioning good role models and the possibility to practice thoroughly the skills, through role-playing with simulated cases and clinical scenarios, facilitated by experts or trained professionals in the area. As such, the examples given here are still the exception and not the rule. The recent reform of medical education with the introduction of European Union standards (the Bologna Treaty) has brought some new opportunities for including regular CST in the medical curricula, as a core-competence that ought to be acquired, developed, and improved throughout the medical education and clinical career. However, as an area that slips out of the main stream of (bio)medical competence into areas typically of Psychology education and field, there is still some conservative attitude into moving it forward. It will require leadership and public demand to make it play a bigger role in the medical education at different levels, undergraduate and postgraduate in our country [3, 28] as it impacts patients' clinical outcomes, satisfaction with care, and healthcare costs.

CST for Cancer Specialists

Regarding CST in the medical education of cancer specialists, the scenario is not much different. It is eventually somewhat worse for surgeons and radiotherapists with no requirement for its inclusion in their training, as these are very technical medical specializations, and eventually somewhat better for medical oncologists since last year their curricula was revised and it mentions communication skills with patients and families to be acquired in their training [29]. The situation is only better for Palliative Care physicians as it is mandatory in their education and training [30].

The area of physician–patient communication in cancer care in Portugal has been examined in terms of physicians' attitudes toward truth-telling with cancer patients [31], patients' desire for information from their doctors [32], and more recently, cancer physicians' communications skills in terms of their own confidence in specific skills and their expectations of outcome of communication with patients and its relation to psychosocial orientation and burnout [1], and their satisfaction with short-training communication skills workshops [33].

Early in our efforts to address this problem, we generated data from the Southern European Psycho-oncology Study (SEPOS)[1] that showed that not only Portuguese cancer physicians but also their colleagues from Italy and Spain reported having received no or minimal training in these skills during their medical education—86 % of the inquired doctors reported no CST. And although they tend to perceive themselves as skilled in communicating with patients, they express less confidence in specific skills such as dealing with denial and managing uncertainty, assessing anxiety and depression, promoting patient-family openness, and BBN [1]. Moreover, the study revealed a relationship between communication skills, expectations of communication outcome, psychosocial orientation, and burnout. Lower confidence in communication skills (poor CS) correlated with higher expectations of a negative outcome following communication with patients, which associated with a lower psychosocial orientation and higher level of burnout. The results suggested training cancer physicians in communication could potentially enhance a psychosocially oriented approach to patients in cancer care, but also positively affect doctors professionally in the Southern European countries (ibid.).

In conducting CST in the studies mentioned above, the SEPOS group developed a specific educational and experiential model (12 h divided into two modules) including formal teaching (i.e., journal articles, large-group presentations), practice in small groups (i.e., small-group exercises and role-play), and discussion in large groups [33]. This training was developed with the aim of improving not only cancer physicians' communication skills but also their ability to identify emotional problems in their cancer patients (e.g., depression, anxiety, and adjustment disorders) and refer them to specialists (e.g., psycho-oncologists). The training course was conducted in hospital settings in Portugal and other southern European countries and was well accepted by most participants, who expressed "general satisfaction and a positive, subjective perception of the utility of the course for clinical practice" (ibidem, pp. 79). The model has proved to be a feasible approach for

---

[1] The Southern European Psycho-oncology Study (SEPOS), a large project entitled "Improving health staff's communication and assessment skills of psychosocial morbidity and quality of life in cancer patients: a study in Southern European countries," has been funded by the European Community (Agreement SI2.307317 2000CVGG2-026—between the European Commission and the University of Ferrara) coordinated by L. Grassi, University of Ferrara, Italy, having L. Travado from Portugal and F. Gil from Spain as main partners.

oncologists and cancer physicians and is easily applicable to various hospital settings (ibidem).

This model has been piloted by the author and used in teaching communication skills in Portugal since 2004. The first group of trainees consisted of general surgeons who were responsible for the treatment of breast and other types of cancer patients and was the pilot training group. They were skeptical in the beginning of the workshop, but during its training activities surrendered themselves to the usefulness of the techniques as important tools for their clinical practice with cancer patients. Due to the positive response of the group to the training, the chief surgeon and team leader of the breast cancer multidisciplinary treatment unit at Hospital S. Jose–Central Lisbon Hospital Centre has been advocating this training for every doctor. He claims its importance in gaining more confidence in dealing with difficult communication situations with patients and family, particularly in "breaking bad news" to patients with cancer, in a more sensible humanistic way, tailoring the approach to each patient's needs.

In an effort to reach more physicians and provide an easy-to-use learning tool (for self-learning and/or use in workshops) to disseminate this training, in 2006 together with Prof. Joaquim Reis, we made a two-DVD set on *Communication and Relationship Skills for Health Professionals*[2]—which included basic and advanced skills and an introduction to the SPIKES BBN protocol [34]. This DVD was launched in a GIST Symposium organized by the Society for Gastrointestinal Stromal Tumors in Portugal with Prof. Walter Baile giving a conference on "*The importance of good communication skills in clinical oncology and its training*," and its first edition was offered to the oncologists' community.

The formal SEPOS training was then modified to include a module on how to break bad news (BBN) to patients and some illustrations of the DVD, on doctor–patient communication scenes played by actors, were also used. In 2007, our group in collaboration with the Portuguese Oncology Society rolled out this new format of CST for oncologists, which was very well received by the attendants.

CST National Pilot Program

In 2009, a Pilot Program on CST for cancer physicians was launched at the national level. The National Coordination for Oncological Diseases (CNDO—http://www.acs.min-saude.pt/cndo/), a department under the Ministry of Health in Portugal, responsible for the implementation of the National Program for the Prevention and Control of Oncological Diseases, undertook this program with the aim of improving

---

[2] Some video clips of the DVD are accessible online at the MDACC—I*CARE Program website at: http://www.mdanderson.org/education-and-research/resources-for-professionals/professional-educational-resources/i-care/teaching-and-learning-communication-skills/communication-relationship-skills-health-professionals.html (last accessed March 28, 2011).

communication with cancer patients and families in clinical oncological settings. In an effort to improve cancer care and also respond to European and international recommendations that suggest CST is a core skill for medical practice, particularly relevant for oncology doctors [7], this program also attempted to provide an opportunity to address this gap in medical professionals education. The program was launched nationally with a Symposium in which international experts—Leslie Fallowfield, Luigi Grassi, and Walter Baile—were invited speakers to talk about the "*Importance of communication skills training in clinical oncology.*" Oncologists, hematologists, cancer surgeons, radiotherapists, and palliative care physicians from all over the country—the target population for this training—attended the Symposium. They were directly invited by letter from the National Coordinator of Oncological Diseases to attend the Symposium with a rationale about this new program and its relevance. The Symposium was presided over by the High Commissioner of Health and the National Coordinator of Oncological Diseases. Nationally, high-profile oncologists, hematologists, palliative care physicians, and the president of the Medical Oncologists College were invited as chairs and moderators of the different sessions. More than 100 physicians attended this Symposium and the 33 that returned the anonymous evaluation form rated it as very satisfactory and very relevant to their clinical practice. All of the respondents considered that "the methods discussed in the symposium will facilitate communication with patients and families in their clinical practice." The respondents had an average age of 46 years and 15 years of clinical practice and were mostly oncologists and surgeons. The program presentations are accessible at: http://www.acs.min-saude.pt/2009/02/13/treino-aptidoes?r+16 (last accessed March 21, 2011). As a result, more than 80 doctors expressed their interest and signed up for the training courses.

The communication skills interactive program of this Pilot program on CST for cancer physicians—free of charge—was subsequently begun and included three programmed workshops in Lisbon and Oporto (main cities) throughout 2009, and an additional one in 2010 in Viseu (countryside interior city). The SEPOS-modified CST model described previously was used by the author, who was also responsible for the development and implementation of this program. Twenty-nine doctors attended the workshops, mostly oncologists, surgeons, radiotherapists, and other physicians working in the cancer clinical settings directly with patients and families.

This initiative and its preliminary results were presented recently at a Symposium [35]. Results indicate a high satisfaction and a positive effect with the workshops. More specifically, the attendants rated the course globally as highly satisfactory (4.7 in 5), having made many favorable comments on its methodology, its dynamic and interactive practice as its most positive aspects, and most participants (78 %) firmly believed that they would be able to introduce some of the techniques trained in the workshop in their clinical practice. Their main communication skills difficulties as well as their psychosocial orientation and burnout were similar to the ones obtained in the SEPOS study mentioned above [1]. The effects of CST on participants' beliefs, attitudes, and choices in communicating with patients and their confidence in CS were significantly improved ($p<0.01$). The positive results from this program, the satisfaction and interest from learners to acquire CS and use them in their clinical settings, and their request for an advanced course have shown a clear interest and motivation from cancer care physicians for the acquisition of these skills, which encourages the continuation of this program and extending it to other health professionals.

Other initiatives in providing CST to cancer care professionals have been undertaken. The Portuguese Academy of Psycho-Oncology (http://www.appo.pt), for several years, has organized short workshops for multiprofessional groups with invited foreign expert speakers (e.g., Prof. Darius Razavi, Jules Bordet Institute, Cancer Centre of Université Libre, Brussels, Belgium). The postgraduation course in Psycho-Oncology, 1 year long, at Independent University of Lisbon, for healthcare professionals, had a module of 20 h dedicated to CST, provided by the author. All major postgraduate courses, masters or education in Palliative Care, also include CST. At Central Lisbon Hospital Centre-Hospital S. José, Prof. Walter Baile, co-author of the SPIKES protocol on BBN from the MD Anderson Cancer Centre, University of Texas, USA, conducted two workshops on communication in Palliative Care (basic and advanced skills; which the author had the pleasure of co-facilitating) included in the education and training program in Palliative Care of a multidisciplinary team of 17 health professionals (including six medical doctors), to foster the development of this area of care at the hospital.[3]

The needs of other healthcare professionals in this area were not addressed here, as traditionally they have CS embedded in their educational curricula (e.g., nurses, physiotherapists, social workers, etc.), and also they do not give clinical bad news. However, all healthcare professionals need to improve their knowledge and practice in CST, as to better relate to patients and families and address their concerns and needs, in aiming for a patient-centered model of care.

Conclusion

In conclusion, CST in Portugal has made progress in the last decade, with some interesting initiatives; however, its inclusion in formal and continuing medical education is still scarce and far from mandatory. Further initiatives like the ones reported here need to continue to cascade this process. The learners can market its usefulness with residents and other colleagues and increase its demand. Also, it is useful to do more 'training the trainers' courses, so as to have certified professionals to conduct this training locally, including it in the clinical sessions and continuing educational programs of hospitals and primary care centers. Portuguese CST teachers and

---

[3]This project and program entitled "Organization and development of Palliative care at Hospital S. José", in Lisbon was supported by a grant of the *Gulbenkian Foundation* in Portugal (2003–2007) (http://www.gulbenkian.pt), which the author, who has written the application and was responsible for its implementation, would like to acknowledge and thank.

facilitators will also need to take the publication of the design and results of their programs in Portuguese journals more seriously, as an important way to disseminate the valuable benefits of CST for clinical practice with patients and families, as in reducing burnout, and positively influence the medical community as well as other health professionals to do CST. Last, it will require leadership to make the necessary changes to consider communication and relationship skills as a core-competence for clinical practice in the health professions, particularly in the medical profession, and CST as a requirement for certification, as suggested by the Accreditation Council for Graduate Medical Education in North America.

References

1. Travado L, Grassi L, Gil F, Ventura C, Martins C and the Southern European Psycho-Oncology Study Group (SEPOS). Physician-patient communication among Southern European cancer physicians: the influence of psychosocial orientation and burnout. Psychooncology. 2005;14:661–70.
2. Carvalho IP, Ribeiro-Silva R, Pais VG, Figueiredo-Braga M, Castro-Vale I, Teles A, Almeida SS, Mota-Cardoso R. [Teaching doctor-patient communication – a proposal in practice][article in Portuguese]. Acta Med Port. 2010;23(3):527–32.
3. Ribeiro PR. A comunicação na prática médica: seu papel como componente terapêutico [Communication in medical practice: its therapeutic role] [article in Portuguese]. Rev Port Clin Geral. 2008;24:505–12.
4. Salgueira AP, Frada T, Aguiar P, Costa MJ. [Jefferson scale of physician lifelong learning: translation and adaptation for the portuguese medical population][article in Portuguese]. Acta Med Port. 2009;22(3):247–56.
5. Carvalho-Teixeira JA. Comunicação em contexto clinico. [Communication in clinical context] [article in Portuguese]. Rev Port Clin Geral. 2007;23:151–4.
6. Reis JC. O Sorriso de Hipócrates: a integração biopsicossocial dos processos de saúde e doença. (Hippocrates' smile: a biopsychosocial integration of health and disease processes). Vega: Lisboa; 1998.
7. Grassi L, Travado L. The role of psychosocial oncology in cancer care. In: Coleman MP, Alexe DM, Albreht T, McKee M, editors. Responding to the challenge of cancer in Europe. Ljubljana: Slovenian Institute of Public Health; 2008.
8. Stewart MA. Effective physician-patient communication and health outcomes: a review. Can Med Assoc J. 1996;152:1423–33.
9. Kinnersley P, Stott N, Peters TJ, et al. The patient-centredness of consultations and outcomes in primary care. Br J Gen Pract. 1999;49:711–6.
10. Pereira AV, Jorge GP, Guerra NC, Branco PR. O Médico de Família Ideal – perspectiva do utente [The ideal family doctor GP – the patient's perspective][article in Portuguese]. Rev Port Clin Geral. 2008;24:555–64.
11. Agostinho C, Cabanelas M, Franco C, Jesus J, Martins H. Satisfação do doente: Importância da comunicação médico-doente [Patient satisfaction: the importance of the doctor-patient communication in clinical context][article in Portuguese]. Rev Port Clin Geral. 2010;26:150–7.
12. Baile WF, Lenzi R, Kudelka AP, Maguire P, Novack D, Goldstein M, Myers EG, Bast Jr RC. Improving physician-patient communication in cancer care: outcome of a workshop for oncologists. J Cancer Educ. 1997;12:166–73.
13. Baile WF, Kudelka AP, Beale EA, Glober GA, Myers EG, Greisinger AJ, Bast Jr RC, Goldstein MG, Novack D, Lenzi R. Communication skills training in oncology. Description and preliminary outcomes of workshops on breaking bad news and managing patient reactions to illness. Cancer. 1999;86:887–97.

14. Fallowfield L, Lipkin M, Hall A. Teaching senior oncologists communication skills: Results from phase I of a comprehensive longitudinal program in the United Kingdom. J Clin Oncol. 1998;16:1961–8.
15. Fallowfield L, Jenkins V, Farewell V, Saul J, Duffy A, Eves R. Efficacy of cancer research in communication skills training model of oncologists: a randomised control trial. Lancet. 2002;359:650–6.
16. Razavi D, Delvaux N, Marchal S, De Cock M, Farvacques C, Slachmuylder JL. Testing health care professionals' communication skills: the usefulness of highly emotional standardized role-playing sessions with simulators. Psychooncology. 2000;9:293–302.
17. Razavi D, Merckaert I, Marchal S, Libert Y, Conradt S, Boniver J, Etienne AM, Fontaine O, Janne P, Klastersky J, Reynaert C, Scalliet P, Slachmuylder JL, Delvaux N. How to optimize physicians' communication skills in cancer care: results of a randomized study assessing the usefulness of posttraining consolidation workshops. J Clin Oncol. 2003;21:3141–9.
18. Nunes JMM. Comunicação em Contexto Clínico [Communication in Clinical Context]. Lisboa: Edições Bayer Healthcare; 2007.
19. Brandão J. Relação e comunicação médico-doente na Revista Portuguesa de Clínica Geral [Doctor-patient relationship and communication in the Portuguese journal of general practice] [article in Portuguese]. Rev Port Clin Geral. 2008;24:503–04.
20. Carvalho IP, Ribeiro-Silva R, Pais VG, Figueiredo-Braga M, Castro-Vale I, Teles A, Almeida SS, Mota-Cardoso R. O ensino da comunicação na relação medico-doente: uma proposta em prática. [Teaching communication in the doctor-patient relationship: a proposal in practice] [Article in Portuguese]. Acta Med Port. 2010;23:527–32.
21. Carvalho IP, Pais VG, Almeida SS, Ribeiro-Silva R, Figueiredo-Braga M, Teles A, Castro-Vale I, Mota-Cardoso R. Learning clinical communication skills: outcomes of a program for professional practitioners. Patient Educ Couns. 2011;84(1):84–9.
22. Faculdade de Ciências Médicas da Universidade Nova de Lisboa: Gabinete de Estudos Pós-Graduados. Retrieved from http://www.fcm.unl.pt/gepg/index.php?option=com_content&task=view&id=404&Itemid=423. Accessed 30 March 2011.
23. Associação de Estudantes do Instituto de Ciências Biomédicas Abel Salazar. Retrieved from http://www.aeicbasup.pt/index.php?option=com_k2&view=item&id=1064&Itemid=232. Accessed 30 March 2011.
24. Salgado R. O que facilita e o que dificulta uma consulta. [What facilitates and what compromises a clinical consultation?] [Article in Portuguese]. Rev Port Clin Geral. 2008;24:513–18.
25. Lopes RG, Santos F. Intencionalidade na comunicação em Grupos Balint [Communication intentionality in the Balint groups] [Article in Portuguese]. Rev Port Clin Geral. 2008; 24:519–25.
26. Brandão J. Relação médico-doente: sua complexidade e papel dos grupos Balint [Doctor-Patient relationship: its complexity and the Balint groups] [Article in Portuguese]. Rev Port Clin Geral. 2007;23:733–44.
27. Cunha E. Portfolio de incidentes críticos: os relatos de consulta como instrumentos de aprendizagem [Portfolio of critical incidents: the consultation reports as learning tools] [Article in Portuguese]. Rev Port Clin Geral. 2003;19:300–03.
28. Santos I. Recensão do livro: Comunicação em Contexto Clínico [Welcoming the book: communication in the clinical context]. Rev Port Clin Geral. 2007;23:147–50.
29. Ordem dos Médicos. Colégio da Especialidade de Oncologia Médica. Retrieved from https://www.ordemdosmedicos.pt/?lop=conteudo&op=bcbe3365e6ac95ea2c0343a2395834dd. Accessed 30 March 2011.
30. Faculdade de Medicina da Universidade de Lisboa. 2010. Investigação e Formação Avançada: Curso de Mestrado em Cuidados Paliativos. Retrieved from http://news.fm.ul.pt/Content.aspx?tabid=61&mid=379&cid=861. Accessed 30 March 2011.
31. Ferraz Gonçalves J, Castro S. Diagnosis disclosure in a Portuguese oncological centre. Palliat Med. 2001;15:35–41.
32. Pimentel FL, Ferreira JS, Vila Real M, Mesquita NF, Maia-Goncalves JP. Quantity and quality of information desired by Portuguese cancer patients. Supp Care Cancer. 1999;7:407–12.

33. Grassi L, Travado L, Gil F, Campos R, Lluch P, Baile W. A communication intervention for training southern European oncologists to recognize psychosocial morbidity in cancer patients I—development of the model and preliminary results on physicians' satisfaction. J Cancer Educ. 2005;20:79–84.
34. Reis J, Travado L. (2006). Communication and relationship skills for Health Professionals and Introduction to the breaking bad news protocol [2 set DVD] Psicolis, Ltd. (Producer). Available from: http://www.psicolis.com/.
35. Travado, L. (2010, September). Promoting communication skills for cancer doctors in Portugal: matching process and content. In W. Baile Chair, Teaching key communication skills for optimizing cancer care in Southern Europe: opportunities and obstacles. Symposium conducted at the international conference on communication in healthcare, of the European Association for Communication in Healthcare, Verona, Italy.

Chapter 26
Communication between Cancer Patients and Oncologists in Japan

Maiko Fujimori, Yuki Shirai, and Yosuke Uchitomi

Abstract In the Japanese clinical oncology setting, truth-telling has still not become common enough, although patients desire a lot of information related to their disease. Japanese patient preferences with regard to communication of bad news have been investigated and shown to consist of four components: setting, manner of communicating bad news, what and how much information to provide, and emotional support. Based on the patients' preferences, a new communication skills training program for oncologists and a train-the-trainer program have been developed and provided in Japan. For cancer patients, we developed a question prompt sheet and reported that it helps patients prepare questions and organize their information needs. In Japan, it is expected that these efforts will further communication between patients and their physicians.

Keywords Truth-telling • Patients-preferred communication • Communication skills training • Question prompt sheet

---

M. Fujimori, PhD (✉)
Psycho-oncology Division, National Cancer Center Hospital,
5-1-1 Tsukiji, Chuo-ku, Tokyo 104-0045, Japan
e-mail: fujimorimaiko@gmail.com

Y. Shirai, RN, PhD
Human Resource Development Plan for Cancer, Graduate School of Medicine,
The University of Tokyo, 7-3-1 Hongou, Bunkyo-ku, Tokyo 113-0033, Japan
e-mail: yukishirai-tky@umin.ac.jp

Y. Uchitomi, MD, PhD
Department of Neuropsychiatry, Okayama University Graduate School
of Medicine, Dentistry and Pharmaceutical Sciences,
2-5-1 Shikata-cho, Kitaku, Okayama 700-8558, Japan
e-mail: uchitomi@md.okayama-u.ac.jp

The Truth-Telling Situation in Japan

Since the hospice movement was introduced to Japan in the late 1970s, cancer-care policy has been slowly changing. The movement was led mainly by nurses and a limited number of physicians. They were concerned with issues related to providing aggressive treatment for terminally ill patients who had not been informed of their diagnosis of cancer. This situation was resulting in impaired communication between the patients and their families, and poor symptom management of cancer patients in pain and distress [1].

In 1989, a Japanese Ministry of Health and Welfare (JMHW) task force recommended the practice of telling the truth to terminally ill patients. In 1995, the JMHW promoted the practice of obtaining patients' informed consent before every medical procedure. A 1994 survey of bereaved family members showed that only 20.2% of cancer patients had been told their true diagnoses [2]. Since 1996, physicians have been permitted to charge a fee for giving patients information about their cancer treatment plans. The above reports did not recommend that obtaining patients' informed consent or telling the truth to cancer patients should be made a legal requirement, because a balance has not yet been established in Japan between the patients' desire for detailed information on their illnesses and the families' and physicians' beliefs that providing patients with such information is beneficial. Therefore, only 65.9% of physicians at 1,500 hospitals told cancer diagnoses to cancer patients and only 30.1% discussed life expectancy with cancer patients even in 2009 [3], although 75% of cancer in-patients treated at cancer center hospitals in Japan had been informed of their diagnosis of cancer in 1997 [4].

Kai et al. [5] studied patient–physician communication about terminal care in Japan and reported that the concordance between a patient's preference and the physician's estimation of it was close to the figure expected by chance alone. Japanese healthcare planners may prefer advances in truth-telling practice in cancer care to be slow, because they are uncertain about the psychological impact of the diagnosis of cancer on the patient and wish to respect the family's and physician's decisions, as well as the patient's preference. There are advanced-cancer diagnoses, recurrences, and treatment failures in clinical oncology settings, which are referred to with respect to truth-telling as "bad news." *Bad news* may be defined as "any information likely to drastically alter a patients' view of their future" [6]. The manner in which oncologists communicate bad news concerning cancer can affect the degree of the patient's distress in response to the news [7–9]. Significant associations have been founded between oncologist support, low levels of distress and helplessness/hopelessness, and a high level of "fighting spirit" [10]. On the other hand, the problems oncologists face when communicating bad news to their patients include a lack of sufficient time, being honest without causing distress [11], dealing with the patients' families, responding to the patients' emotions [11, 12], and discussing life expectancy [12].

Patient Preferences for Communication of Bad News

Because of the above issues, communication between patients and their oncologists in Japan needs to be facilitated further [13]. In Japan, there is a lack of guidance for physicians with regard to the optimal way to approach communication, though the literature in Western countries has suggested guidelines on communication between patients and their oncologists, especially when disclosing bad news.

In addition, most of the recommendations have been written from the physician's perspective, with less attention focused on the patient's perceptions and preferences. Because giving unfavorable news is a two-way communication between the physician and the patient and because the patient is the one whose life is directly affected, it is particularly important to consider and understand the patient's perspective on communication [14]. Furthermore, since patients' preferred manner of communication by physicians has recently been shown to be related to a lower level of psychological distress and a higher level of patient satisfaction [8], some studies have focused on preferences regarding communication style, such as what information to give and how to convey it.

The value of providing individualized communication with patients has been recognized; it is also important to understand medical and psychosocial predictive variables that are associated with patients' preferences [14–16]. Cultural as well as social variables pertaining to both patients and oncologists determine the oncologists' communication style. Some cultural aspects concerning the patient–oncologist relationship in oncology settings differ between Western and Asian countries [11, 17]; for example, family-centered decision-making processes, the use of euphemisms, and physician paternalism are more common in Japan [18, 19]. Therefore, we need to know the optimal way to communicate bad news in Japan.

There are an in-depth interview survey in which 42 cancer patients and seven oncologists participated and a questionnaire survey based on the results of the interview survey in which 529 cancer patients participated in Japan [19, 20]. The results of those surveys showed that Japanese cancer patients' preference with regard to communication with their physician consists of four components:

(a) Setting: spend sufficient time to discuss their illness with them
(b) How to deliver the bad news: discuss the impact of their disease and treatment on their daily activities
(c) Additional information: give information and facilitate their understanding about the impact on daily activities and alternative therapy
(d) Reassurance and emotional support: encourage and allow expression of their emotions

Four Components of Patients' Preferred Communication

Setting

The *setting* component included face-to-face consultation (the rate of patients who responded to prefer: 90.7%), sufficient consultation time (87.0%), and privacy (81.1%). Seventy-eight percent of patients wanted to be told the bad news while their relatives were present. Very few patients (17.5%) desired the presence of other health professionals. Physicians should be trusted by (84.0%) and familiar to their patients (69.7%), would be better off turning off their beepers to avoid interruptions (56.3%), and should greet the patient and family members politely (83.0%) before beginning the consultation.

How to Deliver the Bad News

The *how to deliver the bad news* component deals with how oncologists should communicate bad news to their patients during consultations. Most patients preferred that their physicians look into their eyes (78.4%) and communicate the bad news clearly (95.7%) and honestly (96.6%), in a manner that facilitates the patient's full understanding (98.0%); this includes choosing words carefully (91.1%), avoiding medical jargon (82.9%), showing actual X-ray films and laboratory data (92.0%), writing on paper to explain (79.4%), and providing written explanations as needed (84.7%).

Additional Information

The *additional information* component refers to the nature and amount of information provided by oncologists during consultations in which bad news is communicated. Many patients (79.2%) wished to receive all the information available, both good and bad. Most patients wanted to know about their chance of a cure (92.1%). However, because patients who wished to discuss their life expectancy remained at 50.4%, oncologists should not talk about the topic with every patient.

Furthermore, patients wanted to receive information regarding their treatment— e.g., information regarding all available treatment options (93.2%), the recommended treatment option (95.1%), the latest treatment and research (95.1%), the future treatment plan (97.3%), adverse effects and risks of treatment (93.2%), information regarding supportive care resources and services (e.g., rehabilitation and psychosocial counseling) (78.3%), as well as information regarding the impact of their disease and treatment on their daily activities (e.g., work, food, and lifestyle) (84.9%).

Reassurance and Emotional Support

The *reassurance and emotional support* component refers to the supportive aspects of communication and includes offering comfort and support to patients.

When communicating bad news, patients desired that physicians considered the patients' (81.9%) and family members' (84.1%) feelings by imagining themselves in their patient's situation (89.3%), speaking gently and softly (85.8%), talking in a way that inspires hope (87.5%), and without touching or hugging (58.8%). After communicating the bad news, patients desired that physicians use supportive expressions to relieve the patients' emotional distress (76.0%), allow the patient to express their feelings (73.3%), and reassure them. Telling the patient not to abandon hope until the end was also considered valuable by patients (96.6%).

The results provide some guidance with regard to physicians' attitudes and behaviors when communicating bad news. Four commonly observed components of cancer patients' preferences were identified: setting, how to deliver the bad news, additional information, and reassurance and emotional support. Cancer patients' preferences suggested that the elements of nonverbal communication, such as setting, manner, and emotional support, are important to cancer patients when physicians communicate bad news to them. These four components of patients' preferences should be assessed before communicating bad news. Information regarding these components would be valuable to physicians, as it would enable them to provide cancer patients with information about their disease in a manner that best meets the patients' needs. In family-centered cultures, such as Japanese culture, patients preferred that relatives be present more than patients in Western cultures did; and comparatively fewer patients preferred to discuss life expectancy in Asian cultures. This preference regarding discussion of prognostic information may be related to a study on what is considered a good death conducted in Japan by Miyashita et al. [22], according to which "unawareness of death" was one of the major contributors to a good death, which is very important in Japan.

The communication styles preferred by the majority of the patients might be recommended to physicians delivering bad news to patients; physicians should deliver both positive (e.g., treatment plan and what the patient can hope for) and negative (e.g., risk and side effects of treatment) information pertaining to the disease and its treatment and should also adopt a supportive attitude. Continuing physician responsibility for patient care and future treatment plans were the most-preferred attitudes, and vagueness was the least-preferred attitude from the patients' perspectives. These findings suggest that engagement between the patients and their physicians is important when bad news is being broken.

It is important to understand communication in which patients responded with interindividual variation. While patients preferred to be clearly told of their diagnosis, half of them preferred that physicians use euphemisms and 33.5% of them preferred that physicians do not repeatedly use the word *cancer*. The use of euphemisms may give patients the impression that their physician is supporting them emotionally; these items were included in the emotional support factor. Interestingly, 84% of the patients preferred to have their physicians show the same concern for the feelings of their family as for themselves. In Japan, families and physicians have been accorded a larger role in clinical decision making, and a patient's family is usually informed of an incurable cancer diagnosis before the patient has been notified [17]. That is to say, the family might experience distress before the patient does. Therefore, patients might desire their physicians to show concern for the feelings of their family. Because 78% of the patients preferred to be with their family when the bad news was being broken and 14% of the patients preferred to receive bad news at their physicians' pace, physicians need to recognize that many Japanese cancer patients prefer to play a collaborative role in the decision-making process, rather than assuming active and passive roles, and will respect the physicians' opinion even if the physicians' recommendation conflicts with their own wishes.

Factors Associated with Patient Preferences for the Communication of Bad News

The value of providing individualized communication to patients has been recognized. Therefore the associations between the dimensions of patients' communication style preferences and demographic, medical, and psychological adjustment variables were explored.

Results showed that preferences varied according to demographic and psychological variables but not according to disease variables. Younger patients, female patients, more highly educated patients, patients who have a high fighting spirit, and patients who have high-anxiety preoccupation desired to receive clear explanation and as much detailed information as possible. Female patients, patients who a have high fighting spirit, patients who have high-anxiety preoccupation, and patients who have high psychological distress desired to receive emotional support. Female patients, more highly educated patients, patients who have a high fighting spirit, and patients who have high-anxiety preoccupation also desired oncologists to provide a considerate setting for their discussion. These results indicate that balancing hope and honesty is an important communication skill.

Cross-cultural differences were indicated by some patients' preferences [21]. Only 30% or fewer of patients in Asian studies preferred to discuss life expectancy, whereas 60% of patients in Western studies preferred to do so. While 78% of patients in Japan were found to prefer to be told with family members present, only 40% in Ireland, 53–57% in Australia, and 61% in Portugal preferred to be told with family members present; and 81% of patients in the United States did not wish anyone else to be present when they received bad news.

Preferred Communication of Bad News in Japan

The findings in the surveys suggested the following implications for physician communication of bad news to patients:

1. Before consultations in which physicians plan to communicate bad news to a patient, they should spend sufficient time to discuss the disease with the patient and their relatives and leave their beepers with another medical staff member to avoid interruption.

2. Physicians should communicate detailed information regarding bad news clearly and honestly, in a manner that facilitates patients' full understanding.
3. When communicating bad news, physicians should consider the patients' and their relatives' feelings by imagining themselves in their patient's situation, speaking gently and softly, talking in a way that inspires hope, without touching or hugging the patient.
4. After communicating bad news, physicians should use supportive expressions to relieve patients' emotional distress, allow patients to express their feelings, reassure patients, and sustain patients' hope.
5. Physicians should discuss information regarding treatment and the impact of the disease and treatment on daily activities with their patients.
6. Younger, female, and more educated patients as well as patients with higher level of distress or anxiety and those with a fighting spirit were found to prefer to be given as much detailed information as possible and to receive emotional support. Patients with moderate income desired more information than low-income patients. Physicians should ask patients about their own preferences, because the existence of individual differences was reported in these studies.

The Effort to Strengthen Oncologists' Communication in Japanese Medical Education

In June 2006, the Cancer Control Act was approved, and the law has been in force since April 2007. Under the law, the Basic Plan to Promote Cancer Control programs was discussed by the Cancer Control Promotion Council and approved by the Japanese Cabinet in June 2007.

Based on the Basic Plans for National Cancer Strategy, communication skills training (CST) workshops for oncologists have been held in Japan since 2007. The CST program aims that oncologists learn to perceive preferences and needs for communication with each patient and to provide suitable communication in the three situations of breaking bad news to patients: diagnosis of advanced cancer, recurrence, and stopping an anticancer treatment. This program adopted the conceptual communication skills model consisting of four dimensions as developed in previous surveys (referred to as SHARE: S, setting up the supporting environment of the interview; H, considering how to deliver the bad news; A, discussing additional information; and RE, providing reassurance and addressing the patient's emotions with empathic responses) [19, 20]. The program stressed RE, because it is the most important patient preference and also one of the most difficult communication skills for physicians [12].

The 2-day program consisted of a didactic lecture, role-plays, and discussions. The participants were divided into groups of four, each group with two facilitators. The facilitators were psychiatrists, psychologists, and oncologists, all of whom had had clinical experience in oncology for 3 or more years and had participated in specialized 30-h training workshops on facilitating workshops on communication skills in oncology. The simulated patients, who had had experience in medical school for 3 or more years, also participated in 30-h training workshops.

For these 5 years, 623 oncologists participated in the workshop. They showed improvement in confidence on communication with cancer patients after the workshop.

A train-the-trainers program for facilitators of CST has also been developed, and these workshops are held as well as the CST workshops. The facilitating CST program was developed to focus on the facilitation process, such as management of small-group workshops, especially role-playing. The program consisted of a 3-h didactic lecture, role-plays and discussions for 27 h, an orientation, an "ice-breaking" session, and a workshop summary—a total of three 2-day workshops. After the large group orientation, the participants were divided into groups of six each, and a facilitator was assigned to each group; then the lecture and role-plays were done. In role-play, one participant volunteered to play the facilitator, another the subfacilitator, and the other participants volunteered to play the CST participants. The "facilitator" managed a simulated interview with a simulated patient in the small group. The facilitators of the train-the-trainer workshop, who had experience as a facilitator of CST and studied communication between patient and healthcare providers for 5 or more years, managed and guided the training process. The simulated patients, who had had experience in medical school and hospital for 3 or more years, also participated in role-playing. Following the 30-h facilitator workshop, all trainee facilitators facilitated CST under the supervision of the experienced facilitators. During these 5 years, 96 oncologists and psychooncologists participated in the training workshop, and they have conducted the CST workshop as facilitators. Further, increasingly widespread efforts toward promoting education on communication for medical staff members are expected.

Support for Patients' Decision Making after Bad News

The patient-centered approach is important in improving communication between patients and physicians. A question prompt sheet (QPS) is a structured list of questions covering the items a patient may want to ask their physicians regarding their illness and treatment. Patients are given the QPS before consultation for them to read and use to determine what questions they would like to ask. In the cancer setting, randomized controlled trials have been performed to evaluate the effectiveness of QPS in encouraging cancer patients regardless of their cancer stage to obtain more information about their illness and its treatment. Patients who received QPS asked more questions [23, 24] and rated the QPS as significantly more helpful than its absence in aiding communication with their physician compared with a control group [25].

Decision making in patients at the time of initial diagnosis of advanced cancer is quite different than for patients with early-stage cancer who are receiving treatments with curative intent or for those with advanced cancer who are already approaching the terminal phase of their illness [26]. Patients who have just been diagnosed with advanced cancer are stunned by the news of having incurable cancer and by the prospect of limited life expectancy [25]. Nevertheless, they are often obliged to make urgent decisions, and this may require an exhaustive search for information about their condition. When deciding on the initial treatment, good communication between an advanced cancer patient and a physician is very important to achieve a better understanding of the medical condition and for the patient to take a more autonomous role in medical care. Therefore, it is important to investigate whether QPS can help advanced cancer patients to ask questions and to collect information when making decisions.

Moreover, there is little research examining the use of QPS by non-English-speaking cancer patients [27]. Our previous surveys in Japan found that some patients preferred that physicians give them a chance to ask questions, while others did not know what questions to ask and wanted to know the questions most frequently asked by other patients [19, 20]. In Japan, it might prove helpful to provide cancer patients with a QPS containing sample questions commonly asked.

Therefore, Japanese patients' perception of the usefulness of a QPS provided to patients newly diagnosed with advanced cancer in helping them decide on their initial treatment was investigated [28].

The Question Prompt Sheet in Japan

The QPS was designed: 10 A4 sheets containing 53 questions grouped into ten topics; diagnosis, condition of a disease, symptom, test, treatment, life, family, psychological issues, prognosis, and other issues and a space for new questions based on previous QPS studies [29–32], a previous study on the preferences of Japanese cancer patients regarding the disclosure of bad news [19], and a pilot survey.

The Usefulness of the Question Prompt Sheet in Japan

Patients with advanced cancer were randomly assigned to either the intervention group (received QPS and Hospital Introduction Sheet, HIS) or the control group (received HIS only). Patients in both the groups were instructed to read the material(s) before the consultation with an oncologist at the thoracic or gastrointestinal oncology division to discuss the treatment plan. Following the next consultation, patients in both groups were asked to complete a questionnaire that assessed the usefulness of the material(s) and their level of satisfaction with the consultation. In addition, the patients were asked about the number and content of the questions for their physician.

Sixty-three (72.4%) of 87 eligible patients participated in the study.

Approximately 75% of the patients in both groups read their respective material(s) prior to consultation. Forty-four percent of the patients in the intervention group and

23% of the patients in the control group decided on their questions in advance ($p=0.075$).

We found that, compared with supplying the HIS only, advanced-cancer patients who received both the HIS and the QPS rated the materials significantly more favorably with regard to the materials' usefulness in helping them ask questions of the physician and for future consultations.

The mean usefulness rate (a numerical rating scale of 0–10) of the material(s) in helping the patients to ask questions was significantly higher in the intervention group than in the control group (4.4 ± 3.6 and 2.7 ± 2.8, respectively; $p=0.033$). The mean score of usefulness of the material(s) in helping the patients to understand the treatment plan tended to be higher in the intervention group than in the control group (4.9 ± 3.6 and 3.3 ± 2.8, respectively; $p=0.051$). The mean score of willingness to use the material(s) in the future was significantly higher in the intervention group than in the control group (5.3 ± 3.8 and 2.8 ± 2.8, respectively; $p=0.006$).

The levels of satisfaction with the ability of the physicians to answer the patients' questions, asking questions, understanding the condition of the disease, comprehending the treatment plan, as well as the overall level of satisfaction with the consultation were high in both groups, although not significantly different.

During the consultation, 63% of the patients in the intervention group and 71% of the patients in the control group asked question(s) (no significant difference). Patients in both groups asked a median of 1.0 question (interquartile range, 2.0) (no significant difference). The majority of questions were related to information about treatment.

The QPS was perceived by the patients as useful for helping them ask relevant questions of their physician and for future use without an increase in the number of questions during the consultation. There are several possible explanations for this. First, communication may be better when patients are able to ask their most meaningful questions rather than just more questions [31]. In our study, patients in the intervention group might be able to consider the information they need to know in advance from the QPS and thereby ask questions that better address their main concerns than simply asking more questions. Second, a QPS might be helpful for advanced-cancer patients in collecting and organizing information. Advanced-cancer patients have high levels of unmet needs in the areas of psychological and medical communication/information and experience difficulty in obtaining sufficient information during consultation [36–38]. During the interview in our study, some patients emphasized their expectations for the future use of the QPS, since they had decided not to ask any questions in the first consultation because they believed that they must first listen to the physician's explanation. Previous QPS studies also reported that the level of satisfaction showed a poor correlation with the number or duration of questions asked [29, 30].

In conclusion, the QPS seemed to be a moderately useful tool for Japanese advanced-cancer patients. Compared with controls, patients rated the QPS more favorably in terms of enabling them to ask relevant questions and for future use. The QPS seemed to help patients prepare questions, and it may help patients articulate and organize their information needs. However, the QPS did not seem directly to promote patient confidence to ask questions. In Japan, active endorsement of QPS by physicians and/or CST for physicians might be effective for promoting question-asking behavior.

Cultural Characteristics of Patient Behavior during Consultation in Japan

Unexpectedly, the use of the QPS did not seem to promote question-asking behavior. The total number of questions asked by the patients in the intervention group (median: 1.0) in our study was smaller than that in the intervention group in previous studies of patients seeing an oncologist for the first time (mean/median: 8.5–14.0) [23, 30, 31], although nearly half of the patients in the intervention group had decided on their questions in advance. One of the reasons behind the fewer questions in the study was assumed the unique patient–physician relationship in Asian culture. The views in Japan on individuality and personal rights are distinctively different from those in North America and Western countries [33, 34]. In Japan, the dominant patient–physician relationship is as follows: "the relationship between a Japanese physician and a patient is clearly asymmetrical, since the patient seeks help and care from a medical expert whose diagnostic evaluations have to be accepted by the patient without discussion" [35]. Patient–physician relationships in Japan have traditionally been based on a paternalistic and hierarchical culture that discourages patients from questioning doctors. For this reason, cancer patients in Asian countries might need more intervention to make them feel comfortable asking questions of their physicians. In our study, the physicians were not asked to refer to or endorse the QPS; however, considering the interactive nature of communication, a combination of QPS and active endorsement of the QPS by physicians and/or CST for physicians might be needed to promote question-asking behavior. Indeed, results from some previous studies suggest that physician endorsement of a QPS seems to enhance its effectiveness [24, 32].

Conclusion

In the Japanese clinical oncology setting, truth-telling still has not become common enough, although patients desire a lot of information related to their disease. Because of these issues, communication between patients and their physicians needs to be facilitated further, but there is a lack of guidance for physicians in regard to the optimal way to approach the communication of bad news in Japan. Therefore, Japanese patient preferences with regard to communication of bad news have been investigated and shown to consist of four components: setting, manner of communicating bad news, what and how much information is provided, and emotional support. Patient preferences were found to be associated with demographic factors. Younger patients, female patients, and more highly educated patients consistently desired to receive as much detailed information as possible and to receive emotional support.

Based on the patients' preferences, we have developed a new CST program for oncologists and a train-the-trainer program. Since the National Cancer Control Act implemented in 2007, 499 oncologists have participated in the CST program, and 84 oncologists and psychooncologists have obtained certification as a facilitator of the CST program. For cancer patients, we developed a question-asking prompt sheet and report that it helps patients prepare questions and organize their information needs. In Japan, it is expected that these efforts will further communication between patients and their physicians.

References

1. Uchitomi Y, Sugihara J, Fukue M, et al. Psychiatric liaison issues in cancer care in Japan. J Pain Symptom Manage. 1994;9:319–24.
2. Japanese Ministry of Health and Welfare. FY 1994 report on the socioeconomic survey of vital statistics; malignant neoplasm. Statistics and Information Department, Minister's Secretariat, Japanese Ministry of Health and Welfare, Tokyo; 1995 (in Japanese).
3. Matsushima E. Survey on informed consent and truth telling. In: Matsushima E, editor. Annual report of the cancer research (8–12) of the Japanese Ministry of Health and Welfare FY 2010. Japanese Ministry of Health and Welfare, Tokyo, Japan; 2010 (in Japanese).
4. Sasaki J. Survey on informed consent and truth telling. In: Sasaki J, editor. Annual report of the cancer research (8–12) of the Japanese Ministry of Health and Welfare FY 1997. Japanese Ministry of Health and Welfare, Tokyo, Japan; 1998. p. 105–20 (in Japanese).
5. Kai I, Ohi G, Yano E, et al. Communication between patients and physicians about terminal care: a survey in Japan. Soc Sci Med. 1993;36:1151–9.
6. Buckman R. Breaking bad news: why is it still so difficult? Br Med J. 1984;288:1597–9.
7. Takayama T, Yamazaki Y, Katsumata N. Relationship between outpatients' perceptions of physicians' communication styles and patients' anxiety levels in a Japanese oncology setting. Soc Sci Med. 2001;53:1335–50.
8. Schofield PE, Butow PN, Thompson JF, et al. Psychological responses of patients receiving a diagnosis of cancer. Ann Oncol. 2003;14:48–56.
9. Morita T, Akechi T, Ikenaga Y, et al. Communication about the ending of anticancer treatment and transition to palliative care. Ann Oncol. 2004;15:1551–7.
10. Uchitomi Y, Mikami I, Kugaya A, et al. Physician support and patient psychologic responses after surgery for nonsmall cell lung carcinoma: a prospective observational study. Cancer. 2001;92:1926–35.
11. Baile WF, Lenzi R, Parker PA, et al. Oncologists' attitudes toward and practices in giving bad news: an exploratory study. J Clin Oncol. 2002;20:2189–96.
12. Fujimori M, Oba A, Koike M, et al. Communication skills training for Japanese oncologists on how to break bad news. J Cancer Educ. 2003;18:194–201.
13. Uchitomi Y. Psycho-oncology in Japan: history, current problems and future aspect. Jpn J Clin Oncol. 1999;29:411–2.
14. Parker PA, Baile WF, de Moor C, et al. Breaking bad news about cancer: patients' preferences for communication. J Clin Oncol. 2001;19:2049–56.

15. Butow PN, Kazemi JN, Beeney LJ, et al. When the diagnosis is cancer: patient communication experiences and preferences. Cancer. 1996;77:2630–7.
16. Butow PN, Maclean M, Dunn SM, et al. The dynamics of change: cancer patients' preferences for information, involvement and support. Ann Oncol. 1997;8:857–63.
17. Ruhnke GW, Wilson SR, Akamatsu T, et al. Ethical decision making and patient autonomy: a comparison of physicians and patients in Japan and the United States. Chest. 2000;118:1172–82.
18. Sekimoto M, Asai A, Ohnishi M, et al. Patients' preferences for involvement in treatment decision making in Japan. BMC Fam Pract. 2004;5:1.
19. Fujimori M, Akechi T, Akizuki N, et al. Good communication when receiving bad news about Cancer in Japan. Psychooncology. 2005;14:1043–51.
20. Fujimori M, Akechi T, Morita T, et al. Preferences of cancer patients regarding the disclosure of bad news. Psychooncology. 2007;16:573–81.
21. Fujimori M, Uchitomi Y. Preferences of cancer patients regarding communication of bad news: a systematic literature review. Jpn J Clin Oncol. 2009;39:201–16.
22. Miyashita M, Sanjo M, Morita T, et al. Good death in cancer care: a nationwide quantitative study. Ann Oncol. 2007;18:1090–7.
23. Butow P, Devine R, Boyer M, et al. Cancer consultation preparation package: changing patients but not physicians is not enough. J Clin Oncol. 2004;22:4401–9.
24. Clayton JM, Butow PN, Tattersall MH, et al. Randomized controlled trial of a prompt list to help advanced cancer patients and their caregivers to ask questions about prognosis and end-of-life care. J Clin Oncol. 2007;25:715–23.
25. Tattersall MH, Thomas H. Recent advances: oncology. Br Med J. 1999;318:445–8.
26. Gattellari M, Voigt KJ, Butow PN, et al. When the treatment goal is not cure: are cancer patients equipped to make informed decisions? J Clin Oncol. 2002;20:503–13.
27. Dimoska A, Tattersall MH, Butow PN, et al. Can a "prompt list" empower cancer patients to ask relevant questions? Cancer. 2008;113:225–37.
28. Shirai Y, Fujimori M, Ogawa A, et al. Patients' perception of the usefulness of a question prompt sheet for advanced cancer patients when deciding the initial treatment: a randomized, controlled trial. Psychooncology; 2011, in press.
29. Butow PN, Dunn SM, Tattersall MH, et al. Patient participation in the cancer consultation: evaluation of a question prompt sheet. Ann Oncol. 1994;5:199–204.
30. Brown R, Butow PN, Boyer MJ, et al. Promoting patient participation in the cancer consultation: evaluation of a prompt sheet and coaching in question-asking. Br J Cancer. 1999;80:242–8.
31. Bruera E, Sweeney C, Willey J, et al. Breast cancer patient perception of the helpfulness of a prompt sheet versus a general information sheet during outpatient consultation: a randomized, controlled trial. J Pain Symptom Manage. 2003;25:412–9.
32. Brown RF, Butow PN, Dunn SM, et al. Promoting patient participation and shortening cancer consultations: a randomised trial. Br J Cancer. 2001;85:1273–9.
33. Blackhall LJ, Murphy ST, Frank G, et al. Ethnicity and attitudes toward patient autonomy. J Am Med Assoc. 1995;274:820–5.
34. Mitchell JL. Cross-cultural issues in the disclosure of cancer. Cancer Pract. 1998;6:153–60.
35. Nomura K, Ohno M, Fujinuma Y, et al. Patient autonomy preferences among hypertensive outpatients in a primary care setting in Japan. Intern Med. 2007;46:1403–8.
36. Rainbird KJ, Perkins JJ, Sanson-Fisher RW. The Needs Assessment for Advanced Cancer Patients (NA-ACP): a measure of the perceived needs of patients with advanced, incurable cancer. A study of validity, reliability and acceptability. Psychooncology. 2005;14:297–306.
37. Rainbird KJ, Perkins JJ, Sanson-Fisher RW, et al. The needs of patients with advanced, incurable cancer. Br J Cancer. 2009;101:759–64.
38. Teno JM, Lima JC, Lyons KD. Cancer patient assessment and reports of excellence: reliability and validity of advanced cancer patient perceptions of the quality of care. J Clin Oncol. 2009;27:1621–6.

Part IV
Cultural and Social Context

Chapter 27
Multicultural Aspects of Care for Cancer Patients in Israel

Miri Cohen

Abstract Care for cancer patients from diverse cultural groups requires cultural competence, including cultural awareness, knowledge, and specific skills. Israel, a multicultural state with many subgroups of Jews and Arabs, displays diverse degrees of religiosity and variety along the continuum from traditional to Western lifestyle. This chapter draws on the very few existing studies of multicultural aspects of care for cancer patients in Israel. It focuses mainly on two specific and culturally distinct groups in Israel: Arabs and ultra-orthodox Jews. It describes perceptions of cancer in the familial and societal context and elaborates aspects of psychosocial interventions in the multicultural context. It concludes with thoughts on how to use cultural knowledge to promote the care of cancer patients.

Keywords Cancer patients • Cultural competence • Ethnic diversity • Religion • Psychosocial care • Arabs • Ultra-orthodox Jews

Introduction

Ethnic and cultural diversity of populations in Western countries poses a unique challenge for the various health care professionals involved in the care of cancer patients. Scholars term this challenge *cultural competence* [24, 54]—professionals' ability to provide health care to patients of diverse backgrounds, tailoring it to each patient's social, cultural, and linguistic needs. Cultural competence includes possession of the knowledge, attitudes, and skills to establish effective communication with cancer patients from diverse cultural groups [24, 25, 54] and thus promote

M. Cohen (✉)
Department of Gerontology and School of Social Work,
University of Haifa, Haifa 31905, Israel
e-mail: cohenm@research.haifa.ac.il

satisfaction, well-being, and better health outcomes [24, 56] and decrease disparities in cancer care [6, 48, 56].

Oncology centers in Israel are an excellent example of multicultural diversity of patients and of healthcare professionals; patients and professionals are a composite of the various Jewish and Arab subgroups in Israel. Understanding the unique cultural aspects of the beliefs, perceptions, and attitudes to illness and treatment of the diverse cultural groups and of their decision making and emotions is an initial and essential step toward providing culturally competent care.

The aim of this chapter is to assemble existing knowledge on various aspects of multicultural cancer care in Israel. Several general cautionary comments should be noted. First, culture and ethnicity are not identical constructs; this chapter will refer to cultural differences among ethnic groups. Second, culture is a dynamic structure, with diverse aspects within each cultural group, rather than a unified and fixed set of beliefs [5]. Ethnic groups in Western countries, furthermore, experience major modernization processes, where modern perceptions of health exist alongside traditional beliefs [5]. These processes include adopting the Western biomedical view and often merging it with traditional beliefs through dynamic and ever-changing processes. In addition, when referring to culture or ethnicity, we actually discuss a range of beliefs, attitudes, and lifestyles from an extreme traditional pole to an extreme Western pole, with most individuals spread along the continuum [46]. Any discussion of cultural differences must therefore suffer from overgeneralization. The chapter describes general characteristics that should be carefully examined when applying this knowledge to an individual.

A third relevant comment concerns culture and religion, which are, indeed, different constructs [19]. Culture goes far beyond religion (e.g., Americans of different faiths identify with the American culture). However, different groups exhibit certain similarities according to level of religiosity: the more devout of different faiths tend to lead a more conservative way of life, and they hold somewhat similar sets of beliefs—for example, about the relationship of God to the individual or the role of fate (or God) as against personal responsibility in one's life. In the case of Israel, most Arabs hold traditional beliefs and attitudes, but in the Jewish population these are mostly evident in the orthodox and ultra-orthodox Jews; the majority of the Jewish people hold a Western orientation [46]. The present review will focus largely on two distinct cultural groups: Arabs and ultra-orthodox Jews. Where data are available, we will also refer to immigrants from the former Soviet Union and elderly Holocaust survivors.

Background: The Population of Israel

Israel is a relatively small country, with a population of approximately 7.7 million people [57], but it holds a great variety of cultures, languages, religions, and ethnicities. The two major groups in the Israeli population are the Jews (75.5%) and the Arabs (20.3%), while the remaining 4.2% consists of many ethnic and religious minorities such as Armenians, Assyrians, and Circassians. Neither the Jews nor the Arabs are homogeneous groups. The Arab population consists of Muslims (83.8%), Christians of various denominations (7.9%), and Druze (8.2%) [57]. The Jewish people in Israel are of widely different backgrounds: There are immigrants and descendants of immigrants from all over the Diaspora who came before the establishment of the state of Israel in 1948; others have continued to arrive ever since. The greatest immigration wave was from 1990 to 1999, when almost a million immigrants entered Israel (enlarging the population by 14%), most of them (87%) from the former Soviet Union.

There is a high level of religiousness in Israeli society; only 21% of Arabs and 42% of Jews define themselves as secular, although for those who claim to be religious the degree varies from ultra-religious to observing various religious traditions [57].

The Israeli population is young compared with Western countries; people aged 65 years and older constitute only 9.8% of the whole population, and children and youth younger than 19 make up 31% of the Jewish population. The Arab population is younger than the Jewish; only 3.9% of the Arabs are over 65 while 46.2% are under 19 years of age [57].

The Jewish People in Israel

According to attitude toward religion, the Jews in Israel can be divided roughly into five groups: secular, who constitute about 42%; mildly religious (25%); traditional (13%); religious (12%); and ultra-orthodox (8%) [57]. The groups differ in the degree of their religious observance, on a continuum from the secular Jews, who lead mostly a Western lifestyle and keep none of the laws of Judaism, to the ultra-orthodox Jews. The latter lead a segregated way of life and pursue only Jewish studies; obeying the Jewish commandments is central to their lives. To preserve the religious way of life, television, the Internet, and secular newspapers are strictly forbidden. They live puritan lives and assign high value to modesty (e.g., women wear long dresses with long sleeves, men and women remain separate) [40]. The traditional and religious Jews maintain the Jewish laws to varying degrees, participate in the secular world, and usually have a fully secular education.

Arab People in Israel

Arab people in Israel share cultural similarities with Arabs in other countries of the Middle East, but they differ from them due to processes of change related to being a minority in a predominantly Jewish and Western democratic state [9]. The Arabs in Israel undergo faster modernization processes than their counterparts in the neighboring countries [14].

The modernization processes encompass many aspects of Arab society, including higher education and a shift in labor patterns, changes in societal values and norms, and the adoption of Western lifestyles [7, 9, 13]. There is also a gradual transformation from a collectivist to an individualistic cultural orientation [9]. Although the Arab people in Israel form a continuum from secular to very religious, the majority of them rank themselves as religious to very religious [29]. Moreover, even the less religious tend to keep some of the religious rituals and laws and largely uphold traditional beliefs, such as those regarding the causes of illness or the role of fate in life [11].

Epidemiology of Cancer in Israel

The age-adjusted rate of cancer is 301.52 per 100,000 in the Jewish population and 179.46 per 100,000 in the Arab population, but the rate of increase is much higher in the Arab population [42]: in the Jewish sector the rise in the number of cancer cases over the years 1982–2002 was 27.7%, and in the Arab population it was 65.6%. Moreover, while between 1995 and 2002 there was a decrease in the cancer rate of 0.8% in the Jewish sector, this rate still increased in the Arab sector, by 3.2% [42].

The most recent 5-year relative survival rates for Israeli cancer patients were estimated for 1999–2002; they were 61.4% for Jewish males and 67.3% for females. For Arabs, the percentages were lower: 50.7% for males and 64.9% for females [42]. This gap is ascribed, among other factors, to late diagnosis due to higher barriers to attendance of screening procedures [10, 12, 28]. The most common malignant tumors in males are of the prostate (20.48%), colorectal (14.17%), and lung (10.11%) [42]. In females, the most commonly encountered cancer is breast cancer (29.73%), followed by colorectal (13.49%), while lung cancer is less frequent than in males (4.93%) [42].

Cultural Beliefs and Perceptions of Cancer

Culture can affect perceptions related to cancer, its causes, course, and meaning [11, 28]. The secular Jewish population mostly perceive genetic, family, and lifestyle factors as causes of cancer, as found in a study with focus groups [11, 17, 18]. Religious Jewish and Arab people tend to ascribe the onset of illness to the will of God or to fate [11, 19, 39]. Recent findings among Muslim and Christian Arab women in Israel showed that perceptions of the causes of cancer are deeply rooted in these beliefs [19, 28]; likewise among ultra-orthodox Jewish women [38]. The Arab women expressed their belief that fate is not a matter of chance, but comes from God in response to their deeds and behaviors; one participants stated, "I believe in God, and believers are not afraid of dying. Everything is in God's hands, and our destiny is to return to God, at some time." Some participants explained that cancer is a way of punishment by God due to improper or unfaithful behaviors. Other women believed that cancer is a kind of test by God of their devotion and personal strength, and therefore should be seen as a challenge [11]. For example, "God tests our patience, just as what happened to Job"; or "It is a test by God. God sends troubles to the ones He loves, to test their patience."

The ultra-orthodox Jewish women stressed more the view that the person, his/her family, or community did something wrong, so the occurrence of cancer in someone in the community necessitates a searching look deep within (Hebrew *heshbon nefesh*— "reckoning of the soul"). However, according to these women, an individual with cancer should accept the illness without asking "Why has it happened to me?" [38]

However, discussions in focus groups with Arab women and ultraorthodox Jewish women revealed that perceptions of causes of cancer as God's will coexist with perceptions of personal, environmental, and lifestyle causes—such as hereditary factors, but also radiation, air pollution, chemicals in foods, a high-fat diet, and hormones in meat [11, 38]. Several women expressed a combination of modern biomedical and traditional views as to the cause of cancer. For example, most participants agreed that giving birth and breast-feeding are protective factors against breast cancer. This notion was explained by information obtained from various biomedical sources, but also from religious sources. An example of the latter is the text "Every Arab woman should breast-feed her babies. Our religion tells us to do so. According to the religion, breast-feeding should last 30 months. In return, it reduces our risk of breast cancer. If we do it, we can protect ourselves." This view was also related to the traditional outlook of raising children as the major role of women in society. The protective quality of breast-feeding was perceived as a reward for fulfilling this role: "God blesses women who give birth to many children, so giving birth and breast-feeding can reduce the chances of cancer" [11].

Focus groups were also conducted with Bedouin women [11]. Bedouins are a distinct Muslim ethnic group. Until several decades ago, the Bedouin were nomads living mostly in the desert. They underwent urbanization processes, and now most of them are settled in urban communities. However, they still constitute a conservative society, with lower education levels than the other Arabs in Israel [21].

Bedouin women in the focus groups voiced much more traditional views of the causes of cancer than other Muslim women. They perceived that among other factors, cancer can occur due to the "evil eye" of envious neighbors. A few women still adhered to an old common belief that cancer is contagious.

Beliefs about the curability of cancer also proved divergent. In a study of Jewish participants in focus groups, most of them probably secular, a range of beliefs about cancer was found, from its being fatal to curable or chronic [18]. A study of 1,550 Jewish and Arab women in Israel revealed especially high fatalistic perceptions in the Arab women and the ultra-orthodox Jewish women, in contrast to secular and traditional Jewish women [17].

In two focus group studies conducted with healthy Arab women [11, 19] and a study with ultra-orthodox women [38], participants expressed strong fatalism regarding the outcomes of cancer. They still perceived cancer as an incurable disease, a certain death sentence [29]. In contrast to these studies with healthy participants, in a qualitative study with in-depth interviews with 20 Arab breast cancer patients, all were optimistic about the outcome of their disease and confident that they would defeat it, with God's help [39].

The Cancer Patient: Individual, Family, and Social Perspective

Western society generally assumes an individualistic orientation, stressing values of individual autonomy and the individual's right to self-determination and her own decision making regarding her own body [55]. Medical decisions are made by the individual and his/her partner, sometimes in consultation with selected members of the family [55]. While these perceptions are held by a majority of Jewish people in Israel, they are less valid for traditional groups such as ultra-orthodox Jews and most Arabs in Israel.

The Arab people in Israel still live in a society that is basically collectivist, albeit shifting toward a more individualistic lifestyle [9, 34]. Scholars argue that personality theories developed in Europe and North America are not relevant for people of traditional-collectivist societies. They postulate that individuation, self-determination, and free will are inapplicable to traditional people. Decisions regarding the individual are a matter of the extended family, often directed by the male family members (husband, father, brothers, and uncles). Decisions on health care are also taken by the family [2]. For example, the health care of breast cancer patients who are widows is often overseen by the male members of the extended family: her father, brothers, brothers-in-law, and adult sons. Issues such as informed consent to treatment are accordingly more complicated in these situations. Information about the disease and treatment choices must often be imparted to several family members.

As a patriarchal society, traditional hierarchical familial roles are strict, even in more modern Arab families [2]. However, a recent study with 56 Arab breast cancer survivors (stages I–III) and 66 age- and education-matched women showed that in cases of women treated for breast cancer, the husbands take on many of the household chores previously done by the women [31]. Participation in household chores was found to be substantially higher for the husbands of the breast cancer survivors than for the husbands of the healthy matched controls, even years following termination of the oncological treatments [31]. Whether the experience of coping with cancer initiates a more profound and lasting change in patterns of spousal relationships is a question that should be further studied. Still, these findings are of special importance, as they contrast sharply with previous findings that a major source of fear of cancer in healthy Arab women is their belief that husbands abandon wives diagnosed with cancer, and these women lose their social status as wives and mothers once they are diagnosed with breast cancer [11, 19].

The breast cancer survivors in this study [31] also reported that their husbands were the main source of support for them. This perception accords with other studies of the Arab population in Israel [9] and is seen as a manifestation of the modernization process, in which the traditional systems of the extended family fail to provide the needed support [9].

Empirical knowledge about the family context of coping with cancer in orthodox Jewish families is almost nonexistent. The family structure is based mostly on the nuclear family, but in decisions about health care orthodox Jews usually rely on the advice of their rabbi. They usually approach him before any oncological or other treatment is taken [38, 49]. In focus groups, orthodox women reported that even in a decision to undergo screening for breast cancer, women seek their rabbi's approval [38].

In both the Arab and ultra-orthodox Jewish societies, a powerful stigma is attached to cancer. Attitudes to cancer that prevailed in the West 40 or 50 years ago [41] still predominate in these traditional groups [11, 38, 39]. People avoid uttering the word "cancer," saying "the disease" instead. Discussing cancer arouses strong fears and the resolve to avoid talking about it. Family members of ultra-orthodox Jewish and Arab cancer patients request that the patient not be told his or her diagnosis, as he or she will not be able to handle it. Also, due to the strong stigma regarding cancer and the shame patients and the family experience, they try to keep the diagnosis within the family circle.

Coping with Cancer

Several studies were conducted in Israel to assess coping strategies used by cancer patients, mostly those from the general Jewish population (e.g. [23, 27]). Diverse strategies emerged, including problem-focused, emotion-focused, seeking social support, and denial. A few studies assessed coping strategies used in specific groups in the Jewish population—recently, for example, elderly Holocaust survivors hospitalized due to acute conditions such as orthopedic trauma, urology-related problems, or internal and heart problems [44]. The Holocaust survivors' appraisal of hospitalization as a threat was much higher, and appraisal of hospitalization as a challenge was much lower, than those of matched controls. The Holocaust survivors reported higher use of emotion-focused and lower use of problem-focused coping strategies than the controls. In another study, breast cancer patients who were Holocaust survivors were found to use less partial denial (measured by the Impact of Events Scale) as a coping strategy than matched controls [15]. They reported higher distress, but a similar functional adjustment level. Cancer patients who were the second generation of Holocaust survivors reported using coping strategies similar to those of matched controls, but nevertheless were more distressed [16].

Coping patterns with stressful encounters may be related to cultural context, while they are also related to situational characteristics [1]. New immigrant cancer patients experience the enormous stressors of being newcomers [51] and the multiple stressors of coping with cancer. Immigration often imposes many stressors on the individual, such as the experience of being uprooted from entire systems of meaning, communication difficulties, changes in the family system, economic stress, diminished professional status, intolerance by the host society, social isolation, anxiety, and uncertainty regarding the future [60]. Most immigrants undergo a temporary process of marginalization in the host society, and many have little chance of regaining their former status [53].

Two studies assessed coping with cancer in recent immigrants to Israel from the former Soviet Union. Surprisingly, the immigrants evinced higher psychological adaptation to illness than veteran Israeli women [22]. Further, a qualitative study with a small sample of eight women with ovarian cancer reported a high fighting spirit in the immigrant women [48]. They perceived the immigration to Israel as an opportunity for better care, although they experienced the cumulative effect of the disease and their immigrant status.

A few studies examined coping with breast cancer by Arab women in Israel. In a recent qualitative study, 20 Arab women aged between 30 and 75 years were interviewed [39]. They were 1–6 years post-chemotherapy and/or radiation treatment due to breast cancer stage I–III, and currently free of disease. Among the various coping strategies, most women emphasized religious coping. They prayed a great deal and read verses from the Quran or the Bible as means of healing. Many reported that their faith in God was strengthened on account of their disease. They also reported their belief that God would guard them against a recurrence. Several women reported that the prayer sessions brought with them valuable feelings of peacefulness and relaxation.

While today it is widely acceptable that expressing and sharing emotions of fear, anxiety, and distress has some value in the coping process [58], these Arab cancer patients invested much effort and energy in "being strong" for their families, especially their children. They perceived expressions of fear, pain, and distress as signifying weakness and suppressed them; moreover, they strove to function and perform many of their tasks as mothers, to show the children "business as usual." Only when alone did they allow themselves to be sad or to cry. The women were encouraged not to betray emotion by their spouses and extended family members. This coping style can be understood in light of the cultural characteristic of Arab society as a collectivist one [9], prioritizing the needs of the family and the social group over personal needs. Dwairy [34] states that Arab people experience more other-focused emotions (e.g., sympathy and shame) than self-focused emotions. Moreover, the expression of negative feelings such as depression or anxiety is not well accepted in the Arab culture, hence emotions are kept deep within the self [2]. So beyond suppression of negative emotions, Arab cancer patients deny their existence or tend to experience them as somatic symptoms [34]. A recent study found that Arab cancer patients reported substantially lower levels of distress, as measured on the distress thermometer, than Jewish cancer patients [32].

Another aspect of coping found unique to the Arab women was the struggle to hide the disease from neighbors, friends, and the various social circles. Breast cancer patients who participated in the above qualitative study [39] reported that in Arab society cancer was still viewed as a death sentence. People react to cancer patients with pity and sometimes by keeping their distance. The women made a great effort to hide the disease from everyone except their family. Several women described the unease of cancer patients entering the oncology unit for fear of being seen by an acquaintance. They were impressed by the way Jewish women felt perfectly comfortable being seen by others in the clinic, socializing with other patients and joining in supportive conversations; at times they envied the Jewish women. By contrast, they described themselves and the other Arab patients as feeling ashamed to come to the clinic and making an effort not to be seen by each other.

Several participants created close relationships with Jewish cancer patients, finding them supportive and comforting, a connection that was not to be found with Arab cancer patients.

Psychosocial Care in a Multicultural Perspective

The expanding area of psycho-oncology has accumulated a wealth of knowledge on psychological reactions to cancer, adaptation processes, psychological distress, and psychosocial interventions [37]. This invaluable knowledge has been acquired mostly through research and clinical experience with Western cancer patients. True, cultural awareness of and sensitivity to cancer are called for [48, 59], but psycho-social and psycho-therapeutic evaluation and intervention methods have developed on the notion of their universality and general applicability to cancer patients. However, empirical and clinical evidence increasingly shows these interventions developed with Western patients are not entirely applicable to people of non-Western societies [33, 34].

Psycho-social evaluation should pay special attention to cultural background. Cohen et al. [32] showed that the distress thermometer is less accurate in identifying distressed Arab cancer patients than Jewish. Dwairy [34] states, "Many normative behaviors in collective cultures could fit within definitions of some psychopathology according to *DSM-IV.*" For example, many people in collective cultures could fit the diagnosis of "dependent personality disorder." Another example concerns symptoms of depression or anxiety. In Western culture, which separates mind and body, distress is typically expressed in psychological complaints. Arab patients, as well as ultra-orthodox Jewish patients, tend to avoid expressing emotions, albeit for different reasons. The Arab collectivistic society has little room for individualism or individual emotions [34], while ultra-orthodox Jews stress the obligation for positive thinking and feelings [38]. Presumably, not only are emotions not expressed, their experience is also suppressed; hence, the clinical picture of psychological symptoms such as distress, depression, or anxiety may be different across cultures [36]. A tendency to experience and express depression and anxiety by somatic complaints has been noted [30]. These complaints are often wrongly diagnosed as somatization by Western-oriented professionals [34].

Accordingly, probing in the diagnostic interview for feelings, thoughts, or psychological symptoms of anxiety or depression probably will not be fruitful and may lead to incorrect evaluation of patients' emotional state [30]. Non-conventional evaluation techniques are needed to understand patients from traditional collective societies. Also, the evaluation should focus on understanding the individual within his/her family and culture [34].

Psycho-social interventions in oncology generally work with individuals' emotions and thoughts. They often focus on expression of emotions, dealing with intra- and interpersonal conflicts, and aim at self-actualization and personal growth [37, 50]. Negative emotions are not acceptable in collective societies, so any form of therapy that encourages the expression of feelings, clarifying personal needs or conflicts, or focusing on self-actualization arouses fear of social disapproval, which is unbearable for a person in a collective society. The need for developing culturally adapted interventions has often been noted [30, 34, 36]. Dwairy [34] suggests that interventions should be concrete, direct, short-term, and problem-focused.

Arab patients may be reluctant to ask for psychological help and may refuse to accept it when it is offered. This should be understood as the norm in Arab culture: problems are to be solved and help offered and received from within the extended family, not from outside [20]. In contrast to traditional psychotherapy, the concept of self-help groups was suggested as a possible efficient mode of helping and supporting Arab patients [8]. Azaiza [8] argues that this accords well with the idea of community support that is familiar to Arab society. He suggests that self-help groups can blend the traditional concepts of support with professional help.

Ultra-orthodox Jewish patients, too, are often reluctant to receive professional help. They resist Western psychology and are suspicious of psychosocial professionals [26, 47]. They may feel ashamed to need professional help from a psychologist or social worker [47], as this may be perceived as failure to cope with the disease according to religious requirements. These patients often seek their rabbi's approval to engage in psychological or supportive therapy [26, 47]. To establish rapport and trust, respect for the strict modesty laws is of primary importance. For example, the helping professional should be of the same sex as the patient; otherwise, the door of the consulting room must be left open during the session. The proper physical distance must be maintained, and hands may not be extended. The presence of a chaperone at sessions has to be accepted [47]. Therapists should acquire a basic knowledge of Jewish laws, as well as the religious background of the specific religious group to which the patient belongs [26, 47] because of the substantial differences in strictness of observances among different ultraorthodox groups. It is essential, but not sufficient, that the therapist be knowledgeable of, sensitive to, and respectful of the patient's religious beliefs; he/she should direct the therapy in directions that suit the religious way of thinking and in which the patient will feel at ease. The therapist should find religiously approved channels for giving professional help [26].

Cultural Competence: Using Culture to Mobilize Change

The importance of cultural sensitivity, cultural awareness, and cultural competence in treating individuals with cancer or other diseases has often been stressed [41, 43, 45, 56]. That professionals must know and be aware of clients' varied perceptions, values, and norms and must accept and respect cultural diversity are widely discussed in the literature. But the focus is mostly on responding to cultural diversity in such a manner as to prevent its being an obstacle in medical or psychosocial treatment. Here, I propose that the concept of cultural competence should be developed a step farther—to a more active approach: to actively use cultural knowledge as a means to promote coping, well-being, and health in patients of ethnic/religious groups. This can be accomplished by embracing cultural aspects within the patient–physician communication or in psychosocial interventions. A start toward achieving this aim could be identifying components in the different cultures that might enhance motivation for treatment, reduce anxiety and depression, and magnify positive emotions, hope, and belief in one's strengths.

Cohen and Azaiza [29] describe an intervention with Arab women to promote attendance of screening for breast cancer. The intervention was directed to reducing barriers, using cultural aspects or religious writings that may promote screening, such as the commandments in each of the three main religions concerning personal responsibility for one's health. This small study bore fruit.

The studies outlined throughout this chapter show the tendency of the religious person (Jew, Muslim, or Christian) to perceive cancer as ordained by God [11, 17–19]. However, opinions and beliefs varied in regarding cancer as God's punishment or a trial [11, 38]. Perceiving one's cancer as divine punishment may reinforce feelings of shame, guilt, and helplessness and exacerbate the sense of lack of control over the disease's course and outcome. But the view of cancer as a trial by God may promote feelings of hope, strength, and control, which are so important for patients' well-being. If they can be encouraged to adopt this view of cancer as a trial, which is a belief in each of the religions, they may be able to replace the notion of punishment by the notion of a trial.

Second, healthcare professionals often emphasize the value of patients' taking an active approach to the treatment process. Studies stress the importance of their being involved in decision making, being knowledgeable of the medical treatment they receive, taking active steps to preserve their health during chemotherapy and afterwards, and so on [4, 59]. However, ethnic patients, especially those belonging to collectivist societies, take on a passive position due to their socialization in respecting authority figures or professionals' expertise [35]. To promote self-responsibility and an active approach to the treatment process, ethnic and religious patients can be reminded of scripture's view that the body is given to persons as a gift or a deposit, and each individual has a duty of care and nurturance for his or her body and of active promotion of its health. The writings thereby encourage believers to take an active role in maintaining their health.

A third example concerns ways to deal with feelings of fear, hopelessness, anxiety, and depression. The Western approach encourages patients to express and share their emotions with important others and mental health professionals, or in support groups [58]. As expressing negative emotions is unacceptable to varying degrees among Arab people or ultra-orthodox Jews, alternative ways of coping should be suggested to and encouraged in these patients. Examples are the use of metaphoric language to avoid confrontation with negative feelings and promotion of coping through prayer, meditation, or reading verses from the holy books.

Social support is widely acknowledged as one of the most important factors related to cancer patients' psychological well-being, severity of symptoms, and quality of life [3]. A foremost aim of psycho-social intervention should, therefore, be to foster support by social networks. However, social support is hindered in societies where the diagnosis is kept secret within the family, where cancer is related to stigma and shame, and where friends and neighbors sometimes keep their distance from the cancer patient. This situation can sometimes be ameliorated by intervening to lower barriers and fears about cancer in patients' social networks.

The role of the extended family should be examined for each patient individually. When applicable, and according to the patient's wish, it may be preferable for the diagnosis, information, decisions about treatment, or about stopping treatment in cases of advanced disease to be conveyed in family sessions rather than individually.

These are some examples of how culture can be used as a tool to improve patients' well-being. However, this approach still needs to be developed with research and clinical experience.

Discussion

Cultural or ethnic groups are characterized by wide diversity within each group and by an extensive spread of individuals along the conservative–modern continuum. Cultural competence, therefore, entails an individualized approach and avoidance of stereotyping, so this chapter should be read as a general conceptualization of the cultural perspective in oncology. Each patient's perceptions and attitudes should be carefully examined. Traditional cultural values and views are often sustained to varying degrees along with modernization. One should be aware of the different patterns of integration that may emerge [5].

Cultural competence in oncology is a construct that entails orientation, values, attitudes, knowledge, and skills [56]; yet it should be understood as a dynamic process of professional development through continuous learning and increasing awareness. Health care professionals should make an effort not only toward increasing cultural competence as individuals and teams, but also on the services and health policy levels.

An essential step toward enhancing cultural competence is enlargement of the scope of research in this area [6]. Efforts to broaden knowledge are to be directed toward better understanding the cultural aspects of cancer and cancer care and the psycho-social aspects of coping with cancer in specific cultural groups. More research is needed into processes of modernization and the way they integrate with traditional systems. Longitudinal design and interventional studies can establish more profound psycho-social interventions. However, most research tools have been designed and validated for Western populations. It is not enough to translate measures into a specific language. Serious concerns have been raised regarding the validity of diagnostic instruments translated from English into other languages. Linguistic equivalence attained by the established methods of expert translation and back-translation may be insufficient. Cultural equivalence—"the way members of different cultural and linguistic groups view or interpret the underlying meaning of an item" ([52], p. 1258)—has to be ensured. Additional obstacles to multicultural research are the existence of confounders, which are hard to control. For example, it is difficult to distinguish cultural aspects from the effect of socioeconomic status (SES), as large proportions of certain ethnic groups may be of low SES. Ashing-Giwa and Kagawa-Singer [6] use the term "culturally competent research" as including "culturally appropriate research designs and methods and culturally suitable study instruments that have been appropriately translated into and validated in other languages."

In closing the chapter, several limitations of this review should be underscored. Research on cultural aspects of cancer in Israel's multicultural society is sparse, while cultural diversity in Israel is enormous, even within individual ethnic groups. Accordingly, this review is partial and possibly only superficially relates to some of the cultural issues raised. Many related topics have not been addressed, such as ethical aspects and end-of-life decisions, as they are beyond the scope of this chapter; yet they are of major importance. The main conclusion is that more specific knowledge is urgently needed. It is hoped that attention will be drawn to the importance of extending knowledge of the many aspects and facets of the multicultural aspects of cancer care.

References

1. Aarons GA, Sawitzky AC. Organizational climate partially mediates the effect of culture on work attitudes and staff turnover in mental health services. Adm Policy Ment Health. 2006;33(3):289–301.
2. Al-Krenawi A, Graham JR. Culturally sensitive social work practice with Arab clients in mental health settings. Health Soc Work. 2000;25(1):9–22.
3. Albrecht TL, Goldsmith DJ. Social support, social networks, and health. In: Thompson TL, Dorsey AM, Miller KI, Parrott R, editors. Handbook of health communication. Mahwah, NJ: Lawrence Erlbaum Associates; 2003. p. 263–84.
4. Andersen MR, Bowen DJ, Morea J, Stein KD, Baker F. Involvement in decision-making and breast cancer survivor quality of life. Health Psychol. 2009;28(1):29–37.
5. Angel RJ, Williams K. Cultural models of health and illness. In: Cuellar I, Paniagua FA, editors. Handbook of multicultural mental health. San Diego, CA: Academic; 2000. p. 27–44.
6. Ashing-Giwa K, Kagawa-Singer M. Infusing culture into oncology research on quality of life. Oncol Nurs Forum. 2006;33:31–6.
7. Azaiza F. Patterns of labor division among Palestinian families in the West Bank. Global Dev Stud. 2004;3:201–20.
8. Azaiza F. Meanings of the concept "Self-Help" among Jewish and Arab students living in Israel. J Hum Behav Soc Environ. 2005;11(1):23–35.
9. Azaiza F. The perception and utilization of social support in times of cultural change: the case of Arabs in Israel. Int J Soc Welfare. 2008;17(3):198–203.
10. Azaiza F, Cohen M. Health beliefs and rates of breast cancer screening among Arab women. J Womens Health. 2006;15(5):520–30.
11. Azaiza F, Cohen M. Between traditional and modern perceptions of breast and cervical cancer screenings: a qualitative study of Arab women in Israel. Psychooncology. 2008;17:34–41.
12. Azaiza F, Cohen M. Colorectal cancer screening patterns, intentions, and predictors in Jewish and Arab Israelis. Health Educ Behav. 2008;35(4):198–203.
13. Azaiza F, Abu-Baker K, Hertz-Lazarowitz R, Ghanem A. Arab women in Israel: current status and future trends. Tel Aviv: Ramot Publishing; 2009.

14. Azaiza F, Cohen M, Awad M, Daoud F. Factors associated with low-screening for breast cancer in the Palestinian Authority. Cancer. 2010;116(19):4646–55.
15. Baider L, Peretz T, Kaplan De-Nour A. Effect of the Holocaust on coping with cancer. Soc Sci Med. 1992;34(1):11–5.
16. Baider L, Peretz T, Hadani PE, Perry S, Avramov R, De-Nour AK. Transmission of response to trauma? Second-generation Holocaust survivors' reaction to cancer. Am J Psychiatry. 2000;157(6):904–10.
17. Baron-Epel O. Attitudes and beliefs associated with mammography in a multiethnic population in Israel. Health Educ Behav. 2010;37:227–42.
18. Baron-Epel O, Klin A. Cancer as perceived by a middle-aged Jewish urban population in Israel. Oncol Nurs Forum. 2009;36(6):E326–34.
19. Baron-Epel O, Granot M, Badarna S, Avrami S. Perceptions of breast cancer among Arab Israeli women. Women Health. 2004;40(2):101–16.
20. Ben Ari A, Azaiza F. Associated meanings of the concept 'self-help': a comparison between Jewish and Arab populations living in Israel. Soc Dev Issues. 1995;17(2/3):127–40.
21. Ben-David Y. The Bedouin in Israel. Resource document. Israel Ministry of Foreign Affairs. 2011. http://www.jewishvirtuallibrary.org/jsource/Society_&_Culture/Bedouin.html. Accessed 2 March 2011.
22. Ben-David A, Gilbar O. Family, migration, and psychosocial adjustment to illness. Soc Work Health Care. 1997;26(2):53–67.
23. Ben-Zur H. Your coping strategy and my distress: inter-spouse perceptions of coping and adjustment among breast cancer patients and their spouses. Fam Syst Health. 2001;19(1): 83–94.
24. Betancourt JR, Green AR, Carrillo JE, Ananeh-Firempong OII. Defining cultural competence: a practical framework for addressing racial/ethnic disparities in health and health care. Public Health Rep. 2003;118:293–312.
25. Bhui K, Warfal N, Edonyal P, McKenzie K, Bhugra D. Cultural competence in mental health care: a review of model evaluations. BMC Health Serv Res. 2007;7:15.
26. Bilu Y, Witztum E. Working with Jewish Ultra-Orthodox patients: guidelines for a culturally sensitive therapy. Cult Med Psychiatry. 1993;17:197–233.
27. Cohen M. Coping and emotional distress in primary and recurrent breast cancer patients. J Clin Psychol Med Settings. 2002;9(3):245–51.
28. Cohen M, Azaiza F. Early breast cancer detection practices, health beliefs and cancer worries in Jewish and Arab women. Prev Med. 2005;41:852–8.
29. Cohen M, Azaiza F. Increasing breast examinations among Arab women using a tailored culture-based intervention. Behav Med. 2010;36:92–9.
30. Cohen M, Arad S, Lorber M, Pollack S. Psychological distress, life stressors, and social support in new immigrants with HIV. Behav Med. 2007;33(2):45–54.
31. Cohen M, Abdallah Mabjish A, Zidan J. Comparison of Arab breast cancer survivors and healthy controls for spousal relationship, body image, and emotional distress. Qual Life Res. 2011;20(2):191–8.
32. Cohen M, Gagin R, Cinamon T, Stein T, Moscovitz M (2011). Adapting of the distress thermometer to screening for emotional distress in multicultural groups of cancer patients in Israel. Qual Life Res. [Epub ahead of print].
33. Comas-Díaz L. Multicultural approaches to psychotherapy. In: Norcross JC, VandenBos GR, Freedheim DK, editors. History of psychotherapy: continuity and change. 2nd ed. Washington, DC: American Psychological Association; 2011. p. 243–67.
34. Dwairy M. Foundations of psychosocial dynamic personality theory of collective people. Clin Psychol Rev. 2002;22:343–60.
35. Dwairy M, Achoui M, Abouserie R, Farah A. Adolescent-family connectedness among Arabs: a second cross-regional research study. J Cross Cult Psychol. 2006;37:248–61.
36. Eshun S, Caldwell-Colbert T. Culture and mood disorders. In: Eshun S, Regan AR, Gurung BA, editors. Culture and mental health: sociocultural influences, theory, and practice. Hoboken: Wiley-Blackwell; 2009. p. 181–95. doi:10.1002/9781444305807.ch9.

37. Fawzy FI, Fawzy NW, Arndt LA, Pasnau RO. Critical review of psychosocial interventions in cancer care. Arch Gen Psychiatry. 1995;52(2):100–13.
38. Freund A, Cohen M, Azaiza, F (in preparation). Perceptions of barriers to screening of ultra-orthodox Jewish women in Israel.
39. Goldblat H, Cohen M, Azaiza F, Rimon M (in press). Perceptions, emotional reactions and ways of coping of Arab and Jewish women with breast cancer. Psychooncology.
40. Greenberg D, Kalian M, Witzum E. Value-sensitive psychiatric rehabilitation. Transcult Psychiatry. 2010;47(4):629–46.
41. Holland JC, Lewis S. The human side of cancer. New York: Harper Collins; 2000.
42. Israel National Cancer Registry. Cancer incidence tables. All sites combined. Resource document. 2010. http://www.health.gov.il/pages/default.asp?maincat=22&catId=183&PageId=3088. Accessed 2 March 2011.
43. Kagawa-Singer M, Blackhall LJ. Negotiating cross-cultural issues at the end of life. J Am Med Assoc. 2001;286:2993–3001.
44. Kimron L, Cohen M (under review). Coping and emotional distress during acute hospitalization of older persons experiencing earlier trauma: the case of elderly Holocaust survivors. Qual Life Res.
45. Kreitler S. The effects of cultural diversity on providing health services. EDTNA ERCA J. 2005;31:93–8.
46. Lavee Y, Katz R. The family in Israel: between tradition and modernity. Marriage Fam Rev. 2003;35(1–2):193–217.
47. Margolese HC. Engaging in psychotherapy with the Orthodox Jew: a critical review. Am J Psychother. 1998;5(1):37–53.
48. Mizrahi I, Kaplan G, Milshtein E, Reshef BP, Baruch GB. Coping simultaneously with 2 stressors: immigrants with ovarian cancer. Cancer Nurs. 2008;31(2):126–33.
49. Mor P, Oberle K. Ethical issues related to BRCA gene testing in Orthodox Jewish women. Nurs Ethics. 2008;15(4):512–21.
50. Newell SA, Sanson-Fisher RW, Savolainen NJ. Systematic review of psychological therapies for cancer patients: overview and recommendations for future research. J Natl Cancer Inst. 2002;94:558–84.
51. Patterson M, Malley-Morrison K. Cognitive-ecological approach to elder abuse in five cultures: human rights and education. Educ Gerontol. 2006;32:73–82.
52. Peña ED. Lost in translation: methodological considerations in cross-cultural research. Child Dev. 2007;78:1255–64.
53. Remennick LI. "Women with a Russian accent" in Israel: on the gender aspects of immigration. Eur J Womens Stud. 1999;6(4):441–61.
54. Shaya F, Gbarayor CM. The case for cultural competence in health professions education. Am J Pharm Educ. 2006;70(6):124.
55. Stirrat GM, Gill R. Autonomy in medical ethics after O'Neill. J Med Ethics. 2005;31:127–30.
56. Surbone A. Cultural aspects of communication in cancer care. Support Care Cancer. 2008;16:235–40.
57. The Israel Central Bureau of Statistics. Israel in figures. Resource document. 2010. http://www1.cbs.gov.il/publications/isr_in_n10e.pdf. Accessed 2 March 2011.
58. Walker LM, Bischoff TF, Robinson JW. Supportive expressive group therapy for women with advanced ovarian cancer. Int J Group Psychother. 2010;60(3):407–27.
59. Weingart SN, Zhu J, Chiappetta L, Stuver SO, Schneider EC, Epstein AM, et al. Hospitalized patients' participation and its impact on quality of care and patient safety. Int J Qual Health Care. 2011;23(3):269–77.
60. Yakhnich L. Immigration as a multiple-stressor situation: stress and coping among immigrants from the Soviet Union in Israel. Int J Stress Manage. 2008;15:252–68.

Chapter 28
Cancer Diagnosis Disclosure: The French Experience

Sylvie Dolbeault and Anne Brédart

Abstract The way patients are informed of an initial diagnosis of cancer in France has improved thanks to the introduction of a procedure referred to as the "Diagnostic Disclosure Procedure," which is part of the first national *Plan Cancer*. This procedure requires the disclosure of a cancer diagnosis to be conducted in accordance with evidence-based recommendations of good communication practices (longer period spent with the oncologist, presence of a specialized nurse, consideration of psychosocial needs, traceability of information exchanged between the parties to ensure improved care coordination). Although three surveys conducted to assess satisfaction with the diagnostic procedure have revealed high levels of satisfaction, they indicate that there are still areas for improvement. These relate primarily to the fact that medical aspects are still presented in a way that is too technical and that there are no information documents relating to the disclosed diagnosis. These observations emphasize the need to pursue and further develop the initiatives present in France, although as yet on an insufficiently widespread basis, designed to assist communication through the use of psychosocial assessment tools within the context of clinical practice. They also indicate that it is necessary to promote training in doctor–patient communication and provide systematic access to high-quality information. Furthermore, the existence of patients at risk due to their age, socioeconomic status, or the presence of physical or psychosocial comorbidities is as yet

---

S. Dolbeault (✉)
Supportive Care Department, Institut Curie, 26 rue d'Ulm, 75006 Paris, France

Inserm, U 669, Paris, France

Univ Paris-Sud and Univ Paris Descartes, UMR-S0669, Paris, France
e-mail: sylvie.dolbeault@curie.net

A. Brédart
Supportive Care Department, Institut Curie, 26 rue d'Ulm, 75005 Paris, France

Supportive Care Department, Institut Curie, 26 rue d'Ulm, 75006 Paris, France
e-mail: Anne.bredart@curie.net

inadequately acknowledged in France. These groups deserve special attention due to the fact that they frequently have greater needs when diagnosed and treated for cancer.

Keywords French disclosure process • Breaking bad news • Cancer • Communication • Doctor–patient interaction • Distress

Introduction

The care offered to patients with cancer and their families has improved greatly over the last 20 years, both in terms of medical and scientific development as well as advances in the provision of global care that focuses on the patient and his or her family members [1–3]. In the light of inadequacies observed in the organization of cancer-related health care in France, complaints made by cancer patients, and the developments observed in other cultures, our country has developed its own healthcare system in order to improve the quality of cancer care provided and enhance cancer patient satisfaction. Special attention has been paid to the processes used to provide information to patients and their loved ones concerning the disease, its treatment and potential side-effects or sequelae, and the prognosis.

The aim of the present chapter is to describe the changes that have taken place in this oncological field in France. After presenting the reasons underlying the changes observed in our country over the last 10 years and describing the new regulations associated with the design of our two national *Plans Cancer* (hereinafter referred to as Cancer Plans), we shall examine the model represented by the "Diagnostic Disclosure Procedure." We shall attempt to point out both the benefits and limitations of this mode of organization, based primarily on the various surveys that have examined patient satisfaction. We shall then point out areas for improvement, illustrated by clinical examples taken from field observations.

Historical Development of the Field in France

In recent years, oncology in France has benefited from the fruits of a genuine effort at the structural level to develop resources for basic and translational research, optimize clinical practices, and organize the health-care trajectories of cancer patients. The founding of the Institut National du Cancer (INCA) (http://www.e-cancer.fr/) and regional organizations known as "cancéropôles" (http://www.e-cancer.fr/recherche/structuration-de-la-recherche/les-canceropoles) has made a great contribution to this endeavor [4].

The general public and, in particular, popular organizations including patients' or expatients' associations such as the *Ligue Nationale Contre le Cancer* (http://www.ligue-cancer.net/), currently France's most highly organized nonprofit association, have also helped to give these developments real impetus. This latter association was responsible for the organization at the national level of the first "Etats Généraux du cancer" (national cancer forum) in 1998. These were the first attempts to form an effective partnership between the country's governmental bodies and representatives of the population at large. Two subsequent national events organized in 2001 and 2003 continued the task of identifying the difficulties encountered by cancer patients and articulating the needs they feel at the various stages of the cancer-care trajectory.

It was as a result of these efforts that France's first Cancer Plan was developed in 2003. This national 5-year plan (2003–2007) (http://www.ladocumentationfrancaise.fr/rapports-publics/094000084/index.shtml) (*Plan Cancer* 2003–2007) reports on the current state of affairs and sets out a series of recommendations relating to cancer care. Given the success of the first Cancer Plan and the results that have already been achieved, France has gone on to develop a second Cancer Plan (2009–2013) (http://lesrapports.ladocumentationfrancaise.fr/BRP/104000350/0000.pdf) [5] with the aim of building on the efforts that have already been made and setting new goals.

One of the many aims of the Cancer Plan is to improve the conditions under which the diagnostic disclosure is made and patients enter into the care process through the development of a "Diagnostic Disclosure Procedure" (item 40 of the Cancer Plan). This defines the roles of each professional and the way they coordinate in caring for the patient, improves the way information is communicated, and provides for the early evaluation of the difficulties exhibited by patients, thus theoretically making it possible to direct patients toward the available supportive care services [6–8]. In many countries, these supportive care services are integrated into the oncology department (http://www.mascc.org) and underpinned by the concepts of multidisciplinary work, coordination, and cooperation between professionals [7, 9] in a way that is reminiscent of the consultation-liaison psychiatry model [10]. However, as yet this organizational model has made little headway in the French professional care context [11].

Along with improvements to the structures underpinning communication and the provision of information, the medical model also seems to be changing in the light of theoretical considerations and clinical experiments conducted in Anglo-Saxon countries [12]. While the idea of sharing decision-making responsibilities in the medical field is far from new, it can be argued that it has only gradually been introduced into French medical practice. Some health-care situations are more suitable than others for the integration of this type of model and can act as pilot projects, making it possible to experiment with new communication methods. As far as oncology is concerned, the most suitable areas lie in the field of predictive medicine (oncogenetics), therapeutic trials, or adjuvant treatments, where several different therapeutic options are conceivable because they offer equivalent levels of efficacy, but may be associated with different toxicity profiles and repercussions.

A number of studies have already shown that the patient's level of satisfaction with the consultation, the information concerning treatment, and the support provided is greater when he or she is involved in the therapeutic decision. At the time when the cancer diagnosis is disclosed, a certain number of attitudes on the part of the clinician are thought to be of help: in particular, the use of the correct tone of voice, the attention paid to the patient's own needs and preferences, an appropriate choice of words, and a supportive attitude that helps the patient maintain hope [13, 14].

The health-care professionals who have been questioned on the subject seem to favor a shift away from the paternalistic care model—in which the clinician alone is responsible for making care-related decisions—toward shared medical decision-making—in which patients are asked about the information they need or wish to receive or their desire to participate in the medical decisions that need to be made. Despite this, these health-care professionals are also aware of the difficulties that this care mode brings with it in terms of communication with the patient. In effect, the sharing of medical decisions does not involve only cognitive operations (for example, providing information about the available choices), but also emotional challenges (for example, being able to perceive indicators that reveal patients' needs); and these two dimensions may affect the way the patient experiences medical decisions [15]. The current literature reveals that in the field of oncology there is frequently a discrepancy between the patient's expectations and the role adopted by health-care professionals with regard to decision-making [16].

A recent survey conducted in France among women who had undergone breast cancer operations reveals the importance of their need for information [17]. This need seems to be met, in particular, with information about the diagnosis and the secondary effects of treatment; but to a lesser extent with information about the consequences of the therapy on the patient's daily life. Within the context of breast cancer care, there are many situations in which treatments have a similar effect in terms of survival but a very different effect at the level of daily life, with the result that patients may well want to be more involved in the decision-making process.

The Diagnostic Disclosure Procedure Developed as Part of the First Cancer Plan

As pointed out in the introduction, the time at which the diagnosis is disclosed is a very important symbolic step for the patient and in itself represents a therapeutic act of significance that frequently goes far beyond what health-care professionals may believe. While many approaches designed to improve this disclosure have been tested in the different locations in which health care is provided, in different medical contexts, and in very different cultures, clinicians and researchers tend to agree that success in this operation is a subtle and complex affair [18–20]. The drafting of the first National Cancer Plan by INCA was largely inspired by recommendations of good practices [21] already developed in a number of other countries, such as the United States (NCCN) (www.nccn.org), Canada (CAPO) (http ://www.capo.ca), Australia (Australian National Breast Cancer Centre and National Cancer Control Initiative) (www.nhmrc.gov.au/publications, 2003), and the United Kingdom (NICE). Many of the recommendations relate to the concept of "breaking bad news." They set out in detail the specific characteristics of the relationship between a patient suffering from cancer and the corresponding medical specialist ("specialist-patient" communication), the nurse participating in the disclosure ("nurse-patient" communication) [22], and also the accompanying person—friend or family member of the patient—whose presence is encouraged in all cases [23].

Definition and Aims of the Organization of the Diagnostic Disclosure Consultation in France

Since 2004, a diagnostic disclosure procedure has been tested in approximately 50 "pilot" health-care establishments [24]. This takes the form of a special consultation referred to as the "consultation d'ancrage" (or "anchor consultation"). This is an extended meeting that promotes the exchange of questions and information between the clinician and the patient, as well as a period of consultation with a so-called "disclosure nurse," who goes over the supplied information with the patient once more and explores his or her need for additional information and the psychosocial difficulties that may be experienced. The nurse also provides information about sources of assistance and makes sure that the dialog conducted with the patient during this consultation is properly recorded in order to improve the coordination of the health care provided. In France, these capabilities are now an integral part of the criteria required in order to gain authorization to perform clinical oncology in health-care establishments [8].

As an example, we present here the experimental use of the diagnostic disclosure procedure during the therapeutic decision phase in the Institut Curie [25]. During the 7–10 days following the surgeon's postsurgical final diagnosis, patients are invited to attend a multidisciplinary consultation where, on the same day, they are seen by both a chemotherapist and a radiotherapist who, in turn, present the envisaged treatment and explain the expected benefits, advantages, and drawbacks and the care administration procedure. Each patient is then seen by a nurse specifically dedicated to the conduct of the corresponding consultation. During a clinical interview, the nurse goes back over the information presented by the doctors, checks that this has been understood correctly, and answers any additional questions raised by the patient. However, this interview also represents an opportunity to perform an initial assessment of the patients' needs and, if necessary, direct them to other professionals in the supportive care field working in close cooperation with, and as a complement to, the specialists in the specific treatment to be administered. It also provides an opportunity to organize coordination between the hospital and those responsible for care of the patient outside of the hospital. This procedure is conducted with the help of assessment tools and serves as the basis for the initial training and subsequent follow-up of the dedicated nursing staff.

During the following days, this stage is complemented by meetings with other doctors and nurses, who provide the patients with additional information, in particular during the initial interview at the chemotherapy clinic and then subsequently at the initial radiotherapy interview. Whenever the therapeutic decision does not reflect a decision described in our reference documents, the patient's file is presented at a multidisciplinary coordination meeting. Both doctors and carers often make use of written documents, which are given to patients following these consultations in order to help them identify and explore in more detail the most important information given to them verbally during the consultation. The patients are regularly encouraged to attend these consultations in the company of a friend or relative.

Evaluation of the Procedure: Benefits and Limitations

This method of organization has been evaluated in the various health-care establishments in which it has been employed: in a sample of public and private establishments, excluding specialist cancer centers; and in specialized cancer centers, which take the form of private establishments within the public system and which, in France, are organized as a federation of 20 regional centers covering the whole of the country.

Two consecutive surveys of satisfaction levels (conducted first in 2005–2006 and then in 2006–2007) used anonymous, self-administered questionnaires, which were given to patients who had experienced the procedure and were designed to evaluate the following points: conduct of the disclosure procedure, inadequacies, possible areas for improvement [26]. They involved 2,583 patients and 64 health-care establishments (excluding specialist cancer centers). Sixty percent of the patients said they were satisfied or very satisfied with the information provided to them, and 95% said that they had confidence in the health-care establishment responsible for their care. The mean score for overall care was 8.2 in the first survey and 8.6 in the second; the only factor identified as influencing satisfaction was the length of the consultation. The feeling that the meeting was of suitable length significantly influenced whether or not the patients considered the information provided to be appropriate in nature. The factors leading to a perceived lack of information included the absence of documents given to the patients, lack of time on the part of the doctor, and the overtechnical nature of the medical explanations provided. The level of convergence between the fields covered by the consultation was high for therapeutic explanations, but less so in the case of emotional aspects, prognosis, and the treatment of symptoms; 30% of the patients thought their expectations in these fields had been met, whereas 73% of oncologists believed that they had responded to them.

The second survey revealed an improvement in certain areas. Despite this, 8% of patients still declared themselves to be dissatisfied in this second survey, and analysis of their responses made it possible to identify certain areas for improvement: the possibility of obtaining a second medical opinion; dictation of the doctor's report in the patient's presence; the value of meeting other health-care professionals, in particular a nurse specializing in the disclosure procedure.

It should also be pointed out that in 90% of cases, the initial diagnosis of cancer is made by a doctor who is not an oncologist. This indicates the need to extend the disclosure procedure to the entire medical community, rather than restricting it to oncology specialists.

Another French survey evaluated the satisfaction of more than 1,600 patients concerning the initial disclosure of the diagnosis of a first cancer and its treatment. This took the form of a telephone survey conducted exclusively among patients treated in specialist cancer centers [27]. High levels of satisfaction with the overall care received were found in 77% of the patients (very satisfied patients) — or 97% if both satisfied and very satisfied patients are included; and the corresponding level was 63% with regard to the disclosure procedure. This level is consistent with that obtained using varying methods in a number of other studies conducted both in France (50–65%) and elsewhere [24]. A model based on a partial least squares regression analysis identified four main dimensions and their respective weights in the patients' global levels of satisfaction: the quality of the patient–doctor relationship (64%); the nature of the communicated information (14%, strongly influenced by information on the type, duration, and practical organization of the envisaged treatment); the timetable (14% greatly influenced by the time spent in the diagnostic disclosure consultation); and finally, accompanying persons (this dimension was influenced equally by information on the role of support provided by family and friends on the one hand, and by associations or similar organizations on the other). First and foremost, the feedback provided by the patients emphasizes inadequacies in certain areas such as administrative aspects and psychological information concerning the existence of patients' associations or focus groups.

One of the limitations of the study lies in the level of participation, which was 70%, due perhaps to the issues addressed by the survey — information communicated during the announcement of bad news. Nevertheless, this type of survey makes it possible to define a baseline, identify areas to be improved, and then assess changes in patient satisfaction as a function of the measures implemented with the aim of bringing about these improvements. In effect, satisfaction is one of the key elements of the quality of the administered health care, even though it is not the only relevant indicator. The literature also reveals a link between satisfaction and long-term quality of life, thus highlighting the importance that should be attributed to this criterion [28].

Structure of the Diagnostic Disclosure Procedure: What Are Its Benefits and Limitations?

The way this disclosure period is structured offers a number of advantages that have been identified both by patients and their relatives, and also by the doctors and nurses involved [25]. First of all, it offers practical benefits: patients need arrange only one visit, they receive all the information on the same day and, in principle, go away from the consultation with the corresponding therapeutic decisions having been made, with their own personalized care schedule, having already met all the doctors who will be responsible for their care. At the psychological level, it is important to emphasize the quantity of medical and organizational information that patients receive during the course of this day. However, the multidisciplinary structure of this disclosure period obliges the health-care professionals involved to cooperate in developing a common vision of the care to be provided to the patient. It makes it necessary to improve the consistency of the information communicated by the various professionals through the explicit coordination of the doctors responsible for the treatment and precise identification of their respective roles. The therapeutic decision is entered at a multidisciplinary level in the patient's medical record, thus ensuring subsequent traceability. This means that patients and their relatives can anticipate the overall care strategy as of the date of the consultation and, in principle, gives patients time to react and ask questions throughout the consultation. The time spent with the nurse following the meeting with the clinician may provide an opportunity to identify the patient's psychosocial needs and refer him or her to other professionals in the supportive care field. The activities of these professionals complement those of the referring doctors, with whom they cooperate closely in the provision of certain aspects of care. Finally, the contribution of this mode of organization to facilitating patient inclusion in therapeutic trials should not be forgotten.

It is very probable that this model brings about a global improvement in the quality of care received and the satisfaction felt by the patients who benefit from it. However, we must also examine its limitations. We shall emphasize three of these here [19]. The model is, in effect, highly focused on the information given to patients and their relatives.

First of all, it should be remembered that informing is not synonymous with communicating, and this is precisely the point of this therapeutic decision consultation: to convey to patients the information they require in order to achieve a correct understanding of their state of health and their health-care needs. While doing this, it is also necessary to continuously monitor the patients' ability to digest and assimilate this "raw" information and make sure there is no other kind of obstacle that might prevent them from accepting the therapeutic proposals and impair their cooperation in the health-care project. However, the risk of things going wrong is well known, and such difficulties may be due to either of the partners: in the patient's case, there is a risk of being submerged in an excess of information or of discordance between the doctor's and the patient's respective agendas, with the result that considerable misunderstandings may arise. For the doctor, there is the risk of "taking refuge" in a process that consists exclusively of transmitting information, when the need to deal with patients as complete human beings, capable of expressing their distress, their uncertainty, feelings of vulnerability, or the disintegration of their "life project" represents too great an interpersonal danger for the clinician.

Another point that deserves to be emphasized is that this method of organization is still very traditional and leaves health-care professionals with the entire responsibility for making therapeutic decisions before actually meeting the patient. We are, therefore, still at a very far remove from the emerging models of shared—or informed—decision-making, in which patients are given considerable freedom to express their own values and preferences in cases where different types of treatment are conceivable.

Finally, it is necessary to point out that during the conduct of this therapeutic decision consultation, there remains a clear division between the objective physical aspects addressed by the doctors and the psychological and social aspects that are left to the appraisal of the nurse as the person who has been trained, to a greater or lesser degree, to evaluate this type of need. However, in principle, the patient's hierarchy of needs does not conform to our traditional medical classification, which always gives the highest priority to physical symptoms at the risk of underestimating or even completely masking other types of difficulty (psychological, social, material, spiritual). Nevertheless, it is well known that an acute psychological state (anxious or depressive adjustment disorders, derealization, and even depersonalization) of the type that is frequently encountered at the time of disclosure may totally block out the benefits of the consultation, and it is essential to take this fact into account in order to achieve the desired aims.

Offering a Systematic Approach to the Identification of Distress and Supportive Care Needs within the Framework of the Diagnostic Disclosure Procedure

Although there can be no doubt that the structured clinical interview helps to identify the patient's psychosocial and information-related needs, further help can be provided through the use of simple screening tools to assist health-care professionals who are not specialists in this field [21, 29–31]. This screening approach consists in identifying not only those patients who need to be referred to another specialist (e.g., a psycho-oncologist), but also those whose most pressing stated needs point to a difficulty in communicating with the oncology staff.

By using these tools for the self-evaluation of the patient's needs when preparing for the medical consultation, it is possible to base the approach on the needs as identified from the patient's own perspective rather than that of the health-care professional. This difference in the way needs are perceived is of vital importance. However, this approach is of value only if a certain number of conditions are satisfied: it has to be used and its results have to be drawn on as the consultation progresses; it should not be thought of as a replacement for dialog; it is necessary to agree to share tasks with the other professionals who will be approached for assistance following this evaluation [32].

The validated tools that are currently in use consist primarily of quality-of-life questionnaires as well as more recently developed questionnaires designed to evaluate the respondent's needs or, more specifically with regard to psychological issues, to determine the appropriate screening tools to identify psychological distress. In clinical practice, quality-of-life evaluations are used primarily to promote better communication and the sharing of medical decisions between the patient and clinician; to evaluate the patient's overall state of health before starting therapy and treat the corresponding problems if necessary; to identify the sources and scale of any physical, emotional, or social dysfunctioning; and to detect the secondary effects of treatment [33, 34]. This type of initiative is being implemented increasingly frequently in North America and Europe, and systems for the reimbursement of medical expenses for this type of consultation involving quality-of-life tools are being examined.

As an example, we present the main results of a pilot experiment recently conducted in connection with the disclosure procedure in our institution [25]. We administered the psychological distress thermometer (PDS) and a problem checklist to 255 patients before nurse consultation, thus helping the nurse manage the clinical interview; explore each patient's distress and supportive care needs; and refer the patients in need to the relevant supportive care units. This pilot study helped us gain a better understanding of patients' most frequent needs at the time of the disclosure. Thirty-five percent of the patients in our sample were referred to the social unit, and 19.6% of patients to the psycho-oncology unit. In cases of significant distress (43% patients with PDS>3), the percentage of patients referred to the psychosocial units increased (44% referred to the social unit, 35% to the psycho-oncology unit). However, the main interest of our screening procedure resides in its qualitative and didactic dimension, based on clinical training and cooperation with health-care professionals during the process of investigating patients' distress and supportive care needs.

We concluded that this first clinical experiment conducted among dedicated nurses involved in a therapeutic decision consultation in a French cancer center provided evidence in support of the idea that nonspecialist professionals are able to identify patients' distress and their supportive care needs (particularly in the psychosocial field) provided that they have received appropriate training.

Other Areas for Improvement

A number of other areas in which improvement in doctor–patient communication and relations are possible also deserve to be mentioned.

Extension of the Disclosure Procedure Model to Other Stages of the Health-care Trajectory

In this chapter, we have described the disclosure stage as conducted at the onset of the illness. However, this model could also be used at many other stages during the patient's health-care trajectory, since the volume of disclosures that occur between the referring doctor and the patient during the period of care administration is well known. For example, the announcement of a disfiguring treatment, of irreversible sequelae, of a recurrence, or of the fact that no further etiological treatments are available, as well as the announcement of the end of the period of care all represent intense periods of this relationship. There can be no doubt that the subjective experience of these periods often has a profound impact on patient and doctor alike [18, 23] and, in each case, is associated with a specific form of distress and psychological challenge. Thus, for example, when the recurrence of an illness is announced, the communication is no longer focused on the hope of a cure but on the possibility of stabilizing the disease. The information to be conveyed in this case is particularly complex (notion of regional or metastatic invasion), and patients may appear ambivalent when faced with this new information or asked to participate in the ensuing medical decisions. The communication of bad news concerning the recurrence of illness must be an interactive process in which both doctor and patient acquire a shared understanding of the content and quantity of the information to be exchanged [35].

That is why it is important to be able to transpose the diagnostic disclosure procedure to other periods involving the communication of news that may be objectively "good" or "bad" from a strictly medical point of view, but that is always emotionally charged due to the many other dimensions involved—dimensions that it is useful to identify and take into account in order to achieve an optimally adapted patient–doctor relationship.

Improvements to the Conduct of the Doctor–Patient Relationship through Communication Training Measures

There is now a large body of literature relating to the doctor–patient relationship; the recommendations resulting from these works provide doctors with guidelines to help them break bad news. They also identify the stages that are essential for the gradual disclosure of this news in a way that is informative but adapted to the patient's knowledge and receptive capabilities and attempt to reduce the risk of psychological destabilization at a time in the subject's life that is already very charged. The most important facets have been described many times and can readily be found in this body of work. They are based on many different recommendations of good practices (e.g., National Breast Cancer Centre, National Cancer Control Initiative, 2003, http://www.nhmrc.gov.au) (National Institute for Health and Clinical Excellence, 2004, http://www.nice.org.uk).

They also form the basis for communication training programs that are conducted in medical and paramedical environments [36, 37] with the aim of optimizing the task performed by doctors in their attempt to inform their patients better, a task which may fail to bear fruit if the emotional dimension experienced by the patient and the communicative aspects that govern the interaction between health-care professionals and their patients are not taken into account. This point is crucial for the success of the therapeutic decision model as it is considered here. To consider it a marginal issue that any health-care professional's intuitive feeling for his or her relationship with the patient will be able to cope with would represent a major danger threatening to cancel out all the benefits that are hoped for at the relational level.

In France, certain institutions have developed this type of training program, ideally in the form of modules focusing on the acquisition of relational and communications skills conducted within the framework of ongoing professional training. Such programs use interactive formats based on discussions of individual cases, Balint groups, as well as recorded or filmed clinical interviews, followed by exercises in the analysis of sequences of patient–carer communication [36–38]. These training modules have gained somewhat in popularity due to the increased level of initial and further training in various higher education (university diplomas, postgraduate degrees), assimilated (*Ecole de Formation Européenne en Cancérologie*), or private establishments (EPAC program: *Ensemble parlons Autrement du Cancer* ("An Alternative Way of Talking about Cancer," financed by a pharmaceuticals company)) [37, 38].

It should be emphasized that this type of training can help reduce professional burnout [39]. However, it is necessary to realize that this type of training has met with only a low level of acceptance in many health-care establishments and that both doctors and institutions have frequently exhibited resistance to it as an element capable of improving the quality of health care. The same comment applies to initial medical training: such programs are still only rarely proposed within the framework of medical studies. Thus, while these training activities are increasing at the national level, their overall number is still moderate and their prevalence varies greatly as a function of location.

Ensuring Coordination at the Level of Multidisciplinary Work

While the presence of multiple actors at the time of disclosure of the diagnosis has many advantages, it also creates additional organizational difficulties and greatly increases the effort involved in coordinating the different parties. It is particularly important that the messages conveyed by the various health-care professionals at this point are consistent and coherent, and this imperative becomes all the more crucial the greater the number of professionals involved. Whereas the attention paid to these considerations improves the patient's ability to assimilate the provided information in the best possible way, discrepancies between the received messages, in contrast, have the risk of increasing the patient's distress and reducing his or her cognitive capabilities.

One of the challenges involved in this activity of coordination consists in enabling the health-care professionals involved to share the task of providing information among themselves in order to prevent any of them from feeling the frequently observed, irrepressible need to "say everything, immediately, all by myself." In contrast to a consultation in clinical practice in which doctors see their patients on a genuine one-to-one basis, hospital work brings with it the ability and desire to collaborate with fellow professionals, while also giving up the desire to do everything oneself in an attempt to adopt a holistic approach, which risks excluding the other actors.

Correct understanding of the roles of each of the personnel (doctors, nurses, supportive care professionals, health-care professionals outside of the hospital environment), together with the acceptance of the principle of task distribution, makes it possible not only to limit such departures from the desired approach, but also to focus on the aim of reducing opposition between the various fields that determine the patients' quality of life and avoid any a priori determination of the patients' needs. A survey recently conducted in France shows just how much the failure to achieve this understanding can negatively affect the satisfaction expressed by patients with regard to the care received [40].

Development of Therapeutic Education Programs in the Field of Oncology

Since this subject is still largely neglected in the field of oncology, it should be possible to draw inspiration from models of therapeutic education that have been developed in connection with other chronic somatic diseases and that have helped patients come to a more balanced, partnership-based relationship with their doctors and care teams and have encouraged them to contribute to the decisions that had to be made. These are facets that must be taken into consideration from the very beginning of the care period. They relate to a variety of aspects, of which we will cite only a few examples here: encouraging patients to come to consultations in the company of a relative; encouraging them to prepare for consultations and to draw up a list of questions; explaining to them that they will be given a lot of information during the initial period of their health-care trajectories and that this information will be returned to at various points; encouraging the use of media that complement verbal communication, such as printed documents provided in addition to the consultation or voice recordings of these documents [41].

At the same time, cancer care institutions must improve patient access to information by providing a documentary base or information technology resources that enable patients to consult medical sites or by developing interface structures such as the "Espaces Rencontre Information" (ERI=Information and Meeting Forums). These have been set up by the French national and regional specialist cancer centers at the initiative of the *Ligue Nationale Contre le Cancer*. Run by professionals who are not themselves carers, these provide an informal structure in which visitors can obtain a variety of informative documents or be helped to contact the relevant associations.

Continuation of the Assessment of the Measures Taken

The various surveys of the level of satisfaction with regard to oncological care conducted in France both among hospitalized patients [9] and those having attended the initial diagnostic disclosure consultation [26, 27] have revealed that there are areas in which patients would still like to see improvements in the care provided. These observations should result in the adoption of measures designed to improve the quality of care; the effects of these measures must be monitored.

Furthermore, these surveys should make it possible to identify the factors that can lead to dissatisfaction with the care provided. A variety of international studies have stressed the need to pay particular attention to patients of modest educational levels, coming from non-Western cultures or belonging to older age groups. In France, although the care offered to elderly patients suffering from cancer takes particular account of their psychosocial needs [42], we have only inadequate knowledge of the specific nature of these needs among patients from other cultures (North Africa, Africa, overseas territories and departments, or Asia) who are living in France or among patients from disadvantaged sociocultural backgrounds. This is despite the fact that these latter groups experience less favorable outcomes in terms of survival [43] and should therefore benefit from a greater level of care in terms of the information provided and the psychosocial support received, thus helping to reduce inequalities at the level of the treatment received.

Conclusion

The cancer care landscape is changing rapidly; a number of initiatives have been implemented in France in order to improve the interaction between the doctor and the patient, which forms the foundation for good quality of care. Although these initiatives have focused primarily on the disclosure of the diagnosis of cancer, they may nevertheless be extended to many other moments during the cancer-care trajectory. A number of surveys have made it possible to highlight areas of patient dissatisfaction and identify scope for further improvement.

In French cancer centers, these innovations are still only tentative; their value must first be acknowledged by the professionals who play a major role in cancer care. This process is underpinned by a change of mentality that places the patient more directly at the center of the care process and focuses on his/her expectations and preferences, skills, and decision-making choices. Only in this way is it possible to guarantee respect for the patient's autonomy.

References

1. Fallowfield L. The challenge of interacting with patients in oncology. Eur J Cancer. 2009;45 Suppl 1:445–6.
2. Arora NK, Street Jr RL, Epstein RM, Butow PN. Facilitating patient-centered cancer communication: a road map. Patient Educ Couns. 2009;77(3):319–21.
3. Venetis MK, Robinson JD, Turkiewicz KL, Allen M. An evidence base for patient-centered cancer care: a meta-analysis of studies of observed communication between cancer specialists and their patients. Patient Educ Couns. 2009;77(3):379–83.
4. Plan Cancer 2003–2007. République Française, Mission Interministérielle pour la Lutte contre le Cancer. 2003. http://www.plancancer.gouv.fr/historique/plan-cancer-2003-2007.html.
5. Plan Cancer 2009–2013. République Française, Mission Interministérielle pour la Lutte contre le Cancer. 2009. http://www.plancancer.gouv.fr

6. Krakowski I, Chardot C, Bey P, Guillemin F, Philip T. Coordinated organization of symptoms management and support in all the stages of cancer disease: putting in place pluridisciplinary structures of supportive oncological care. Bull Cancer. 2001;88(3):321–8 (French).
7. Krakowski I, Boureau F, Bugat R, Chassignol L, Colombat P, Copel L, et al. For a coordination of the supportive care for people affected by severe illnesses: proposition of organization in the public and private health care centres. Bull Cancer. 2004;91:449–56 (French).
8. Bergerot P, Rodde-Dunet MH. Ten years of reflection around the announcement of cancer: from the patients' questions to implementation. Bull Cancer. 2010;97(10):1195–6 (French).
9. Brédart A, Robertson C, Razavi D, Batel-Copel L, Larsson G, Lichosik D, et al. Patients' satisfaction ratings and their desire for care improvement across oncology settings from France, Italy, Poland and Sweden. Psychooncology. 2003;12(1):68–77.
10. Strain JJ, Blumenfield M. Challenges for consultation-liaison psychiatry in the 21st century. Psychosomatics. 2008;49(2):93–6.
11. Dolbeault S. La détresse des patients atteints de cancer: prévalence, facteurs prédictifs, modalités de repérage et de prise en charge. Thèse de doctorat de l'Université Paris VI Pierre et Marie Curie; 2009. p. 259.
12. Moumjid N, Gafni A, Brémond A, Carrère MO. Shared decision making in the medical encounter: are we all talking about the same thing? Med Decis Making. 2007;27(5):539–46.
13. Gattellari M, Butow PN, Tatterhall MH. Sharing decisions in cancer care. Soc Sci Med. 2001;52:1865–78.
14. Thorne S, Oliffe J, Kim-Sing C, Hislop TG, Stajduhar K, Harris SR, et al. Helpful communications during the diagnostic period: an interpretive description of patient preferences. Eur J Cancer Care (Engl). 2010;19(6):746–54.
15. Smith A, Juraskova I, Butow P, Miguel C, Lopez AL, Chang S, et al. Sharing vs. caring—the relative impact of sharing decisions versus managing emotions on patient outcomes. Patient Educ Couns. 2011;82(2):233–9.
16. Tariman JD, Berry DL, Cochrane B, Doorenbos A, Schepp K. Preferred and actual participation roles during health care decision making in persons with cancer: a systematic review. Ann Oncol. 2010;21(6):1145–51.
17. Moumjid N, Charles C, Morelle M, Gafni A, Brémond A, Farsi F, et al. The statutory duty of physicians to inform patients versus unmet patients' information needs: the case of breast cancer in France. Health Policy. 2009;91(2):162–73.
18. Baile WF, Aaron J, Parker PA. Practitioner-patient communication in cancer diagnosis and treatment. In: Miller SM, Bowen DJ, Croyle RT, Rowland J, editors. Cancer control and behavioral science. Washington: APA; 2009. p. 327–46.
19. Dolbeault S, Bredart A. Announcing cancer diagnosis: which communication difficulties from professional and from patient's side? Which possible improvements. Bull Cancer. 2011;97(10):1183–94 (French).
20. Costantini A, Baile WF, Lenzi R, Costantini M, Ziparo V, Marchetti P, et al. Overcoming cultural barriers to giving bad news: feasibility of training to promote truth-telling to cancer patients. J Cancer Educ. 2009;24(3):180–5.
21. Brédart A, Dolbeault S, Razavi D. *Psycho-Oncology*. In Boyle P & Levin B (Eds) World Cancer Report 2008 of IARC (International Agency for Research on Cancer), section 1 Global Cancer Control, chapter 1.9, p. 74–83. http://www.iarc.fr/en/publications/pdfs-online/wcr/
22. Gilbert JE, Green E, Lankshear S, Hughes E, Burkoski V, Sawka C. Nurses as patient navigators in cancer diagnosis: review, consultation and model design. Eur J Cancer Care (Engl). 2011;20(2):228–36.
23. Liénard A, Merckaert I, Libert Y, Delvaux N, Marchal S, Boniver J, et al. Factors that influence cancer patients' and relatives' anxiety following a three-person medical consultation: impact of a communication skills training program for physicians. Psychooncology. 2008;17(5):488–96.
24. Ganem G. Management of patients with cancer. Introduction. Bull Cancer. 2010;97(10):1151–2 (French).
25. Dolbeault S, Boistard B, Meuric J, Copel L, Brédart A. Screening for distress and supportive care needs during the initial phase of the care process: a qualitative description of a clinical pilot experiment in a French cancer center. Psychooncology. 2011;20(6):585–93. doi:10.1002/pon.1946.

26. Ganem G, Krakowski I, Rixe O, Batt M, Brocvielle AL. Initial management in oncology: results of CPRIM surveys on 2,583 patient's perceptions and expectations (outside anticancer centers). Bull Cancer. 2010;97(10):1153–62 (French).
27. Grenier C, De Jésus A, Farsi F, Marx G, Brédart A, Peixoto O, et al. Communication around the cancer diagnosis: patient satisfaction and process quality in French comprehensive cancer centers. Bull Cancer. 2010;97(10):1163–72 (French).
28. Brédart A, Bouleuc C, Dolbeault S. Doctor-patient communication and satisfaction with care in oncology. Curr Opin Oncol. 2005;17(4):351–4.
29. Ryan H, Schofield P, Cockburn J, Butow P, Tattersall M, Turner J, et al. How to recognize and manage psychological distress in cancer patients. Eur J Cancer Care (Engl). 2005;14(1):7–15.
30. Jacobsen P, Donovan K, Swaine Z, et al. Management of anxiety and depression in adult cancer patients: toward an evidence-based approach. In: Chang AE, Ganz PA, Hayes DF, et al., editors. Oncology: an evidence-based approach. New York: Springer; 2006. p. 1552–79.
31. Mitchell AJ, Kaar S, Coggan C, Herdman J. Acceptability of common screening methods used to detect distress and related mood disorders-preferences of cancer specialists and non-specialists. Psychooncology. 2008;17(3):226–36.
32. Rosenbloom SK, Victorson DE, Hahn EA, Peterman AH, Cella D. Assessment is not enough: a randomized controlled trial of the effects of HRQL assessment on quality of life and satisfaction in oncology clinical practice. Psychooncology. 2007;16(12):1069–79.
33. Velikova G, Booth L, Smith AB, Brown PM, Lynch P, Brown JM, et al. Measuring quality of life in routine oncology practice improves communication and patient well-being: a randomized controlled trial. J Clin Oncol. 2004;22(4):714–24.
34. Lipscomb J, Reeve BB, Clauser SB, Abrams JS, Bruner DW, Burke LB, et al. Patient-reported outcomes assessment in cancer trials: taking stock, moving forward. J Clin Oncol. 2007;25(32):5133–40 (review).
35. Step MM, Ray EB. Patient perceptions of oncologist-patient communication about prognosis: changes from initial diagnosis to cancer recurrence. Health Commun. 2011;26(1):48–58.
36. Razavi D, Merckaert I, Marchal S, Libert Y, Conradt S, Boniver J, et al. How to optimize physicians' communication skills in cancer care: results of a randomized study assessing the usefulness of posttraining consolidation workshops. J Clin Oncol. 2003;21(16):3141–9.
37. Merckaert I, Libert Y, Razavi D. Communication skills training in cancer care: where are we and where are we going? Curr Opin Oncol. 2005;17(4):319–30.
38. Stiefel F, Barth J, Bensing J, Fallowfield L, Jost L, Razavi D, et al.; participants. Communication skills training in oncology: a position paper based on a consensus meeting among European experts in 2009. Ann Oncol. 2010;21(2):204–7.
39. Armstrong J, Holland J. Surviving the stresses of clinical oncology by improving communication. Oncology (Williston Park). 2004;18(3):363–8.
40. Moret L, Rochedreux A, Chevalier S, Lombrail P, Gasquet I. Medical information delivered to patients: discrepancies concerning roles as perceived by physicians and nurses set against patient satisfaction. Patient Educ Couns. 2008;70(1):94–101.
41. Rodin G, Mackay JA, Zimmermann C, Mayer C, Howell D, Katz M, et al. Clinician-patient communication: a systematic review. Support Care Cancer. 2009;17(6):627–44.
42. Sifer-Rivière L, Saint-Jean O, Gisselbrecht M, Cudennec T, Girre V; on behalf of Programme d'OncoGériatrie de l'Ouest Parisien (POGOP). What the specific tools of geriatrics and oncology can tell us about the role and status of geriatricians in a pilot geriatric oncology program. Ann Oncol. 2011;22(10):2325–9.
43. Menvielle G, Leclerc A, Chastang JF, Luce D. Socioeconomic inequalities in cause specific mortality among older people in France. BMC Public Health. 2010;10:260.

Chapter 29
Communication with Patients with Hematological Malignancies in Argentina

Astrid Pavlovsky, Lourdes Bertolino, Victoria Patxot, and Carolina Pavlovsky

Abstract Argentina is a country of immigrants and Buenos Aires, its capital city, one of the largest urban areas in the world. The country in which we live with all its cultural background together with the characteristics of the institution where we work, are important factors influencing our communication with patients.

Although the clinical information we give to our patients as well as the effort we take into communicating adequately are important therapeutic tools, in our country, there is no formal education on these topics. Most doctors learn to communicate with patients, guided by a model they choose and by personal intuition.

The time and effort dedicated to each patient regarded as an individual with all their personal characteristics, is of paramount importance throughout their new life situation facing a hematological diagnosis.

Chronic diseases with no necessary immediate treatment, others in which the overall survival can depend on the treatment compliance, and other cases needing aggressive chemotherapy with bad prognosis are some of the scenarios and challenges of communication with patients with hematological malignancies in Argentina.

A. Pavlovsky (✉)
Centro de Hematologia, Department of Hematology, FUNDALEU, Buenos Aires, Argentina
e-mail: astridp@intramed.net

L. Bertolino • V. Patxot
FUNDALEU, Psicologia, Caba, Buenos Aires, Argentina
e-mail: lourdesbertolino@yahoo.com.ar; vpatxot@yahoo.com.ar

C. Pavlovsky
FUNDALEU, Hematology, Buenos Aires, Argentina
e-mail: cpavlovsky@fundaleu.org.ar

Prologue

The author selected by the editors to write this chapter was originally Dr. Santiago Pavlovsky. Dr. Pavlovsky was a highly recognized hematologist in Argentina, renowned around the world, founder of various oncohematology organizations, and member of the most prestigious international associations. He published nearly 150 articles in international journals and was contributor to more than 78 books.

Dr. Santiago Pavlovsky was also my father and my mentor.

The responsibility of writing this chapter was probably the last one he assumed. He accepted this challenge in June 2009, was diagnosed with lung cancer in November 2009, and died in September 2010.

The last thing he wrote on his computer was the first paragraphs of this chapter he never finished:

> Argentina is a country that was at the beginning of the 20th century one of the richest of the world, with a strong agricultural industry and a strong middle class with a high rate of literate inhabitants. Medicine had a high standard, at the beginning of the 20th century with a close communication with France, and in the second half of the century with the United States. Reflecting this fact, most of the professors of medicine before the sixties were fluent in French. Later on most of the young physicians who were willing to do training abroad chose to do a residency or fellowship in academic centers in the USA. Three Nobel Prizes in Medicine (physiology, biochemistry, and immunology) were awarded to Argentine doctors graduated and trained in Argentina. Unfortunately, many facts contributed to the deterioration of the economy, especially politics and corruption.
>
> I graduated in medicine at the University of Buenos Aires in 1964, doing my training in internal medicine and later in hematology in Buenos Aires. I completed my training in hematology at the Centre Hayem in the Hospital Saint Louis, whose director was the world-renowned Professor Jean Bernard. My chief was Aggregate Professor Dr. Jacques Luis Binet, who worked in cytopathology mainly in chronic lymphocytic leukemia. He later on became a well-known expert in chronic lymphocytic leukemia. During 1966–1967 I worked with Binet in immunology and cytopathology, but at the same time participated in the care of patients with hematological malignancies as outpatients as well as admitted to the hospital. I was lucky to participate in the first symposium of a new drug, Daunorubicin, which, in combination with Vincristine and Prednisone, produced a high rate of complete remission in childhood acute lymphoblastic leukemia. To this symposium Jean Bernard invited most of the leaders of the world in acute leukemia. At that time Argentina had no clinical trials, and I was impressed with the cooperation between the Hospital Saint Louis and the Cancer and Acute Leukemia Group B (CALGB) of the USA, with Dr. James Holland as acting chairman. We were lucky that two other young physicians trained with Jean Bernard and another in Detroit, USA. Coming back to Buenos Aires…

As mentioned, Dr. Santiago Pavlovsky was a very qualified hematologist with an excellent academic background; but this is not what made him so special. After his death, we received hundreds of e-mails and letters honoring him for his human qualities, his ability to give confidence, hope, and peace to his patients. The time and effort he dedicated to communicate with his patients made each of them feel special and unique. The kind and warm relationship he achieved with his patients was an important part of the treatment he gave them. These are just a few of the comments his patients wrote:

"… a great one, a doctor with a huge heart, an incredible human being, a father to his patients…"

"He was our calm guide through the hard walk to cure…"

"Thank you for everything, but mainly for that virtue only great ones have: to transmit even in the worst of times that everything would be fine, that everything would get better…"

"He was a great doctor and an exceptional person who gave me hopes to keep on fighting…"

The way he is remembered by his patients shows us that the doctor–patient relationship can be just as important as making the right diagnosis or offering the correct treatment. Many can have the correct approach to a *disease*, but we must all try to have the best approach to our *patients*.

Throughout the following chapter, I along with other coworkers of my father will guide you on what we think are important points in the challenges in communication with patients with hematological malignancies in Argentina (Fig. 29.1).

—Astrid Pavlovsky

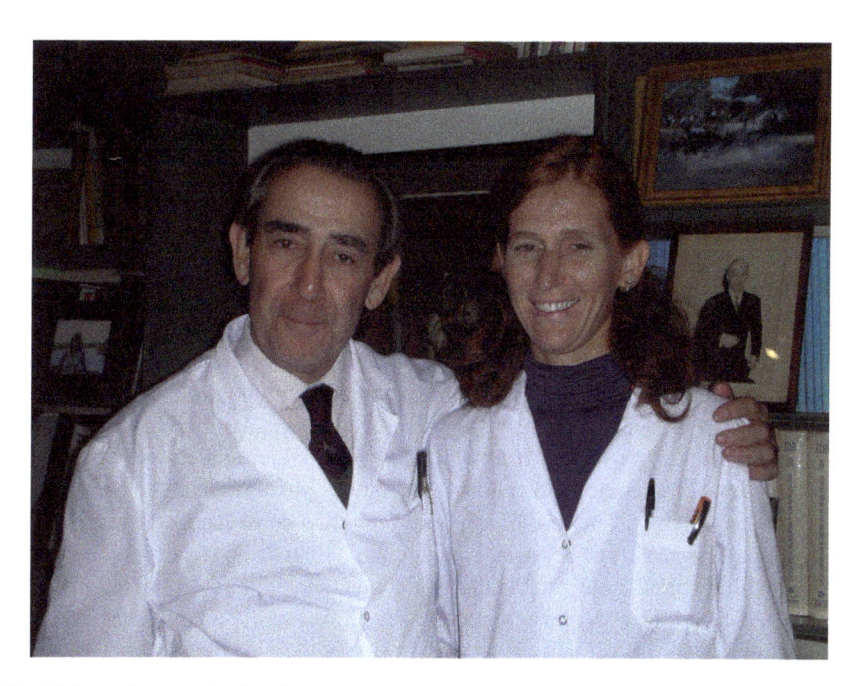

Fig. 29.1 Dr. Santiago Pavlovsky and Dr. Astrid Pavlovsky

Argentina, a Country of Immigrants

Argentina is the second largest country in South America. Highly urbanized, ten metropolitan areas account for half of the population; fewer than 1 in 10 live in rural areas. Approximately three million people live in Buenos Aires City and around 13 million in Greater Buenos Aires, making it one of the largest urban areas in the world. As with other areas of the New World, Argentina is considered a country of immigrants. Most Argentines descend from colonial-era settlements and nineteenth- and twentieth-century European immigrants. Eighty-six percent of Argentina's population self-identify as being of European descent, mostly Spanish or Italian. An estimated 8% of the population is "mestizo" (people of mixed European and Native American heritage or descent), and 4% of Argentines are of Arab or Asian descent. In addition, illegal immigration has been a recent factor in Argentine demographics, with most immigrants coming from Bolivia or Paraguay.

The Constitution guarantees freedom of religion, but also requires the government to support Roman Catholicism economically. According to the World Christian Database, 92% of Argentines are Christians, the majority of whom are Roman Catholics.

In Argentina, health care is provided through a combination of employer- and labor union-sponsored plans, government insurance plans, public hospitals, clinics, and private health insurance plans. The high-complexity healthcare institutions are centralized in the large capital cities (mainly in Buenos Aires), making access to medical resources unevenly distributed. As a result, in many cases the patient needs to move from his or her home to one of these cities in order to receive adequate treatment, thus adding difficult variables to the diagnosis and treatment itself.

A Hematological Institution in Buenos Aires

FUNDALEU (Foundation for the Fight against Leukemia) is an institution located in the city center of Buenos Aires City. It has 18 beds and no more than 15 doctors, 2 psychologists, and a group of highly specialized nurses. At FUNDALEU, we are dedicated to the diagnosis and treatment of hematological malignancies, including autologous and allogeneic stem cell transplantation. Most of our patients have labor union-sponsored or private health insurance plans and come from all over the country. Each patient has his or her own treating hematologist. This is usually the hematologist with whom the patient had the first contact and who informed him or her of the diagnosis and the necessary treatment. "Their doctor" is the one that sees them as outpatients and almost on a daily basis as inpatients. This physician takes part in deciding and communicating every important aspect of the patient's disease.

The country in which we live, with all its cultural background, and the institution where we work are important factors influencing our communication with our patients.

The clinical information we give our patients as well as the effort we take to communicate adequately are important therapeutic tools. Good doctor–patient communication is essential for the patient's and the family's acceptance of the disease, for compliance with the treatment, and for hoping for a good outcome; it thus helps to reduce the stress encountered in this new situation and provide a better quality of life [1].

Challenges in Communication with Patients with Hematological Malignancies in Our Daily Practice

The psychological damage caused by communicating the wrong way may be just as harmful as giving the wrong diagnosis or treatment.

In our country, most doctors learn to communicate with patients at the beginning of their careers, guided by a teacher or professor and by personal intuition. There is no formal education on this topic at the universities, only a few isolated projects with the intention of improving this aspect of medical studies [2].

This lack produces great insecurity and feelings of anxiety and unease at the moment of having to face the job. Having to communicate, for instance, the negative aspects of a disease or its treatments produces stress and different types of fears, such as of causing more pain, destroying hope, being rejected for giving bad news, committing a mistake, and making the patient have to go through unjustified trauma; and the fear of producing emotional decompensation in the patient and being unable to resolve it.

Every day and with every patient in our small institution, we face different challenges of communication characterized by our idiosyncrasies, cultural backgrounds, health policies, and in many cases by our religious beliefs.

Communication is encompassed within the doctor–patient relationship and acquires special significance in patients suffering from oncohematological diseases. The best care for these patients must take cultural variables into account [3, 4].

Culture can be defined as a series of learned models, behaviors, beliefs, and shared values by a particular social group, which give the individuals an identity and a frame of reference to interpret experience. Cancer is, nevertheless, a disease feared in every culture. The attributable causes of cancer, the role of the family in the care of the patient, the transmission process of the medical disease, and attitudes facing pain and death as well as mourning rituals are just a few of the cultural variables influential in the adaptation of the oncological patient.

The needs of cancer patients and the types of intervention used are similar in almost every culture, with the main difference being the availability of the latter.

In our country, different models of doctor–patient relationship coexist that correspond to different historical phases of the relationship.

Even though these days most medical decisions are made taking the patient's needs into consideration, respecting his or her autonomy, and under consensus, it is still common to find paternalistic models in which the doctor's authority prevails, to the detriment of the patient's autonomy.

Moreover, the doctor–patient relationship is certainly asymmetrical, not because one is more valuable than the other — both are equal in dignity, but rather because of the circumstances they find each other in: one needs help, and the other is able to offer it. It is an encounter between someone with a need and someone who can satisfy that need. Throughout history until a few decades ago, paternalism was the most common form of doctor–patient relationship; the doctor acted practically without the patient's opinion [3].

The changes in the past century emphasized the importance of individual rights, making the patients' autonomy take on enormous relevance. Autonomy requires the patient to have the ability to make decisions according to his or her own values and preferences, and based on information provided by the doctor, so that the decision may be as accurate as possible.

In the clinical practice at our Center, the decision-making process is shared: the doctor provides information and guidance to the competent patient so that the patient may actively participate in the decision, which will affect him or her according to personal preferences, values, and objectives.

Treating a patient is not simply an act of giving a diagnosis and indicating a treatment; it also means that the professional has understood the physical, mental, economic, and social effects an ailment has on the person who is ill and is sensitive to these effects. This standpoint requires the capacity for effective communication with the patient, the patient's family, or the social environment. It is much more than a mere service agreement. A style of doctor–patient relationship that focuses on the patient's needs, stimulates his or her personal and social resources, and reduces levels of stress benefits the quality of assistance. Additionally, this style affects the patient's mood, implies good empathy between the parties, including the professional's acceptance of the fears and worries of the patient, and generates trust and mutual respect.

The definition of communication tells us that it is a process in which messages are exchanged between individuals through a common code of signals such as language, gestures, or signs. It is a two-way process that includes speech and goes beyond it [5]. Communication with the patient is especially important in the context of life-threatening diseases such as the oncohematological diseases, in which the information conveyed is potentially anxiogenic.

Many are the situations, in which the right communication generates a change in the course of the disease in patients with hematological malignancies. Through examples and reflections on situations experienced in our practice in FUNDALEU, we would like to point out the following:

- The challenge of communication with patients with chronic or indolent diseases.
- Communication in difficult situations: refractory patients, end of life.
- Communication in the interdisciplinary team.

How Communication Affects Patients with Chronic or Indolent Oncohematological Diseases

The Importance of How the Diagnosis Is Given in Oncohematological Diseases Requiring No Treatment

Chronic and indolent hematological malignancies are a common cause for consultation. In many of these cases, such as chronic lymphocytic leukemia, different histological subtypes and stages of lymphoma or smoldering myeloma, no therapy is needed. The "watch and wait" strategy is an accepted approach. Patients leave the hematologist's office with an oncological diagnosis and the medical indication that no treatment is necessary.

In these cases, the most important responsibility the hematologist has is to communicate the diagnosis and give the necessary reassurance in order for the patient (with a new life situation) to be able to continue his or her life without fear and with the possibility of future plans.

This is the case of Stella, a 59-year-old woman diagnosed with chronic lymphocytic leukemia almost 11 years ago and still with no need for treatment.

> In the beginning of 1999 as I did every year, I took my children for routine blood tests and decided to get tested myself as well. When we got the results, our PCP recommended repeating mine because—and I quote him—"according to these tests you should be in the hospital, repeat them and come back to see me with the results."
>
> I thought the tests would be fine, but they weren't. I can still remember how the look on my doctor's face changed as he read the test results while he was speaking to me. He told us that according to what he observed the diagnosis would surely be cancer or leukemia and that we shouldn't waste any time. He was harsh and decisive, and for a long time I thought he should have given me the news differently…it destroyed me.
>
> Leukemia, that terrible word we are so afraid of, cannot be digested. You think that it's over, that you are dying tomorrow, that everything is finished. My world fell apart, I was so sad I couldn't do a thing. I was paralyzed, me and my whole family. You may understand why I felt like a time bomb…. And that was how I came to make an appointment to meet Dr. Pavlovsky….
>
> From the moment I entered his office I felt at peace, cared for. He had the ability to make you feel secure. He took all the necessary time to look at everything, to listen to me, and examine me until he started speaking. Undoubtedly he knew so much, but not just about leukemia; he knew how to take care of a person with a disease, how to make you feel secure, that feeling of security that never comes back after receiving a diagnosis like mine. He always told me, always, every time I went in to see him, that I was lucky I didn't need treatment; his positivity and knowledge always calmed me….

There are many ways of arriving at an oncohematological diagnosis. One way is with the appearance of a bothersome symptom, the etiology of which must be investigated. This requires a series of progressively more complex tests, which finally lead to a diagnosis.

Another is through an unexpected finding in a routine medical checkup, such as the case mentioned earlier, without the patient having ever experienced a symptom.

This is frequent in hematological diseases and causes disbelief. As the disease is not visible through symptoms, the patient is incredulous of the tests and repeats them over and over in different places and seeks second and third opinions.

A diagnosis of indolent and chronic hematological disease and the possibility of receiving aggressive and invasive treatments in the future evoke the thought of dying, of losing one's health, one's identity (not being the same person anymore), of losing control and one's lifestyle, of losing one's life project and the feeling of equality with others, and loss of one's scheme of values. These diseases, in particular, give the feeling of living in a constant "time bomb" state—with the threat of having to start aggressive treatment from one day to the next.

How a person faces this situation depends on the intersubjective evaluation of the threat posed to reality. This reaction will become more intense as the person perceives that his or her resources are insufficient to control the negative consequences of the prognosis. The valuation of the occurrence as loss produces a feeling of sadness, which may trigger other pathologies, such as depression.

The two foremost expected reactions upon a diagnosis are:

- Great anxiety: initial shock, despair, insomnia, inexplicable crying, social withdrawal, irritability, and the feeling of being overwhelmed by unmanageable circumstances
- Self-control: emotional distance, intention of minimizing the information, and the appearance of a certain degree of denial

In this phase of the diagnosis, communication has particular characteristics. This is the time when doctor and patient are getting to know one another; thus, information must be given clearly, respecting the patient's timing, using language in accordance with the patient's level of education, and avoiding technicalities. Also, the information must be transmitted while giving hope, indicating the steps that should follow and making it possible for the patient to express his or her unease, doubts, feelings, and emotions. Quite often, it is necessary to repeat the information given [6].

As in Stella's case, successful communication is associated with the doctor's willingness to listen to the patient and his or her family, as well as the ability to understand and relate to the patient's emotions, thus encouraging them. When diagnoses of indolent hematological diseases are given, the anxiety and concerns of the patient usually diminish as the doctor–patient relationship becomes stronger. The ability and experience of the doctor to communicate with each individual, taking into consideration each particular situation, makes a life difference to many patients.

At this stage, the doctor–patient communication is focused on encouraging the continuation of the checkups and calming the anxiety that appears prior to screenings in fear of a worsening situation of the disease. Adaptation to the new circumstances and improvement of quality of life are the main objectives of the meetings between doctor and patient.

Communication in these indolent chronic diseases becomes a process: the continuation of the visits to the hematologist with the repetition of the same concepts regarding the lack of a need for treatment and limitations in everyday life allows the patients, who at first feel "paralyzed," to be able to go on with their daily routine. We frequently hear things like: "Every time you tell me my blood counts are stable, I start feeling better" or "Now that you say everything is fine, I feel fine again."

As hematologists, we should be aware in these cases of the need to put emphasis on the necessary checkups and the criteria to initiate treatment; but we also must be mindful of the great influence our words have on the psychological and spiritual health of our patients.

The Attitude the Hematologist Adopts with Patients with Chronic Myeloid Leukemia Can Have an Impact on Their Overall Survival

How we communicate a diagnosis of chronic leukemia can leave an erroneous message with a patient who hears the word *leukemia* for the first time and is unaware that, in a diagnosis such as chronic myeloid leukemia (CML), the prognosis has changed since the introduction of imatinib.

CML is caused by a chromosomal abnormality (the Philadelphia [Phi] chromosome) associated with the creation of BCR-ABL fusion oncogene [7]. The hyperactivity of the BCR-ABL kinase causes an uncontrolled proliferation and survival, leading to CML. In the absence of treatment, CML is inexorably fatal. Imatinib is a tyrosine kinase inhibitor (TKI) that blocks the ATP binding site of the BCR-ABL, suppressing downstream signaling [8]. The treatment of CML with imatinib mesylate selectively inhibits the Philadelphia (Phi) clone.

Regarding CML, in the TKI era what had been a fatal disease is now considered a chronic one. The reason for obtaining different responses in different patients is not well known. Though a combination of different factors surrounding the patient can lead to treatment failure, treatment adherence is definitely important.

Adherence has been defined by the WHO as the extent to which a person's behavior corresponds with agreed recommendations of a healthcare provider. Different studies show that adherence rates vary between 0 and 83% [9]. Marin et al. conducted a study with CML patients in complete cytogenetic response (CCyR), measuring adherence with a microelectronic chip (MEMS). It was shown that no complete molecular response (CMR) was observed when adherence was ≤90%, and no major molecular response (MMR) was observed when adherence was ≤80%.

Nonadherence is a frequent problem in patients with CML under treatment with imatinib. Marin reports that 26% of CML patients on long-term imatinib have an adherence lower than 90%, which has an unfavorable impact on achieving MMR. Why patients are not fully adherent is not known, yet the healthcare professional has an important role and work to do to improve patients' adherence to >90%.

The ADAGIO [10] study (Adherence Assessment with Glivec: Indicators and Outcomes) examined over a 90-day period in a "real practice" setting the prevalence of imatinib nonadherence in patients with CML in Belgium and studied whether the treatment response was associated with adherence levels. The doctor–patient relationship must always be reinforced, because nonadherence is the responsibility of the doctor as well as the patient. In this study, physicians' experience, practice patterns, and practice environment influenced adherence. Good adherence was related to an active CML practice, spending more time with the patient at the time of diagnosis, and practice as a hematologist in a teaching hospital. Patients with a lesser response had taken between 74 and 76.8% of the prescribed dose, compared to 89.9 and 92.7% for patients with a better response. The most common reason for intentional nonadherence was to deal with side effects, and the unintentional reason was that they forget to take the drug.

If the physician does not communicate the impact that adherence has on response, the patients may believe that their clinical responses have not been affected by nonadherence. It is, therefore, important to know how to transmit this to our patients. Sometimes patients feel uncomfortable talking about adherence; they feel judged or not trusted.

CML Clinical Case

This is one of Dr. Santiago Pavlovsky's cases, to whom he applied everything mentioned, in his daily clinical practice. A 52-year-old male patient with no comorbidities was diagnosed with CML in 2004. He had an intermediate Sokal risk score and was treated with hydroxyurea for a few days and later with noninterrupted 400 mg of imatinib per day.

The patient had been informed that he had leukemia by his first doctor with a quick and unclear explanation of his disease and prognosis. He was left worried and thinking he did not have many treatment possibilities available and was dying. Under the circumstances, he decided to get a second opinion. With a clear explanation and taking the necessary time for it, this hematologist gave the patient new hope. He told him about "fantastic" drugs such as TKI, known as "target therapy," which had been discovered in this new era for this type of leukemia. The doctor said,

> This type of leukemia has excellent prognosis. Many drugs have been developed lately. If you don't respond to one of them, don't worry; there are two or three more being tested. If I had to choose a type of leukemia, I would definitively choose this one because of its excellent prognosis—that is, if you comply with treatment as indicated.

Having heard this, the patient left Dr. Santiago's office full of hope and happiness. He trusted his physician and this allowed him to go on with future plans.

Adherence to Medication

While on imatinib, the patient experienced some grade 1–2 adverse events. His doctor took the time to point out that even though this was a chronic leukemia with an excellent prognosis, "it was cancer" nonetheless, and there should be no interruption unless grade 3–4 adverse events were experienced. Therefore, palliative treatment for the events caused by imatinib was indicated, with good response.

The persistent message of the importance of adherence to treatment given during every visit to the doctor kept this patient aware; and this had a direct impact on the treatment response. At first, adherence was simply checked by asking the patient in every visit if he had interrupted imatinib. But since 2009, we started measuring adherence with a daily medication diary to be kept by each patient.

In this particular case, the patient's adherence showed to be 100%. CCyR was achieved at 6 months and MMR at 18 months of treatment. At 24 months, he showed persistent complete response including CMR, monitored every 6 months in the same institution by an international standardized molecular laboratory. Today, he is still alive and doing well.

This is a chronic disease; the time and effort we dedicate to our patients in each visit has a direct impact on achieving longer survival.

Communication in Difficult Situations: Refractory Patients, End of Life

The role and responsibilities of the treating hematologist change along with the stage of the disease. The first communication challenge is to give the diagnosis in the best possible way, always telling the truth but giving hope. As the disease becomes refractory and the chances for cure decrease, the message to the patient and the family becomes harder to give [11]. In our specialty, refractory diseases and death are real facts. The doctor must have the ability to understand the patient, the family, and their particular situation as well.

This is an example of a 55-year-old woman refractory to four lines of treatment. Susana was a widow with a 23-year-old son and a 21-year-old daughter. She lived with her daughter and was the economic and spiritual support for her children and her father. In addition, she could not count on her sister, who was emotionally unstable.

Susana came in for consultation with a stage IV Diffuse Large B Cell Lymphoma with pleural effusion, splenomegaly, tricytopenia with transfusional requirements, and B symptoms.

At diagnosis, the patient was angry and did not want to accept her disease; she even considered the possibility of not doing any invasive treatment. She needed time to accept this new life situation, but the aggressiveness of her disease did not give us this time; we could not take long before starting chemotherapy. Susana's difficulty in accepting her disease was also reflected on her children, who did not accompany her enough during this stage because they did not understand the seriousness of the situation.

She received treatment, achieving complete remission and, due to the high possibilities of relapsing, underwent autologous stem cell transplantation. Throughout these 10 months of treatment, she maintained a close relationship with her doctor, hoping to be "cured." Nevertheless, 3 months after her transplant she relapsed, with the same signs and symptoms as when diagnosed. A second line of treatment was then offered. With high toxicity from chemotherapy, she completed three cycles and achieved a second complete remission. This lasted only 4 months, until she once again started experiencing shortness of breath, anemia, and an enlarged spleen. By then, the chances for a cure were almost nil, but the patient was young and hoped to continue treatment. She therefore received another line of chemotherapy; yet the symptoms came back as soon as we stopped.

Susana knew she had no chance. She wanted to keep on fighting. Her primary worry was the suffering of her children, who had already lost their father. Communication at this time was effective through gestures or by simply listening to her questions. Her physician encouraged and scheduled many visits in quiet offices and offered enough time to listen to her questions. She felt new adenopathies and was scared to feel pain or sudden symptoms while she was alone. By then, the patient asked questions about the end of life and was satisfied with short answers.

She accepted palliative treatment to be able to go back home and avoid future admissions to the hospital. She died after almost 3 months at home.

In a case in which the expected recovery is not achieved, doctor–patient communication is faced with a new challenge. The patient must undergo a new process of adaptation in which the initial fears and anxiety of the diagnosis reappear with greater potency. Feelings such as frustration, anger, and discouragement appear. In Susana's case, the initial anger transformed into cooperation during the treatment; she was always hoping for a cure. Once the disease became refractory, the doctor's speech had to focus on the continuity of palliative care and accompaniment until the last moments of life. This was difficult for the doctor, because the patient was young [12, 13].

The good relationship established with the professional helped when it came time for Susana to accept palliative care and decide to stay home as long as possible, avoiding hospitalization. Also helpful was the fact that her children became aware of the gravity of the situation and stayed by her side.

The psychological state of mind of patient and family revolves around symptoms of deterioration, ever more visible, and the perception of dying. The reality of death interferes in everyone's life more than ever. Even though some people go through this process with acceptance and serenity, it is frequent for the patients and their families to have to endure moments of great suffering. Emotional reactions range from minor expressions of anxiety and distrust to proposing a change of therapy. Usually, though with greater hopelessness, patients choose to accept other lines of treatment, adapting to each new circumstance. Even in the last stages, Susana accepted oral chemotherapy.

The concomitant emotions go from desperation to sadness to psychopathological conditions such as depression, and generalized anxiety disorders, which require specific psychotherapeutic treatments.

Persons constantly aware of the approach of death are few. Usually the habit of not talking directly about death can be a useful relief upon which to rest. Arguing against denial is not beneficial, since denial is usually a method of adaptation. Another common method is ambivalence: persons affected by a disease may present a limited capacity to accept death, often protecting themselves by making plans [14].

Perhaps one of the most important challenges for physicians who work with oncohematological patients is informing the patient that the disease is refractory to treatment. This moment will depend largely on the relationship established previously. It is necessary to ask oneself what the patient is ready to know and what not. Transmitting this type of information implies the commitment to accompany, to not abandon, the other person at this time.

Patients are more receptive to comments about their own evolution than to statistics; setting limits or schedules usually does not help the patient's situation. Giving bad news is not a single act; it is gradual and progressive and changes from day to day. The criterion that should be followed is that of communicating the bearable truth—information the patient can handle and accept, which changes according to the moment in the evolution of the disease and the information received.

Often by the time the disease becomes refractory, the patient needs specialists in palliative care or is in an intensive care unit. Nevertheless, the treating hematologist should be there. The simple presence of the treating hematologist throughout the last moments is important for both the patient and the family.

The criteria that bear on communication with the patient must also apply to their closest friends or relatives. Family members and friends also suffer the emotional impact of this moment, and each person does so in a different way and at different moments, according to their personality, experience with disease, age, relationship with the patient, and capacity to confront adversity [15, 16].

Communication in the Interdisciplinary Team

Nowadays, the effectiveness of the oncological treatments require the participation of several specialized professionals in order for the treatment to be an integral one. Interaction becomes essential, not only because of the multiple dimensions of the human being, but also because of their interrelations.

The characteristics that define the interdisciplinary team are the existence of a work methodology, the coordination and cooperation between members, and the presence of common objectives. In the same way that doctor–patient communication is fundamental for better development of the treatment, so is communication between members of the multidisciplinary team.

The formal meetings of the entire team, where patient cases are presented and discussed, enable the unification of criteria, the incorporation of more ideas and alternatives for decision making, and the possibility of doing so under consensus. This encourages shared responsibility and mutual support, especially in difficult situations; helps to avoid contradictions that could be transmitted to the patient; and increases efficiency by avoiding the overlapping of efforts. In our institution, the treating hematologist is usually the person in charge of communicating with the patient and the one who gives information on matters concerning the evolution of the disease, decisions, possible treatments [16], etc. As the Institution is relatively small, informal exchange is encouraged among the entire staff—physicians as well as personnel from the administrative, housekeeping, maintenance, hemotherapy, and pharmaceutical areas.

Summed up in a patient's words: "Despite the fact that the hospitalization is due to a serious disease, the friendly and kind environment of the entire institution helps one feel well."

The development of assistance in teams for the diseases described, presents us, on one hand with the challenge of having to share the patient's information among several professionals, and on the other of having to strengthen the treating hematologist's communication with his or her patient in order for there to be coherence and consistent objectivity in the information given.

Conclusion

In Argentina, information concerning the patient's suffering is usually handled verbally and directly by the treating physician, who is in charge of this task almost exclusively. Access to the treating physician is quite facilitated. Even if the patient establishes a relationship with the rest of the team and a specific institution, the relationship with the treating physician continues to be paramount. Each professional develops a very particular style of communication. There are no systematized protocols for the giving of information, and so there are patients who choose or change their doctor according to the level of communication and relationship they are able to establish, notwithstanding the physician's professional training.

Although for the time being there is no formal education on these communicational aspects of medical treatment, there is great interest in exploring them further and not leaving communication to depend simply on intuition and personal professional experience. The formal education of these topics should take into account the particular characteristics of the doctor–patient relationship in our country (personal, emotional, and direct) as well as adapt to the new challenges presented by the diseases and their various treatments.

References

1. Sanchez N, et al. Preferencias de comunicación y apoyo de pacientes oncológicos españoles. [Preferences of communication and support in Spanish oncology patients]. Psychooncology. 2005;2(1).
2. Isola L, et al. Medicina interna: la formación clínica inicial [Internal medicine: initial clinical education]. Buenos Aires: Editorial Losada; 2009.
3. Vidal y Benito M. La relación médico paciente [Doctor-patient relationship]. Buenos Aires: Editorial Lugar; 2010.
4. Gonzalez Baron M, et al. La relación médico paciente en oncología [Doctor-patient relationship in oncology]. Barcelona: Editorial ARS Médica; 2002.
5. Die Trill M. Psiconcologia [Psycho oncology]. Madrid: Editorial Ades; 2003.

6. Vidal y Benito M. Psiquiatría y psicología del paciente con cáncer [Psychiatry and psychology in cancer patients]. Buenos Aires: Editorial Polemos; 2008.
7. Bartram CR, de Klein A, Hagemeijer A, et al. Translocation of c-abl oncogene correlates with the presence of a Philadelphia chromosome in chronic myelocytic leukaemia. Nature. 1983;306:277–80.
8. Druker BJ, Tamura S, Buchdunger E, et al. Effects of a selective inhibitor of the Abl-tyrosine kinase on the growth of Bcr-Abl positive cells. Nat Med. 1996;2:561–6.
9. Partridge AH, Avorn J, Wang PS, et al. Adherence to therapy with oral antineoplastic agents. J Natl Cancer Inst. 2001;94:652–6.
10. Noens L, van Lierde M-A, De Bock R, et al. Prevalence, determinants, and outcomes of non adherence to imatinib therapy in patients with chronic myeloid leukemia: the ADAGIO study. Blood. 2009;113:5401–11.
11. De Simeone G. El final de la vida: situaciones clínicas y cuestionamientos éticos [End of life: clinical situations and ethical questions]
12. Bayes R. Psicología del sufrimiento y de la muerte [Psychology of suffering and death]. Barcelona: Editorial Martinez Roca; 2001.
13. Gomez Sacho M. Como dar las malas noticias en medicina [How to give bad news in medicine]. Madrid: Editorial Aran; 2006.
14. Arranz P, et al. Intervención emocional en cuidados paliativos. Modelos y protocolos [Emotional intervention in palliative care. Models and protocols]. Barcelona: Editorial Ariel; 2005.
15. De Simone G. Final de Vida: situaciones clínicas y cuestionamientos éticos. Cuadernos del Programa Regional de Bioética OPS/OMS [End of life: clinical situations and questions. Journal of the Regional Bioethics Program PAHO/WHO]. Acta Bioethica. 2000;VI(1):47–62.
16. Gonzalez Baron M, Lacasta M, et al. El sindrome de agotamiento profesional en oncologia [Syndrome of professional exhaustion in oncology]. Madrid: Editorial Panamericana; 2008.

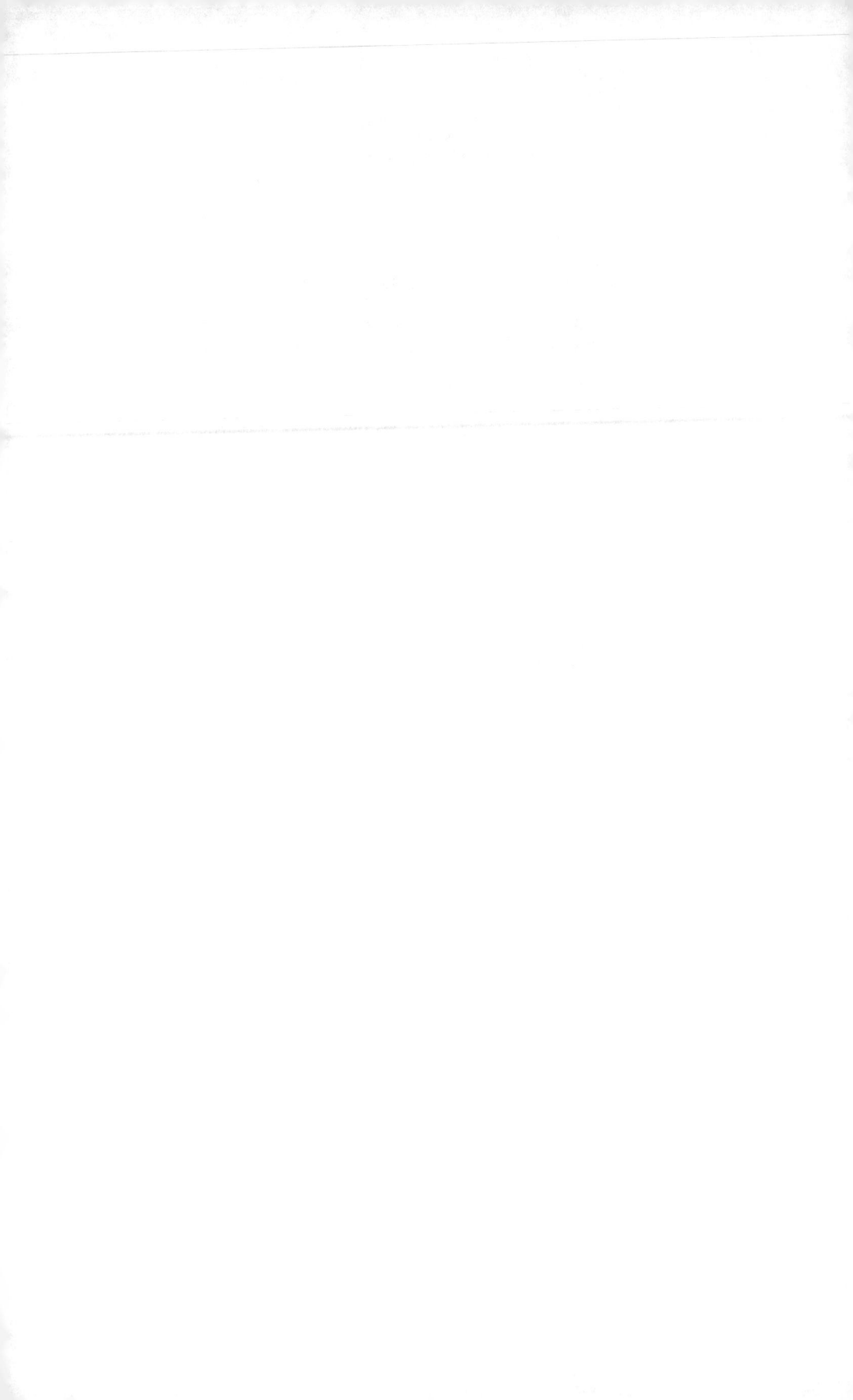

Chapter 30
Teaching Culturally Competent Communication with Diverse Ethnic Patients and Families

Marjorie Kagawa-Singer

Abstract Cultural competence is a critical skill set for improving the quality of health care, working toward equity in its availability, and eliminating health disparities among diverse population groups. Eliminating sociocultural, language, and health literacy barriers to effective clinician/patient and family communication could significantly improve the quality of appropriate and acceptable cancer care provided along the entire cancer care continuum from screening and early detection, timely and state-of-the art treatment, quality palliative care, long-term follow-up, and supportive end-of-life care.

This chapter will define culture and cultural competency, and then provide suggestions to conduct more culturally based communication strategies to build trust between the patient and his or her family members and the clinician. Once trust has been established, it will be easier respectfully to create the basis for more productive dialogue and enable the patient, family, and clinician to negotiate more mutually agreeable goals for care.

Keywords Culture • Cultural competency • Cross-cultural communication • Race and ethnicity • Cancer care • Continuum of care

Two major demographic changes have occurred globally that necessitate changing the nature of the delivery of cancer care: (1) As of 2010, cancer has been the number one cause of death globally [47]; and (2) the globalization of the world's population has exponentially increased cross-cultural encounters clinically. However, our professional training in providing quality care in a multicultural society has not kept pace with these changes.

M. Kagawa-Singer, PhD, MA, MN, RN, FAAN (✉)
Department of Asian American Studies, UCLA School of Public Health,
Los Angeles, CA 90095, USA
e-mail: marjorie.kagawasinger@gmail.com; mkagawa@ucla.edu

In the US, we have some of the most sophisticated technical care to treat cancer available in the world, but we also have unnecessary inequity in access to these treatments by diverse segments of our population, which result in growing disparities in outcomes for cancer by income and ethnic/cultural background. The inequities in the quality of care according to insurance or income status are social and policy problems that will not be addressed in this paper. The focus of this paper is on the inequities that are created by the lack of cultural competence in our healthcare system and the clinicians who work within this system. These issues can and should be addressed immediately to have an impact on the quality of care provided to all Americans in order to bring equity to the care for all cancer patients. For example, the state of California, with a population of over 37 million residents, was the first state of the contiguous US to have no ethnic majority. In Los Angeles County, California, the population distribution of its 9.7 million residents is 55% Latinos/Hispanics, 29% non-Hispanic Whites, 16% Asian Americans and Pacific Islanders, 15% African Americans, 10% two or more race/ethnicities, and 1% American Indians. This combination is predicted to become the face of the US by 2042 [45]. The lessons learned in our multicultural society would likely be of value to others worldwide in developing their own responses to the changing demographics.

One of the major strategies to respond to the impact on communication effectiveness with the growing diversity of cultures of both patients and clinicians is the development of cultural competent skills in patient/family/clinician communication. However, in most curricula on this topic, clear definitions for and understandings of culture itself seem to be missing. Without a definition, practitioners are challenged to know whether or not they are meeting the criteria of competence. Therefore, a clear and strong basic understanding of culture is necessary before we can discuss strategies to overcome cross-cultural misunderstandings and develop culturally competent skills.

Defining Culture

Culture affects every aspect of cancer care for the patient, family, and clinician, but is the least studied of any of the variables that impact health [38]. This omission hinders our ability to ascertain how to measure it and its impact. Table 30.1 lists the major areas of variation due to cultural differences of the patient and family as well as that of the clinician and the healthcare delivery system. Each of the variations can differentially impact communication patterns and the meaning of and discussions about the diagnosis of cancer.

Most often *culture* is used either synonymously with *race* or is reduced to one or two beliefs or values [28]. None of these strategies is correct. Race is a scientific myth [9]. No genetic basis exists for the differentiations currently used to separate groups by racial categories. Genetic polymorphisms exist between population groups, but the distributions of these variations are geographically and environmentally based.

Table 30.1 How culture affects the clinical encounter

Personal and social norms	Clinical effects
Concepts of health and death	Decision-making styles
Mechanistic	Concepts of autonomy
Spiritual	Family member
Metaphysical	Head of the household/clan/village elder or chief as decision-maker
Attitudes toward pain and suffering	Dependency expressions
Meaning of cancer	Communication etiquette
Experience personally	Gender roles
Experience socially	Age
Concepts of "privacy"/individuality	Education
Drug metabolism due to genetic polymorphisms	Class
Fast/slow	Communication patterns
Pharmacodynamics	Silence/nonverbal
Pharmacokinetics	Direct or third-person focused
Appropriate emotional responses	Truth-telling
Anger	
Resignation	
Expressive or stoic	
Social support: who, what, and when	

For example, triple-negative breast cancers (TNBC) are defined as breast cancer that is negative for estrogen receptor, progesterone receptor, and human epidermal growth factor receptor 2; they portend poor outcomes. This variant of breast cancer, found in African-American women, is not unique to African-American women as had commonly been thought. Similar incidence of this aggressive cancer is also found among low-income women in Scotland [5], leading to speculation that this occurrence may be part of a gene-environment phenomenon exacerbated by conditions of poverty. A recent study found that the prevalence of TNBC for Hispanic women was higher than that reported in White women with breast cancer [31].

Ethnicity is defined as one's sense of identity as a member of a cultural group within a power structure of a multicultural society and is identified by others as a member of that group based upon sociohistorical context. Thus, ethnicity is socially constructed, contextual, and dynamic [27]. How individuals identify with their ethnicity can be separate from their phenotypic experience, but it is essential to their sense of self and the lifestyles they choose. For example, consider a middle-aged woman of Korean heritage who was adopted as an orphan by a non-Hispanic White family of German heritage in Wisconsin. She never experienced Korean culture and ethnically identified completely as non-Hispanic White. Therefore, she had none of the behavioral risk factors typical of her Korean ancestry, such as pickled or fermented foods, smoking, or drinking behaviors. Her social experience as someone who looks "different" from her community, however, may impact how she responds to health professionals or how the healthcare system reacts to her.

Culture is the core, fundamental, dynamic, responsive, adaptive, and relatively coherent organizing system of life designed to ensure the survival and well-being of its members and to provide common ways of finding meaning and purpose throughout their lives and to communicate caring and need. Culture, has two major functions. It serves as a tool to (1) assure the survival and well-being of its members and (2) provide the meaning of and for life and the means to make predictable and controllable the unpredictable and inevitable. The most recognizable elements of culture are its beliefs, values, and lifestyle. However, the other elements of culture actually mold the beliefs, values, and lifestyle of its members, but are less visible and usually not acknowledged as part of culture. The seven nested elements of culture begin with its environment, which determines its economy and technology [22]. From this emanates its worldview, religion, and language. Together, these elements inform the social structure that connects the preceding five elements; and then the beliefs, values, and lifestyle are formed to integrate the seven elements into a coherent whole. The environment is a critical element in assessing the culture of a population group, for it differentially affects populations due to social, political, and geographic variations [4]. For example, various tools implements are used by every cultural group to provide shelter and facilitate work.

Thus, culture is a multilevel, multidimensional, and dynamic biopsychosocial ecological system in which a population of people exists and enables them to manipulate the environment for food and shelter, to make cognitive and emotional sense of the chaos of reality around them, to find meaningful, structured modes of social interactions interpersonally and institutionally to support the well-being of its members, and to provide the rules of behavior that define a good person and prescribes the means to live a life worth living. Importantly, culture provides ways to make sense of life events, especially at times of trial, such as when a person develops cancer, through its worldview or construction of reality [17, 26].

Culture enables its members to make sickness and death more comprehensible and manageable through specific beliefs, values, and rituals. It shapes appropriate emotional reactions and behavioral responses to the disease and how one's social network communicates caring and provides safety and social support. Thus, diet, marriage rules, social roles, and means of livelihood that influence gene expression, health status, and disease prevalence are largely culturally prescribed or proscribed [6, 14].

Culture, then, is not merely a collection of beliefs and values interchangeable on the same template as that of the culture of the northern European-American dominant culture [4]. Since these factors vary and develop dynamically due to geographic, social, and political circumstances, cultures evolve differently. Efforts to apply the concept of culture in medical practice would require an assessment of the critical elements within the system and across time [26]. The current lack of precision in this regard results, at best, in misleading assumptions or stereotypes about individuals [37, 40] and impedes our ability to recognize the contribution of each component and culture to cancer outcomes along the entire continuum of care [15, 33].

Notably, definitions of health also differ by culture. For example, in one study, Japanese-Americans with end-stage cancer saw themselves as healthy according to their definition which was the ability to work towards life objectives and full and fulfilling lives as an essential part of their social network [21]. Their physical health framed their definition, but was not part of their definition; the criterion used was social function—fulfilling their role in their social network.

Thus, a more accurate definition of culture requires this holistic understanding of the dynamic nature of culture that is designed to adapt to changing time and place to maintain the well-being of its members. The velocity of change today and the exposure to a multitude of alternatives, however, is much greater than most cultures can adapt to as an integrated system; so different aspects are changing at different rates, creating tensions and contradictions within any of the systems. Therefore, stereotypical assumptions about any culture will likely be wrong, and clinicians must be open-minded and skilled enough to elicit the information needed to interact effectively with patients and families from diverse backgrounds.

Cultural Competency

Cultural competency describes a means to work more effectively in culturally discordant encounters and ultimately provide quality care and achieve optimal health outcomes [42]. Cultural competency enables researchers and practitioners to communicate more effectively with individuals of backgrounds different from their own [11, 25]. Using a skill set that ranges on a five-point continuum from culturally destructive to skilled, with three stages in between. One's skill level differs with each culture; therefore, complacency is not an option if we want to deliver quality care to all patients and families with cancer.

Culturally competent care enables the practitioner in a culturally discordant encounter respectfully to elicit (from the patient and family) the information needed to (1) make an accurate diagnosis and—a critical point—(2) negotiate mutually satisfactory goals for treatment. Both goals require ongoing discussions with patients and families as they are able to absorb the information and as clinical conditions change. The practitioner systematically integrates this knowledge and understanding to make an accurate diagnosis, take acceptable and appropriate action for care, develop credibility with the patient and family, and ultimately create a relationship of trust, acceptance, and mutual respect for one another's values, beliefs, and practices, especially when they may not be in agreement [7, 13].

The Economic Burden of Health Disparities in the United States

Notably, the persistence of health disparities in the US is not only an issue of equity and social justice, but it is also an enormous and avoidable economic burden. The US spends $2.2 trillion (>16% of GNP) on health care. LaVeist et al. [32] used three measures to calculate the cost of health disparities: (1) direct medical costs of health inequalities, (2) indirect costs of health inequalities, and (3) costs of premature death [32]. Indirect costs include lost productivity, lost wages, absenteeism, family leave to deal with avoidable illness, and lower quality of life. Premature death imposes significant costs on society in the form of lower wages, lost tax revenue, additional services and benefits for families of the deceased, and lower quality of life for the survivors. They found that between 2000 and 2006, the combined costs of health inequalities and premature death in the US were $1.24 trillion. Eliminating health disparities for African Americans, Asian Americans, and Hispanics would have reduced direct medical care expenditures by $229.4 billion dollars. Elimination of the indirect costs noted above would have more than tripled this saving.

Changing Demographics

For all countries, the globalization of the economy also brings large waves of new immigrants. This has implications for health education and clinical awareness as well, because the sites and incidence of cancers change as immigrants adapt to the host countries' lifestyles, such as in food, parity, and age of marriage. Within 10 years, the cancer sites and rates for new immigrants to the US begin to mirror those of the host country [1, 18, 41]. For example, the fastest growing rate of breast cancers is among Asian-American women. Japanese-American women, who have been in the US the longest, with the fewest new immigrants, now show rates of breast cancer about equal to non-Hispanic White women, who have the highest rates of breast cancer in the US [12, 34]. Thus, clinicians cannot assume that a particular cultural or ethnic group has the same cancer rates as they do in their home countries. These communities also need education about their increasing need for screening and early detection strategies in the host country and the changing disease incidence rates. Another example is a study of the top five cancers for Filipino men in Manila and in the US. Prostate cancer is now the leading cause of cancer for Filipino men in the US, whereas in the Philippines it is number three and lung cancer is the leading site for cancer. Both clinicians and the Filipino community should be aware of these differences [39].

Culturally Competent Practice

Culturally competent practice requires more than knowledge and skill building by clinicians; it also requires health delivery systems to be culturally competent [11, 25].

This requires attention to three main areas: a business model that integrates stewardship of resources to translate efforts into savings and integrates consumer choice; second the legal realm, which requires meeting the new JAHCO requirements for cultural competency [44], the federal Culturally and Linguistically Appropriate

Services requirements according to the Office of Civil Rights; and Title VI, which addresses language access with trained medical interpreters and risk management [46]. For example, one of the highest sources of lawsuits is lack of language concordance. The third area, healthcare outcomes that directly address the elimination of disparities in outcome for cancer care, was outlined in the 2002 Institute of Medicine Report on Unequal Care, which clearly shows that health disparities are due primarily to biased or differential care, prejudice, the operation of healthcare systems, and the legal and regulatory climate [19]. Genetic differences are not part of this equation. The identified barriers are all under our control as health professionals to eliminate disparities in cancer outcomes among diverse population groups.

Universally, it appears that patients and families all want the same thing from their clinicians: (1) not to be abandoned, (2) to be respected as an individual, and (3) to be understood and cared for and to have their fears addressed. Their disease-specific concerns revolve around knowing their prognosis and the effect on their own life as well as their family's life; then they can determine if the treatments will preserve a life worth living [23].

However, the one area that makes cross-cultural interactions most difficult and problematic in the US is probably the issue of truth-telling [2, 3, 8, 10, 16, 20, 24, 36]. Many physicians today do not remember that prior to 1976 physicians in the US did not give the diagnosis of cancer to their patients. Giving the diagnosis of cancer was thought to be unethical because it would take away hope. However, with the patients' rights movement and better treatments, this practice changed completely over the next several years. Yet notably today, the practice of giving the diagnosis to all patients exists in only a handful of countries besides the US, such as England, Germany, the Netherlands, and the Scandinavian countries. For most of the rest of the world, the diagnosis is given to varying degrees and usually for only a few cancer sites. Thus, for many of our newer immigrant families, giving the diagnosis is felt to be cruel and unethical. For some, effective treatments for cancer are not available in their home countries, and cancer is still, almost always, a death sentence. For others, giving such potentially bad news is culturally just not condoned. The phrase, "…and the truth shall make you free" is a Judeo-Christian concept from the Book of John and is not of equal validity as a moral belief in other cultures. Desire for such truth differs individually as well. However, what is most important is that the "truth" has different meanings and often can be told indirectly. Many cultures are highly skilled in tangential, inferential styles of communication. The message is the same, but the means may be quite different [43].

One example is Japan. A young couple wished to marry, but wanted the blessings of their respective parents. The girl's parents were supportive, but the young man's mother was not. The young couple beseeched the girl's mother to speak to the young man's mother. She acquiesced and scheduled a tea at the young man's mother's home. After the meeting, the mother reported that the other mother would not give her approval. When asked how the conversation unfolded, the young couple was told that the mothers did not speak about the couple at all. When asked how she then could possibly know the intent of the young man's mother, the young woman's mother said that when the young man's mother served her tea, she accompanied the tea with two small cakes. Each of the cakes had different cultural meanings, but when served together, were totally incompatible. Therefore, without a word being spoken about the subject at hand, the young woman's mother knew that the issue was closed. The young man's mother had clearly communicated her feelings. Information and intention can be powerfully and clearly communicated nonverbally. Notably, only about 7% of communications of feelings and attitudes are verbal [35]. Most cultures in the world place more value on what is communicated nonverbally than verbally in assessing the veracity of the information exchanged. This is usually not stressed in clinical training. How one communicates is as important as what is communicated in words, and the how varies immensely cross-culturally.

Suggested Practice Strategies

The goal of good cross-cultural communication requires that the message delivered has the desired impact. This seemingly simple goal is fraught with difficulties when discussing cancer diagnoses and treatment choices with those of one's own culture, and the difficulties are magnified when the encounters are across cultures. Thus, effective cross-cultural communication requires the elimination of cultural and structural barriers that restrict the healing process. Importantly, these cultural and structural barriers are not just those of the patient and family, but include the cultural assumptions of the clinician, the support staff, and the healthcare system [25].

One of the first steps in communication about cancer is the fundamental fact that this disease is a family condition, not only a condition of the patient with the diagnosis. As such, communication about diagnosis, treatment, and follow-up care should, with the patient's consent, include the family members he or she designates as essential to the conversations. Kleinman developed a list of questions for clinicians to use in assessing what the patient and family understand and what their expectations are of the diagnosis and treatment—the patient's Explanatory Model for his/her condition [30]. These questions elicit the patient's world view and enable the clinician to probe more deeply into the responses to understand what the meaning of cancer is to the patient and how the condition will affect the patient him-/herself and, as importantly, how it will affect the family. Notably, the family carries different definitions cross-culturally, and this information should also be elicited. The patient or family also indicates how much information should be communicated and, importantly, to whom; for some patients, it may not be a biological family member, but a clan or tribal leader.

Table 30.2 lists Kleinman's seven questions [29]. The clinician must not use the term *cancer* initially, until the patient indicates that he or she knows or is open to knowing. Kleinman purposely begins with the term *condition* and then uses the patient's response to determine subsequent questions, then leads into the clinical discussion according to the guidelines established by the patient. This strategy serves two purposes: The clinician learns about the patient's understanding of

Table 30.2 Beginning the conversation with an explanatory framework [29]

What is your understanding of your condition?
What is your understanding of what you can expect from the treatments?
Tell me what the time frame is for you with this condition?
What kinds of changes would you like us to consider in your treatment?
What are the most important results you hope to receive from this treatment?
What are the chief problems the treatments have caused for you and your family?
What can we provide for you and your family to help you make the decisions you are facing?

appropriate treatment of the illness, which can then serve as a basis for negotiation regarding the communication of information. Second, the patient feels that the clinician truly wants to know about his/her feelings and understanding. The patient will feel listened to, heard, and cared for as an individual. This is the bedrock of trust, especially in such a frightening situation as having cancer. Knowing that your doctor truly wants to hear and listen and respects your personal and cultural individuality is an extremely powerful basis to build on to effectively reduce the unequal burden of cancer and to eliminate unnecessary mortality and suffering from cancer. Our goal is to optimize care. Effective and caring communication is the key.

References

1. Babey SH, Ponce NA, Etzioni DA, Spencer BA, Brown ER, Chawla N. Cancer screening in California: racial and ethnic disparities persist. Policy Brief UCLA Cent Health Policy Res. 2003;PB2003-4:1–6.
2. Back AL, Arnold RM, Baile WF, Tulsky JA, Fryer-Edwards K. Approaching difficult communication tasks in oncology. CA Cancer J Clin. 2005;55(3):164–77.
3. Baider L, Surbone A. Cancer and the family: the silent words of truth. J Clin Oncol. 2010;28(7):1269–72.
4. Bourdieu P. In other words: essay towards a reflexive sociology (M. Adamson, Trans.). Stanford, CA: Stanford University Press; 1990.
5. Brawley OW, Smith DE, Kirch RA. Taking action to ease suffering: advancing cancer pain control as a health care priority. CA Cancer J Clin. 2009;59(5):285–9.
6. Bronfenbrenner U, Ceci S. Nature-nurture reconceptualized in developmental perspective: a bioecologic model. Psychol Rev. 1994;101(4):568–86.
7. Burgess DJ, Ding Y, Hargreaves M, van Ryn M, Phelan S. The association between perceived discrimination and underutilization of needed medical and mental health care in a multi-ethnic community sample. J Health Care Poor Underserved. 2008;19(3):894–911.
8. Chiu LQ, Lee WS, Gao F, Parker PA, Ng GY, Toh CK. Cancer patients' preferences for communication of unfavourable news: an Asian perspective. Support Care Cancer. 2006;14(8):818–24.
9. Collins FS. What we do and don't know about 'race', 'ethnicity', genetics and health at the dawn of the genome era. Nat Genet. 2004;36:S13–5.
10. Costantini A, Baile WF, Lenzi R, Constantini M, Ziparo V, Marchetti P, et al. Overcoming cultural barriers to giving bad news: feasibility of training to promote truth-telling to cancer patients. J Cancer Educ. 2009;24(3):180–5.

11. Cross TL, Bazron BJ, Dennis KW, Isaacs MR. Towards a culturally competent system of care: a monograph on effective services for minority children who are severely emotionally disturbed. Washington, DC: Child and Adolescent Service System Program (CASSP), CASSP Technical Assistance Center, Georgetown University Child Development Center; 1989.
12. Deapen D, Cockburn ME. Cancer in Los Angeles County: trends by race/ethnicity, 1976–2000. Los Angeles: Los Angeles Cancer Surveillance Program, University of Southern California; 2003.
13. Dovidio JF, Penner LA, Albrecht TL, Norton WE, Gaertner SL, Shelton JN. Disparities and distrust: the implications of psychological processes for understanding racial disparities in health and health care. Soc Sci Med. 2008;67(3):478–86.
14. Dressler W. Culture and the risk of disease. Br Med Bull. 2004;69(1):21–31.
15. Epstein R, Street Jr RL. Patient-centered communication in cancer care: promoting healing and reducing suffering. Bethesda: National Cancer Institute; 2007.
16. Freedman B. Offering truth. One ethical approach to the uninformed cancer patient. Arch Intern Med. 1993;153(5):572–6.
17. Hartigan J. Race in the 21st century: ethnographic approaches. New York: Oxford University Press; 2010.
18. Institute of Medicine. In: The unequal burden of cancer: an assessment of NIH research and programs for ethnic minorities and the medically underserved. Haynes MA, Smedley BD, editors. Washington, DC: National Academy Press; 1999. p. 339.
19. Institute of Medicine. In: Unequal treatment: confronting racial and ethnic disparities in health care. Smedley BD, Stith AY, Nelson AR, editors. Washington, DC: National Academy Press; 2002. p. 768.
20. Jotkowitz A, Glick S, Gezundheit B. Truth-telling in a culturally diverse world. Cancer Invest. 2006;24(8):786–9.
21. Kagawa-Singer M. Bamboo and oak: differences in adaptation to cancer between Japanese-American and Anglo-American patients. Unpublished dissertation. Los Angeles: University of California; 1988.
22. Kagawa-Singer M. From genes to social science: impact of the simplistic interpretation of race, ethnicity, and culture on cancer outcome. Cancer. 2001;91(1 Suppl):226–32.
23. Kagawa-Singer M, Chung R. A paradigm for culturally based care for minority populations. J Community Psychol. 1994;22(2):192–208.
24. Kagawa-Singer M, Emmons KM. Behavioral theory in a diverse society: moving our field forward. Health Educ Behav. 2009;36(5 Suppl):172S–6.
25. Kagawa-Singer M, Kassim-Lakha S. A strategy to reduce cross-cultural miscommunication and increase the likelihood of improving health outcomes. Acad Med. 2003;78(6):577–87.
26. Kagawa-Singer M, Valdez-Dadia A, Yu MC, Surbone A. Cancer, culture, and health disparities: time to chart a new course? CA Cancer J Clin. 2010;60(1):12–39.
27. Kagawa Singer M. From genes to social science: color coding cancer care. Cancer. 2000;91(1):226–32.
28. Kagawa Singer M. Where is culture in cultural tailoring? In: McMullin J, Weiner D, editors. Confronting cancer: metaphors, inequality, and advocacy. Santa Fe: School of American Research; 2009. p. 207–29.
29. Kleinman A. Patients and healers in the context of culture: an exploration of the borderland between anthropology, medicine, and psychiatry. Berkeley: University of California Press; 1980.
30. Kleinman A, Eisenberg L, Good B. Culture, illness, and care: clinical lessons from anthropologic and cross-cultural research. Ann Intern Med. 1978;88(2):251–8.
31. Lara-Medina F, Perez-Sanchez V, Saavedra-Perez D, Blake-Cerda M, Arce C, Motola-Kuba D, et al. Triple-negative breast cancer in Hispanic patients: high prevalence, poor prognosis, and association with menopausal status, body mass index, and parity. Cancer. 2011;117(16): 3658–69.
32. LaVeist TA, Gaskin DJ, Richard P. The economic burden of health inequities in the United States. Washington, DC: Joint Center of Political and Economic Studies; 2009.

33. Maly RC, Umezawa Y, Ratliff CT, Leake B. Racial/ethnic group differences in treatment decision-making and treatment received among older breast carcinoma patients. Cancer. 2006;106(4): 957–65.
34. McCracken M, Olsen M, Chen Jr MS, Jemal A, Thun M, Cokkinides V, et al. Cancer incidence, mortality, and associated risk factors among Asian Americans of Chinese, Filipino, Vietnamese, Korean, and Japanese ethnicities. CA Cancer J Clin. 2007;57(4):190–205.
35. Mehrabian A. Silent messages: implicit communication of emotions and attitudes. Belmont: Wadsworth; 1981.
36. Moy B, Polite BN, Halpern MT, Stranne SK, Winer EP, Wollins DS, et al. American society of clinical oncology policy statement: opportunities in the patient protection and affordable care act to reduce cancer care disparities. J Clin Oncol. 2011;29(28):3816–24. doi:10.1200/JCO.2011.35.8903.
37. Group NP. Illuminating BiDil. Nat Biotechnol. 2005;23(8):903.
38. Oppenheimer GM. Paradigm lost: race, ethnicity, and the search for a new population taxonomy. Am J Public Health. 2001;91(7):1049–55.
39. Prehn A, Lin S, Clarke C, Packel L, Lum R, Lui S, et al. Cancer incidence in Chinese, Japanese and Filipinos in the US and Asia 1988–1992. Union City: Northern California Cancer Center; 1999. p. 24.
40. Sankar P, Kahn J. BiDil: race medicine or race marketing? Health Aff (Millwood). 2005;Suppl Web Exclusives:W5-455-63.
41. Smith BD, Smith GL, Hurria A, Hortobagyi GN, Buchholz TA. Future of cancer incidence in the United States: burdens upon an aging, changing nation. J Clin Oncol. 2009;27(17): 2758–65.
42. Surbone A. Cultural competence in oncology: where do we stand? Ann Oncol. 2010; 21(1):3–5.
43. Surbone A, Ritossa C, Spagnolo AG. Evolution of truth-telling attitudes and practices in Italy. Crit Rev Oncol Hematol. 2004;52(3):165–72.
44. The Joint Commission. Advancing effective communication, cultural competence, and patient- and family-centered care: a roadmap for hospitals. Oakbrook Terrace, IL: The Joint Commission on Accreditation of Healthcare Organizations; 2010. p. 102.
45. U.S. Census Bureau. State and County quick facts. 2010. http://quickfacts.census.gov/qfd/states/06/06037.html. Accessed 14 Aug 2011.
46. U.S. Department of Health and Human Services Office of Minority Health. National Standards on Culturally and Linguistically Appropriate Services (CLAS). 2007. http://minorityhealth.hhs.gov/templates/browse.aspx?lvl=2&lvlID=15. Accessed 14 Aug 2011.
47. World Health Organization. World cancer report 2008. Lyon: International Agency for Research on Cancer; 2008.

Chapter 31
Breaking Bad News and Truth Disclosure in Australia

Phyllis Butow, Martin H.N. Tattersall, Josephine Clayton, and David Goldstein

Abstract Effective communication is a core component of quality cancer care, yet is challenging for patients and doctors alike. Many doctors find that "breaking bad news" consultations are particularly difficult and stressful. This chapter addresses how truth-telling within bad news consultations is approached in Australia. The cultural norm is for open disclosure and truth-telling, yet there are many situations in which physicians still struggle to break bad news, with little support or training. Unique features of the Australian environment, and Australian government policy, clinical practice guidelines, and training opportunities for breaking bad news, are reviewed. Evidence on current practice in Australia is presented. Cultural issues,

P. Butow (✉)
Centre for Medical Psychology and Evidence-based Medicine (CeMPED), School of Psychology and Department of Medicine, University of Sydney, Sydney, NSW 2006, Australia

Psycho-Oncology Co-operative Research Group, University of Sydney,
Sydney NSW 2006, Australia
e-mail: phyllis.butow@sydney.edu.au

M.H.N. Tattersall
Centre for Medical Psychology and Evidence-based Medicine (CeMPED), School of Psychology and Department of Medicine, University of Sydney, Sydney, NSW 2006, Australia
e-mail: martin.tattersall@synde.edu.au

J. Clayton
Centre for Medical Psychology and Evidence-based Medicine (CeMPED), School of Psychology and Department of Medicine, University of Sydney, Sydney, NSW 2006, Australia

HammondCare Palliative and Supportive Care Service, Greenwich Hospital,
Sydney, NSW 2006, Australia
e-mail: josephine.clayton@sydney.edu.au

D. Goldstein
Department of Medical Oncology, Prince of Wales Hospital, Randwick Sydney, NSW 2031, Australia
e-mail: d.goldstein@unsw.edu.au

which are of great importance in a multi-cultural society such as Australia, are discussed. Finally, Australian-developed tools to facilitate bad news discussions are described, and recommendations for the future are made.

Keywords Oncology • Breaking bad news • Truth disclosure • Cross cultural

Introduction

Patients and doctors confront the diagnosis of cancer with grave discomfort. Challenges for patients throughout the time course of cancer include existential concerns, dealing with uncertain outcomes, grappling with unfamiliar concepts, fear of tests, and treatments, coping with problematic side effects of treatment, difficulties in adjusting to physical changes in body appearance and functioning, social disruption, and financial concerns. Many doctors find that "breaking bad news" consultations are particularly difficult and stressful, even when the news they are delivering is relatively hopeful. This chapter addresses how truth-telling, within a context of patient-centered care delivery, is approached in Australia.

Demographic Factors Influencing Communication with Cancer Patients in Australia

Australia is a modern, developed country that has a relatively small population of approximately 20 million people, living in eight states and territories, in an area approximately the size of Western Europe. Health care is funded at both the federal and state levels and includes a mixture of public and private health service delivery. Australia has a national health insurance system (Medicare) that provides universal access to health services. Private health insurance covers fees for private hospitals and selected doctors in public hospitals, in addition to allied health services and optical and dental care. Thus in general, high-quality health care is easily accessible.

While most people live in an urban environment, 31% live in rural and remote areas [1], thus making access to health care more difficult. Rural people often have to travel a long way to medical facilities and appointments, making telephone communication of bad news more likely and desired.

While free public education is widely available and most Australians now complete at least 12 years of schooling, of Australians aged between 15–74 years in 2006–2007, fewer than half (41%) have an adequate or better level of health literacy [2]. This can make communication of complex information, such as prognosis, more challenging.

Australia is very multicultural. In 2006, 24% of people living in Australia were born overseas, 44% had at least one parent born overseas, and over 560,000 people (3% of the total population) spoke a language other than English and spoke English poorly or not at all [3]. Immigrants often report that they struggle with language difficulties, that they lack information, and that health professionals do not understand them [4–7]. Communicating bad news is particularly challenging in this context, because immigrants may come with expectations based on the norms of their home country, which may include nondisclosure or disclosure through the family, and communication may be either hampered by language difficulties or forced to occur through an interpreter.

Policy Factors Influencing Communication with Cancer Patients in Australia

In Australia, a culture of disclosure of the diagnosis of cancer is widely endorsed and practiced, on the basis of medical ethics and patient autonomy. Australian policy makers have strongly endorsed patient-centered care and shared decision making over the past 20 years. The Australian Council for Safety and Quality in Health Care recently developed an *Australian Charter of Healthcare Rights* [8], which stipulates among other things that all Australians have the right to:

- Receive care that shows respect to them and their culture, beliefs, values, and personal characteristics;
- Receive open, timely, and appropriate communication about their health care in a way they can understand;
- Join in making decisions about their care and health service planning.

The Australian Government Department of Health & Aging receives advice and recommendations from the National Health & Medical Research Council (NHMRC). The NHMRC has published a series of booklets on doctor-patient communication. One [9], *Communicating with Patients: Advice for medical practitioners,* states that:

> Information should not be withheld from patients. There are very few exceptions to this principle, but these include:
>
> - Situations in which a patient expressly directs the doctor or another person to make the decisions, and does not want the offered information.
> - Even in these situations, the doctor should give the patient basic information about the illness, proposed treatments and the risks involved, and be satisfied that the patient understands both their right to receive information and that this right is being waived.
> - Situations where a patient has impaired decision-making capacity, and the legally appropriate person requests that information not be provided either to the patient or to that person.
> - Situations where there is good reason for the doctor to believe that the patient's physical or mental health might be seriously harmed by the information. Information should not be withheld simply because the patient might be disconcerted or dismayed, or because the doctor finds giving particular information difficult or unpleasant. The doctor needs to identify and address the concerns of family and carers about perceptions that the patient will be harmed by full disclosure.
> - Situations where there is good reason for the doctor to believe that another person's physical or mental health might be seriously harmed by the information. Examples include issues such as domestic violence and intrafamilial child abuse.

Guidelines and Training

In the past 20 years there has been growing recognition in Australia that communication, and in particular breaking bad news and truth-telling, is challenging and requires specific guidance and training. This has led to a proliferation of communication research and the development of specific guidelines addressing these topics. For example, the authors of this chapter have been involved in research in the discussion of prognosis [10, 11] and end-of-life (EOL) issues [12, 13], shared decision-making [14], and strategies to promote patient involvement in decision-making [15, 16]. Australia produced some of the first guidelines internationally on breaking bad news in 1995 [17]. The NSW Cancer Council published several Interactional Skills Manuals in 1997, including one on "Breaking Bad News" [18] and others addressing adherence, smoking cessation, and preparing patients for aversive procedures.

In addition, the Australian National Breast Cancer Centre published *Clinical Practice Guidelines for the psychosocial care of adults with cancer* in 2003 [19]. These summarize the research evidence relating to means of maintaining cancer patients' emotional health. The guidelines encourage doctors to use supportive communication skills in their interaction with patients, to provide adequate and tailored information, to elicit patients' preferred role in treatment decision-making, and to use strategies that are likely to aid patients in their recall and understanding of information. Finally, Australian guidelines for communicating prognosis and EOL issues with adults in the advanced stages of a life-limiting illness and their caregivers were published in 2007 [20].

Australian Clinical Practice Guidelines for specific tumors also emphasize patient-centered care. For example, the Clinical Practice Guidelines for the Management of Melanoma in Australia and New Zealand published in 2008 [21] state in their Executive Summary that: "Approved communication skills training should help promote patient-centered care, shared decision-making, empathy and support where desired."

These guidelines and policy documents have stimulated the development of communication skills training courses in medical schools, and the establishment of training courses particularly for oncologists. The Oncology Education Committee of the Cancer Council Australia recently launched the *Ideal Oncology Curriculum for Medical Schools: Knowledge, Skills and Attitudes of Medical Students at Graduation* [22], in which communication skills are identified as one of the core skills and competencies in oncology that graduating medical students should possess. The Australian Medical Council's Accreditation Standards for Medical Schools [23] advise that all medical graduates should involve patients in formulating a management plan, and should be good listeners and be able to provide information in a manner that allows patients and families to be fully informed. At a more senior level, the National Breast and Ovarian Cancer Centre developed and offered communication skills training to a variety of cancer health care professionals over many years, while several professional groups, such as the Medical Oncology Group of Australia and the College of Physicians Chapter of Palliative Medicine, have made communication skills training compulsory for junior medical staff training as specialists. Communication skills workshops are now running regularly at the annual meeting of the Medical Oncology Group of Australia and by the College of Physicians. Nevertheless, most training in both medical schools and at a senior level is very limited, comprising 0.5–3 day courses with little follow-up to consolidate learning.

Truth-Telling in Australia

Breaking bad news includes communicating not only the original diagnosis, but the prognosis, news of recurrence, treatment failure, the futility of further active anticancer treatment, the transition from curative to palliative care, bad test results, and approaching end of life. Australian research has documented that a clear majority of cancer patients, both with early and late stage cancer, report a preference for detailed information about their disease and prognosis and that this information be given in a direct and honest manner [11, 24].

With an increased culture of open disclosure, comfort with breaking the news of diagnosis has increased. In 1997, a survey of Australian surgeons showed that 80% felt the need for further training in breaking bad news [25]. However, in a similar survey of 134 cancer specialists conducted in 2008 [26] (see Table 31.1), fewer than five reported having a lot of difficulty with any task involving communicating bad news, and only 32% reported *any* difficulty with disclosing the diagnosis. More reported some to quite a bit of difficulty in discussing treatment failure (67%), the transition from curative to palliative care (60%), recurrence of cancer (60%), and bad test results (59%); and being completely honest about prognosis (38%).

Table 31.1 The level of difficulty reported by cancer specialists associated with various consultation tasks

Item	Not at all	Somewhat	Quite a bit	A lot
I find it difficult to:				
Tell patients they have cancer	91 (68)	38 (28)	5 (4)	0
Tell patients they have a cancer recurrence	51 (38)	66 (49)	15 (11)	2 (2)
Discuss bad test results with a patient	55 (41)	68 (51)	11 (8)	0
Discuss treatment failure	44 (33)	74 (56)	14 (11)	1 (1)
Discuss transition from curative to supportive care with patients	50 (38)	68 (51)	12 (9)	3 (2)
Bring up the topic of do-not-resuscitate	49 (37)	61 (46)	19 (14)	4 (3)
Respond to patients when they are emotional	53 (41)	63 (48)	13 (10)	2 (2)
Be completely honest about a patient's prognosis	81 (61)	45 (34)	5 (4)	2 (2)
Discuss high-cost drugs with patients I know cannot afford them	28 (22)	56 (44)	26 (21)	17 (13)
Discuss complementary therapies with patients	75 (57)	44 (33)	11 (8)	2 (2)
Deal with patients when I have problems at home	57 (44)	62 (47)	10 (7)	2 (2)

Interestingly, the communication task they found most difficult, was "discussing high-cost drugs with patients I know cannot afford them," with 13% reporting having a lot of difficulty with this and 65% reporting some to quite a bit of difficulty with this (Table 31.1).

Communication with Family Members

Disclosure is potentially more complex if family members prefer less or more information than the patient. Most studies have found that patients favor complete openness with the family [27], while some have found that patients favored openness with family members but rejected unconditional disclosure of information without their consent and rejecting their family influencing what information they would be given [28, 29].

In one Australian and Canadian study, 21 patient–family dyads of primarily Anglo–Australian origin recruited from Perth, Western Australia and 14 dyads and 2 patients in Winnipeg noted that the timing, management, and delivery of information and the perceived attitude of practitioners were critical to the process at all stages of the illness. All patients, regardless of origin, wanted information about their illness and wanted it fully shared with relatives. Almost all patients requested prognostic information, and all family members respected their wishes. Information was perceived as important for patient–family communication. The information needs of patient and family changed and diverged as illness progressed, and communication between them became less verbally explicit. The study concluded that information delivery for patients needs to be individualized, with particular attention to the process at all stages of illness.

We discussed communication with patients and families in focus groups and individual interviews with 19 patients with far-advanced cancer and 24 caregivers from 3 palliative care (PC) services in Sydney and 22 PC health professionals from around Australia [30]. A desire to restrict the patient's access to information by the caregiver or vice versa was reported by the health professionals to be one of the most challenging issues they faced when discussing prognosis and EOL issues. The participants had varying views regarding whether patients and caregivers should be told different information concerning prognosis and EOL issues. Some felt it was important to communicate all information to patients and family members together, to encourage open discussion, so that they all had the same information, and to avoid coalitions forming between any of the parties. However, several health professionals said that although it is important not to give conflicting information, it may be very helpful to have separate one-to-one discussions with patients and their caregivers regarding prognosis and EOL issues, because this makes it easier to explore their unique concerns and informational needs. Having separate conversations was thought to allow honesty without worrying about what the other party was feeling. Some nurses said it is useful to have the discussion initially with both the patient and caregiver present and then a separate discussion with only the caregiver that focused on the caregiver's needs. The importance of obtaining the patients' permission first to discuss their condition with family members was emphasized, unless the patient was gravely ill or incapacitated.

The situation in which a family asks the health professional to withhold the diagnosis or prognosis from the patient was described by health professionals as a delicate balance of the family's vs. the patient's rights to information, autonomy, maximal well-being, and confidentiality. Information regarding prognosis and diagnosis was viewed not as being owned by the patient but rather as having an effect on the entire family. Most participants said that they tried to negotiate openness or consented to nondisclosure only if the patient did not ask a direct question, reassuring the family that they would respond only to direct patient questions with the family present.

All participants thought these discussions were particularly challenging if the family and patient were of a different culture from that of the doctor.

Cultural Issues

Since Australia is so multicultural, consideration of cultural issues is particular salient in this country. The evidence suggests that, while Australian patients of Anglo-Saxon background prefer disclosure [24], those from other cultural backgrounds tend to vary more, with a tendency to favor nondisclosure [6, 31].

Members of some cultures may prefer that the family have a high level of involvement in medical consultations and in some cases that the family be informed first of the diagnosis and prognosis and that the patient be either told gradually or not at all. Australian research [6, 31] suggests that family members of immigrant cancer patients may censor information that is provided during consultations, and also may act as principal decision-makers on behalf of patients. Another Australian study [32] found that in many cultures, such as Chinese, Filipino, and Greek, families prefer the doctor to discuss the diagnosis and treatment of cancer with the eldest son rather than with the patient. The family will then decide what the patient should be told, and when. The family would then prepare and emotionally support the patient before telling him/her the bad news. Conversely Dutch, Poles, and Muslims interviewed for this qualitative study believed the patient should be told, whereas Macedonians and Croatians did not want to be told at all.

In our own work, we recently interviewed 73 patients with metastatic cancer (31 Anglo-Australians, 20 Chinese, 11 Arabic, and 11 Greeks) and 65 relatives (25 Anglo-Australians, and 23 Chinese, 11 Arabic, and 7 Greek) regarding their experience of and views on truth-telling [33]. We found that, contrary to previous research, immigrant patients often expressed a desire for open disclosure. However, discordance was common between immigrant patients and their families. Family members often wanted to protect their relatives from emotional distress by meeting with oncologists separately beforehand and directing the oncologists on what and how information should be conveyed to patients. Thus the oncologist faces a complex scenario, with potentially differing preferences and needs within families. In addition, our research has identified the added complexity of the role of and interaction with the interpreter within that dialogue [34]. Initiatives to enhance the interaction of interpreters and health professionals are currently being researched [35]. The need for doctors to avoid possible cultural stereotypes when discussing diagnosis and prognosis in cancer has also been noted [32].

Equally unexpected was our finding that a higher proportion than expected of those with Anglo-Saxon backgrounds requested nondisclosure or more limited disclosure of prognostic information. This reinforces an emerging theme regarding the need to probe the individual's wishes and tailor information disclosure to individual preferences. The initial challenge was to overcome the previously routine tendency to limit disclosure. A much more nuanced approach that moves beyond a new paternalism of insisting on full disclosure is likely to be the challenge of the next decade.

Tools to Assist Doctors and Patients Discuss Bad News

Given the complexity of discussing bad news, resources, and strategies to assist doctors and patients to clarify the information needed and negotiate the process may be helpful. Australian researchers have evaluated a number of interventions to assist at this time, notably question prompt lists (QPLs). These are lists of questions derived from patients, health professionals, and carers that patients and family members may want to ask. The questions are organized into categories for simplicity, and cover areas such as diagnosis and prognosis. The value of QPLs is that they give patients explicit permission to ask questions, knowing that the doctor endorses and welcomes any questions listed on the QPL. Further, patients can choose which questions they want to ask and when to ask them, and thereby control the flow of information they receive. Several randomized controlled trials of QPLs in the Australian context have demonstrated that provision of QPLs increase patient question-asking, particularly regarding prognosis, without increasing consultation duration or patient anxiety, particularly if doctors endorse them [36–38] (Fig. 31.1).

Summary and Conclusions

In summary, while the cultural norm in Australia is for open disclosure and truth-telling, there are many situations in which physicians still struggle to break bad news. The skills required are great, and the training provided is still minimal. There is a continued need for properly conducted randomized trials of communication strategies and interventions to inform evidence-based guidelines for complex disclosure scenarios. Ongoing training should be provided not only at the junior level, but for senior clinicians, who are more likely to be delivering grave news. Guidelines and training in culturally competent care are urgently needed in this area.

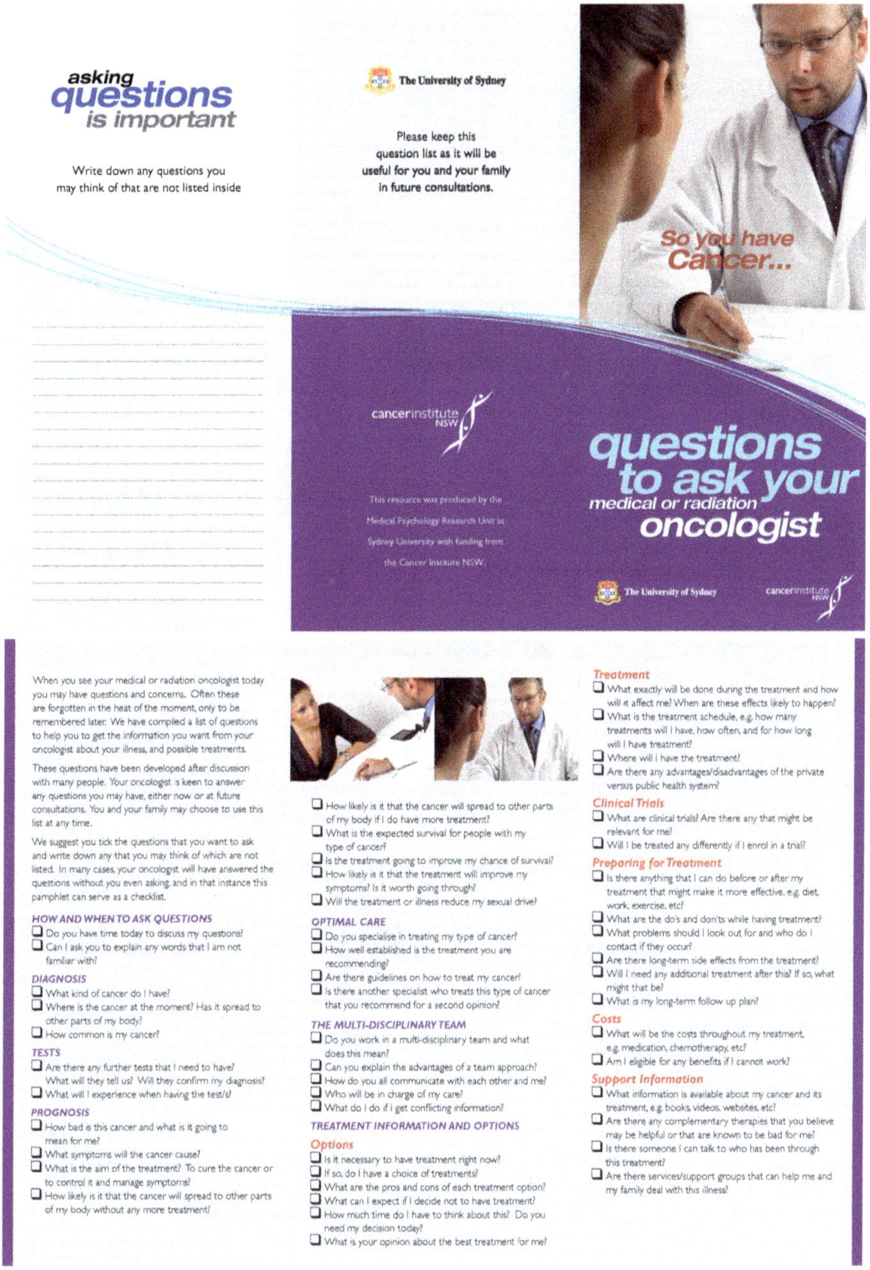

Fig. 31.1 An exemplar question prompt list (QPL)

References

1. Australian Bureau of Statistics: http://www.abs.gov.au/ausstats/abs@.nsf/Latestproducts/3218. Accessed 16 Sept 2010.
2. Australian Institute of Health and Welfare. Australia's Health 2010. The twelfth biennial health report of the Australian Institute of Health and Welfare. Canberra, 2010. ISSN 1032–6138.
3. Australian Bureau of Statistics. Australian social trends799 (4102.0). Canberra: AGPS; 2006.
4. Moore R, Butow P. Culture and oncology: impact of context effects. In: Speigel D, editor. Cancer, communication and culture. New York: Kluwer Academic/Plenum Publishers; 2005.
5. Butow P, Sze M, Dugal-Beri P, Mikhail M, Eisenbruch M, Jefford M et al. From inside the bubble: migrants' perceptions of communication with the cancer team. Support Care Cancer. 2010. Doi: 10.1007/s00520-010-0817-x.
6. Goldstein D, Thewes B, Butow P. Communicating in a multicultural society II: Greek community attitudes towards cancer in Australia. Intern Med J. 2002;32:289–96.
7. Ngo-Metzger Q, Massagli MP, Clarridge BR, Manocchia M, Davis RB, Lezzoni LI, et al. Linguistic and cultural barriers to care: perspectives of Chinese and Vietnamese immigrants. J Gen Intern Med. 2003;18:44–52.
8. http://www.safetyandquality.gov.au/internet/safety/publishing.nsf/content/Priorityprogram-01. Accessed 3 April 2012.
9. NHMRC Communicating with patients: advice for medical practitioners. http://www.nhmrc.gov.au/guidelines/publications/e58. Accessed 3 April 2012.
10. Butow PN, Dowsett S, Hagerty R, et al. Communicating prognosis to patients with metastatic disease: what do they really want to know? Support Care Cancer. 2002;10(2):161–8.
11. Hagerty RG, Butow PN, Ellis PA, et al. Cancer patient preferences for communication of prognosis in the metastatic setting. J Clin Oncol. 2004;22(9):1721–30.
12. Clayton JA, Butow PN, Tattersall MHN. When and how to initiate discussion about prognosis and end-of-life issues with terminally ill patients. J Pain Symptom Manage. 2005;30(2):132–44.
13. Clayton JM, Butow PN, Arnold RM, et al. Discussing end-of-life issues with terminally ill cancer patients and their carers: a qualitative study. Support Care Cancer. 2005;13(8):589–99.
14. Gattellari M, Butow PN, Tattersall MHN. Sharing decisions in cancer care. Soc Sci Med. 2001;52(12):1865–78.
15. Brown R, Butow PN, Boyer MJ, et al. Promoting patient participation in the cancer consultation: evaluation of a prompt sheet and coaching in question asking. Br J Cancer. 1999;80(1–2):242–8.
16. Butow P, Devine R, Boyer M, et al. Cancer consultation preparation package: changing patients but not physicians is not enough. J Clin Oncol. 2004;22(21):4401–9.
17. Girgis A, Sanson-Fisher RW. Breaking bad news: consensus guidelines for medical practitioners. J Clin Oncol. 1995;13(9):2449–56.
18. Cancer Council. How to Break Bad News: An Interactional Skills Training Manual for General Practitioners, Junior Medical Officers, Nurses, Surgeons. Copyright NSW Cancer Council, December 1997. ISBN 1 875591 85 0. Published online in Wiley Online Library (wileyonlinelibrary.com). DOI: 10.1002/pon.1923.
19. National Breast Cancer Centre and the National Cancer Control Initiative. Clinical practice guidelines for the psychosocial care of adults with cancer. Syndey: National Breast Cancer Centre; 2003. ISSN 1 74127 000 6.
20. Clayton J, Hancock K, Butow P, et al. Clinical practice guidelines for communicating prognosis and end-of-life issues with adults in the advanced stages of a life-limiting illness, and their caregivers. Med J Aust. 2007;186(12):S77–108.
21. Cancer Council Australia/Australian Cancer Network/Ministry of Health, New Zealand. Clinical practice guidelines for the management of Melanoma. Syndey: Cancer Council Australia/Australian Cancer Network; 2008. ISBN 978-0-9775060-7-1.

22. Oncology Education Committee, Cancer Council Australia. Ideal oncology curriculum for medical schools: Knowledge, skills and attitudes of medical students at graduation. The Cancer Council Australia. 2007. ISBN: 0-9775060-4-5.
23. Australian Medical Council Incorporated. Assessment and accreditation of medical schools: standard and procedures 2002. Australian Medical Council Incorporated: Canberra; 2006. ISBN 1875440232.
24. Lobb EA, Kenny DT, Butow PN, Tattersall MHN. Women's preferences for discussion of prognosis in early breast cancer. Health Expect. 2001;4:48–57.
25. Girgis A, Sanson-Fisher RW, McCarthy WH. Communicating with patients: surgeons' perceptions of their skills and need for training. Aust N Z J Surg. 1997;67(11):775–80.
26. Dimoska A, Girgis A, Hansen V, Butow PN, Tattersall MH. Perceived difficulties in consulting with patients and families: a survey of Australian cancer specialists. Med J Aust. 2008; 189(11–12):612–5.
27. Kirk P, Kirk I, Kristjanson LJ. What do patients receiving palliative care for cancer and their families want to be told? A Canadian and Australian qualitative study. BMJ. 2004; 328(7452):1343.
28. Benson J, Britten N. Respecting the autonomy of cancer patients when talking with their families: qualitative analysis of semistructured interviews with patients. Br Med J. 1996;313(7059): 729–31.
29. Kaplowitz SA, Campo S, Chui WT. Cancer patients' desire for communication of prognosis information. Health Commun. 2002;14(2):221–41.
30. Clayton JM, Butow PN, Tattersall MHN. The needs of terminally ill cancer patients versus those of caregivers for information regarding prognosis and end-of-life issues. Cancer. 2005;103(9):1957–64.
31. Huang X, Butow P, Meiser B, Goldstein D. Attitudes and information needs of Chinese migrant cancer patients and their relatives. Aust N Z J Med. 1999;29(2):207–13.
32. Norman C. Breaking bad news. Aust Fam Physician. 1996;25(10):1583–7.
33. Mitchison D, Butow P, Sze M, Aldridge L, Hui R, Vardy J et al. Prognostic communication preferences of migrant patients and their relatives. Psycho-Oncology. In Press
34. Butow PN, Lobb E, Jefford M, Goldstein D, Eisenbruch M, Girgis A, et al. A bridge between cultures: interpreters' perspectives of consultations with migrant oncology patients. Support Care Cancer. 2012;20(2):235–44.
35. Lubrano di Ciccone B, Brown RF, Gueguen JA, Bylund CL, Kissane DW. Interviewing patients using interpreters in an oncology setting: initial evaluation of a communication skills module. Ann Oncol. 2010;21(1):27–32.
36. Butow PN, Dunn SM, Tattersall MHN, et al. Patient participation in the cancer consultation: evaluation of a question prompt sheet. Ann Oncol. 1994;5(3):199–204.
37. Brown RF, Butow P, Dunn SM, et al. Promoting patient participation and shortening cancer consultations: a randomised trial. Br J Cancer. 2001;85(9):1273–9.
38. Clayton JM, Butow PN, Tattersall MHN, et al. Randomized controlled trial of a prompt list to help advanced cancer patients and their caregivers to ask questions about prognosis and end-of-life care. J Clin Oncol. 2007;25(6):715–23.

Chapter 32
Defining the Possible Barriers to Communication with Cancer Patients: A Critical Perspective from Turkey

Tolga Güven

Abstract In this chapter, I aim to define and examine the factors that may have a negative impact on communication with cancer patients in Turkey, where a move towards a patient autonomy-centered health care service has recently been observed, although paternalism still appears to be the dominant approach shaping health care professional–patient communication. Based on case reports, research findings, legal regulations, and authors' arguments from Turkey, I focus on a number of separate but interrelated factors and argue that all of these have the potential to become barriers to communication with cancer patients. In addition, I examine two other factors—namely, therapeutic privilege and family involvement in cancer communication—and claim that they are also strongly associated with the paternalist tradition. I conclude that neither the paternalist perspective, which can impose helplessness and silence on patients, nor the legally imposed minimalist approach, in which communication is reduced to disclosure of information, is adequate to define and meet the communication needs of cancer patients. I assert that health care professionals in Turkey need to make a fresh start by abandoning the paternalist perspective and interpreting the legal criteria as a minimal ethical framework in order to understand communication as a process of continuous interaction, in which providing support and care for the cancer patient should be paramount.

Keywords Cancer • Paternalism • Therapeutic privilege • Cultural differences

---

T. Güven, MD (✉)
Department of Medical Ethics and History of Medicine, Marmara University, Istanbul, Turkey
e-mail: tolgaguven@hotmail.com

Introduction

The patient–physician dialogue has been a topic of interest throughout the history of medicine. Bioethics texts generally acknowledge that until the second half of the twentieth century, medical paternalism was the dominant doctrine shaping the dialogue between the two parties and that this doctrine advocated that information judged to be "harmful" by the physician was to be hidden from patients.

Contemporary bioethics has questioned and examined paternalism meticulously and has heavily criticized its implications. Authors such as Katz have even asserted that there has not been significant emphasis on establishing a dialogue between patient and physician throughout history, as is also implied by the title of the author's landmark text, *The Silent World of Doctor and Patient* [1]. Paternalism has usually been criticized as incompatible with the concept of patient autonomy and, particularly, with the ethicolegal doctrine of informed consent, which asserts that, as autonomous individuals, patients have the right to self-determination. In this perspective, communication between the parties is considered first and foremost an obligation to ensure that "truthful disclosure" to patients has taken place, while the other purposes communication may serve appear to be overlooked. Still, the emphasis on patient autonomy is known to have improved patient–physician dialogue, and it should be noted that this improvement was directly related to the practice of oncology. The results of two studies from the USA, first published by Oken in 1961, then repeated after almost 20 years by Novack in 1979, are frequently compared in the bioethics literature as proof of the dramatic change in the attitude of physicians towards the disclosure of the diagnosis of cancer [2]. Therefore, it is reasonable to conclude that there is a strong connection between the concept of disclosure of information to patients in bioethics and the practice of clinical oncology. The fact that terms such as "truth-telling" and "truthful disclosure" frequently come up in the analysis of cancer cases in the bioethics literature can be considered further proof of this connection, even though the ethical dilemmas that can be associated with these terms are definitely not specific only to the practice of oncology.

However, despite the recent improvements summarized above, communication in oncological practice continues to be a very challenging issue, and this challenge concerns the practice not only of the clinician, but also of the bioethicist. There are a number of reasons for this situation. First of all, although the idea of a patient autonomy-centered health care service is now well established in North America, this does not indicate that the concept has been embraced in other parts of the world; paternalism is probably still common in many other regions. Furthermore, those concerned about "ethical imperialism" note that individual autonomy is mainly a concept of the Western cultures and implementing this concept in other cultural settings may be unjustified. In addition, the concept of respect for autonomy itself is reported to "continue to be misunderstood and perhaps even deliberately misrepresented" [3], while some authors also point out the problems in the patient–physician relationship associated with the so-called independent choice model, which confuses autonomy with independence [4].

These problems are magnified by the dominance of legal concerns in the regulation of medical practice. Despite the controversies regarding the compatibility of the Western concept of individual autonomy with other cultural contexts, the legal norms of informed consent have been "transplanted" by many countries into their health care legislation. As a result, health care professionals are becoming increasingly concerned about legal liability issues in their practice rather than with the ethical aspects of patient–physician interactions; and they become prone to thinking that satisfying a set of legal requirements and simply disclosing information to patients may also be adequate to fulfill their ethical duties and ensure good communication. However, in this so-called age of information, through the Internet and other sources patients today can access all kinds of specific medical information, including prognostic data. This not only means that withholding information from patients may no longer be a realistic option, but also suggests that "truthful disclosure" to oncology patients may no longer be adequate to meet their expectations with regard to communication.

Turkey's health care scene has been undergoing rapid change in the last decade, and this transformation appears to have created a rather eclectic environment, further complicated by the existence of various social, cultural, and economic differences among the different regions of the country. Almost all of the problematic issues summarized above can now be observed in patient–health care professional communication in Turkey. On the one hand, there are still many physicians who have been trained in line with the teachings of the paternalist tradition; but on the other hand, there are also others—probably the younger generation of physicians—trying to adapt to the recent patient rights implementation policies, particularly the requirements of informed consent. Furthermore, while access to health care is still a major issue for Turkey, the practice of family medicine in primary health care is now encouraged by the new health care policies, and these policies appear to have been met with enthusiasm, at least by some. In addition, the Ministry of Health has been taking concrete measures to implement certain patient rights in the last 4–5 years; and we now observe that patient rights is becoming an increasingly popular concept in Turkey, an observation confirmed by the recent establishment of a number of nongovernmental patient rights organizations in several cities. Although the efficiency of some of the governmental measures is questionable, all the recent developments appear to support a more patient autonomy-centered approach in health care. For this reason, it would be logical to expect these changes to be reflected in discussions of communication in oncological care, and at least one recent study from Turkey suggests that cancer patients may have rather high expectations with regard to information: 92.3% of 104 cancer patients were reported to think that physicians should inform patients about their diseases and treatment choices [5]. However, in a previous study, conducted with health care professionals participating in a national oncology meeting in Turkey, a considerable percentage of physicians stated that they never (9%) or rarely (39%) disclose the diagnosis to their patients [6]; this suggests that there may be serious discrepancies between the expectations of patients and the practice of professionals. As a matter of fact, another study from Turkey reported a rather high percentage (63.4%) of uninformed cancer patients [7].

In the light of this background, I aim here to define and focus on a number of separate but related concepts as possible barriers to communication in cancer care in Turkey. Although the examples will be drawn mostly from Turkey's health care scene, I believe the critical perspective provided here can also be useful in other settings, particularly in those where a transition from the paternalist tradition to a more patient autonomy-centered approach is taking place.

Medical Paternalism as a Barrier to Communication in Cancer

In the modern bioethics literature, paternalism is usually analyzed as a problematic approach because it assumes that the physician "knows best" for each patient and it fails to respect the patient's autonomy by not recognizing him/her as the decision-maker. Here, however, I will analyze paternalism specifically as a barrier to communication between health care professionals and patients in general, and in cancer cases in particular, as seen in the excerpt of the case description below:

> …[The patient] said he was going to be operated on for his gastric ulcer. He told me the decision to perform surgery was made after he was examined with a tube inserted from his mouth. He asked me questions such as "What are they going to do to me?" "Do I have cancer?" When I told him he should ask his doctor, he expressed his distrust of his physician by saying "I did ask; he told me I do not have cancer, but I do not believe him, because the patient in the next room was also told he did not have cancer, but his son told us his father has cancer." The patient insisted that I look at his file. He said: "Please tell me, wouldn't you understand [the terms]? If I have cancer, so be it; what is done is done. Do not worry, I would not be scared. If I cannot find out, I will die of curiosity anyway."
>
> (Translated by the present author; words in brackets were added to clarify the meaning.)

This excerpt was translated from a case reported by Ersoy in one of the first doctoral dissertations on informed consent in Turkey (an unpublished study, available only in Turkish) [8]. The researcher later found out that the man (a 47-year-old technician with two children) had, indeed, been diagnosed with gastric cancer.

In this particular patient's situation, the negative effect of paternalism on the patient–health care professional interaction is clearly seen. The patient's concern about receiving correct information is only part of the problem; the patient does not *trust* that his physicians will be truthful. We do not know for certain whether the patient's willingness to find out his diagnosis is an indicator of his desire to become involved in the decision-making process. Still, it is clear that the communication between the parties is problematic and the patient is definitely not satisfied with his current status.

At this point, it could also be argued that the patient's assumption about the professionals' possible response should be questioned. However, the real issue here is the presence of distrust for the professionals, rather than the accuracy of the patient's assumption. In a sense, the lack of communication here causes the patient to experience a form of "learned helplessness," because he is not willing to try to communicate with his physicians any more. He seems to have lost hope that health care professionals can be truthful about the diagnosis of cancer, and therefore he is trying to receive information from other sources.

Perhaps the most striking feature of the case description above is its illustration of the possible role of medical paternalism as a factor that shapes not only the health care professionals' behavior, but also the *patients'* behavior. Paternalism can become a significant barrier to communication by causing a vicious cycle: paternalist health care professionals can choose to hide information from their patients because they believe the information will harm them; consequently, patients who understand that physicians will not tell the truth may choose not to demand information at all, and this in turn supports the paternalist misconception that patients do not want information. Unfortunately, health care professionals can fail to recognize this effect of paternalism and mistakenly think that patients approve their approach; whereas the "silence" of the patients could, indeed, be masking the real expectations of the patients and even their distrust towards health care professionals.

Misconceptions Arising from the Debate on Cultural Differences: Another Barrier to Communication

Although the concept of patient autonomy has been instrumental in exposing the problematic aspects of the paternalist tradition, bioethicists have also been voicing their concerns about the "cultural compatibility" of this concept, arguing that individual autonomy is mostly a product of Western thought and culture, and questioning whether implementing this concept in other cultural contexts can be justified. These concerns are addressed under several terms in the bioethics literature, including ethical imperialism [9], cultural imperialism, and value absolutism [10]. In the context of oncology, the argument becomes particularly important when health care professionals trained in accordance with the requirements of the informed consent doctrine encounter patients with a cultural background that differs significantly from the so-called Anglo-American cultures; examples of such encounters in the literature involve patients from various cultures, such as Far Easterners [11] and Native Americans [3].

As a bioethicist, I believe that these concerns—which I refer to as *the cultural difference argument*—should not be taken lightly. However, I also think that the practical implications of the argument for respecting cultural differences need to be clarified. In the case description reported by Ersoy presented above, for instance, there are no health care professionals trying to impose the so-called Western norms of autonomy on the patient, but it is clear that there is a serious ethical issue that prevents the patient from communicating with his health care professionals. How the cultural difference argument would apply here may not be obvious.

One way of looking at this issue is to refer to the main concern behind the argument—preventing ethical imperialism. If imposing the norms of a certain culture on another is unethical, then one can argue that by refusing to provide information to patients, health care professionals are imposing the norms of the medical culture—which have obviously been shaped by the paternalist tradition—on the patients here, and this cannot be justified. It should be noted that this claim does not necessarily rely solely on the concept of individual autonomy to counter the paternalist perspective;

in fact, the patient in the case cited does not seem to be interpreting autonomy in such a manner either. His use of the term *us* suggests that he is acting together with at least one of his family members, and they appear to be functioning as a single unit. Yet, they are having communication problems due to the environment created by the paternalist approach.

I should note that the use of the term *culture* in this analysis could be open to debate. Macklin, for instance, argues that there is a difference between professional and cultural norms, asserting that "not every set of norms deserves to be a culture" and that medicine does not actually match the anthropological meaning of the term *culture* [12]. Therefore, it would be more accurate to say that paternalist health care workers are imposing their "professional," rather than "cultural," norms in this case. However, for the purpose of this argument, what really matters is not whether the term *medicine* comes under a certain theoretical definition, but the fact that medical professionals have the power to uphold and impose the teachings of medical paternalism, regardless of whether this has been demanded or approved by their patients. Furthermore, while distinguishing between the professional and cultural norms of an individual health care worker may be important and possible, recognizing the complex interaction between these two factors may be more important than separating them. In the case reported above, for instance, one could refer to the patient's action as an indicator of a certain cultural response towards cancer, but it is the professional norms that shape this reaction. Macklin also recognizes the power professionals possess and acknowledges that "nondisclosure to patients appears to have been a nearly universal customary practice *dictated* by medical professionals throughout the world" (italic emphasis added) [12]. As a matter of fact, this was the reason why medical paternalism was condemned in the first place by the prominent critics of this tradition such as Veatch, who is reported to have noted the "morally indefensible" position created by "the arrogance of the medical professional claiming that he or she (mostly 'he') had the authority to decide, even against a patient's wishes, what was best for the patient..." [13].

At this point, it should be clear that the cultural difference argument in essence shares the same concern with antipaternalist arguments that health care professionals can exert a certain degree of authority to impose their professional norms on their patients. Therefore, both arguments in fact strive to limit and control the use of such authority. However, when the cultural difference argument is formulated with a one-sided perspective—that is, in a fashion that focuses exclusively on the possible problems of imposing the requirements of individual autonomy on patients—it can easily be distorted so as to justify paternalism and ironically become just another authoritarian rhetorical device. A general surgeon from Turkey, for instance, opposes open disclosure of prognosis and diagnosis to patients in Turkey by referring to "dominance of emotions" and "blending with Eastern cultures" in the community [14]. A concern to emphasize the cultural difference of patients in Turkey is rather evident in his statements, but, as compassionate as his claim may sound, it is a seriously misconceived and distorted version of the cultural difference argument. I have argued in detail elsewhere that such "cultural incompatibility" claims may harbor paternalist concerns, particularly when they are endorsed by physicians and voiced by them on behalf of patients [14]. Such attempts to define the good for patients by health care professionals alone are a typical aspect of paternalism; and when paternalism is allowed to distort the concerns for respecting cultural differences, the resulting environment is very likely to become another barrier to communication. The physician in question and the policy he advocates actually fail to embrace the possibility that cancer patients in Turkey may have diverse cultural backgrounds and that their expectations may differ widely. He simply expects his formula to work for all patients; or, to be more precise, he expects all cancer patients to comply with his terms, which have been determined by him beforehand. Therefore, his claims totally miss the mark and fail to grasp the essence of the concerns about cultural differences.

There is a second problem that may arise when using the cultural difference argument: if not used with caution, it can easily combine with stereotyping attitudes and prejudices, which can then become further barriers to communication. Consider this statement: "However, in Turkey, the general ability to squarely face the prognosis in severe cases is very limited when compared to that of the patient population in Europe" [15].

This claim by a radiation oncologist from Turkey shows a paternalistic attitude, for which I have already criticized it in a previous article [14]. It also contains other problems that are worth noting. For instance, there is no factual evidence for this bold statement, and there are no study findings cited in the original text to support the comparison. Therefore, the strength of the claim appears to rest solely on the fact that it is an "expert opinion." So, what we are reading is, at best, a very problematic generalization derived from the author's professional experience in two different settings, Europe and Turkey. The claim becomes much more confusing, however, when the author writes that "Though it is not a routine procedure to pronounce the exact diagnosis to the patients in Turkey…" [15]. While this observation is, indeed, compatible with study findings from Turkey and its paternalist environment, it also renders the former claim rather absurd. One cannot help but wonder how the "ability to face the prognosis" of patients in Turkey can be known, let alone compared with that in Europe, if even disclosure of diagnosis is not "a routine procedure" in the country.

It should be obvious at this point that the author's claim includes some degree of prejudice, which appears to be masked under a misconceived cultural difference argument. Equally problematic, however, is the fact that the nature of the statement does not appear to have been questioned further by the editor(s) and the reviewer(s) of an international academic publication. I doubt if such a comparison could be published without any cited evidence if it involved, for instance, comparing the incidence of a certain type of neoplasm. A possible explanation that comes to mind here is *orientalism*, a term that is used to refer, among other things, to a stereotyping Western perspective on Eastern cultures. However, stereotyping is always problematic, regardless of its origin and is certainly not an issue exclusive to "Westerners." In a national ethics congress I attended in Turkey in 2003, the speaker (a surgeon) clearly opposed the disclosure of the diagnosis to cancer patients in the context of Turkey's health care, and one of the ethicists in the audience wanted to know why.

The answer he gave was not only stereotypical in nature, but also embarrassing. He said: "Because, we are not Americans. We are emotional people." Apparently, such stereotyping perspectives not only can become a barrier to communication, but also have the potential to alienate the members of different cultures from one another.

If these problems associated with the misrepresentation and distortion of the cultural difference argument are to be avoided, health care professionals should first be able to see that the cultural difference argument itself does not provide any justification for paternalism and it certainly does not grant the professionals any authority to declare what is "culturally appropriate." What the argument really implies is that health care professionals should not assume that their current *modus operandi* meets all cultural expectations adequately and they should strive to be more self-critical of their own practice in order to become more aware of the cultural differences among their patients. In short, this argument should facilitate, rather than discourage, heath care professional–patient communication.

Patient Autonomy as a Legally Imposed Concept in Turkey: Disclosure vs. Communication

The concept of informed consent has recently been gaining popularity in Turkey. However, when one considers the heavily paternalist history of the patient–physician relationship in this country, it does not seem realistic to think that this recent interest in the issue originated from members of the medical profession. The emphasis on consent and disclosure of information as one of the relevant components of consent has been most notably observed in the Regulation on Patient Rights (RPR) (*Hasta Hakları Yönetmeliği*), issued in 1998. On the other hand, it should be noted that consent in medical interventions is hardly a new concept in Turkish law; the Law on the Practice of Medicine and Its Related Arts (*Tababet ve Şuabat-ı Sanatlarının Tarz-ı İcrasına Dair Kanun*), dating from 1928, addresses the issue in its Article 70 and emphasizes the importance of consent, while further noting that consent for major surgical interventions has to be documented in written form. Interestingly, although this law, enacted by the parliament, has a much higher standing in the hierarchy of norms in Turkish legal doctrine than the RPR, which was issued by the Ministry of Health and serves essentially administrative purposes for regulating health care services, RPR's provisions appear to have had a far more influential impact with regard to informed consent.

This may be due in part to the fact that RPR is a rather recent document that has detailed provisions regarding informed consent and particularly the content of information to be disclosed to patients. In that sense, the document can be considered a milestone in Turkish medical law. However, RPR's influence has probably been enhanced by other recent developments, including the efforts of the Ministry of Health to implement certain patient rights in health care in the last 4–5 years and the growing popularity of the concept of patient rights in Turkey. Furthermore, medical malpractice and mandatory professional liability insurance (medical malpractice insurance) are now the topics of heated debates among Turkey's health care professionals, due to a recently enacted law that contains provisions on these issues. All of these developments, which were not present during the enactment of earlier laws and regulations in health care, suggest that there is now a move towards a patient autonomy-centered health care service in Turkey.

Unfortunately, these changes by themselves do not show that paternalist practices have been abandoned in Turkey, because, as already noted above, the changes have originated mostly from sources outside the profession. Although the current environment in Turkey expects health care professionals who have been trained and practiced medicine with paternalist teachings for years to comply with legal requirements for informed consent, that does not necessarily mean that the problems of paternalism have been critically examined and understood by the professionals involved. Therefore, for the time being, it is not realistic to expect the concept of patient autonomy to have a practical meaning for the majority of Turkey's health care professionals. Under these circumstances they may at best try to satisfy the legal requirements for informed consent. This, however, may hardly be enough to ensure good communication and may even do more harm than good: when legal concerns take priority over ethical ones, professionals may become prone to deliver cancer-related information in an insensitive or callous manner.

This pessimistic but possible future scenario for Turkey's health care scene suggests that the recent attempts to impose patient autonomy can easily become another barrier to communication that will be highly relevant to cancer care, particularly if informed consent is treated simply as a legal concept.

It could be argued that the legal emphasis on disclosure of truthful information is nevertheless an improvement over the "silence" dictated by the paternalist tradition. Furthermore, "the right not to know" has also been recognized in the aforementioned Regulation's Article no. 20, under the title "Forbidding Disclosure"; and this can at least prevent the "force feeding" of information to patients who do not want to be informed about their situation. However, the utilization of this right is also heavily dependent on the sensitivity of the health care professionals. Furthermore, this right alone is not adequate to eliminate the problems that may arise as a result of equating disclosure with communication. It is undoubtedly true that communication involves the disclosure and exchange of information between parties in many instances, but in the care of chronically and terminally ill individuals, communication can serve many other purposes. It can play a vital role, for instance, in addressing the patient's possible fears and letting him/her know that he/she is not alone, that the professional will be responsive to the suffering of the patient and is willing to care and help. Even patients who prefer "not to know" will probably welcome and perhaps expect the use of communication for such purposes, and reducing this process to a simple operational directive such as "Inform only those who wish" can create a significant communication barrier. For all these reasons, health care professionals should be encouraged to take legal provisions as a starting point and interpret the legal criteria as a minimal, rather than the optimal, ethical framework.

Other Factors That May Influence Communication in Cancer

Therapeutic Privilege

Despite the developments summarized above, it should be noted that the well-known paternalist doctrine of therapeutic privilege is still present in Turkey's legislation and most notably in Article 14 of the Medical Deontology Regulation (*Tıbbi Deontoloji Tüzüğü*). From a purely historical point of view, however, this is hardly surprising for a regulation dating from the year 1960; apparently, this paternalist doctrine was not challenged even in North America before the 1960s. Veatch notes that while the landmark Nathanson-Kline decision dates from 1960, a number of landmark court decisions were made between 1969 and 1972 [16].

From Turkey's perspective, a more problematic fact is the existence of this doctrine in the much more recent RPR discussed above. Addressing this "privilege" recognized for physicians in a patient rights document, where detailed provisions on informed consent have also been defined, can at best be regarded as frustrating, if not tragicomic. I have translated the article in question below; the words in brackets have been added where necessary to clarify the meaning:

> Conditions where disclosure is inappropriate and precautions that should be taken—Article 19:
> It is appropriate to hide the diagnosis in cases where [such information] has the possibility of worsening the disease by causing a harmful effect on the spiritual condition of the patient, and when the course and the prognosis of the disease are considered to be poor.
> Informing the patient or his relatives about the medical condition of the patient is up to the physician's decision within the conditions defined in the paragraph above.
> A diagnosis [of a disease] with no treatment can only be disclosed or implied by a physician. Unless the patient has indicated otherwise or if the person to be given such information has not been determined beforehand, such diagnosis is to be disclosed to the patient's family.

I believe this text, dating from 1998, speaks volumes about the strength of the paternalist tradition in Turkey; considering the rich literature on paternalism and particularly on the doctrine of therapeutic privilege in bioethics, a detailed criticism of these provisions appears to be unnecessary at this point. The Ministry of Health has recently been preparing an updated version of the Regulation in question, but although an extensive update in the informed consent section has been proposed, the therapeutic privilege section was left untouched. This suggests that the negative impact of paternalism on communication, as well as on the informed consent process, has still not been adequately understood by the administrative authorities of health care services in Turkey. However, to my knowledge, the doctrine of therapeutic privilege has not yet been challenged with a lawsuit in Turkey, so whether it can serve as a legitimate justification for withholding information from a patient in a court case remains to be seen.

Families vs. Patients: A Cultural Barrier?

As already noted by bioethicists from Turkey, such as Oguz [17] and Aksoy [18], the family in Turkish society is a significant social unit. The fact that families may play an important role as caretakers as well as decision-makers during the care of chronic disease and particularly of cancer is a well-known issue in bioethics, and Turkey is no exception. Families frequently want to be involved in these processes in an effort to support the patients in the best way they can. Unfortunately, such support does not necessarily involve families and patients acting together. Anecdotal evidence suggests that families may attempt to prevent the disclosure of cancer-related information to the patient and may demand to be informed instead of the patient. However, whether such demands can be justified is an issue that needs to be examined carefully. Empirical evidence from Turkey suggests that family members may not be using a consistent criterion in this process. In one study, 66% of the relatives of patients recently diagnosed with cancer were found to oppose the disclosure of truth to patients, but 71% would request such information for themselves if they were suffering from a lethal disease [19]; similar findings have been reported in another study by Aksoy, who indicates that families may be using a double standard [18]. Furthermore, the inevitable question of why physicians choose to communicate with the family instead of the patient in the first place also needs to be answered. In a previous article, we have examined two different dramatic cancer cases from Turkey, reported by Ersoy [20] and Buken [21], and argued that the involvement of family members instead of the patients themselves was a choice made primarily by the physicians [22]. Bearing these points in mind, I assert that the influence of paternalism and the possible role of health care professionals in similar cases must also be taken into consideration before one considers the involvement of families in Turkey simply as a cultural barrier to communication in cancer. Other reasons that may be contributing to the situation, such as the lack of the necessary skills for communicating cancer-related information to patients, should also be kept in mind. The role physicians may play in cancer communication is also supported by empirical evidence from Turkey. Ozdogan et al., a group of Turkish oncologists investigating communication issues in cancer, have defined the medical training of physicians as one of the factors determining the truth-telling practice of professionals [6]. In another study, which specifically examined the involvement of the patient's relatives in "honest disclosure," the researchers also emphasized the importance of effective communication skills and noted that physicians "should find ways to overcome cultural barriers to adopting honest disclosure in daily practice" [19], although the vital question of why physicians choose to communicate with relatives in the first place was not addressed. Similarly, Sen, who reported a very high percentage (88%) of cancer patients who were informed about their diagnosis, stressed the possible effect of the efforts of the department on communication and of the "largely European-trained" staff on the results, while noting that "this very likely does not represent a general trend in the Turkish medical population" [15].

Conclusion

As a leading cause of mortality throughout the world, cancer is frequently associated with pain, suffering, and death—terms that may have a frightening ring to them even when only on paper. These also make the task of examining cancer communication at the normative level a very difficult one; setting out to establish a formula that will work in all cases seems to be an impossible task. However, denying the need for communication, particularly when it is understood as an instrument for expressing emotions and thoughts and connecting with others—rather than simply as a means of exchanging information—appears to be equally impossible. For this reason, in this chapter I have chosen to assume that communication as a basic human need will always be demanded by patients; rather than attempting to define a set of strict rules or conditions to be satisfied, I have focused on a number of possible obstacles that could be blocking the way. This makes practical sense for Turkey, where recognition and removal of these problematic factors should be a high-priority goal.

Among all the factors I have defined in the text, medical paternalism still appears to be the most problematic barrier of all. Unfortunately, this tradition has enjoyed an uninterrupted reign for a very long time. While we are now aware of many of the ethical issues it causes, we can only guess how profound an effect it has on the way we perceive the ethical aspects of medical practice. Paternalism can impose helplessness, silence, compliance, and even obedience on patients; any of these influences alone certainly has a negative effect on communication. Sadly enough, these effects of paternalism are dismissed all too readily by some, who may prefer to blame the "cultural aspects" of a society and overlook or deliberately disregard the fact that such cultural aspects are also shaped and nurtured by the practice of professionals and the norms they impose. If health care professionals genuinely want to improve communication in cancer, they should be ready to question their possible role in the situation at hand. As a matter of fact, when one considers the role health care professionals have played in upholding the teachings of the paternalist tradition, it seems only fair to say that health care professionals should take some responsibility to "undo" these possible harmful effects of paternalism, rather than simply trying to maintain the *status quo*. However, the paternalist motto "the doctor knows the best" hardly encourages self-criticism, and perhaps this is why legal intervention will be inevitable at some point.

On the other hand, an issue as complicated as communication is almost impossible to address in detail in legal documents, where only general standards can be defined. While legal norms must be learned by all professionals, ensuring good communication should be understood as an ethical duty that involves a continuous interaction between the parties in which providing support and care for the patient is paramount; such interaction usually requires going beyond the minimal standards defined by the law. During this process, health care professionals should certainly take into consideration the concerns of those who note that "The truth may be 'brutal,' but telling it should not be" [23] and the possible ethical issues related to value absolutism. However, I would like to point out that autonomy can also be interpreted as a concept that requires the recognition of each patient as a unique and particular human being, not necessarily as an isolated individual without social ties and responsibilities. Such recognition is impossible from the paternalist perspective. This is particularly evident in the claims of those who distort the cultural difference argument and succumb to stereotyping while claiming that they know what is culturally appropriate. If these problems are to be avoided, health care professionals should be willing to make a fresh start, abandoning altogether the previous habits and paternalist assumptions regarding the preferences of cancer patients. This is probably the only way to avoid prejudice and to understand truly how cancer patients in Turkey choose to express themselves and how their own social and cultural backgrounds are reflected in their decisions. The other option, where communication may be reduced merely to disclosure of information through court decisions and legal sanctions, does not appear to be promising for patients or for professionals.

Acknowledgments I would like to thank Professor Nermin Ersoy for kindly allowing me to use an excerpt of a case description from her doctoral thesis. I also would like to thank Professor Ray Guillery for editing an earlier draft of this chapter and Dr. Gurkan Sert for the insight he provided regarding the legal status of the regulations cited in the chapter.

References

1. Katz J. The silent world of doctor and patient. Baltimore: The John Hopkins University Press; 2002.
2. Beauchamp TL, Childress JF. Principles of biomedical ethics. 6th ed. New York: Oxford University Press; 2009. p. 290.
3. Macklin R. Ethical relativism in a multicultural society. Kennedy Inst Ethics J. 1998;8(1): 1–22.
4. Quill TE, Howard B. Physician recommendations and patient autonomy: finding a balance between physician power and patient choice. Ann Intern Med. 1996;125(9):763–9.
5. Erer S, Atici E, Erdemir AD. The views of cancer patients on patient rights in the context of information and autonomy. J Med Ethics. 2008;34:384–8.
6. Ozdogan M, Samur M, Artac M, Yildiz M, Savas B, Bozcuk HS. Factors related to truth-telling practice of physicians treating patients with cancer in Turkey. J Palliat Med. 2006;9:1114–9.
7. Samur M, Senler FC, Akbulut H, Pamir A, Arıcan A. Kanser tanısı almış, hastaların bilgilenme durumu: Hekim ve hekim adaylarının yaklaşımları hakkında Ankara Universitesi Tıp Fakultesi İbni Sina Hastanesi'nde yapılan sınırlı bir araştırmanın sonuçları [Information status of patients diagnosed with cancer: results of a limited study on the approach of clinicians and physician candidates in Ankara University Faculty of Medicine Ibni Sina Hospital]. Ankara Univ Tıp Fak Mecm. [J Ankara Univ Fac Med.] (in Turkish) 2000;53(3):161–6.
8. Ersoy N. Cerrahi'de Hastayi Bilgilendirmeye ve Onamini Almaya Iliskin Etik Sorunlar [Ethical problems about informing patients and obtaining their informed consent on surgical treatment]. Unpublished Doctorate Thesis (in Turkish), Istanbul University Institute of Health Sciences, Istanbul; 1991. p. 173.
9. Loewy EH. Textbook of healthcare ethics. New York: Plenum; 1996. p. 2–3, 69.
10. Gbadegesin S. Bioethics and cultural diversity. In: Kuhse H, Singer P, editors. A companion to bioethics. Oxford: Blackwell; 2001. p. 24–31.
11. Lee A, Wu HY. Diagnosis disclosure in cancer patients—when the family says 'No!'. Singapore Med J. 2002;43(10):533–8.
12. Macklin R. Against relativism. Cultural diversity and the search for ethical universals in medicine. New York: Oxford University Press; 1999. p. 86–107.
13. Levine C. Analyzing Pandora's box: the history of bioethics. In: Eckenwiler LA, Cohn FG, editors. The ethics of bioethics. Mapping the moral landscape. Baltimore: The John Hopkins University Press; 2007. p. 7.
14. Guven T. Truth-telling in cancer: examining the cultural incompatibility argument in Turkey. Nurs Ethics. 2010;17(2):159–66.

15. Sen M. Communication with cancer patients—the influence of age, gender, education and health insurance status. Ann N Y Acad Sci. 1997;809:514–24.
16. Veatch RM. Basics of bioethics. Upper Saddle River: Pearson Education; 2003. p. 76–7.
17. Oguz NY. Autonomy: cutting the Gordian knot. Bioeth Exam. 2002;6(1):1–3, 8–9. http://www.ahc.umn.edu/img/assets/26102/BE-2002-spring.pdf. Accessed Mar 2011.
18. Aksoy S. End-of-life decision making in Turkey. In: Blank RH, Merrick JC, editors. End-of-life decision making. A cross-national study. Cambridge: MIT Press; 2005. p. 183–95.
19. Ozdogan M, Samur M, Bozcuk HS, Coban E, Artac M, Savas B, et al. 'Do not tell': what factors affect relatives' attitudes to honest disclosure of diagnosis to cancer patients? Support Care Cancer. 2004;12:497–502.
20. Ersoy N. Case report no. 1. In: Carmi A, editor. Informed consent. Haifa: Israel National CommissionforUNESCO;2003.p.3.http://unesdoc.unesco.org/images/0014/001487/148713e.pdf. Accessed Mar 2011.
21. Buken NO. Truth telling information and communication with cancer patients in Turkey. J Int Soc History Islamic Med. 2003;2(4):31–7.
22. Guven T, Sert G. Advance directives in Turkey's cultural context: examining the potential benefits for the implementation of patient rights. Bioethics. 2010;24(3):127–33.
23. Jonsen A, Siegler M, Winslade WJ. Clinical ethics: a practical approach to ethical decisions in clinical medicine. 4th ed. New York: McGraw-Hill; 1998. p. 66.

Chapter 33
Cancer Disclosure, Health-Related Quality of Life, and Psychological Distress: An Iranian Perspective

Ali Montazeri

Abstract Cancer disclosure has always been difficult for clinicians. Contemporary medicine recommends honest disclosure of the disease. It is argued that timely disclosure of the cancer diagnosis might help patients to have informed treatment choices, cope better, adhere to treatment and tolerate its symptoms, and show improved quality of life. But is this practical everywhere? Do patients and their families and caregivers believe the same? Evidence suggests that there are differences in perceptions among physicians, patients, and families in bad news communication. This chapter gives an account of cancer disclosure as it relates to health-related quality of life and psychological distress in cancer patients, leading the author to propose two hypotheses that should be tested in real practice. Perhaps testing these hypotheses could help search for new grounds in cancer communication and provide evidence-based guidelines for cancer disclosure.

Keywords Cancer disclosure • Knowledge of cancer diagnosis • Quality of life • Psychological distress • Anxiety • Depression

Background

Most existing literature on disclosing cancer diagnosis comes from Western countries, where in most instances physicians disclose the bad news to patients directly and usually no one other than the patient has the right to know the diagnosis unless he or she gives permission to doctors to disclose the diagnosis to family members. As noted in Western culture, this is due to an individualistic philosophy that favors personal autonomy [1]. This approach has been criticized as violating the right of the patient not to know his or her diagnosis, but in general this is currently

---

A. Montazeri, MPH, PhD, FFPH (✉)
Iranian Institute for Health Sciences Research, ACECR, Tehran, Iran
e-mail: montazeri@acecr.ac.ir

the mainstream school of thought in modern medicine [2]. A recent investigation of cancer patients and their family caregivers reported that not only patients and their family knew the diagnosis but also a majority of patients (58.0%) and caregivers (83.4%) were aware of the patient's terminal status. Approximately 28% of patients and 23% of caregivers reported that they guessed it from the patient's worsening condition. The patient group was more likely than the caregiver group (78.6% vs. 69.6%) to prefer that patients be informed of their terminal status. Patients informed of their terminal diagnosis had a significantly better quality of life and fewer symptoms and had a lower rate of emotional distress than patients who guessed it from their worsening condition. The authors concluded that most patients with terminal cancer and their family caregivers preferred disclosure, and patients who knew of their terminal diagnosis had a lower rate of emotional distress and a higher health-related quality of life [3]. However, as many investigators discussed, the assumption that truth-telling is always beneficial to patients can be questioned on several grounds, including cultural diversities, individual differences, some difficulties common to all medical specialties for truth-telling worldwide, and ethical justifications [4, 5]. Here, findings from a study in Iran focusing on patients with gastrointestinal cancer will be provided to illustrate how the issue might differ in various parts of the world. The incidence of esophageal and stomach cancer in Iran is high, well above the world average [6]. It is the first leading cause of cancer-related deaths in men and the second among women [7]. An investigation was carried out to assess health-related quality of life, anxiety, and depression in this group of patients and to investigate whether the knowledge of the cancer diagnosis affects their quality of life and psychological distress. Quality of life was measured using the European Organization for Research and Treatment of Cancer Quality of Life Questionnaire (EORTC QLQ-C30), and the Hospital Anxiety and Depression Scale (HADS) was used to measure psychological distress. A summary of findings followed by a proposal for testing two hypotheses will be presented [8, 9].

Summary of Findings

The mean age of patients was 54.1 ($SD=14.8$) years; most patients were married (86%), male (56%), and illiterate (55%); their diagnosis was related to stomach (30%), esophagus (29%), colon (22%), rectum (16%), and small intestine (3%). Only 48% knew their cancer diagnosis, whereas 52% did not know. They were quite similar in most characteristics. Thus, the comparison was made between the two groups.

Quality of Life

Comparing functioning and global quality of life scores between those who knew their diagnosis and those who did not showed that those who knew their diagnosis reported a significantly lower degree of physical ($P=0.001$), emotional ($P=0.014$),

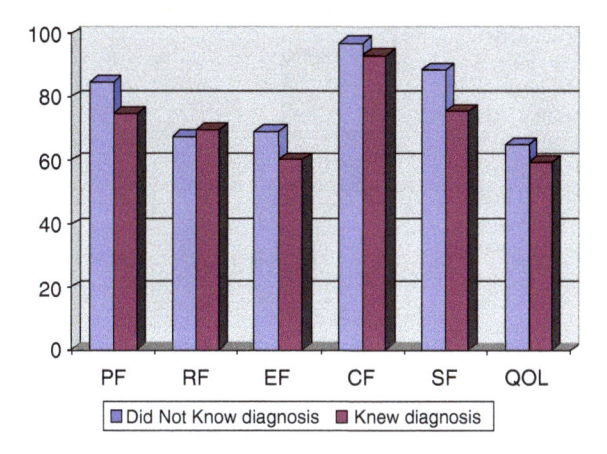

Fig. 33.1 Patients' functioning and global quality of life scores as measured by the European Organization for Research and Treatment of Cancer Quality of Life Questionnaire (EORTC QLQ-C30). *PF* Physical functioning, *RF* Role functioning, *EF* Emotional functioning, *CF* Cognitive functioning, *SF* Social functioning, *QOL* Global quality of life. Possible scores for functioning and global quality of life scores range from 0 to 100 with higher scores representing better conditions

and social functioning ($P<0.001$). Also, the findings indicated that there were no statistically significant differences between the two groups in symptom scores, except for fatigue ($P=0.014$) and financial difficulties ($P=0.005$). Further analysis was carried out to examine whether age, education, and cancer site had any effects on physical, emotional, and social functioning, fatigue, and financial difficulties. Functioning and symptom scores were considered as dependent variables; and knowledge of cancer diagnosis, educational status, and cancer site were considered as fixed factors; and age was considered a covariate. There were no clear patterns for effects of independent variables studied on outcomes that are physical, emotional, and social functioning or fatigue and financial difficulties; but in all instances knowledge of diagnosis showed significant effects on observed differences between the two groups (Fig. 33.1).

Psychological Distress

The mean anxiety score was 7.6 ($SD=4.5$) and for depression this was 8.7 ($SD=3.8$), from highest possible scores of 21. Overall 47.2% and 57% patients scored high on both anxiety and depression. There were statistically significant differences between anxiety and depression and patients' knowledge of their diagnosis. The results indicated that those who knew their diagnosis showed a significantly higher degree of psychological distress (mean (SD) anxiety score: knew diagnosis 9.1 (4.2) vs. 6.3 (4.4) did not know diagnosis, $P<0.001$; mean (SD) depression score: knew diagnosis 9.1 (4.1) vs. 7.9 (3.6) did not know diagnosis, $P=0.05$). Considering patients' demographic status, the findings showed various features indicating that there were

Fig. 33.2 Patients' anxiety and depression scores as measured by the Hospital Anxiety and Depression Scale (HADS). Possible scores for both anxiety and depression range from 0 to 21 with higher scores indicating higher psychological distress

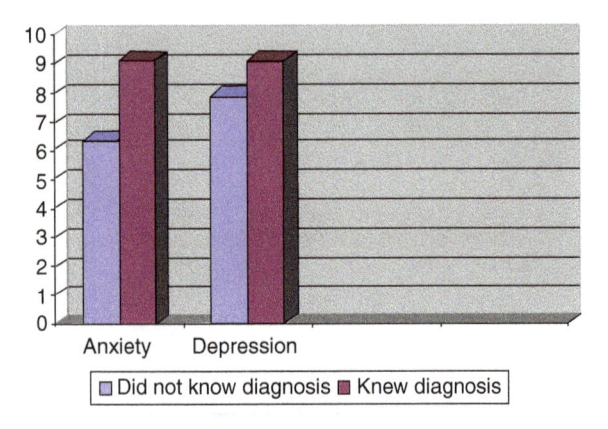

no statistically significant differences between patients' anxiety, depression, gender, educational level, marital status, and cancer site. However, age and anxiety showed a significant relationship ($P=0.005$), indicating that patients aged between 30 and 39 were more anxious compared with others. Finally, performing regression analysis of excess levels of both anxiety and depression showed the strongest association with knowledge of diagnosis (odds ratio for anxiety: 2.7, 95% CI: 1.1–6.8, $P=0.03$; odds ratio for depression: 2.8, 95% CI: 1.1–7.2, $P=0.03$). No other variables studied showed significant results (Fig. 33.2).

Discussion of Findings: Proposing Two Hypotheses

Although contradictory, the findings that in Iran cancer patients who knew their diagnosis reported higher psychological distress and lower quality of life than those who did not are not unique. Similarly in Turkey and India it has been demonstrated that psychiatric disorders occurred to a lesser extent in patients who were not aware of their cancer diagnosis. The authors concluded that these patients had a more hopeful outlook to the outcome of treatment [10, 11]. However, studies from different cultural backgrounds suggested that awareness of cancer diagnosis and prognosis does not itself cause emotional distress, and honest disclosure of truth does not worsen any dimension of quality of life [12–14]. Such mixed observations led the author to propose two hypotheses in order to understand why cancer disclosure might have different effects on different patients.

The Indirect Knowledge of Diagnosis

This hypothesis assumes that since most evidence suggests that sensible disclosure of diagnosis improves quality of life, if in some instances investigators reported that knowledge of diagnosis led to psychological distress and decreased quality of life, this should be attributed not to knowledge of the diagnosis but to the way the patient was informed about his or her cancer diagnosis. As suggested in many traditional cultures (e.g., most Asian countries and a few European cultures), in an effort to protect the patient from despair and feelings of hopelessness, family caregivers more often exclude patients from the process of information exchange. In such societies the family plays an important role in the provision of care and information disclosure, and they usually make decisions on the patients' behalf [15]. Thus, the hypothesis argues that since in some cultures (due to collectivist culture) the diagnosis usually is kept secret from the patients and first-degree family members or close relatives are informed about the diagnosis, this situation causes families to behave artificially in the front of the patients and make them suspicious regarding their own illness. Consequently, patients themselves seek ways to acquire some information about their disease and finally become aware of the illness. The information might be obtained from peer patients, some family members, or other sources. The proposed hypothesis argues that indirect knowledge of cancer diagnosis makes patients experience a higher level of emotional distress and thus a lower self-reported health-related quality of life. In other words, this hypothesis suggests that it is not the knowledge of the diagnosis that makes patients feel emotionally distressed, but the indirect route to the knowledge of the diagnosis that causes such a condition for patients.

Literacy and Knowledge of Diagnosis

This hypothesis assumes that since most evidence suggests that sensible disclosure of diagnosis improves quality of life, if in some instances investigators have reported that knowledge of diagnosis led to psychological distress and decreased quality of life, this should be attributed not to knowledge of diagnosis but to the patients' educational level. It seems that there is a relationship between literacy and knowledge of diagnosis. The relevance of level of education and knowledge of cancer diagnosis might be explained in the following possibilities:

I.   Patients are well educated and have knowledge of their diagnosis
II. Patients are well educated and do not know their diagnosis
III. Patients are less educated and have knowledge of their diagnosis
IV. Patients are less educated and do not know their diagnosis

Accordingly patients in conditions I and IV might report better quality of life, but patients in conditions II and III usually report poorer emotional functioning and quality of life, as illustrated in Fig. 33.3. This hypothesis argues that it is not the knowledge of diagnosis that contributes to decreased health-related quality of life, but it is patients' educational level that determines whether or not the diagnosis should be disclosed to patients.

Fig. 33.3 The hypothetical relationship between level of education and knowledge of diagnosis and its possible outcomes

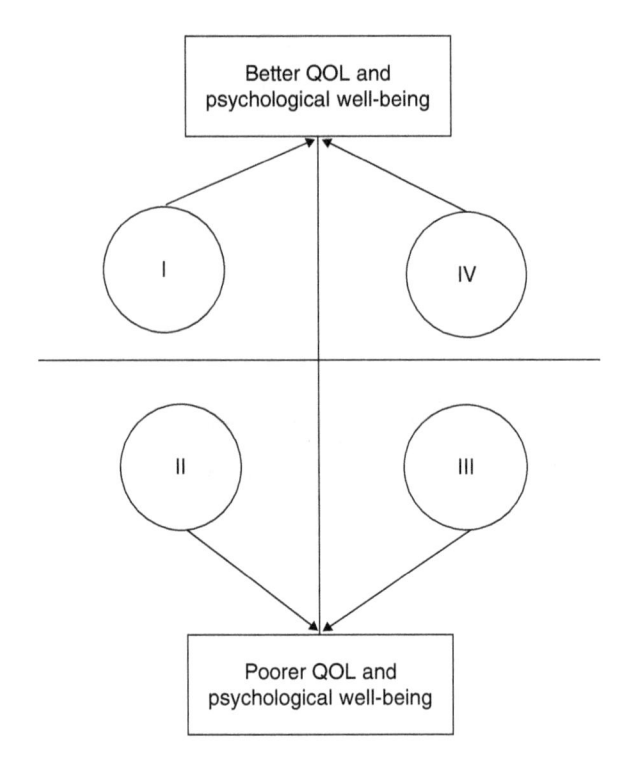

Future Directions: Implications of Findings

The findings from the current study highlight two lines of future research in cancer communication: first, to examine the ways we provide information and disclosure; and second, to investigate the relationship between patients' level of education and their response to bad news. For the purpose of the former hypothesis testing, there is a need to study psychological distress and quality of life in two groups of patients: those who have been informed of their diagnosis by their doctors directly and those who became aware by themselves through indirect channels. The comparison of quality of life and psychological distress then could be made. For the purpose of the latter hypothesis, testing the comparison should be made between well-educated patients and less-educated patients, but divided into two groups, as suggested earlier. Finally, one should be aware that when it is believed that disclosure and knowledge of cancer diagnosis does improve patients' quality of life and psychological well-being, in all circumstances it is assumed that we are referring to effective, adequate, honest, timely, and culturally competent disclosure of the cancer diagnosis. The notion of cultural competence and effective communication in cancer care are discussed elsewhere [16–18] and in this book.

References

1. Dhruva A, Cheng J, Kwong M, Luce JA, Abrams DI. Contrasts, conflicts, and change: a case in cultural oncology. J Support Oncol. 2006;4:301–4.
2. Higuchi N. The patient's right to know of a cancer diagnosis: a comparison of Japanese paternalism and American self-determination. Washburn Law J. 1992;31:455–73.
3. Yun YH, Kwon YC, Lee MK, Lee WJ, Jung KH, Do YR, et al. Experiences and attitudes of patients with terminal cancer and their family caregivers toward the disclosure of terminal illness. J Clin Oncol. 2010;28:1950–7.
4. Surbone A. Telling the truth to patients with cancer: what is the truth? Lancet Oncol. 2006;7:944–50.
5. Kazdaglis GA, Arnaoutoglou C, Karypidis D, Memekidou G, Spanos G, Papadopoulos O. Disclosing the truth to terminal cancer patients: a discussion of ethical and cultural issues. East Mediterr Health J. 2010;16:442–7.
6. Sadjadi A, Nouraie M, Mohagheghi MA, Mousavi-Jarahi A, Malekzadeh R, Parkin DM. Cancer occurrence in Iran in an international perspective. Asian Pac J Cancer Prev. 2002;6:359–63.
7. Mohagheghi MA. Final report of research for cancer registration in Iran. Tehran: Cancer Institute, National Cancer Registry; 2002.
8. Tavoli A, Mohagheghi MA, Montazeri A, Roshan R, Tavoli Z, Omidvari S. Anxiety and depression in patients with gastrointestinal cancer: does knowledge of cancer diagnosis matter? BMC Gastroenterol. 2007;7:28.
9. Montazeri A, Tavoli A, Mohagheghi MA, Roshan R, Tavoli Z. Disclosure of cancer diagnosis and quality of life in cancer patients: should it be the same everywhere? BMC Cancer. 2009;9:39.
10. Atesci FC, Baltalarli B, Oguzhanoglu NK, Karadag F, Ozdel O, Karagoz N. Psychiatric morbidity among cancer patients and awareness of illness. Support Care Cancer. 2004;12:161–7.
11. Chandra PS, Chaturvedi SK, Kumar A. Awareness of diagnosis and psychiatric morbidity among cancer patients—a study from south India. Psychosom Res. 1998;45:257–61.
12. Bozcuk H, Erdoğan V, Eken C, Ciplak E, Samur M, Ozdoğan M, et al. Does awareness of diagnosis make any difference to quality of life? Determinants of emotional functioning in a group of cancer patients in Turkey. Support Care Cancer. 2002;10:51–7.
13. Barnett MM. Does it hurt to know the worst? Psychological morbidity, information preferences and understanding of prognosis in patients with advanced cancer. Psychooncology. 2006;15:44–55.
14. Montazeri A, Hole D, Milory R, McEwen J, Gills CR. Does knowledge of cancer diagnosis affect quality of life? A methodological challenge. BMC Cancer. 2004;4:21.
15. Mystakidou K, Parpa E, Tsilika E, Katsouda E, Vlahos L. Patterns and barriers in information disclosure between health care professionals and relatives with cancer patients in Greek society. Eur J Cancer Care. 2005;14:175–81.
16. Surbone A. Cultural aspects of communication in cancer care. Recent Results Cancer Res 2006;168: 91–104.
17. Surbone A. Cultural aspects of communication in cancer care. Support Care Cancer. 2008;16:235–40.
18. Surbone A. Cultural competence in oncology: where do we stand? Ann Oncol. 2010;21:3–5.

Chapter 34
The Challenges in Communication with Cancer Patients in Contemporary Bosnia and Herzegovina Society

Bakir Mehić

Abstract With the advent of a certain degree of democratization in Bosnia and Herzegovina, the level of disagreement between law and morality has been reduced. The reason is that legislation, which is based on consensus building within the society, leaves much more room for ethical decision-making in the case of controversial issues. Today, in a situation where health care has devolved from the state (society) to the individual and the distribution of cash flow and capital is uneven, health insurance funds have limited financial resources, so that patients often have to buy their own medications, including cytostatics. People are starting to realize that health has monetary value, and patients insist on talking with doctors, wanting to be informed about everything, to participate in decision-making regarding diagnosis and treatment. Officially the view of the medical profession in Bosnia and Herzegovina is that the patient should be told what the expectations are regarding his/her disease; and that for incurable patients, the dignity of their sickness and dying should be respected. However, we cannot say that this kind of dialogue is practiced in all parts of Bosnia and Herzegovina and at all levels of its society.

Keywords Bosnia and Herzegovina • Challenges in communication • Cooperative doctor–patient relationship • Alternative medicine • Informed consent

B. Mehić (✉)
Clinical Center University of Sarajevo, Clinic of Lung Diseases and TB,
Bardakčije 90, Sarajevo, Bosnia and Herzegovina
e-mail: mehicb@bih.net.ba

Introduction: An Example

A 23-year-old man, a smoker, was admitted to the hospital with a suspected lung tumor. Clinical evaluation confirmed the diagnosis of non-small cell lung carcinoma at an early stage of the disease. After consultation with the surgeon, the patient was advised to report to the department of thoracic surgery for surgery.

Although I was not the managing physician for this case, during my regular visit in the course of 24-h duty, I noticed a slightly different behavior in this patient in comparison with others. He was always in bed, Laying still, acted withdrawn, and answered questions with brief negations, in the sense that he is fine and he does not need anything.

Six months later, he was admitted to the department for intensive therapy because of heavy coughing up of blood. He had not reported for thoracic surgery, but gave himself alternative treatment, of which the basis was drinking petroleum. He lost 11 kg in weight, and the tumor shadow in the lung appeared slightly larger. During his stay at the intensive therapy department, during every visit I tried to establish a conversation with him at a somewhat higher level than, "How are you today? How many times did you cough up blood yesterday?" Because additional clinical evaluation showed that his condition required surgical treatment, I tried to influence him to change his mind and give his consent to surgery. However, he was very negative, and I had the impression that he was quite convinced of the correctness of his attitude and commitment that he does not need surgery and that help will arrive from the Creator.

After the cessation of his coughing up blood and the improvement of his general health condition, but without his undergoing surgery or any other treatment, I discharged him from the hospital with the recommendation for symptomatic treatment as deemed necessary by his family doctor.

Fifteen days later, he was readmitted to the hospital because of phlebothrombosis of the right leg below the knee. New enlargement of the mediastinum was found, indicating the loss of conditions permitting surgical resection of the lung. Professional curiosity, but also the fact that this patient still refused any kind of modern treatment, told me that I must devote much more time to him. During the first 24-h duty I attempted to talk with him. In the beginning, he was unwilling to talk; but when we moved away from the topic of his disease and began the story of his past, the conversation started. We talked about his former way of life, his remaining family after the war casualties in Bratunac and Srebrenica, what he was doing, and how he was going through the period since having been told that he had cancer of the lung. After that, I decided to explain to him what lung cancer is, how it occurs, and how it is treated. During my explanation, he repeatedly asked: How often is that successful? How much sense does the treatment that I suggested to him make? and so on. I answered that it is worthwhile, it does make sense, it is more bearable than drinking petroleum. I told him he still has a lot to do in this world, and I suggested that he start with radiation treatment and then continue with chemotherapy.

After almost 4 h of talking on three separate occasions, he clearly let me know that I had gained his trust and he would agree to my proposal—that I can treat him as I think best.

Today, 5 years later, he is still alive; a year ago he got married; 6 months ago he and his wife came to tell me that they want to have a baby. On this occasion he informed me that he decided to stop taking inhibitors of receptors of epidermal growth factor. The shadow on the lung persists, but it is not growing. It is difficult to assess by CT scan whether there is only post-irradiation fibrosis or there are elements of tumor organization.

He is coming for regular follow-ups. He says that he has found a new purpose in life, that he wants to have a child; but that he is not sorry to die, because it seems to him that he has fully justified his existence in this world. To my statement that I am not sure that his disease is gone, he replied: "You're my doctor and are more burdened by it than I am."

The above example shows something of the difficulty and complexity of the relationship between the physician and the oncology patient.

The Challenges in Contemporary Bosnia and Herzegovina Society

Like many other important aspects of life in Bosnia and Herzegovina, the characteristics of the practice of oncology medicine in Bosnia and Herzegovina may be divided between those that existed before the war (1992–1995) and those that exist in the postwar period. Such clearly defined distinctions are the result of differences in social systems: the earlier one, socialist, characterized by a proprietary system that was in the hands of society; the contemporary one, democratic, characterized by the privatization of formerly socially owned property.

With the advent of a certain degree of democratization in Bosnia and Herzegovina, the level of disagreement between law and morality has been reduced. The reason is that legislation, which is based on consensus building within the society, leaves much more room for ethical decision-making in the case of controversial issues. Differences between the health system and the physician–patient relationship in the socialist society of Bosnia and Herzegovina and that in the contemporary society of Bosnia and Herzegovina are shown in Table 34.1.

Challenges in Communication with Cancer Patients

Close to the end of the last century, socialist society developed into a society that ignored the sociopsychological and mental premises of the patient. As a result, until 15 years ago, oncology patients usually did not hear the truth about what they were suffering from in spite of the genuine care and empathy of the medical staff. This was the result of the will of the doctor on the one side and the wishes of the patient's family on the other side. In this way, avoiding open discussion with patients, doctors and close family members were spared from the patient's emotional state and

Table 34.1 Differences between the health system and doctor–patient relations in the socialistic society of Bosnia and Herzegovina and the contemporary B&H society

B&H socialist society	B&H contemporary society
Health insurance fund of republic of B&H	Two entity health insurance funds in B&H
Medications were free and available to everyone	Availability of medications is limited by the "list of cytostatics" at the level of entity funds
Health care was regulated by republic administration	Health care is up to the patient himself/herself
Doctors did not know the price of medications	Doctors are familiar with the prices of medications
Information about diseases, diagnosis, treatment, and medications was not available to the general public	Information about diseases, diagnosis, treatment and medication through the mass media and the internet is accessible to everyone
There were no services for palliative care and treatment of oncology patients	Services for palliative care and treatment of oncology patients are increasingly developing
There was a paternalistic attitude of doctors toward a patient	There is a cooperative doctor–patient relationship
Doctors did not tell the truth to patients or they told only part of it	Doctors tell the truth to patients
Informed consent was not present in the diagnosis and treatment of oncology or any other patients	Informed consent is present in the diagnosis and treatment of every patient [4]
The work of oncologists, surgeons, radiation oncologists, and other specialists in medical oncology was independent	The work of oncologists and other specialists is carried out within an interdisciplinary team
In the work of an oncologist evidence-based medicine was minimally present	Work of oncology team is based on evidence-based medicine
Patients often looked for cure in alternative medicine	Patients less often seek help in alternative medicine
Association of patients suffering from malignant diseases did not exist	There are associations of patients suffering from malignant and many other diseases or syndromes
Clinical research trials of new medications in oncology did not exist or were unavailable	The number of clinical trials and testing of new medications in oncology based on good clinical practice is rising [6]

reactions that followed the knowledge of the truth, that he/she was suffering from an incurable disease. Later in the course of the relationship between doctor and patient, if there was a need for surgical intervention, irradiation, or chemotherapy, the previously silent truth would put physicians in the unenviable situation of lying about the facts that would follow. Thus, the reactions to chemotherapy would be justified by the "stronger therapy" needed to "break" the inflammatory process that could not be healed by the previous antibiotic therapy. If irradiation was needed, then there would be the "warming of the lung," which aims to "expand the blood vessels in the area of inflammation so medications could arrive at the right place." Resection surgery was usually rationalized as the "urgent need to remove part or all of an organ so the infection would not spread to other organs or body parts."

Generally such relationships between doctors and patients were as harmful to the physician as they were to the patient, because to more intelligent and better educated patients the truth soon became clear anyway. This would result in emotional

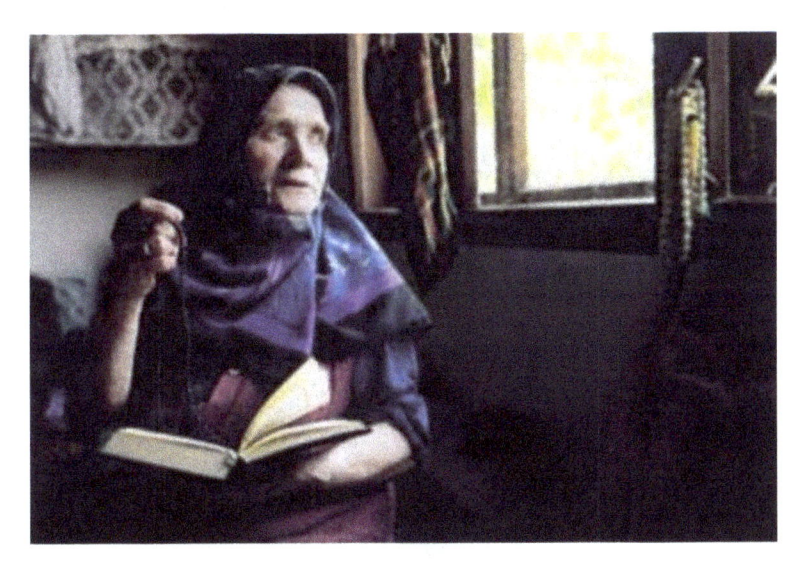

Fig. 34.1 Woman who heals with the help of the holy book

tension, fear, anger, depression, and sometimes resistance and public expression of feelings of vulnerability, refusal to continue treatment, or insisting that treatment be continued in another institution.

Until a few decades ago chemotherapy did not have clear goals and functions. It was not grounded in evidence-based medicine. Often the doctors who administered it did not have a clear conception of the relationship between chemotherapy's benefit and its toxicity, and did not clearly perceive the meaning of such treatment. Recommendations for it could be heard in the form, "Give him a little chemotherapy" and the like. As a result of all this uncertainty, it was not uncommon that oncological patients looked to Eastern medicine for drugs and various forms of alternative medicine—healing herbs, a variety of exotic plants, metals, crystals, bioenergy, and the supposedly sacred words that lead to healing (Figs. 34.1 and 34.2) [1, 2].

Today, in a situation where health care has devolved from the state (society) to the individual and the distribution of cash flow and capital is uneven, health insurance funds have limited financial resources, so patients often have to buy their own medications, including cytostatics. People are starting to realize that health has monetary value, and patients insist on talking with doctors, on being informed about everything, on participating in decision-making regarding both diagnosis and treatment [3]. The availability of information through mass media and the Internet has created a situation in which patients sometimes know more than their doctors about medical resources available elsewhere in the world. Dialogue and communication between doctor and patient has become indispensable for the creation of mutual trust.

The official view of the medical profession in Bosnia and Herzegovina is that the patient should be told what the expectations are regarding his/her disease; and that for incurable patients, the dignity of their sickness and dying should be respected [4]. However, we cannot say that this kind of dialogue is practiced in all parts of

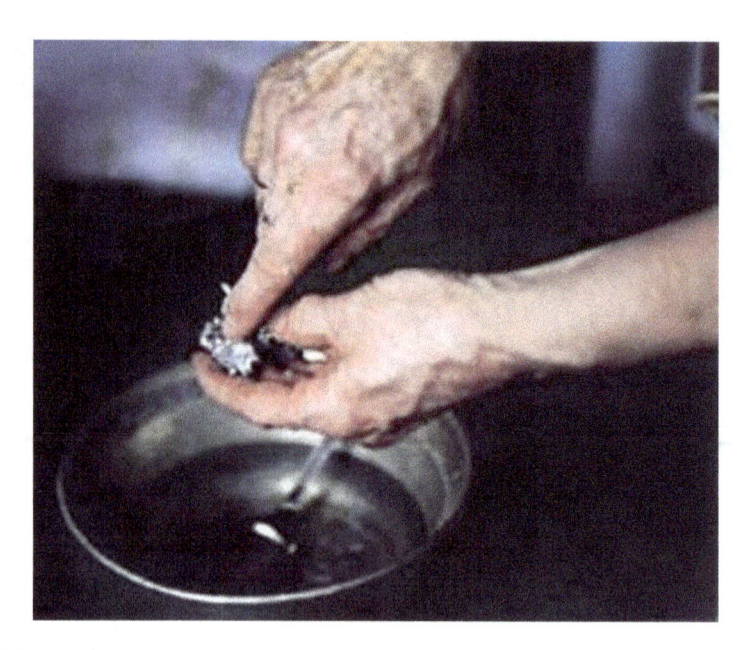

Fig. 34.2 The plumbous which is melted in a spoon and later thrown in a dish with water

Bosnia and Herzegovina and at all levels of its society. The reasons for this may be found in the level of education of patients, their familial status, profession, religion, and the fact that not communicating the whole truth by doctors does not often result in litigation. It should be noted that the interpersonal relationships of doctors and patients are not always at the required level, that they depend in part on the time the doctor spends with the patient, that each patient requires a different amount of time, and that doctors are not always in the mood to provide to each patient the same level of dedication. These interpersonal relationships depend on the ability of doctors to meet their patients' expectations concerning their treatment and care, the doctors' ability to convey properly the necessary information to the patient, but also the doctors' concern for, friendship with, and kindness toward the patient. Doctors in Bosnia and Herzegovina at this time do not feel as compelled to communicate the full truth as do those in such countries as the USA and the UK.

More educated patients are in a better position to understand the situation they are in, and, by virtue of that knowledge of the unpleasant truth, to keep their psychological and mental status under better control. Religious people often reject the idea that the truth should be told to the patient. They see it as in the patient's best interest to be spared psychological pain and insist on "peace" for the patient [5]. However, one must ask how ignoring the truth as the patient's health and life are obviously declining can contribute to peace? And yet, today in Bosnia and Herzegovina most oncology patients are not aware of the roles in which they find themselves or of their rights. As a result, they give up their autonomy, deciding to allow their doctor to do whatever he/she thinks best, often saying something like, "do what you would do if you were in my position" [6].

The use of new drugs in the treatment of patients with malignant disease sometimes enables long-term survival, and conducting long-term therapy requires good communication between patients, physicians, and members of their families. This communication is not just to help the patient deal with bad news or bear the emotional pressure of a life-threatening illness; it also helps the patient understand and remember a lot of information about the disease, treatment, and prognosis. Diagnosis is not the end but the beginning of treatment [7]. The period of uncertainty after the completion of treatment is often long, and often involves changes in the team that is treating the patient. Only communication allows the patient to understand the statistics relating to prognosis and to tolerate uncertainty when there is hope.

Contemporary Bosnia and Herzegovina society does not provide all oncology patients with palliative treatment and care when they are needed, so the majority of oncology patients remains without social or psychological support. Motivational therapy is also often lacking, usually resulting in patient's development of feelings of anxiety and/or depression that can complicate the work of their doctors [8]. Unfortunately, the family quickly becomes burned out in monitoring these patients, because, as the life span of oncology patients is increased, so are the various stages of deterioration and improvement, repeated treatments, and medical interventions. Still, despite the low average educational level of the population of Bosnia and Herzegovina and because, in part, of the frequency of watching movies and TV series in which the life prediction of difficult patients is openly talked about, it is now usual for families at the first meeting with the doctor to insist on a forecast of the survival of oncology patients. They become very disappointed if the doctors do not give a time frame for the life expectancy of their sick members. But they have no sense of whether their behavior is appropriate, whether they are too serious and tense in the period after the diagnosis, or too relaxed when the disease persists. Illness, fear of death, the feeling that death is really possible or is already near initiate the analysis of family relationships in general, as well as those with the patient. Usually it is said that with the disease the whole family gathers together and becomes closer; but in some cases the stress of the disease only deepens misunderstandings and problems that had existed before. It is important to overcome the stressful situations as soon as possible and to maintain communication in order to achieve a new balance that takes into account the new situation.

Finally, when it comes to dying patients, there is often among health professionals a conflict between "affective neutrality" and the need to empathize with the patient. Communication with the dying patient is a great emotional burden, so the health care professionals usually prefer to avoid it rather than to be engaged [9]. In contemporary Bosnia and Herzegovina society there are no teams dedicated to the psychological support of oncology or dying patients, whether through psycho-oncological counseling or through work in the department of oncological treatment and care. We hope that such teams come into use.

References

1. http://www.narodnilijek.com. Accessed 14 Mar 2011.
2. Seksan V. Stravom protiv užasa. Dani. Arhiva dani 211; 2001.
3. Zakon o lijekovima i medicinskim sredstvima BiH. Službeni glasnik BiH 217/08.
4. Ong LM, Visser MR, Lammes FB, et al. Doctor-patient communication and cancer patients' quality of life and satisfaction. Patient Educ Couns. 2000;41(2):145–56.
5. http://www.dusaitijelo.blogger.ba. Accessed 08 Oct 2008.
6. Talanga J. Odnos liječnika i pacijenta prema medicinskoj etici. BS 2006;76(1)47–59.
7. Albrecht TL, Franks MM, Ruckdeschel JC. Communication and informed consent. Curr Opin Oncol. 2005;17(4):336–9.
8. Braš M. Modeli organizacije palijativne medicine. Hrvatsko društvo za palijativnu medicine. Zagreb 2010.
9. www.plivamed.net/clanak/3225/www.plivamed.net/clanak/3224/Komunikacija-liječnika-s-teško-oboljelom-osobom. Accessed 10 Mar 2011.
10. Sorensen JB, Rossel P, Holm S. Patient-physician communication concerning participation in cancer chemotherapy trials. Br J Cancer. 2004;90(2):328–32.

Chapter 35
Evolution of Truth-Telling Practices in Brazil and South America

Gilberto Schwartsmann and Andre T. Brunetto

Abstract Truth-telling practices represent an old dilemma for caregivers, generating controversy in every age of mankind. The twentieth century witnessed the growing supremacy of truth and the gradual decline of merely "instilling hope" regarding the diagnosis and prognosis of cancer. More recently, with the introduction of more effective therapies and easier access to information by the general public, physicians are shifting towards an attitude of disclosing the correct diagnosis to patients. In a culturally, religiously, and socioeconomically heterogeneous population, such as in South America and Brazil, known for cancer health disparities, the development of tailored communication strategies and educational interventions are highly desirable. Here, it was common practice until 2 decades ago for doctors to withhold the diagnosis of cancer from patients. Although cancer prognosis is discussed more openly in some cultures, such as in North America and certain countries in Europe, there seems to be a trend towards disclosure of more detailed information regarding diagnosis and prognosis, at least in the more developed areas of South America and Brazil, compared to the past; although it should be accepted that many differences still remain as part of our cultural and socioeconomic background.

Keywords Truth-telling • Truth disclosure • Communication • Prognosis • Terminally ill • South America • Brazil

---

G. Schwartsmann (✉) • A.T. Brunetto
Hospital de Clínicas de Porto Alegre, Universidade Federal do Rio Grande do Sul,
Rua Ramiro Barcelos 2350, Porto Alegre, RS 90035903, Brazil
e-mail: gilberto.ez@terra.com.br; brunettoandre@hotmail.com

Truth-Telling Practices: An Historical View

Truth-telling practices represent an old dilemma for caregivers, generating controversy in every age of the history of mankind [1, 2]. In Western culture, physicians have witnessed a shift from a deception-friendly attitude towards a more deception-phobic one with regard to cancer diagnosis and prognosis. Even considering that deception is rejected in most human codes of ethics, the acceptability of deception in cancer is still observed in a variety of forms in certain cultures and individual practices [3, 4].

The Hippocratic writings encouraged doctors to be somewhat "economical" with the truth, suggesting that "such honest revelations" about disease outcome could be the cause of the worsening of the patient's prognosis [5]. Plato also was said to draw an analogy between lies and medicines, in the sense that sometimes a lie could act as a medicine to prevent undesirable actions and beliefs in suffering patients [6].

In the early 1800s, the prestigious English physician Thomas Percival was clear in his recommendations that "…the life of a sick person can be shortened not only by the acts, also by the words or manners of a physician. It is, therefore, a sacred duty to avoid all things which have a tendency to discourage the patient and to depress his spirit…" [7].

Furthermore, the first Code of Ethics issued in 1847 by the American Medical Association instructed physicians to avoid making "gloomy prognostications" to patients, leaving the information on cancer diagnosis and bad prognosis to their relatives [8].

Truth-Telling Attitudes in the Twentieth Century

The twentieth century witnessed the growing supremacy of truth and the gradual decline of simply "instilling hope" about the diagnosis and prognosis to cancer patients [9]. Physicians began to question the inability of patients to cope with bad news, believing that the short-term advantages of a lie were outweighed by the long-term benefits of the truth [10].

The prestigious Canadian physician William Osler appeared to favor both truth telling and deception, depending on the patient context. He was quoted as saying "…it is a hard matter and really not often necessary (since nature usually does it quietly and in good time) to tell a patient that he is past all hope…" [11].

In the early 1950s, in a survey performed in the Philadelphia area of the USA, it was observed that 69% of physicians who responded to a mailed questionnaire acknowledged that they never informed or usually did not inform the patient of a diagnosis of cancer. Twenty-eight percent said that they usually informed the patient, while only 3% said that they always informed the patient. The main reasons for not giving clear information to the patient were the fear of an unfavorable reaction from the patient and the family's request not to inform him or her, reflecting a time when relatives often were informed about a cancer diagnosis before the patient [12].

The above-mentioned attitude of nondisclosure of a cancer diagnosis was supported by another observation in the 1960s in a study by Oken and colleagues, which revealed that 90% of a sample of 219 doctors in the Chicago area said that they usually withhold a cancer diagnosis from patients [13]. That was also the case in a different study performed in the UK, showing that three out of four physicians treating terminal patients preferred not to inform them about their dismal prognosis [14].

Until the first decades of the twentieth century, the most important outcome of many medicines was probably the placebo effect. Therefore, a great deal of the success in medical practice was based on the ability of the physician to instill a sense of confidence in the patient [11, 12]. This scenario started to change in the 1950s, when several effective drugs became widely available, and physicians could then count on their positive pharmacological effects [15].

In 1979, an almost identical questionnaire to that applied to physicians in the Philadelphia area was sent to American physicians. Only 40% of them responded to the questionnaire; however, 97% of the responders said they would disclose a diagnosis of cancer to their patients [16]. Although these results were highly provocative, they were not confirmed by others, suggesting that there was a difference between what physicians answer in a questionnaire and their attitude in "real-life" medical practice [17].

With the introduction of more effective therapies and easier access to information on the subject of cancer by the general public, physicians appear to be shifting towards an attitude of disclosing the correct diagnosis to patients [18–20]. In North America and some European countries, especially in Scandinavia, this attitude goes even further in terms of discussing openly the patients' prognosis [21–23].

This truth-telling attitude is far from universal. In the late 1970s, the Deontology Code issued by the Italian Medical Association stated that "A serious or lethal prognosis can be hidden from the patient, but not from the family" [24]. This deception-friendly attitude is still observed today in many countries, as reported in studies conducted in China, Japan, Singapore, and Lebanon, where patients with cancer are often not told their diagnosis and almost never told their real prognosis [25–29].

The Situation in South America and Brazil

In a culturally, religiously, and socioeconomically heterogeneous population, such as in South America, that is known for cancer health disparities, the development of tailored communication strategies and educational interventions is highly desirable [30]. By this approach, knowledge about cancer can be enhanced, helping the physician accurately explain the risks and benefits of treatments, dispel negative beliefs, and promote a better doctor–patient relationship [31].

In South American countries, it was common practice until 2 decades ago for doctors to withhold the diagnosis of cancer from patients. Neither patients, relatives, nor the healthcare team would mention the word *cancer* during the consultation, replacing it by less precise terms or euphemisms. In certain communities, cancer was even considered a potentially infectious disease, which could put the lives of others at risk [32, 33].

There are several reasons to explain this behavior. Until recently, cancer was considered a death sentence, and patients, relatives, and the medical team rarely discussed it openly. Cancer patients were left in complete isolation. In many cases, relatives would first discuss the diagnosis with the medical team and make sure that it would be hidden from the patient [34].

Over the past 4 decades, major advances in the treatment of malignancies have been achieved. In many types of cancer considered to be fatal in the past, such as acute leukemias, lymphomas, and germ-cell tumors, the cure rates have increased significantly. In other malignant conditions, such as breast and ovarian cancer, the survival rates and control of symptoms have also improved dramatically. The improvements in treatment outcome for many malignancies and the significant increase of life expectancy for cancer patients became a valuable tool in the discussion concerning diagnosis and prognosis [35].

In Brazil, the study of oncology as a separate discipline in the curriculum of medical universities is a reality of the last 2 decades. Before, medical students received their training on the management of cancer patients from general surgeons, gynecologists, radiotherapists, and clinicians. Nowadays, oncology is part of the curriculum in several medical schools, but not in all of them. Nevertheless, the establishment of oncology as an independent discipline and the provision of a proper education in this subject have been critical aspects in changing our mentality from a deception-friendly to a more deception-phobic attitude [36].

As elsewhere in the Western world, we are witnessing a tendency towards a truth-telling attitude, especially among physicians working in academic centers of urban areas; while a more deception-friendly attitude is still the rule in most rural and less-developed areas [37].

Physicians can develop psychological defense mechanisms related to the fear of death and the uncontrolled suffering of cancer [38, 39]. These feelings may act as a barrier in the doctor–patient relationship [40], explaining why communication between physicians and cancer patients can sometimes be difficult. It is important that these emotional aspects are handled properly by the medical team.

In several South American countries, there may be a problem of illiteracy, which also creates a barrier in doctor–patient communication. In our view, individuals coming from distinct geographical, cultural, religious, or socioeconomic backgrounds have more emotional aspects to share than differences to separate them. Medical experience suggests that when the word *cancer* cannot be used in a specific medical context, or when it is not technically understood by the patient or relatives, there are alternative expressions, such as "a serious disease that puts life at risk," that can be used instead [41].

Competent physicians can make use of such expressions in order to explain the diagnosis and, sometimes, prognosis to patients and relatives. In other words, there is always an honest and kind way to tell the truth to the patient that can strengthen the doctor–patient relationship—that can establish a bond of trust between the doctor and patient, instead of increasing the feeling of isolation, especially in difficult moments such as the diagnosis of cancer [42].

Currently, in most countries of South America and in Brazil, the Medical Code of Ethics states clearly that a practicing physician must ensure that the patient (or his legal representative) receives proper information on the nature, purpose, and potential consequences of medical actions that will be undertaken for diagnosis, treatment, or research [43–46].

Studies have demonstrated that most North Americans want to know if they have a life-threatening illness and how long they will live [18, 26, 27]. Unfortunately, this kind of information is very limited in peer-reviewed literature for South America [28–30].

Bruera et al. [47] compared the attitudes and beliefs of palliative care specialists regarding communication with the terminally ill in Europe, South America, and Canada. The authors show that palliative care physicians in all three regions believe that cancer patients should be informed of their diagnosis and the terminal nature of their illness. Physicians reported that at least 60% of their patients knew their diagnosis — 52% in South America and 69% in Europe, respectively. While 93% of Canadian physicians stated that at least 60% of their patients wanted to know about the terminal stage of their illness, only 18% of South American and 26% of European physicians said this. Finally, in their daily decision making, South American physicians were significantly more likely to support beneficence and justice as compared to autonomy.

In a recently published Brazilian study, Trindade and colleagues [48] interviewed 38 physicians regarding the disclosure of diagnostic and prognostic information to cancer patients. The majority (97%) informs their patients of the diagnosis, and 50% rely on the family for support. In cases of poor prognosis, 63% tell only the families, while 31% prefer to tell only the patients. In addition, the study revealed that physicians can misunderstand beneficence and paternalism.

Pinto et al. [49] surveyed 239 patients regarding their preferences about cancer information in São Paulo, Brazil. Patients were interested in obtaining information on their health condition: whether they had cancer (95%), the chances of recovery (89%), and the side effects during treatment (94%). Younger patients tended to show more interest in obtaining information than the elderly. No correlation was found between psychiatric morbidity and the desire for information.

A similar Brazilian study was conducted by Gulinelli et al. [50] of 363 patients, evaluating their desire to be informed about the diagnosis of severe diseases and to participate in therapeutic decisions. Ninety-six percent of men and 92% of women showed the desire to be informed in cases of cancer diagnosis, and 87% of men and 84% of women wanted to have their families informed. While 86% of women and 76% of men wanted to be informed in the case of a diagnosis of an abdominal tumor, only 58.5% of women and 39.6% of men wanted to give their opinion regarding different therapeutic alternatives. The desire to participate in therapeutic decisions was significantly lower in men, people older than 60 years, and inpatients.

Although cancer prognosis is discussed more openly in some cultures, such as in North America and certain countries in Europe, there seems to be trend towards disclosure of more detailed information regarding diagnosis and prognosis in developed areas of South America [21–23], although it should be accepted that many differences still remain as part of our cultural and socioeconomic background. As a rule, discussing the prognosis of cancer with patients and relatives is a very difficult task for physicians anywhere in the world, and this surely is the case in Brazil. It is clear from the literature that better communication skills improve patient satisfaction and clinical outcomes, at least in the form of improved quality of life [19, 51, 52].

Establishing prognosis for patients with advanced cancer is generally inaccurate. In a recent survey, physicians' estimates of prognosis for patients in palliative care programs were shown to be overoptimistic [53–55]. It was observed that physicians tend to overestimate survival, being most accurate in those patients with the shortest overall survival [56, 57]. A meta-analysis of these studies suggests that survival is generally 30% shorter than predicted by physician estimates [58, 59]. Survival data for most cancers according to stage are widely available. However, this information is not very useful in assessing the prognosis of an individual patient. Prospective randomized trials that include a "best supportive care" arm could guide doctors in providing information on the impact of a specific type of treatment upon the natural course of a disease [60, 61]. Integrating the effect of various physical symptoms with data from multiple sources of prognostic information improves the ability of a physician to predict disease outcome with more accuracy [62, 63].

What Are We Teaching Young Oncologists in Academic Hospitals in Brazil?

It is our experience that communicating diagnosis and prognosis using a direct and compassionate manner helps patients and relatives cope with the disease and facilitates treatment planning. This attitude is essential for patients to maintain autonomy and tends to strengthen the doctor–patient relationship.

A clear disclosure of diagnosis and prognosis is very important for both treatment and decision making for patients with cancer. Patient desire should be always respected. The art of the doctor–patient relationship resides in developing mutual confidence to provide a sense about the level of information and truth with which each specific patient is to be able to cope [64].

Developing effective communication skills is part of what we consider the training and duty of a good cancer specialist. The competent oncologist should be capable of building a relationship with the patient and his or her relatives, in which the patient should be able to gather the necessary information about the diagnosis, the planned treatment, and potential outcome at the appropriate time [65, 66].

Patients may want to have an approximate idea of their future in order to plan their lives. In these cases, it is desirable to provide survival estimates. Good communication skills can make difficult discussions with cancer patients and relatives easier, providing them with the information necessary to make informed decisions about their treatment [67, 68].

There are general recommendations on how physicians should deal with the truth about cancer diagnosis and prognosis that are applicable to any country in the world, including those of South America. The diagnosis of cancer is a dramatic event in the life of a human being. Therefore, this information should be handled by an experienced, senior member of the medical team. The physician in charge of this difficult task should be familiar with all available information concerning the diagnosis and the treatment options to be offered to the patient in the institution and, preferably, in other centers.

The more experienced physicians would first establish some level of confidence with the patient and his relatives, leaving the discussion about prognosis to a separate visit. A direct presentation of negative figures about cancer survival during the first contact with the patient may be a sign of omnipotence, lack of experience, or poor training in the art of the doctor–patient relationship. In most cases, patients with cancer will first receive accurate but simple information on diagnosis, while the information on (bad) prognosis will be built along future visits and influenced by treatment results [66].

The consultation with the patient and relatives should be done in an appropriate environment, with the level of privacy required for such an important situation. This appointment should be scheduled in a way that patient and family will have the time necessary to clarify doubts and ask questions about the diagnosis, treatment, and prognosis. The medical team should make sure that all cultural and/or idiomatic barriers that could have a negative impact on the communication are solved beforehand [66].

It is critical to establish what and how much each patient wants to know about the diagnosis and prognosis. The way the patient reacts to the questions gives indications about his level of understanding and family dynamics. Each individual handles information differently, depending on cultural, religious, socioeconomic class, or other factors. Patients also have the right to decline to receive information about their disease and may designate another member of the family or a close friend to communicate with the medical team on their behalf.

Not infrequently do relatives ask the physician not to tell the patient the diagnosis. Although it is our legal obligation to inform the patient and to obtain informed consent from him or her before starting treatment, a healthy doctor–patient relationship also requires a congenial alliance with the family. Rather than confronting their request to omit the truth from the patient, it is recommended that their reasons for concern and the advantages of open communication be discussed. In difficult situations, support from the local ethics committee might be helpful. Unless the patient has previously indicated that he or she wishes to receive no information, hiding the diagnosis is neither ethical nor legally acceptable [65].

Cancer patients can express their desire to receive more detailed information about prognosis, because it can influence their decisions regarding future plans. Giving precise details about the life expectancy of an individual patient is a very complex and risky task. Most patients will be satisfied with general information. Patients and relatives react to bad news in different ways. Some respond with sadness, anger, anxiety, or other feelings. Others respond with denial, blame, guilt, or fear or may intellectualize the situation. It is important to give the patient and family enough time to react to and accept the new situation [63, 64].

Some cancer patients do not ask direct questions about their prognosis. Usually in this situation the prognosis is discussed more openly with the relatives. Some family members fear that the information on diagnosis and prognosis will be so distressing that it will affect the patient adversely. Carefully shared information is critical to the patient and family who wish for detailed counsel and advice and minimizes the chance that they will distrust the doctor and the medical team.

In summary, it is important to reassure the patient and his or her relatives that the medical team will be always there to support them during the course of the illness. Medical students and physicians in training in oncology should receive proper guidance from more experienced members of the medical team concerning the importance of building an honest and empathic doctor–patient relationship.

References

1. Fletcher J. Morals and medicine. London: Victor Gollancz Ltd.; 1955.
2. Sokol D. How the doctor's nose has shortened over time; a historical overview of the truth-telling debate in the doctor-patient relationship. J R Soc Med. 2006;99:632–6.
3. Sokol D. Truth-telling in the doctor-patient relationship: a case analysis. Clin Ethics. 2006;1:130–4.
4. Thomsen O, Wulff H, Martin A, Singer P. What do gastroenterologists in Europe tell cancer patients? Lancet. 1993;341:473–8.
5. Jones W, editor. Hippocrates II. London: Harvard University Press; 1988.
6. Plato. The republic [translated by Lee, D.]. London: Penguin; 2003.
7. Thomas WJ. Informed consent, the placebo effect, and the revenge of Thomas Percival. J Leg Med. 2001;22:313–48.
8. Code of Ethics of the American Medical Association. 1847. http://www.ama.assn.org/ama/upload/mm/369/1847code.pdf.
9. Jackson J. Truth, trust and medicine. New York: Routledge; 2001.
10. Cabot R. The use of truth and falsehood in medicine: an experimental study. Am Med. 1903;5:344–9.
11. Osler W. The treatment of disease. Can Lancet. 1909;42:899–912.
12. Fitts W, Ravdin I. What Philadelphia physicians tell patients with cancer. J Am Med Assoc. 1953;153:901–4.
13. Oken D. What to tell cancer patients: a study of medical attitudes. JAMA. 1961;175:1120–8.
14. Kelly W, Friesen S. Do cancer patients want to be told? Surgery. 1950;27:944–7.
15. Schwartsmann G, Ratain MJ, Cragg GM, Wong JE, Saijo N, Parkinson DR, et al. Anticancer drug discovery and development throughout the world. J Clin Oncol. 2002;20(18 Suppl):47S–59.
16. Novack D, Plumer R, Smith R, Ochitill H, Morrow G, Bennett J. Changes in physician's attitudes toward telling the cancer patient. JAMA. 1979;241:897–900.
17. Miyaji N. The power of compassion: truth-telling among American doctors in the care of dying patients. Soc Sci Med. 1993;36:249–94.
18. Kurtz SM. Doctor patient communication: principles and practices. Can J Neurol Sci. 2002;29 Suppl 2:S23–9.
19. Fallowfield L, Jenkins V. Communicating sad, bad, and difficult news in medicine. Lancet. 2004;363:312–9.
20. Maguire P. Improving communication with cancer patients. Eur J Cancer. 1999;35:2058–65.

21. Ashbury FD, Findlay H, Reynolds B, McKerracher KA. Canadian survey of cancer patients' experiences: are their needs being met? J Pain Symptom Manage. 1998;16:298–306.
22. Maguire P. Improving the recognition of concerns and affective disorders in cancer patients. Ann Oncol. 2002;13 Suppl 4:177–81.
23. Thorne SE, Bultz BD, Baile WF. Is there a cost to poor communication in cancer care? A critical review of the literature. Psychooncology. 2005;14:875–84.
24. Surbone A. Letter from Italy. JAMA. 1992;268:1661–2.
25. Hamadeh G, Adib S. Cancer truth disclosure by Lebanese doctors. Soc Sci Med. 1998;47:1289–94.
26. Lee A, Wu H. Diagnosis disclosure in cancer patients: when the family says "no!" Singapore Med J. 2002;43:533–8.
27. Sekimoto M, Asai A, Ohnishi M, et al. Patients' preferences for involvement in treatment decision making in Japan. BMC Fam Pract. 2004;5:1.
28. Seo M, Tamura K, Morioka E, Ikegame C, Hirasako K. Telling the diagnosis to cancer patients in Japan: attitude and perception of patients, physicians and nurses. Palliat Med. 2000;14:105–10.
29. Jadalla A, Sharaya H. A Jordanian view about cancer knowledge and attitudes. Cancer Nurs. 1998;21:269–73.
30. Faria SL, Souhami L. Communication with the cancer patient: information and truth in Brazil. Ann N Y Acad Sci. 1997;809:163–71.
31. Schwartsmann G. Breast cancer in South America: challenges to improve early detection and medical management of a public health problem. J Clin Oncol. 2001;19(18 Suppl):118S–24.
32. Olopade OI, Schwartsmann G, Saijo N, Thomas Jr CR. Disparities in cancer care: a worldwide perspective and roadmap for change. J Clin Oncol. 2006;24(14):2135–6.
33. Carlson RW, Anderson BO, Chopra R, Eniu AE, Jakesz R, Love RR, et al. Treatment of breast cancer in countries with limited resources. Global Summit Treatment Panel. Breast J. 2003;9 Suppl 2:S67–74.
34. Sikora K, Advani S, Koroltchouk V, Magrath I, Levy L, Pinedo H, et al. Essential drugs for cancer therapy: a World Health Organization consultation. Ann Oncol. 1999;10(4):385–90.
35. Ribeiro MM, Krupat E, Amaral CC. Brazilian medical student's attitudes towards patient-centered care. Med Teach. 2007;29:204–8.
36. Victorica MIG, Bertolino L, Pavlovsky S. Argentina: telling the truth to cancer patients in a multicultural society. Ann N Y Acad Sci. 1997;809:152–62.
37. Dolbeault S, Brédart A. Difficultés de l'annonce du côté des professionnels et de leurs patients: Quells obstacles á la communication et quels recours possibles? Bull Cancer. 2010;97:1183–94.
38. Buckman R. How to break bad news: a guide for health care professionals. Baltimore, MD: The Johns Hopkins University Press; 1992. p. 65–97.
39. Garg A, Buckman R, Kason Y. Teaching medical students how to break bad news. CMAJ. 1997;156:1159–64.
40. Quill TE, Arnold RM, Platt F. "I wish things were different": expressing wishes in response to loss, futility, and unrealistic hopes. Ann Intern Med. 2001;135:551–5.
41. Gilbar R, Gilbar O. The medical decision-making process and the family: the case of breast cancer patients and their husbands. Bioethics. 2009;23(3):183–92. doi:10.1111/j.1467-8519.2008.00650.
42. Baile WF, Aaron J, Parker PA. Practitioner-patient communication in cancer diagnosis and treatment. In: Miller SM, Bowen DJ, Croyle RT, Rowland J, editors. Cancer control and behavioral science. Washington, DC: APA; 2009. p. 327–46.
43. Burton M, Watson M. Communication problems. In: Burton M, Watson M, editors. Counselling people with cancer. Chichester: Wiley; 1998. p. 69–94.
44. Back AL, Arnold RM, Baile WF, Tulsky JA, Fryer-Edwards K. Approaching difficult communication tasks in oncology. CA Cancer J Clin. 2005;55:164–77.
45. Stiefel F, Favre N, Despland JN. Communication skills training in oncology: it works! Recent Results Cancer Res. 2006;168:113–9.
46. Brazilian Medical Ethics Code. Novo Código de Ética Médica Brasileiro. version 2010. Accessed by http://www.portalmedico.org.br/novocodigo/index.asp.

47. Bruera E, Neumann CM, Mazzocato C, Stiefel F, Sala R. Attitudes and beliefs of palliative care physicians regarding communication with terminally ill cancer patients. Palliat Med. 2000;14(4):287–98.
48. de Souza Trindade E, de Azambuja LE, Andrade JP, Garrafa V. The physician when facing diagnosis and prognosis of advanced cancer. Rev Assoc Med Bras. 2007;53(1):268–74.
49. Pinto RN, Chaves AC, Lourenço MT, Mari Jde J. Information needs of recently diagnosed cancer patients in Brazil. Int J Psychiatry Med. 2004;34(4):319–29.
50. Gulinelli A, Aisawa RK, Konno SN, Morinaga CV, Costardi WL, Antonio RO, et al. Desire for information and participation in therapeutic decisions concerning severe diseases, in patients of a university hospital. Rev Assoc Med Bras. 2004;50(1):41–7.
51. Baile WF, Buckman R, Lenzi R, Glober G, Beale EA, Kudelka AP. SPIKES: a six-step protocol for delivering bad news: application to the patient with cancer. Oncologist. 2000;5:302–11.
52. Silverman J, Kurtz S, Draper J. Skills for communicating with patients. 2nd ed. Oxford: Radcliffe Medical; 2005.
53. O'Brien MA, Whelan TJ, Villasis-Keever M, Gafni A, Charles C, Roberts R, et al. Are cancer-related decision aids effective? A systematic review and meta-analysis. J Clin Oncol. 2009;27:974–85.
54. Roter DL, Larson S, Fischer GS, Arnold RM, Tulsky JA. Experts practice what they preach: a descriptive study of best and normative practices in end-of-life decisions. Arch Intern Med. 2000;160:3477–85.
55. Vignano A, Doran M, Bruera E, Suarez-Alzamor ME. The relative accuracy of the clinical estimation of the duration of life for patients with end of life cancer. Cancer. 1999;86:170–6.
56. Heyse-Moore LH, Johhnson-Bell VE. Can doctors accurately predict the life expectancy of patients with terminal cancer? Palliat Med. 1987;1:165–6.
57. Justice AC, Covinsky KE, Berlin JA. Assessing the generalizability of prognostic information. Ann Intern Med. 1999;130:515.
58. Parkes CM. Accuracy of predictions of survival in later stages of cancer. BMJ. 1972;2:29–31.
59. Glare P, Virik K, Jones M, et al. A systematic review of physicians' survival predictions in terminally ill cancer patients. BMJ. 2003;327:195–200.
60. Maltoni M, Caraceni A, Grunell C, et al. Prognostic factors in advanced cancer patients: evidence-based clinical recommendations—a study by the Steering Committee of the European Association for Palliative Care. J Clin Oncol. 2005;23:6240–8.
61. Loprinzi CL, Laurie JA, Wieand HS, et al. Prospective evaluation of prognostic variables from patient-completed questionnaires. J Clin Oncol. 1994;12:601–7.
62. Maltoni M, Nanni O, Dermi S, et al. Clinical prediction of survival is more accurate than the Karnofsky performance status in estimating life span of terminally ill cancer patients. Eur J Cancer. 1994;30A:764–6.
63. Maltoni M, Pirovano M, Scarpi E, et al. Prediction of survival of patients terminally ill with cancer. Cancer. 1995;75:2613–22.
64. Hagerty RG, Butow PN, Ellis PM, et al. Communicating with realism and hope: incurable cancer patients' views on the disclosure of prognosis. J Clin Oncol. 2005;23:1278–88.
65. Clever SL, Tulsky JA. Dreaded conversations: moving beyond discomfort in patient-physician communication. J Gen Intern Med. 2002;17:884–5.
66. Girgis A, Sanson-Fisher RW. Breaking bad news: consensus guidelines for medical practitioners. J Clin Oncol. 1995;13:2449–56.
67. Moss AH, Lunney JR, Sulp S, et al. Prognostic significance of the "surprise" question in cancer patients. J Palliat Med. 2010;13:837–40.
68. Finlay E, Casarett D. Making difficult discussions easier: using prognosis to facilitate transitions to hospice. CA Cancer J Clin. 2009;59(4):250–63.

Chater 36
Communication with Cancer Patients in Russia: Improving Patients' Participation and Motivation

Eugeny Demin and Anastasia Gamaley

Abstract The authors present their vision of open communication with cancer patients in Russia in comparison with such interactions in Western Europe and the USA. In Russia, the Western approach to cancer awareness is still uncommon, particularly with regard to truth-telling. Patients who are currently diagnosed with cancer, and healthy people who may be diagnosed at some time, do not know how they should react, because they are not adequately informed about cancer. One of most effective ways to make people not delay visiting a specialist is to involve the various segments of society in communication. Cooperative, honest, and active patient participation is a new challenge in communication with the public and cancer patients in Russia. It is accepted that motivation of people to be responsible for their own life in the case of cancer leads to its earlier detection and to better treatment results. Patients are not indifferent to knowing how long they would live and what their life would be like if they were affected by such a devastating disease, with the spectrum of a possible recurrence at any time. Key tasks following diagnosis are to help patients gradually adapt to new living conditions and to be compliant through full understanding of the suggested scope of treatment. There are millions of individuals who have survived cancer. Most of them were enabled to do so not only because of high-quality treatment, but because of early diagnosis, which was achieved by satisfactory communication between doctor and patient. Only direct, balanced, optimistic interaction among physicians, cancer patients, and healthy people will help those who have been taken ill or may be.

Keywords Communication • Cancer patients • Awareness of cancer • Truth-telling • Quality of life

---

E. Demin (✉) • A. Gamaley
Department of Cancer Control, N.N. Petrov Research Institute of Oncology,
68 Leningradskaya Street, Pesochny 197785, St. Petersburg, Russia
e-mail: doctor-demin@yandex.ru; demin@niioncologii.ru

Introduction

There live among us a number of people who were told, "You have cancer," and their lives divided into two parts, before and after. While many events may divide people's lives, cancer patients differ from other people: all of them have gone an amazing way that taught them to live with cancer, to survive its rather aggressive treatment, and to live under the sword of Damocles because of the disease's unpredictable recurrence.

In Russia, such awareness of cancer is still atypical. Specialists are able to value these circumstances; but ordinary people—patients who are currently diagnosed with cancer and healthy people who may be diagnosed in the future—do not know how they should react, because they are not adequately informed about cancer.

Although paying homage to the wise statements of Professor Nikolai N. Petrov (the founder of Russian oncology at the beginning of the last century) about how not to bruise cancer patients' psychology [1, 2], we must view the problem of communication in cancer from the perspective of today's life. This comes down to whether or not the truth about the disease should be told to a cancer patient and, more generally, whether or not there should be more, and more open, talk about cancer among all people. Taken out of the boundless sea of moral necessity, these questions still remain debatable in Russia, where a polarity of opinions—either "yes" or "no," both given firmly—makes itself quite conspicuous. Sometimes even experienced oncologists are ineffective when talking to their patients. How, then, would young specialists get on with the issue? Avoiding the talk altogether would be to follow a wrong, destructive path. So it is necessary to make a clear decision about what to say and, more important, *how* to say it, how far a specialist should go in furnishing information. Furthermore, the conversation should create minimum uncertainty, with all the patient's questions answered, since any hesitation may well be taken by the patient in a detrimental way [3].

Some Data on Cancer Control and Early Diagnosis in Russia

Cancer has held an important place among threatening chronic noninfectious diseases in Russia. About 500,000 new patients with malignant tumors are registered annually. In men, lung cancer has the leading position, with the second and the third places occupied by cancers of the stomach and prostate, respectively. In women, the first place belongs to breast cancer; malignancies of skin and colon occupy the second and the third places, respectively.

Cancer emerges without any preliminary warning signs. It is often impossible to catch cancer in an early stage. It has no early signs of pathology; its primary clinical evidence may not give any reason to worry. Quite commonly, cancer is disguised under general disorders, which visit us rather often in our lives and can disappear without any assistance. And here we find ourselves in a fairly dangerous situation: cancer cannot be caught on time—except for cases of visible skin parts; and once it *is* detected, it is no longer incipient; it has advanced. Unlike cardiovascular diseases

(CVD), which have the highest death rate, cancer can be lethal, yet it does not tend to lead to sudden death. Cancer takes away the lives of more than 300,000 patients every year in Russia.

Fortunately, science forges ahead. Traditional methods of cancer therapy are being improved, new ones are being developed, and the contingent of patients with lasting remission grows larger. At present, around 2.5 million former cancer patients are registered in Russia. Furthermore, our medical network, from general practitioners and various specialists up to oncology professionals, makes it possible to identify cancer cases throughout the whole country. We have a rather good working organization in oncology; a person diagnosed with cancer can receive adequate assistance at qualified oncology institutions (specialized hospitals, dispensaries, and institutes) located in all the large towns of Russia.

Improvement, however, is still needed in Russia in several ways. First, we must pay strict attention to the Cancer Alarm Approach. In the 1950s, the American Cancer Society (ACS) enunciated seven warning signs of cancer, each of which was supposed to turn one's mind to a possible cancer occurrence. These signs are well known: unusual bleeding or discharges; a lump or thickening in the breast or elsewhere; a sore that does not heal; change in bowel or bladder habits; hoarseness or cough; indigestion or difficulty in swallowing; change in a mole or wart. The list is still of interest and significance and the tests are relatively simple. The ACS's advice was, "If you notice any of these symptoms *go to your doctor without delay*! It may not be due to cancer, but if it is, the sooner treatment begins the greater will be your chance of cure." Disappointingly, in Russia, although our pioneers in oncology tried to implement a similar approach long before the ACS [1], it is not much liked.

The Cancer Alarm Approach can be brought into action in both subjective and objective ways. An example of the subjective way is when a person having unexplained changes in his/her body or a specialist advising such a person at the outset does not consider the possibility of tumor disease; considering this possibility would allow the cancer to be detected before it has reached an advanced stage. So far in our country, both specialists and patients often ignore this timely way of diagnosis. This testifies that there is not enough interaction between professionals and the general public. It is sad that a person with a health problem is examined without the physician taking into account that the problem might itself indicate cancer or could be further transformed into cancer as a result of its biological characteristics.

An objective way of using the Cancer Alarm Approach is through cancer screening programs, which are used extensively in Western Europe and the USA; these increase the likelihood of diagnosing symptomless malignancies. Unfortunately, this method has not been adequately adopted in Russia, because of the significant financial expenditure required as well as indolence on the part of public health officials. Even if expenditures for cancer screening look huge at first sight, those for treatment of advanced cancer are incomparably greater. (In Russia, there has been no official calculation of these numbers.)

Gradually, however, this method of cancer control is entering the consciousness of our specialists. Systematic screening is a way to save many lives and to lower the rate of negative side effects of tumor therapy at earlier stages, when the treatment is less aggressive. Oncologists have been trying to attract the attention and cooperation of the mass media in promoting knowledge about tobacco-related cancer, explaining the danger of smoking and the benefits of screening for lung, breast, colon, prostate, and cervical cancer; and also clarifying that the primary goal of prevention and screening is reducing the mortality rate by means of early diagnosis. Disappointingly, little has changed in Russia over the last few years, particularly in connection with cancer of the lung; despite broad warnings, smoking in public places is still not forbidden, and women smoke as much as men.

Historical Notes on the Development of Communication about Cancer in Russia

All activities and spheres of the former Soviet society were affected by its secrecy. Clinical medicine—oncology in particular—was not an exception, being just a part of the isolated system. Medical ethics were also affected and depended on ideological considerations. This has all changed. Now we cannot picture life without computer, fax, e-mail, and an expansive mass media. We no longer identify people by their class or oppose ourselves to the entire world. Rather, we welcome new illuminating ideas that could enrich and modernize our perceptions regarding interpersonal relations in oncology [4]. We cannot undo history, but we should accept it as what it was and move on, gradually rejecting dated postulates and giving up old habits. Opinions are changing. Nowadays, Russian people approach medical issues differently, as they have access to the large amount of information about a healthy lifestyle and therapeutics that is now available through the Internet and medical literature. It is now difficult to withhold information or to conceal certain facts from patients.

In this regard, large-scale implementation of multicenter clinical trials of new anticancer agents has made oncology a more open discipline. Now it is simply impossible to treat cancer without explaining to patients what is actually happening to them. One cannot help wondering how an author from an earlier era, such as Professor Petrov, cited above, would feel about informed consent, which has become an important instrument of everyday communication between oncologist and patient? In 1945, Petrov wrote: "Tell people the truth about cancer and they will stop being afraid of it. Communicate with people frankly and make them believe that by means of reasonable activities many forms of cancer can be prevented" [2]. This reference shows that already in the early twentieth century some physicians believed in truth-telling and its potential beneficial effects on patients, yet the practice of informed consent as necessary for patients to participate in decision-making would have sounded unthinkable. The pioneers of Russian oncology urged patients and physicians to take very cautiously any dubious symptoms or symptoms that do not fit the common illness-condition scheme, and they taught to see in such symptoms signs of cancer. They considered that in the long run it was better for a suspected tumor not to be confirmed than for it to be missed. It is important not to overleap ourselves in the search for cancer and not to frighten unnecessarily someone who might not have cancer.

Real and Ideal Communication with Cancer Patients in Russia

In the sphere of oncology, communication with either potential or actual patients has a specific character. Unfortunately, the prevailing public opinion about cancer mortality in Russia is getting in the way of constructive interaction. If positive results of cancer therapy depend directly upon the earliest possible detection of neoplasm, general physicians should immediately refer their patients to oncology specialists. Here we encounter a vicious cycle: Usually people who see others suffering from cancer do not take into account that most of them have gone through a certain history of the illness that brought them to their current state. Instead, they see cancer as it is at that particular moment. They tend to ignore that if these sufferers had sought medical attention even a little sooner, their illness might have been less severe and their rehabilitation more effective. In the near future, cancer will not be completely curable. From an economic viewpoint, a public health service can rarely afford extremely expensive medicine to treat incurable illnesses. However, to make after-treatment remission last longer is an attainable task, both medically and economically.

Hence, cancer appears also to be a social problem, not only involving people's health and relationships, but also their own financial well-being, as well as affecting the public health system. We can end the vicious cycle just by communicating with people, not insisting on the negative side of cancer, which could be very frightening and result in fatalism; but rather providing information about modern ways of diagnosing and treating cancer. In order to achieve these ambitious goals in Russia, many stakeholders should be involved in an interactive process: doctors, mass media, patients' relatives, volunteers and patients' advocates, and social organizations. We should also add medical psychologists to the list, consultations with whom are usually initiated by a doctor in charge. Psychologists should be involved as specialists, not merely as substitutes for the oncologist when the latter simply does not want to spend time talking.

These days it is impossible to conceal the truth from a patient who has been hospitalized and has signed the informed consent to various treatment modes. How would it be possible to keep something back from a patient who is going to have surgery that will bring disablement? However, neither informed consent or punctiliously following the instructions of Good Clinical Practice can ever replace direct verbal contact with a cancer patient. And communication demands from the doctor attention and respect towards a patient. The very word "cancer" can frighten any person, not only because of fear of forthcoming treatment and its direct results, but also because people are never indifferent to knowing how long they would live and wonder about what their life would like be if it were struck by cancer—often a devastating disease, which, even being treated, can always recur. Thus, one of the medical team's key tasks is to gradually help patients adapt to new living conditions and to become active participants in their treatment and rehabilitation. As for rehabilitation, there should be no dividing patients into groups—those for whom it is necessary and those who can survive without it (for instance, at an advanced stage).

All patients should be informed from diagnosis about the different potential outcomes of their cancer and the different forms of cancer care—from active treatment to palliative care to end-of-life care—in order to participate in the decision-making process at all stages. Despite early cancer detection and optimal treatment, there is no guarantee of its eradication, and those patients who have been diagnosed with an advanced-stage cancer should be helped to acquire awareness of their status, in order for end-of-life care to be more consistent with the patients' wishes.

A patient must be given clear, understandable information by his/her doctor and be helped to exercise free choice concerning treatment and posttreatment care. Only through the alliance of clinician and patient can positive results be achieved [5]. The old aphorism "treat the patient, not the disease" is certainly applicable where cancer is concerned.

Current Challenges in Communication in Russia

The physician is clearly a key figure in promoting the understanding of cancer. This role is not limited to the oncologist. Any thoughtful doctor should talk about cancer with patients who have come for a consultation to help them learn that no one is immune to cancer, that it need not be frightening but should be faced realistically, that medical science can do many things but is not all-powerful in the face of advanced disease, that the notion of "high-risk groups" works more in retrospect than in prospect. Only with such communication can our scientific discoveries be turned to practical use and general benefit. We are not alone [6] in considering that education of people to be responsible for their own life in case of cancer is as important as education about healthy lifestyles in the general population.

The situation is different for persons who already have cancer. The physician must both treat and communicate with the patient. Who else but a doctor can give a patient the necessary information? Contemporary achievements in medicine and related sciences have already made long-term survival possible. Yet a considerable part of society has not made any effort to understand and accept cancer survivors as "normal" people. In Russia, we are bound to call public attention to the problem over and over again: these cancer survivors are eager to lead a dignified life, satisfying themselves and their loved ones. Cancer survivors also have a right to continuous medical care, according to their past illness and present condition. Oncology professionals involved in the process should make all possible efforts to be:

- Sympathetic and supportive to patients' choices of lifestyle and to their wish to regard themselves as equal members of society
- Willing to keep the information they have confidential
- Considerate to patients regardless of the duration of their life
- Willing to admit that fear of the disease's recurrence is natural
- Direct and communicative in providing patients with the necessary information in order to encourage their conscious coparticipation
- Helpful in finding adequate sources of psychosocial support and rehabilitation, as well as in developing appropriate relationships with family caregivers

Presumably, people in good health who watch others going through cancer treatment and the posttreatment period would become very anxious about malignancy. Medical psychologists can help not only patients, but oncologists themselves, with specific knowledge and role-playing exercises designed to improve their social and communicative skills [7]. It has become the practice in much of the world to create multiprofessional teams for this purpose. Today in Russia, we try to follow such an approach in our work

Open communication between oncologist and patient should never be harmful to the patient or—odd though it may seem—the doctor. The term "Informed Consent" is accepted as regulating mutual relations between specialist and patient, who has a right to know about the character of his/her own disease and to learn about all treatment and rehabilitation modalities. We believe that a patient should be aware not merely of the consequences of the disease, but also of the medical impact on his/her quality of life. Patients who are included in clinical trials are required to sign informed consent to protect the pharmaceutical firms supplying the drugs against accusations on the part of patients that the drugs had an adverse effect. In Russia, participation in a clinical trial is not the only way for a cancer patient to be treated according to modern standards. Up-to-date cancer treatment is available here in most of the main oncology institutions. Usually clinical trials are undertaken when foreign companies make their products available to be checked in several independent medical centers in order to confirm or deny their efficacy and safety. Cancer patients in Russia sign informed consent for regular treatment (surgery, radiotherapy, chemotherapy) as well.

The necessity of patients and doctors dealing with informed consent, which is essentially a legal matter, emphasizes and increases the importance of communication between them. It was once believed that cancer patients do not like talking about their illness with their oncologists. Empirical data now show that the opposite is true and that cancer patients welcome conversations with medical and nursing staff. A patient left alone with only a hunch about his/her illness is quite vulnerable. Such a patient can be very difficult to deal with during the preparatory period, as he/she must agree on the treatment while under the pressure of unresolved problems, may not be or feel able to make a decision, and in effect, may delegate to the doctor the right to act on his/her behalf [8, 9]. Good oncologists, however, need to have a clear sense of the patient's wishes and priorities, in order to provide the best care, while avoiding understatement or uncertainty regarding the treatment and its results. Unfortunately, mutual dissatisfaction cannot always be ruled out within the framework of the patient–oncologist relationship [10, 11].

In our opinion, a careful, considerate oncologist should not become too involved with a patient to the point to feel the patient's problems as his/her own, since it may limit or obstruct the specialist's ability to help the patient make a good decision. Meanwhile, a specialist must not shift the responsibility for choosing a treatment onto the patient. The balance that the oncologist–patient alliance produces should become neither a trap nor a gap; on the contrary, it has to mobilize the specialist to cooperate with the patient actively by providing the patient with adequate information regarding his/her illness, treatment, and outcome. Studies [12, 13] have shown that cancer patients who are provided with a choice of treatments turn out to be more compliant than those who are not.

The following case is a rather extreme example of how the relationship between specialist and patient can go very wrong [14].

> One of his patients came to see him in a nervous condition. He placed a gun upon a table and demanded the truth, having learned from another doctor that he had cancer. He said that if it were true, he would shoot himself dead right there before the doctor's eyes; or if he sensed that he was being deceived, he would kill the doctor. Great resourcefulness was needed on the part of the physician to persuade the man to do neither.

What works in some countries may be unacceptable in others [15]. In general, to ask people who are in good health if they want to know the truth about cancer is inappropriate: a large number of them may not know how to respond; but some persons who tend to be hypochondriacs and are especially worried about developing cancer can react negatively, at times in unpredictable ways. The origins of the phobia can, to a great extent, be attributed to society's mistaken attitude towards cancer [16]. In Russia, mass media dishonesty impresses people with fear, and proper information about the disease is concealed from patients and their relatives. Under such conditions, a cancer patient cannot help taking the disease as "fate" and considering himself/herself an invalid who is excluded from society, emotionally and socially excommunicated. We all must find new ways to converse, seek common ground, and learn to understand one another—doctors and nondoctors, well or sick. This would make it much easier for a cancer patient to think of the disease, its treatment, and his/her life in a constructive way.

Mass media support on this issue would be quite effective if more press and air time were given to it. Use of the Internet for this purpose could be particularly effective: it is now widely available to a large number of people in Russia; there are no language barriers in its use here, as it may be read in Russian. If a celebrity here dies of cancer, the event is widely reported, but the reports usually do not dwell upon the cancer itself and its particular problems. By contrast, if journalists were to tell something about how famous persons deal with their disease, how they survived its different stages, how they communicated with their cancer specialists, and how they were helped by them, this information would be very useful in informing the public. There is no more eloquent example than of a celebrity who, with a personal story, confirms the truth: the sooner cancer is detected, the easier and less traumatically it may be cured and the better the prognosis is. Public talks of professionals and former patients would be also useful. Mass media should tell people about the actual state of things in the realm of cancer rather than concentrating on appalling stories that make the information unbearable for the audience. We cannot stop cancer, but we can and must change people's attitude towards it, so that they do not see cancer only as a death sentence. In today's Russia, we have started doing everything we can to diminish cancer's psychosocial and emotional impact on human beings. For example, when people hear such epithets as "mortal" and "fatal," they are not encouraged to visit a doctor as soon as possible. Human relations, in general, are multifaceted and often fragile, also in the oncology sphere. Cancer often strains such relations even more than in other medical areas. The effectiveness of early cancer detection depends not only on scientific programs, but also on the knowledge and belief that any person diagnosed with cancer remains an equal member of society. Positive information lets people know enough about cancer to keep them from putting off going to a specialist regardless how small the complaint is and to accept the diagnosis and share in treatment decisions, so that their satisfaction, compliance, and quality of life can improve.

Unfortunately, mass media in Russia are still not adequately supportive in this way. For example, once we tried to publish a book written by Moran [17], best known in Great Britain as the Green Goddess, a producer, actress, keep-fit and fashion-show presenter at the BBC, journalist, and model. In her book she told the remarkable story of her life and career as affected by breast cancer. She had had adequate treatment and full recovery. Diana Moran emphasized the following idea: "by disclosing what has been a very close secret I hope to help other women to keep themselves fit in body and mind during the trauma of what has been a difficult exercise." This edition was translated into Russian and offered to several publishing houses in order to demonstrate to our breast cancer patients that nothing needs be lost in their own lives if they accept their disease as it is and continue their survival in an optimistic manner. Also, it could be beneficial for healthy women. The book was rejected by all the publishing houses we applied to. In their opinion, the subject was not of adequate importance and it would not bring enough profit. These days similar stories composed by Russian former cancer patients occasionally appear in shops. Publication of these manuscripts is usually financed by their authors. More often, one finds printed leaflets for patients and their families written and produced by oncology specialists in a limited quantity. These are destined to patients and families and are not produced in sufficient amounts for distribution to the general public.

Usually relatives of cancer patients in Russia report anxiety and helplessness— not only because of their dismay and worry about their loved one, but also as a consequence of their lack of comprehension and of knowledge of how to act and what to do. Relatives of a cancer patient should perceive that:

- Cancer is an illness that lies heavily on the whole family, not only a single person; everyone gets involved in the adaptive process
- Interaction in the family in such critical circumstances is a factor of great importance; it may be supportive or destructive
- Real partnership and communication benefit the patient

Medical psychologists' advice must not be ignored. It is known that psychologists work with relatives of accident (e.g., car, plane, rail) victims. According to what we know about cancer today, it also can be regarded as a catastrophe.

Psychosocial support groups, consisting of specifically selected, educated, and trained former cancer patients who have survived several years after treatment, can be a real help in enlarging cancer patients' knowledge base concerning the disease. Although volunteers cannot be a substitute for professional psychologists, many charitable societies for this purpose exist around the world, including in Russia. In St. Petersburg, the social organization Nadezhda (Hope), the first one established in our country, has already celebrated its 22nd anniversary. Its volunteers assist women affected by breast cancer, providing them with physical, emotional, and cosmetic support in full accordance with the rules of the famous Reach to Recovery Program [18]. Their experience indicates that, regardless of the form of cancer:

- A cancer patient meeting with a survivor who has gone through the same illness and problems tends to feel more optimistic
- Volunteer support assures that health means not only "being free of disease," but also "having a well-deserved quality of life" not later, but now

This activity is good for the volunteers themselves: being involved in the process of supporting others, they are having an active lifestyle, developing their own skills in communication, and increasing their understanding of living with cancer. Years ago, when they needed it, they had no one's support; now they understand better than anyone else all the problems that cancer patients encounter. People who have survived the disease, as well as people who are in good health, are needed for optimal communication about cancer.

Conclusion

We have previously asserted that any further discussion of "to tell or not to tell" the truth about cancer should be ruled out [19, 20]. An entire volume of the *Annals of the New York Academy of Sciences*, published in 1997, was devoted to the problem of communication with cancer patients, and the authors of several articles gave the answer, "to tell" [21]. Oncologists or other professionals who try to evade discussion with cancer patients often do so because they want to spare themselves the discomfort of unpleasant talk and emotions [22]. Any information that a cancer patient gets from a specialist whom the patient does not trust will sound unconvincing [23]. The specialist should not merely thrust the truth upon the patient. Physicians ought to provide only information that the patient is ready to take in. Special training can be useful in helping physicians manage problems in communication with patients [7].

It is important that the following still-too-common attitudes to cancer in Russia be changed:

- The still generally conservative attitude to communication with cancer patients and the public
- Withholding truth from patients, thus preventing their shared participation in the recovery process
- The lack of open discussion with people explaining the benefit of an early visit to a specialist in case of any abnormality in health
- The negative nature of the information about cancer put forth by the mass media, which does not motivate constructive action
- The inadequate awareness on the part of relatives of cancer patients of how they should act under the circumstances

We all must promote balanced communication with cancer patients and healthy people. With such an approach, this interaction will become constructive and motivating. In all parts of the world, cancer remains a stressful problem, not only in its medical aspects. However, the practice of oncology is improving. There are now millions of people who have survived cancer. For the majority of them, it happened not only thanks to high-quality treatment but because of early diagnosis, which was achieved by satisfactory communication among the physicians and patients involved. Only direct, optimistic interaction can motivate people to be responsible for their own life in the case of cancer, and this will also benefit those who do or might become ill.

References

1. Petrov NN. Issues on surgical deontology. Leningrad: State Institute for Advanced Medical Education; 1945. p. 60.
2. Serebrov AI. Nikolai Nikolaevich Petrov (by the 100th anniversary). Probl Oncol (Russ). 1976;22:3–11.
3. Ammann RA, Baumgartner L. Bad news in oncology: which are the right words? Support Care Cancer. 2005;13:275–6.
4. Blokhin NN. Deontology in oncology. Moscow: Medicine; 1977. p. 70.
5. Rodin G, Mackay JA, Zimmermann C, et al. Clinician-patient communication: a systematic review. Support Care Cancer. 2009;17:627–44.
6. Yoo GJ, Aviv C, Levine EG, et al. Emotion work: disclosing cancer. Support Care Cancer. 2010;18:205–15.
7. Gysels M, Richardson A, Higginson IJ. Communication training for health professionals who care for patients with cancer: a systematic review of effectiveness. Support Care Cancer. 2004;12:692–700.
8. Coulter A, Entwistle V, Gilbert D. Sharing decisions with patients: is the information good enough? BMJ. 1999;318:318–22.
9. Meredith C, Symonds P, Webster L. Information needs of cancer patients in the west of Scotland: cross-sectional survey of patients' views. BMJ. 1996;313:724–6.
10. Bartlett EE, Grayson M, Barker R. The effects of physician communication skills on patient satisfaction, recall and adherence. J Chronic Dis. 1984;37:765–72.
11. Steward MA. Effective physician-patient communication and health outcomes: a review. Can Med Assoc J. 1995;152:1423–33.
12. Fallowfield LJ, Hall A, Maguire GP, Baum M. Psychological outcomes of different treatment policies in women with early breast cancer outside a clinical trial. BMJ. 1990;301:575–80.
13. Morris J, Inghman R. Choice of surgery for early breast cancer: psychological considerations. Soc Sci Med. 1988;27:1257–62.
14. Portmann G. L'environnment psychologique des cancereux. Rev Laringol Otol Rhinol. 1973;94:1–10.
15. Surbone A. Communication preferences and needs of cancer patients: the importance of content. Support Care Cancer. 2006;14:789–91.
16. Sauer R. Krebstangst. ZFA Med Stuttgart. 1977;53:923–6.
17. Moran D. A more difficult exercise. London: Bloomsbury; 1989. p. 179.
18. American Cancer Society. Reach to recovery program guide. Atlanta: American Cancer Society; 1985. p. 68.
19. Demin EV. Oncology and ethics: coexistence and collaboration. Probl Oncol (Russ). 2001;47:366–9.

20. Demin EV. Quality of life of cancer patients: an experience of implementation of reach to recovery program. AquaVitae (Russ). 2001;3:34–6.
21. Surbone A, Zwitter M. Communication with the cancer patient: information and truth, vol. 809. New York: Annals of the New York Academy of Sciences; 1997. p. 540.
22. Klocker JK, Klocker-Kaiser U, Schwaninger M. Truth in the relationship between cancer patient and physician. In: Surbone A, Zwitter M, editors. Communication with the cancer patient: information and truth, vol. 809. New York: Annals of the New York Academy of Sciences; 1997. p. 56–65.
23. Annunziata MA. Ethics of relationship. From communication to conversation. In: Surbone A, Zwitter M, editors. Communication with the cancer patient: information and truth, vol. 809. New York: Annals of the New York Academy of Sciences; 1997. p. 400–10.

Chapter 37
Communication with Cancer Patients in Zimbabwe

Ntokozo Ndlovu

Abstract Cancer is still perceived as synonymous with a death sentence in Zimbabwe, due mainly to the consequences of patients presenting late. Most of these patients and their families have a knowledge deficit with regard to cancer prevention, diagnosis, treatment, and palliation. The HIV epidemic and the resultant surge in the prevalence of HIV-related cancers have led to new communication challenges in managing patients with both HIV infection and cancer. These patients face two potentially life-threatening diseases simultaneously, and these diseases both have stigmas within the community. While families can be very supportive to these and other cancer patients, the extended family dynamics need to be understood and taken into account in decisions to involve family in patient management. Cancer treatments themselves are often misunderstood by all. The negative perception of these treatments, radiotherapy in particular, may be the cause of poor uptake of and compliance with treatment out of fear of harm. Future changing communication needs with cancer patients in Zimbabwe will have to be anticipated and planned for as we move into introducing a comprehensive cancer control program and the conduct of clinical trials in cancer. Communicating with cancer patients who have concurrent HIV infection needs further study, since little is known about the special communication needs of such patients and how they can be addressed.

Keywords HIV/AIDS • Cancers • Communication • Radiotherapy • Chemotherapy • Compliance

N. Ndlovu (✉)
Department of Radiology, College of Health Sciences,
University of Zimbabwe, Harare, Zimbabwe

Parirenyatwa Hospital, Harare, Zimbabwe
e-mail: nndlovu@mweb.co.zw

Introduction

It is hard to dispel the perception of cancer as a death sentence, particularly in a limited-resource setting where the general population has been exposed to less-than-optimal cancer care and a large number of cancer patients dying of their disease. The biggest contributing factor to this outcome is patients presenting with late-stage disease. This is known to be typical in the majority of patients in most developing countries, and Zimbabwe is not an exception. The health professional involved in the management of cancer generally encounters the reluctance of the patient and his or her family to be engaged in management decisions for the patient. This reluctance is due mainly to the fear of the treatment itself or of being told that nothing can be done to change the health outcome of the cancer sufferer.

Communication with the patient and his or her family in such a setting therefore involves incorporating cancer education on prevention and early detection all at one sitting, largely for the relatives' or companions' benefit. Even with such a high literacy rate as is found in Zimbabwe and elsewhere in Africa, there is still a knowledge deficit on cancer, its causes, and treatment [1]. Discussing the individual circumstances of the particular patient's cancer diagnosis and management needs also take place at the initial consultation.

Communicating with the Patient with Cancer and HIV/AIDS

A 35-year-old male patient had been recently diagnosed with a MALT lymphoma of the stomach. He was rather frail looking and had lost a lot of weight due to both the cancer and HIV disease, of which the latter had been diagnosed a few years earlier. He had not been compliant with taking antiretroviral therapy (ARV), the reason for which was not clear. This patient was accompanied to the consultation by his father and wife. He was advised on the appropriate management of his condition, which included seeing an HIV specialist physician for review of the antiretroviral treatment prior to chemotherapy for the lymphoma. With correct management, he soon improved until 3 months later, when he suddenly deteriorated. He was brought in very ill and in as poor a general condition as he had initially presented.

Southern Africa has been hard hit by the HIV/AIDS epidemic. Cancer has not been spared from the impact of this epidemic. It is estimated that 70–80% of all cancers that were diagnosed in Zimbabwe during the time of the HIV epidemic were HIV-related, such as non-Hodgkin's lymphoma (NHL), Kaposi's sarcoma (KS), cervical cancer, and squamous cell carcinoma of the conjunctiva [2, 3]. In the majority of these cases, the cancer was the first presenting symptom suggestive of HIV disease that lead the patient to seek help from a health care facility [4–6]. It is also known that many other cancer patients with non-HIV-related cancers are infected by the HIV virus in a proportion that corresponds to the general population's prevalence of HIV infection at that time. With such patients who present with HIV-related and nonrelated cancers, a great communication challenge arises: first, disclosing the cancer diagnosis, and second, explaining the relation that the cancer may have with HIV infection. All that is done at the initial consultation.

What reaction is to be expected from these patients after receiving such news? The first reaction is commonly the patient's being totally overwhelmed by the "double" diagnosis of potentially life-threatening conditions. Indeed, most patients express it as "dying twice in a single space of time." Even to the patient who knows his or her HIV-seropositive status at the time of diagnosis of the cancer, this information is usually not taken very well. The patient then commonly bargains with the oncologists for the focus to be on one or the other diagnosis first, not both at the same time. Cancer is the diagnosis usually preferred, as it is perceived generally to have less stigma than HIV infection. The request for HIV testing would then follow, while simultaneously continuing to fully investigate the patient as appropriate for the staging of the individual's cancer. Avoidance of having an HIV test is usually one of the primary reasons for the patient to want the emphasis to be on cancer management alone. It is common at this point for the patient to agree to undergo all tests, but to refuse to consent to HIV testing.

In other settings, such avoidance behaviors in cancer patients have been shown to be associated with an increased likelihood of depression and anxiety. These patients also tend to have less emotional support and an increase in self-blame [7]. It is therefore important to give such patients the necessary counseling and support to be able to confront their illness realistically.

An oncology professional who has had formal training in HIV pre- and posttest counseling has an advantage in this situation, even if the patient is later referred to a testing center where professional counseling is available. Preliminary counseling in the oncology clinic improves the rate of acceptance of HIV testing. This can be very costly in time for the oncologist, who may already be swamped by many other patients. It has, however, been shown in other palliative care settings that staff members have various preferences for training in communication skills, based on their level of involvement with patients [8]. This would have to be taken into account in addressing the training needs of each group of health-care workers.

Most patients in such a situation cannot mentally assimilate all the information given at this first sitting. Being overwhelmed with information may be another reason for the high default rate at this particular point in patient care in our setting. The chance of the patient refusing continued medical care in this period can be minimized by ensuring that, where possible, the patient is seen with at least one close relative or the spouse. These persons can assist in communicating what the health care giver is conveying to the patient with regard to health care management and encourage the patient to follow the instructed processes after consultation. Even in the best of circumstances, one still frequently has patients coming back for review having all the other test results but not the HIV test results. Such patients then start bargaining on the necessity of the HIV test all over again.

It undoubtedly is very important for the healthcare professional to communicate clearly and consistently about the relationship of the cancer to the immunosuppressive effects of the HIV virus. The need for both conditions to be treated simultaneously must be emphasized. It is also important for the patient to understand that the success of the treatment of the cancer has a close bearing on control of the HIV infection. Not addressing the HIV infection while treating cancer would definitely lead to increased toxicity of the cancer-related treatments and a much poorer outcome, if not fatal consequences.

While it may sometimes be necessary in an emergency, such as upper airway obstruction by a large tumor mass, for the oncologist to start some form of treatment before the HIV test is done, this can send the wrong signal to the patient and relatives that perhaps testing for HIV was not necessary after all. Such cases may need more individual counseling so that the relief of symptoms from the emergency treatment is not taken to indicate complete management of both the cancer and the HIV disease.

Engaging a counselor who is trained in dealing with HIV-infected patients throughout the treatment becomes of paramount importance in the management of patients with HIV-related cancers. All the various aspects of care pertaining to both conditions must be covered. Some aspects of care that need to be addressed include adherence to treatment (for both HIV and cancer), safe sex practices, disclosure to close persons, potential drug interactions, lack of a strong evidence base in the management of HIV-related cancers, as well as other important issues related to this complex dual treatment. These aspects are tied very closely with the outcome of the management of the cancer; without proper attention to them, the actual cancer treatment may be rendered futile.

Successful communication with patients with HIV-related cancers is marked by relief on the part of the cancer sufferer in getting to know their HIV status, as many had entertained the possibility of having HIV/AIDS. When the patient finally has the chance to confirm his or her status and be able to have something done about it, a sense of the purposefulness of seeking health intervention is experienced. This positive benefit of HIV testing increases as the treatment results show a significant improvement in the patient's general physical well-being, income generation, and social acceptability. A negative test result has an equal positive benefit psychologically, since these patients are relieved by knowing their HIV status and are reassured of a better outcome.

Very little has been published on the communication needs of the patient with HIV-related cancer. In a study carried out in Uganda and South Africa, the need for information by both caregiver and patient was found to be one of the major themes. This lack of information was said to reduce the ability of the patients to manage their condition. In this study, of the 90 patients enrolled, only 6 had both HIV and cancer, with the rest of the patients having other progressive life-limiting diseases [9]. This confirms the need for further studies on the communication needs of patients with these dual life-limiting diseases, particularly in an African setting.

The Patient's Relatives and the Health-care Worker

We continue with the 35-year-old patient who had a MALT lymphoma described in the previous section. When he was seen again in a deteriorated state, he was accompanied by his father and a woman who was not previously known to the staff. She later introduced herself as the wife of the patient and went on to request all the information that was provided at the initial consultation, including the basic care, dietary requirements, and medications for the patient. It was then that the cause of the deterioration in this patient's condition became apparent. He was a polygamist, and all the care instructions had been given to only one of his wives; when handing over his care to another wife, she did not pass on all the information she had been given at the healthcare institution. It was later learned by the staff that this man actually had four wives.

This brings us to the question, Who is the next of kin and principal caregiver in such a family setup? How many people should be instructed in the home-based care of our patients, so vital to the patient's well-being? How can we get our patients to disclose polygamous relationships that they may feel embarrassed to talk about, or any other such taboo subjects that may have a bearing on their treatment outcomes?

Zimbabwean people tend to have very large extended families; they take their relationships with one another very seriously. Most of the time, the differences between a mother and an aunt, between a brother and a male cousin are not acknowledged as such, so that one individual can have many "mothers" and many sets of "siblings." It is very important to note this clearly prior to engaging the family in any discussions so as to avoid disclosing any information to a person who is really not considered next of kin. This can be a serious challenge when communicating with relatives about a patient who has impaired verbal communication or understanding.

The relatives also might not want the healthcare provider to communicate directly with the patient, but through them for fear of a negative reaction from the patient once they know the truth with regard to their condition. This is strongly discouraged, as the patient may perceive that his or her condition is being withheld, which can erode the confidence of the patient in his/her caregiver.

Communication with the Patient on Cancer Treatment

A 43-year-old female patient walked into the consultation room looking very pale, in a lot of pain, with a drooping left shoulder and an obvious football-sized mass on her left chest, showing even through the heavy clothing she was wearing. A quick look at her records revealed that this was not her first visit to the oncology clinic. She had been seen only once, 2 years ago, following a biopsy of a 2-cm left-breast mass, which had been found on histology to be invasive ductal carcinoma of the breast. At the time of the biopsy, there were no other obvious abnormalities, and the patient had an excellent performance status. She had expressed doubt as to why she even needed to be seen for the cancer, as she was not in pain and after all the lump had been removed. She had been told by her aunt, who knew a nurse who worked at the local hospital, that cancer treatment was painful and really only for patients who were dying, not her. After all, the local traditional healer was known to treat cancer with just herbs and not all the other treatments that had been suggested she might need, which she perceived as harsh. She even regretted having the excision biopsy and wished she had gone to the healer first; then she would have avoided having the horrible scar on her breast. She also wished she could have more children, and now it would be difficult for her, as traditional belief is against breast feeding with a breast that has been operated on. After some discussion she accepted having staging investigations done and agreed to return for further consultation; but she had not returned until this day.

After a patient has been told that he or she has cancer, more information is given to the patient in a time period that may be perceived by the individual sufferer as very short. Something needs to be done for the good of the patient. Complex processes have to be set in motion to evaluate the patient and plan for appropriate interventions. It is at such a time that a lot of misconceptions about cancer and its treatment can be formed, especially if there is a language barrier as well. Indeed, the language barrier starts with the health care professional, who is competent in one language the patient does not understand—the language of medicine. This calls for translation into a day-to-day form of that language, then into the language that the patient understands.

Such language barriers are common worldwide, wherever there are diverse cultural groupings and large immigrant populations [10, 11]. Butow et al. observed that doctors speak less to patients when using an interpreter with delayed responses and ignored cues from patients. This difference in interaction could well result in compromise of the patients' well-being and decision-making [11].

The common cancer treatments—surgery, chemotherapy, and radiotherapy—can all be misunderstood by patients, their families, and the general population. The mention of radiotherapy conjures up a lot of mostly negative perceptions. Where available, radiotherapy is the most common cancer treatment in Africa as a whole. This is due to the advanced nature of the disease at presentation [12]. It is therefore important that cancer patients understand this form of treatment. In Zimbabwe, the local languages translate radiotherapy as a treatment that uses electricity. Electricity applied to the body is naturally associated with fear, harm, and shock, feelings that can easily be translated into a perception of painful and negative effects.

All this gives the impression of a treatment that has more risk than benefit. So deeply entrenched is this misconception of radiotherapy treatment in the society that even health workers who are not familiar with a cancer treatment unit have it. Such workers are not a rarity either, as there are only two radiotherapy units in the country, and many health-care professionals have not had an opportunity to become familiar with radiotherapy treatments in the course of their normal duties. It remains the lonely task of staff members in these radiotherapy centers to communicate with patients and convince them of the true meaning of radiotherapy and its benefits.

It is not surprising that many patients, on completing treatment, remark that, had they known before that radiotherapy is painless and beneficial, they would have presented for treatment early in the course of their disease. These cancer survivors are a group of individuals with a lot of potential to get the messages of cancer education to the general population. Unfortunately, they are reluctant to share their experiences for fear of social losses—work-related repercussions and stigmas—that can follow such disclosure. The benefits of effective communication with the patient in a way that results in the correct perspective of the treatment accrue not only to the individual patient, but have the potential to be a tool for promotion of early presentation in our communities where late presentation of cancer is a major problem.

In another setting, it has been found that there may be complex interactions between rural/urban residence, race, and income when it comes to the choice of treatment modalities for cancer. A study by Steenland et al. of 516 men with prostate cancer showed that, while White men were more likely to choose surgery than African-American men, more African-American men were likely to chose the option of no treatment at all. More rural patients were likely to have external beam radiation alone and were less likely to receive brachytherapy alone or surgery. Poor communication was recognized as the main cause of poor treatment choices [13].

Patients tend to make the same choices of treatment that someone they know may have chosen in the past. In our setting, there is a large leaning towards alternative therapies with unproved value at the expense of avoiding standard therapies for cancer. This has also been shown to be the case in other African countries, where such choices result in delayed treatment start [14–16]. It becomes very important in our setting to discourage the practice of treatment choices based entirely on what is commonly practiced. Indeed, Zikmund-Fisher et al. made a similar recommendation for choices that may not represent good clinical practice [17].

Fear of harm is equally expressed with chemotherapy treatment; this tends to be nonspecific, with less focus than would be expected on real side effects such as nausea, vomiting, and hair loss. A big challenge that has influenced departmental policy is that of compliance with oral chemotherapy. It has proved difficult to communicate to patients the dangers of oral chemotherapy drugs with respect to storage, administration, and compliance. There have been suspected cases of patients sharing drugs ("It got rid of my lump, yours can shrink too.") and perhaps inadvertently exposing pregnant women and young children to the drugs in their homes inappropriately.

This is an example of where communication has not yet been effective enough, posing a danger to the community at large. A policy of avoiding oral chemotherapy as far as possible and preferred use of intravenous drugs has been the easier way to circumvent the need for increased patient education that goes with administering oral chemotherapy. The problems of administration of and compliance to oral cancer treatment is well recognized even in the developed world [18, 19].

Communication on Compliance to Treatment and Follow-Up

Patients with cancer who are seen at our health institutions tend to present with late stage of disease [6, 12]. By and large, it is the symptomatology that prompts them to seek medical treatment in the first place, due to the cultural perception of disease as a state of discomfort. Perceptions of cancer and its treatment are those of pain and a debilitated look, unlike the perceptions that the consumer magazines have created in the Western world [20].

Where there is no pain or discomfort, treatment is viewed as pointless. Unfortunately for cancer patients, pain is usually a symptom of advanced disease. Any treatment, whether symptomatic or definitive, that results in the patient's being relieved of symptoms before the disease is eradicated has the potential to encourage the patient to stop treatment before it is appropriate to do so. Most cancer treatments fall into this category. This heightens the need to clearly communicate to the patient the aim of any treatment offered and the value of compliance to that and subsequent cancer treatments. It is not uncommon for a patient with brain metastases, for example, whose symptoms have been relieved by high-dose steroid treatment, to be reluctant to go on and have radiotherapy as definitive palliative treatment. Such patients may even question the diagnosis of cancer in spite of clear evidence from brain scanning that proves they do have metastatic disease.

Another big challenge to the health-care provider in our setting is ensuring that patients obtain cancer treatment once they have been seen in the cancer treatment centers. Several factors can be responsible for failure to obtain treatment, such as unavailability of the appropriate treatment, distance to the treatment facility, and the high cost of care for the patient who has to pay for treatment. It is notable, however, that a sizable proportion of patients who are offered cancer treatment will default either before the start of or during treatment. From retrospective analyses of patient records, the figure can be as high nearly 50% of patients with certain diagnoses not attending a second visit at the oncology centers for new patients. This obviously cannot be explained by demise from advanced disease alone, although that has been suggested, particularly for HIV-related cancers in the pre-ARV era. Follow-up is equally deficient, with only about one third of treated patients attending at 3 months. Most patients return only if a new problem develops, as they have not be in pain since the completion of treatment and saw no reason to come back sooner. Cancer patients may find it difficult to accommodate the many instructions and advice they were given at the end of treatment once they have returned to normal life [21].

Aboriginal people in Australia have also been observed in the major hospitals to either not take up or continue with cancer treatments. A higher mortality that is out of keeping with the cancer incidence in this population has been ascribed to this. Some suggested solutions have been the building of respect, relationships, fostering open communication, and attention to practicalities such as costs, transportation, and patients' responsibilities [22].

Chemotherapy treatment is better complied with, and most who default do so mainly for financial reasons. There are patients, however, who stop treatment due to poor management of side effects. Most of these patients do not default if they have grasped the information on how to manage nausea at home, in particular, when they are discharged.

The Future Needs of Communication with Patients in Zimbabwe

As the planned national comprehensive cancer control program comes to reality, communication with the general population on cancer prevention, early detection, treatment, and palliation will have to be addressed as an important element for its success. Many barriers to the success of screening programs have been identified in the populations where screening has become routine. Some of these barriers are patient educational status, lack of trust, poor physician–patient communication, and recommendations made by the physicians [23, 24]. Shah et al., however, found that there was greater use of cervical cancer screening among women who were on ARVs [25].

With the conduct of clinical trials in cancer in Zimbabwe now imminent, new communication challenges have to be anticipated and planned ahead for. As shown elsewhere, the patient's understanding of what clinical trials are and the processes of informed decision-making is very important to the ethical conduct of clinical trials [26]. In cancer trials, these processes can be more complex than others. In this part of the world, such problems can be compounded by local beliefs and practices. Measures of cancer clinical trial understanding are being developed, but they may still need to be adapted to address the developing world [27]. It has been shown that with clear communication and information by the investigators, even those patients who may initially be hesitant to join clinical trials do end up joining [28].

These communication needs are but a few that can be anticipated. As we move away from the debate of whether to communicate the diagnosis and prognosis to our cancer patients and as we openly communicate on all aspects of this disease, new challenges in communication are bound continually to arise. Professionals in cancer care will have to continue to identify these challenges and work on how best to address them.

References

1. Aderounmu AO, Egbewale BE, Ojofeitimi EO, Fadiora SO, Oguntola AS, Asekun-Olarinmoye EO, et al. Knowledge, attitudes and practices of the educated and non-educated women to cancer of the breast in semi-urban and rural areas of SouthWest, Nigeria. Niger Postgrad Med J. 2006;13(3):182–8.
2. Masanganise R, Rusakaniko S, Makunike R, Hove M, Chokunonga E, Borok MZ, et al. A historical perspective of registered cases of malignant ocular tumors in Zimbabwe (1990 to 1999). Is HIV infection a factor? Cent Afr J Med. 2008;54(5–8):28–32.
3. Chokunonga E, Levy LM, Bassett MT, Borok MZ, Mauchaza BG, Chirenje MZ, et al. Aids and cancer in Africa: the evolving epidemic in Zimbabwe. AIDS. 1999;13(18):2583–8.
4. Muguti GI. Experience with breast cancer in Zimbabwe. J R Coll Surg Edinb. 1993;38(2):75–8.
5. Nkrumah FK, Danzo AK, Kumar R. Wilms' tumour (nephroblastoma) in Zimbabwe. Ann Trop Paediatr. 1989;9(2):89–92.
6. Ndlovu N, Kambarami R. Factors associated with tumour stage at presentation in invasive cervical cancer. Cent Afr J Med. 2003;49(9–10):107–11.

7. Donovan-Kicken E, Caughlin JP. Breast cancer patients' topic avoidance and psychological distress: the mediating role of coping. J Health Psychol. 2011;16(4):596–606.
8. Turner M, Payne S, O'Brien T. Mandatory communication skills training for cancer and palliative care staff: does one size fit all? Eur J Oncol Nurs. 2010;15(5):398–403.
9. Selman L, Higginson IJ, Agupio G, Dinat N, Downing J, Gwyther L, et al. Meeting information needs of patients with incurable progressive disease and their families in South Africa and Uganda: multicentre qualitative study. BMJ. 2009;338:b1326.
10. Kagawa-Singer M, Dadia AV, Yu MC, Surbone A. Cancer, culture, and health disparities: time to chart a new course? CA Cancer J Clin. 2010;60(1):12–39.
11. Butow P, Bell M, Goldstein D, Sze M, Aldridge L, Abdo S, et al. Grappling with cultural differences: communication between oncologists and immigrant cancer patients with and without interpreters. Patient Educ Couns. 2011;84(3):398–405.
12. Sharma V, Gaye PM, Wahab SA, Ndlovu N, Ngoma T, Vanderpuye V, et al. Palliative radiation therapy practice for advanced esophageal carcinoma in Africa. Dis Esophagus. 2010;23(3):240–3.
13. Steenland K, Goodman M, Liff J, Diiorio C, Butler S, Roberts P, et al. The effect of race and rural residence on prostate cancer treatment choice among men in Georgia. Urology. 2011;77(3):581–7.
14. Levy LM. Communication with the cancer patient in Zimbabwe. Ann N Y Acad Sci. 1997;809:133–41.
15. Clegg-Lamptey JN, Dakubo JC, Attobra YN. Psychosocial aspects of breast cancer treatment in Accra, Ghana. East Afr Med J. 2009;86(7):348–53.
16. Ly M, Diop S, Sacko M, Baby M, Diop CT, Diallo DA. Breast cancer: factors influencing the therapeutic itinerary of patients in a medical oncology unit in Bamako (Mali). Bull Cancer. 2002;89(3):323–6.
17. Zikmund-Fisher BJ, Windschitl PD, Exe N, Ubel PA. "I'll do what they did": social norm information and cancer treatment decisions. Patient Educ Couns. 2011;85(2):225–9.
18. Hohneker J, Shah-Mehta S, Brandt PS. Perspectives on adherence and persistence with oral medications for cancer treatment. J Oncol Pract. 2011;7(1):65–7.
19. Goodin S, Griffith N, Chen B, Chuk K, Daouphars M, Doreau C, et al. Safe handling of oral chemotherapeutic agents in clinical practice: recommendations from an international pharmacy panel. J Oncol Pract. 2011;7(1):7–12.
20. Phillips SG, Della LJ, Sohn SH. What does cancer treatment look like in consumer cancer magazines? An exploratory analysis of photographic content in consumer cancer magazines. J Health Commun. 2011;16(4):416–30.
21. de Leeuw J, Prins JB, Merkx MA, Marres HA, van Achterberg T. Discharge advice in cancer patients: posttreatment patients' report. Cancer Nurs. 2011;34(1):58–66.
22. Thompson SC, Shahid S, Bessarab D, Durey A, Davidson PM. Not just bricks and mortar: planning hospital cancer services for Aboriginal people. BMC Res Notes. 2011;4:62.
23. Young RF, Schwartz K, Booza J. Medical barriers to mammography screening of African American women in a high cancer mortality area: implications for cancer educators and health providers. J Cancer Educ. 2011;26(2):262–9.
24. Wegwarth O, Gaissmaier W, Gigerenzer G. Deceiving numbers: survival rates and their impact on doctors' risk communication. Med Decis Making. 2011;31(3):386–94.
25. Shah S, Montgomery H, Smith C, Madge S, Walker P, Evans H, et al. Cervical screening in HIV-positive women: characteristics of those who default and attitudes towards screening. HIV Med. 2006;7(1):46–52.
26. Surbone A. Cultural competence in oncology: where do we stand? Ann Oncol. 2010;21(1):3–5.
27. Miller JD, Kotowski MR, Comis RL, Smith SW, Silk KJ, Colaizzi DD, et al. Measuring cancer clinical trial understanding. Health Commun. 2011;26(1):82–93.
28. Jenkins V, Farewell D, Batt L, Maughan T, Branston L, Langridge C, et al. The attitudes of 1066 patients with cancer towards participation in randomised clinical trials. Br J Cancer. 2010;103(12):1801–7.

Part V
The Contribution and Interference of Modern Information Technologies

Chapter 38
The Dialectics of the Production of Printed Educational Material for Cancer Patients: Developing Communication Prostheses

Paulo Roberto Vasconcellos-Silva

Abstract There are substantial knowledge and research gaps about the effects of printed educational material on professional practice. In the last decades, the popularization of low-cost leaflets for health education has helped disseminate information more broadly. Nonetheless, several extensive reviews on this matter have led pamphlet producers to inconsistent results and dubious conclusions. In view of the debate on the effectiveness and usefulness of this kind of material, we conducted a review of studies published over the past 54 years (1957–2011), selecting those that brought critical assessments of the role of education through printed materials in health care. Qualitative perspectives were applied to the readings, considering the definition of "efficiency" used by each author. We selected the papers that involved some kind of "value judgment" about this activity, either by quantification of their results or by proposing methods of improving its effectiveness, which illustrated a pattern of rationality behind the production, use, and evaluation of this type of resource. We selected 79 works that were considered a representative sample of the epistemological premises depicted above; from these, 22 were produced by professionals dealing with cancer care. In general, health care leaflets invest in the power of "ideal printed information" as efforts to produce the "perfect information package"—one that efficiently describes its technical content for several purposes. They are used for alleviation of anxiety in imminence of painful procedures as well as for unidirectional persuasion as a kind of "educational strategy" or "health promotion." Under these perspectives, printed material is frequently used as "communication prostheses"—an artificial support constructed for professionals who lack time, have a great volume of information to transmit, are not able to engage in closer interaction

---

P.R. Vasconcellos-Silva (✉)
Oswaldo Cruz Foundation – IOC. Laboratory of Therapeutic Innovation,
Education and Bioproducts—LITEB

Federal university of the state of Rio de Janeiro; Gaffrée e Guinle School Hospital,
Rio de Janeiro, Brazil
e-mail: pr@ioc.fiocruz.br

with their patients, or are overconfident in the information resources available on the Internet. These materials are supposed to inform patients by transmitting the adjusted "dose" of information by efficient routes of administration.

In synthesis, information is prepared as an active principle with peculiar assessment methods based on cognitivist premises—which are central in biomedical rationality. With the exception of a few cases, communication prostheses are used without any kind of research on message reception, a specialized tool used by communication experts. These gaps pose the need for a deconstruction of the systems of instrumental thinking, so peculiar to health professionals. The present narrative review addresses the relevance of information through printed material and adds a contribution to the understanding of its use in assisting professionals working with cancer patients.

Keywords Communication • Communication barriers • Hospital–patient relation • Communication media • Patient education • Interprofessional relations

An Introduction to a Complex Scenario

Printed educational materials (PEMs) are widely used with passive dissemination strategies to improve knowledge, awareness, attitudes, skills, professional practice, and patient outcomes. Traditionally, they are presented in paper formats such as brochures, flyers, and booklets, which seem to be the most frequently adopted method for disseminating information. In the hospital environment of cancer care, professionals are daily faced with the need to meet the demand for information from patients regarding chemotherapy, surgery, and other important issues that, obviously, cannot be provided merely by Internet access. The need to keep patients informed is widely recognized and practiced in a diversity of cancer treatment situations, usually guided by and adapting to technical imperatives.

In Brazil, the popularization of low-cost leaflets edited and illustrated on personal computers has helped disseminate information for patients in a very specific way, but not much different from other countries, as we shall see in the conclusion. Certainly, information technology is a very successful tool for formatting printed material and disseminating relevant content by electronic media. Personal computers have provided, for the first time, the opportunity to write, edit, and publish information on a large scale directly for patients and their families. In the hospital environment, material made by health professionals is profuse and is distributed with leaflets created by public bodies for promoting health care campaigns and other texts created with subtle commercial intentions. Rozemberg et al. [21] analyzed strategies, interests, assumptions, and concerns among producers of PEM on infectious diseases in a public hospital in Rio de Janeiro. Leaflets were generally linked to the professional experience of providing health care, but the lack of pertinent research prior to the production of PEMs leads to simplifications and generalizations concerning the patients' most common doubts and questions. Illustrations were seen as an important aspect of this material, considering the limits of written

Table 38.1 Optimistic authors (PEMs are essential to provide relevant information)

Main author	Year of publication	Title of the article
Robinson	2011	Efficacy of an educational intervention with kidney transplant recipients to promote skin self-examination for squamous cell carcinoma detection
David	2010	Effectiveness of "palliative care information booklet" in enhancing nurses' knowledge
Weintraub	2004	Suitability of prostate cancer education materials: applying a standardized assessment tool to currently available materials
Harvey	2000	The health promotion implications of the knowledge and attitude of employees in relation to health and safety leaflets
Macfarlane	1997	Reducing reconsultations for acute lower respiratory tract illness with an information leaflet: a randomized controlled study of patients in primary care
Chung	1999	Long-term benzodiazepine users—characteristics, views, and effectiveness of benzodiazepine reduction information leaflet
Frost	1999	Importance of format and design in print patient information
Jackson	1995	Reducing anxiety in new dental patients by means of leaflets
Murphy	1995	Information for family carers: does it help?
Tourigny	1998	Effects of a preoperative educational intervention on the behavior of parents of 3- to 6-year old children having day surgery
Fallowfield	1990	Psychological outcomes of different treatment policies in women with early breast cancer outside a clinical trial

language for an illiterate patient population. They concluded that such material followed a "linear communication model," according to which health messages are effective in producing a single effect on their users.

More recently, a bibliographic survey performed by Freitas et al. [9] studied communication models, users' representations, and the dynamics of content selection and assessment of PEM in health care settings in Brazil. The analysis of 11 articles surveyed indicated that the communication was characterized by the same linear model referred to by Rozemberg. The patients were considered to be mere consumers of scientific concepts. In most cases, health professionals were the only people responsible for the selection of content. In the articles surveyed could be found a clear conflict between the needs of patients and the perspectives of printed materials producers.

Reviews and a Second-Order Review

Several extensive reviews have led printed material producers to inconsistent results and dubious conclusions. In the field of evaluation methodologies of PEM production for patients, there have been problems whose solutions, suggested by various authors, are complex and even contradictory (Tables 38.1 and 38.2). In this context, a second-order review—a qualitative analysis of previous analysis—can disclose a

Table 38.2 Skeptical authors (about difficulties in producing of PEMs)

Main author	Year of publication	Title of the article
Helitzer	2009	Health literacy demands of written health information materials: an assessment of cervical cancer prevention materials
Shieh	2008	Printed health information materials: evaluation of readability and suitability
Kline	2007	Cultural sensitivity and health promotion: assessing breast cancer education pamphlets designed for African American women
Galaal	2007	Interventions for reducing anxiety in women undergoing colposcopy
Hunter	2005	Cervical cancer educational pamphlets: do they miss the mark for Mexican immigrant women's needs?
Paul	2003	Print material content and design: is it relevant to effectiveness?
Humphris	2001	Immediate knowledge increase from an oral cancer information leaflet in patients attending a primary healthcare facility: a randomized controlled trial
Chung	2000	Oral cancer educational materials for the general public: 1998
Freemantle	2000	Printed educational materials: effects on professional practice and healthcare outcomes
Richard	1999	Humor and alarmism in melanoma prevention: a randomized controlled study of three types of information leaflet
Humphris	1999	The experimental evaluation of an oral cancer information leaflet
Luck	1999	Effects of video information on precolonoscopy anxiety and knowledge: a randomized trial
Street	1998	Interactive multimedia information program for use by breast-care nurses—a patient acceptability study
Drossaert	1996	Health education to improve repeat participation in the Dutch breast cancer screening program: evaluation of a leaflet tailored to previous participants
Meredith	1995	Comparison of patients' needs for information on prostate surgery with printed materials provided by surgeons
Murphy	1993	Crutches, confetti, or useful tools? Professionals' views on and use of health educational leaflets
Doak	1980	Patient comprehension profiles: recent findings and strategies
Cole	1979	The understanding of medical terminology used in printed health education materials

different point of view centered on the way of thinking about the communication process among health professionals. Some aspects that occasioned inconsistency at the first-order level can be partially resolved by inquiring at the second-order analysis into the nature and scope of the rationality applied. Our intention was to put forward an analysis that took as its starting point the primary studies performed by health care professionals in their professional environment and context, stressing the articles on cancer care. In our study, it was assumed that limitations eventually observed at the first-order questions (or even in systematic reviews) could provide a privileged access to an alternative standpoint. We consider this review as a necessary preliminary

Table 38.3 "Anti-information" authors (excesses could trigger anxiety) in contrast with "dialogic" authors

Main author	Year of publication	Title of the article
Garrud	2001	Impact of risk information in a patient education leaflet
Kruse	2000	A randomized trial assessing the impact of written information on outpatients' knowledge about and attitude toward randomized clinical trials
Entwistle	1998	Disseminating information about health-care effectiveness: a survey of consumer health information services
Nelson	1997	Why are you waiting? Formulating an information pamphlet for use in an accident and emergency department
Lamb	1994	Can a physician warn patients of potential side effects without causing fear of those side effects?
Pratt	1957	Physicians' view on the level of medical information among patients
Dialogic authors		
Ibrahin	2010	The effect of printed educational material from the coroner in Victoria, Australia, on changing aged care health professional practice: a subscriber survey
Schreiber	1997	Duty of information, patient's leaflet, and physician's data sheet from the juridical point of view
Granitza	1997	Patient education responsibility, specialty and administration information from the viewpoint of the pharmaceutical industry
Fawdry	1994	Prescribing the leaflets

to answering issues raised from the observation of the communication phenomena within health care teams.

Among descriptions of successes and failures, the publications selected for the following narrative review were those that gave a more detailed description of their assessment strategies. The educational emphasis was stressed, since the publications followed the same guiding rationality for production, utilization, and evaluation. Many studies were not selected because they were considered redundant in relation to others with a greater degree of detail. Editorials and opinion letters were also excluded, as were papers describing experience with the process of compiling leaflets that did not, however, add any kind of evaluation.

The information search was limited to PEMs aimed at the lay public; those related to professional training, information, or updating were excluded. Studies on communication among patients with cognitive disorders or any other type of disability were excluded, since that topic, which is more specific and technically complex, deviates from the theme that was being pursued. A list of studies was drawn up (Tables 38.1–38.3) according to qualitative approaches and thematic analysis of contents that represent the rationality behind the production, use, and evaluation of pamphlets.

On the Efficacy of Leaflets in Health Education

Thesis: Printed Materials Are Efficient in Delivering Information

According to several government health agencies, all patients should have improved access to high-quality information, health professionals should communicate more effectively with their patients, and there should be a rational approach to producing and delivering information [3]. Patient information leaflets are a good example of how this can be achieved, for several important reasons. Printed materials allow better communication between doctors and patients, which is especially useful in reducing patients' fear and anxiety concerning poorly understood procedures, which are common in the diagnosis and treatment of cancer. Furthermore, physicians, nurses, and other professionals have to act under technical imperatives that are complex and time-demanding; cancer treatment poses a level of complexity that did not exist some decades ago.

Printed materials are widely used in cancer education, and there are a remarkable number of guidelines in the literature on their content. The National Cancer Institute [2] conducted a comprehensive needs assessment to identify key design elements of cancer education programs and created a cost-effective process that would ensure consistency in the development of materials. Format, design, and placement of materials for patient access need to be considered as a priority for their efficacy in delivering information. However, outcome-based evidence about materials containing ideal attributes under real-world conditions is considered ambiguous. Despite the description of many failures, as we shall see, the power of information to lessen patients' anxiety when imminently faced with the invasive processes of cancer care has always been recognized, even if only intuitively, by health care teams. In this context, cognitive impairment caused by emotional stress can easily create conditions adverse to diagnostic and treatment procedures. Evidence suggests that women with breast cancer who had received chemotherapy experienced cognitive problems. Although these are largely subtle deficits, they can negatively impact a patient's quality of life, ability to work, and subsequently, employment decisions [20]. High levels of anxiety negatively affect how information is received by patients with cancer with decreasing comprehension, retention, and satisfaction. Despite evidence about cognitive problems associated with therapy, support for the emotional distress associated with several situations is clearly needed.

Research has repeatedly shown that, after a careful assessment of individual needs, information delivered after the initial phase of diagnosis and treatment can reduce fear, improve self-care decisions, decrease side effects of treatment, and enhance quality of life [18]. Many factors may interfere (for example, the availability of Internet access and educational level) with the ability of patients newly diagnosed with cancer to cope with treatment and decrease their comprehension of procedures. Several authors are unanimous in stating that health care teams should be aware of patients' informational needs during this critical phase. Emotional, social, and physical limitations have been identified as most important in dealing with breast cancer treatment [22]. Fear of recurrence and anxiety regarding postoperative cancer treatments, which could be lessened by informational material, seem to be major factors of concern. Doctors can improve the quality of care for women with breast cancer and their families by providing additional informative support services and post-treatment information during the follow-up call period.

The need for understandable materials is also especially useful for men diagnosed with early-stage prostate cancer. They are usually faced with the challenge of choosing among several options of treatment. These men need to participate knowledgeably and confidently in the treatment decision-making process, and those at later stages of the disease need to understand how to manage symptoms and adjuvant therapy side effects. Satisfying information needs can also improve patient outcomes, including perception of control, level of distress and psychological well-being, sense of participation, as well as awareness of everyday life changes. The research conducted by Wong et al. [25] about understanding the needs of breast cancer patients provides good reasons to help them better understand their treatment options. In summary, PEMs can represent invaluable support in circumstances of diagnosis, treatment, or follow-up that raise concern about future complications or adverse prognoses. Most cited authors conclude that closer contacts with the health team are essential for patients to share concerns and needs.

Antithesis: Development of PEMs Is Complex: Outcomes Are Ambiguous and Do Not Meet Expectations

Other authors are skeptical about printed material used to help patients under any conditions. PEMs must be evaluated under an economy of efficiency: cost-benefit analysis, systems analysis, and budgeting in terms of providing pertinent information in an understandable and meaningful way. The production, distribution, and evaluation of printed material under such circumstances may or may not provide worthwhile results. A review conducted by Arthur [1] performed a historical synthesis of studies concerning PEMs at that time, recalling that, notwithstanding the great investments, there are few in-depth studies in relation to the significant volume of printed material for these purposes. Like others, he questioned the usefulness and applicability of this resource when not preceded by demand and understandability studies. Studies in the field ought to be more profound for reasons that are as much economic as ethical.

People at all literacy levels prefer simple written materials over complex ones [4]. This is especially true at moments of "existential stress," such as having received a cancer diagnosis. Weintraub et al. [24], assessing material for prostate cancer patients, found that 90% of materials assessed scored "not suitable" for their reading grade level, and 55% of the materials could not be rated on cultural appropriateness because of lack of cues about the intended audience. Also, many of the materials scored poorly on content, graphics, self-efficacy, learning motivation, and stimulation. Overall, the findings pointed to the need to carefully assess materials used for multicultural audiences with low reading ability. According to the authors, further research is needed to establish evidence regarding optimal presentation of key elements of PEMs. Culture is an important variable, affecting the retention and use of information. Nonetheless, the majority of the PEMs described in the literature are culturally insensitive, with the visual message being the weakest component of all the materials. Effective cancer education materials can be achieved by employing strategies that aim to enhance patient understandability, usability, relevance, and motivation. Learner verification is a quality control process and a technique that helps ensure that materials are suitable for the intended audience and better matched to patients' learning needs [4].

Several systematic reviews (mentioned in Table 38.2) analyzed works that described the use of informative leaflets with various purposes and contexts; these reviews bring out more doubts than clarifications. The authors provided a broad synthesis concerning an activity that is widely employed in current practice in health care services of various conditions and specialties throughout the world. The study conducted by Freemantle et al. [8] (Table 38.2) involved 1,848 physicians from 11 works comparing PEMs with nonintervention controls. The benefit from the printed material ranged from −3 to 243.4% for process outcomes and from −16.1 to 175.6% for patient outcomes. The practical importance of these changes was considered, at best, small; and the author concluded: "The effects of PEMs compared with no active intervention appear small and of uncertain clinical significance. These conclusions should be viewed as tentative due to the poor reporting of results and inappropriate primary analyses...."

In other terms, when compared with control groups, the results triggered by printed material were insignificant and had little practical importance and uncertain clinical relevance (justified by methodological limitations on the evaluation of primary sources). The additional impact caused by other information transfer strategies (speeches and workshops) was considered small, although the role of educational visits and the influence of "opinion-formers" merited highlighting and were considered to have probable value.

More recently, Farmer et al. [6] showed similar results: PEMs appear to have small beneficial effects on professional practice. The author concluded:

> ...when compared to no intervention, printed educational material when used alone may have a beneficial effect on process outcomes, but not on patient outcomes. Despite this wide of range of effects reported for PEMs, clinical significance of the observed effect sizes is not known. There is insufficient information about how to optimize educational materials. The effectiveness of educational materials compared to other interventions is uncertain.

Although recognizing that the use of leaflets is an economically accessible practice, the authors questioned the idea that the mere transfer of information would be capable of influencing behavior and decisively modifying the course of therapeutic action. This statement was emphatically supported by Lundberg, for whom these data call into question the whole dogma that PEMs used by physicians have a net beneficial effect on patients [17].

Meredith et al. [19] (Table 38.2) conducted a study on deficiencies in leaflets distributed by urologists to patients in the prostatectomy preoperative phase. Among the 4,226 questionnaires answered by patients and 807 supplementary comments, the problems most frequently indicated related to the omission of relevant information on cancer recurrence and sexual life. Only one of the leaflets studied had information concerning the malignant potential of prostatic diseases, while 29% of the patients felt a lack of such information. The study concluded that, in addition to a lack of uniformity of form and content, the standards of printed information did not meet patients' demands in that field and context. A qualitative evaluation of educational material on cancer distributed by two American institutions [7] pointed out the demand among patients for content related to emotions and sex—absent in the leaflets, but accessible through personal contacts.

Synthesis: Information as a Drug and Communication Prosthesis

The "One-Size-Fits-All" Approach

Kreuter [15] observed that printed materials frequently consist of mass-produced brochures, booklets, or pamphlets developed with a "one-size-fits-all approach" that might be appropriate under certain circumstances. Even with small changes produced at relatively modest cost, they cannot address the unique needs, interests, and concerns of unique individuals. With the advent and dissemination of new communication technologies, our ability to collect information from individuals and provide feedback tailored to the specific information collected has become not only possible, but practical. It can be seen that, although apparently contradictory in results and conclusions, the converging point among the studies that have assessed the leaflets is fundamentally cognitivist and "readability-centered." In other words, it is focused on a kind of "universal comprehensibility" and "one-size-fits-all perspective" about the patients' content assimilation. Even if leaflets were plentifully endowed with illustrations, culturally adjusted, and cognitively well implanted, they did not unequivocally attain the objectives that had been proposed for them. (Nevertheless, we have to recognize that such attributes were rarely encountered at the same time among the consulted works.) The mere fact that the text and graphics were comprehensible, with careful evaluation by specialists and readability scores, was not a guarantee of the attitude changes desired. All the reviewers seem to appeal to a sort of reductionist bias that underestimates the complexity that surrounds the matter. Direct correlations between cognition and behavioral changes are usually made without contextualization of scenarios.

It is well known by common sense that, in regard to old, ingrained habits, people do not always act according to knowledge. On the other hand, cognitive impairment caused by emotional stress can easily create adverse conditions to diagnostic and treatment procedures. Depending on the situation, the mix of desires, fears, beliefs, and conveniences seems to be stronger than information acquired from brochures.

The phenomenon is well known by social psychology as "cognitive dissonance." People are biased to think of their choices as correct, despite any contrary evidence. This bias gives dissonance theory its predictive power, shedding light on otherwise puzzling, irrational, and self-destructive behavior.

In cancer care, we usually have to deal with multiple and complex factors that pose an individual (to professionals) and collective (to the health team) challenge. Sometimes the "transmission tactic" does not reach its objectives and fails in the statistical validation processes that it is subjected to. In certain contexts, it is not possible to advocate the absolute abolition of such tactics or to prescribe them unconditionally from such disappointing results. From this impasse we believe that, depending on the context in question—the presence or absence of unique needs attended to only by personal contact or even emotional factors interfering with the process of cognitive gain—such tactics will be doomed to failure.

Most of the works cited here illustrate the superimposition of a cognitivist bias over the informative demands perceived in the cancer care context: dissemination of information (instead of interpersonal interaction); the imperative to systematically measure the achieved information; and subsequent studies for validating the whole process. Upon these models, the cognitive assumptions mentioned above are articulated as drawn, perhaps intuitively, from educational models of school environment. With the exception of qualitative studies applied in specific contexts, the present review of literature reveals the dominance of the epistemological models classically used in clinical trials. Under such frameworks, printed information is evaluated under the randomized controlled trial perspective. Changes in behavior or good scores in cognitive validation questionnaires are considered "positive outcomes" equivalent to behavioral changes. Compared to control procedures, information leaflets are considered a kind of "medicine" with an "active principle" for ignorance treatment. Under the premises of this metaphor, information is tested as a kind of pharmaceutical preparation that exerts a distinct effect from the inert fillers and placebo.

The rationality of these studies recalls the methodology for evaluating the efficacy of medications. Studies on drug absorption and their bioavailability (the proportion of the dose that becomes available in the plasma to cause effects) may be compared with the linear association made with readability and clinical outcomes. In the same way, the need for associations with other adjuvant cognitive agents could be compared to a "drug prescription" of databanks and multimedia resources for disseminating knowledge.

The discussion regarding the selection of the most important subjects and the prescriptive competence of doctors raises questions about their paternalistic tendencies in the choice of information considered pertinent. Several studies have pointed out the challenge of the "ideal information dose" and the risks of collateral effects on overinformed patients. In this respect, some curious premises have been highlighted, such as "the impression that the more informed the patient is, the more he will feel imaginary complications." Entwistle and Watt [5] (Table 38.3) described similar phenomena regarding the early detection of prostate cancer. They described some reluctance to distribute informational material due to the belief that information excesses could trigger anxiety among those it was destined for. In the same way, a belief among professionals is described [11] (Table 38.3) that detailed information on the risk of laparoscopy would induce patients to decline to undergo the surgery procedure. As a result of these premises, mostly in environments overloaded with the weight of extreme emotions, papers consider excess of information as risky or in some other way disadvantageous. In short, by means of leaflets with different "doses" of information—from the most laconic to the most detailed—the most detailed could interfere by increasing the degree of anxiety or influencing the decision concerning invasive procedures. Garden et al. [10] (Table 38.3) also devoted study to the "ideal information dose" on anesthesia offered before surgeries. To discover the appropriate quantity of information, they distributed leaflets with three levels of content: complete and detailed information; standard information; and the minimum content necessary. It is noteworthy that, when the leaflets were distributed separately, patients showed themselves satisfied with the level of explanations offered in a similar way for the three groups. However, when they had access to a set of the three types of leaflet, they began to consider the "minimal discourse" as insufficient, demanding information that previously they had not perceived to be absent. In Kruse et al. [16] (Table 38.3), we also find emphasis on the dose of subject matter and concern with "pharmaceutical forms." To evaluate the knowledge acquired and the changes in patients' attitudes, they compared different formats for carrying information: leaflets or booklets (with increasing levels of detail regarding the matter dealt with) and concluded that the best results were gathered from information carried via booklets. More than a half-century ago, with the same perspective of "absorptive competence" or "information bioavailability," [26] (Table 38.3) observed that doctors generally overestimate patients' capacity for information retention.

Taking the reading of these works as a whole, we could state that, according to the authors, ideal PEMs should transmit large doses of "good information" to be adjusted "in terms of its posology," according to individual capabilities for assimilation. The study and recognition of cognitive and cultural profiles would add complexity to the challenge of producing ethnicity-adjusted data, and this should lead to a high bioavailability of useful information. In the production process, it is not uncommon to observe demands for omitted ingredients in the construction of the informational pieces. It is relevant to point out that the majority of the work described above tends to characterize the activity of supplying patients with information as a complementary activity of poor relevance to the therapeutic intervention. Thus, PEMs are employed as "communication prostheses," occasionally used to shorten direct interactions and rarely taking into account all the diversity of content and emotional contexts, ignoring the multivoiced nature of human communication. The ritual of information transmission is taken here to be a standard procedure in professional interaction, wasting moments that would be suitable for mutual enrichment.

Whether as a substitute for or complement to this interaction, PEMs are exhaustively dismantled, redefined in their communicative attributes, and finally considered of ambiguous efficacy. Their impact can oscillate among these studies due to the peculiar conditions in which they are developed. In methodological terms, the authors compare the same instrument in different and unpredictable circumstances permeated by factual conditions and cultural and emotional modulators (enhanced by difficulties of linguistic communication). Leaflets for cancer patients that are sufficiently informative and deal with issues of dying, mutilation, pain, and loss pose an insurmountable challenge to their producers. On this scenario, blatant lapses point to a poorly satisfied demand: the discussion regarding emotions and death, domains that are accessible only by closer personal approaches. Health care professionals with distinguished expertise and coming from various health care environments have improved their scales and scores instruments for stratifying educational differences and cognitive impairments. From their results, communication prostheses are developed and used to support deficiencies that professionals actually do not have: human interaction and listening skills.

Conclusions

Nobody can deny that Internet information resources provide a great amount of relevant and useful information to millions of patients under various circumstances. On the other hand, the proliferation of health websites and the emergence of self-diagnosis sites, as we have pointed out [23], may confirm the hypothesis that communication between doctors and patients is not satisfactory. There is a growing demand for information poorly covered by usual formats of communication. In cancer care settings, far beyond the comprehensibility of information, there are emotional conditions and feelings of existential threat that should not be ignored. Even in the Internet era, PEM production has never been so prolific in hospitals. The healthcare teams are deeply involved with the development of material that, in the recent past, was shared only among communication professionals. As expected, a remarkable increase in the number of articles for evaluation and validation of these materials has been observed. However, the results have led to ambiguous conclusions. There are many works that encourage this kind of project, along with skeptical assessments of its importance [12–14]. Recent systematic reviews (although they are not clear about the importance of PEMs in cancer care) are skeptical about their usefulness. Nonetheless, a decline in production of these leaflets has still not been observed.

The vast majority of the PEMs strive to convey practical knowledge. According to the evaluation articles, the cognition attribute seems to be the most valuable; reception studies are rarely used to validate content in the subjective dimension. In cancer prevention, the most disappointing results are usually found among the materials produced to change ingrained habits. Contrary to the success of educational leaflets in the school environment (in which prominent results are achieved through dialog in the teacher–student relationship), such an impact has not been observed, in a qualitative perspective, on cancer prevention. In that sense, we may distinguish several levels of impact. When discussing "intended" and "liquid" impacts, it is necessary to ask what we mean by "influence" or "impact." Is it an attempt to guide people's behavior, a "soft imposing" of health standards for healthy individuals, or does it aim at an internalization of medical standards to improve people's health?

After reading the present reviews, we could state that the concept of "impact" is related to the process of cognitive transmission of technical imperatives in such a way that lay people may become acquainted with them (and perhaps reproduce them). It is argued that when assessing impact, authors used the resources of a pre-idealized "clinical rationality"—concepts about randomization, control groups, and controlled trials. These premises and the expected outcomes for PEMs mutually influence one another. It is relevant to keep in mind that their effects were not confined to factual phenomena, in terms of actions, but also in terms of subjective encoding, which is not measurable by clinical trials. Besides, it is also quite conceivable that several "levels" of cognition, motivation, and action can also operate simultaneously in an intangible dimension in clinical trials. Nevertheless, leaflets have repeatedly been produced and sent out as instruments voicing a monologue, developed to transmit information unilaterally defined as relevant, without subsequent reception studies.

Several authors believe that brochures cannot provide or be a substitute for a discursive approach. Such an approach goes beyond the mere transmission of information by reaffirming the ethical objectives of the discussion in a context of a relationship, in which leaflets may have only adjuvant relevance. Weak as communication prostheses and disconnected from personal approaches, leaflets fail to influence those for whom they are designed, who are necessarily equalized in their culture, biography, and subjective demands. Such leaflets, although excessively technical, are read attentively by cancer patients, even when they are without illustrations or other adornments. This interest can be attributed to the anxiolytic function of information, whether given by text or speech, on invasive procedures that involve high complexity and risks in an emotional context of "life or death" such as is frequently observed in moments of cancer diagnosis, postsurgery, or in follow-up after treatment. These perspectives do reaffirm the importance of these materials on cancer care, assuming the premise that an essentially cognitive evaluation may not be the most appropriate way to assess their usefulness.

The point of discussion regarding PEMs is not simply, Yes, it works, or No, it doesn't work. In cancer care contexts, an equally irrelevant issue is: Who might benefit from PEMs? Do educated cancer patients nowadays really need leaflets, with all the information available on the Internet? Are PEMs developed primarily for the uneducated, for whom they must be simple, easily readable, and understandable? Patients are not passive message receivers; their reactions to information provided might change according to their needs and individual reactions. As stated before, information is crucial for people with cancer—for their successful treatment and rehabilitation; to promote their involvement and informed decision making; to reduce negative perceptions. There are several investigations concerning information use by cancer patients, and they confirm that printed media is an important contributor to knowledge and a facilitator for decision making. Nonetheless, the subjective coding of relevant elements depends on patients' unique needs and their trust in the sources. There is a great demand for information by the population suffering from chronic conditions that impose significant limitations on their quality of life. We stress here that under these circumstances the results are encouraging when interpersonal interactions are combined with leaflet distribution. Therefore, we conclude that the apparently contradictory results of systematic reviews may be associated with: inadequate comparison of noncomparable instruments; use of these instruments under noncomparable circumstances; overall evaluation under the same methodological perspectives. The exposure conditions are ignored, and the information (as a protection factor) is linearly related to the outcomes (cognitive effects), not necessarily linked to the expected impact that could be the result of cognitive dissonances.

From an anthropological point of view, the rationality of such assessments reveals more about the reviewers than about what is reviewed. This way of thinking, so familiar to the biomedical sciences, is based on statistical validation guided by epistemological concepts usually applied on studies about medicines. Such a theoretical framework has permeated a half-century discussion. Drug attributes are intuitively applied: "dose" (more or less detailed pamphlets); "administration routes" (by mail or distributed personally); "bioavailability" (proportion between what is delivered and what is retained); "adjuvant elements" (supported by illustrations, humorous style and slang); "adverse effects" (fear, anxiety, and risk of giving up procedures); and "validity period" (need of new information and continuous updating). Many of the unsuccessful experiments used what we call "communication prostheses," defined here as artifacts developed to deliver impersonal information. Knowledge is a kind of "active principle"—independent of other forces that govern human action, such as culture, values, ingrained habits, and fears. Moreover, in contexts of ultra-specialization and distance in the doctor–patient relationship, such information prostheses can easily become a surrogate for interaction.

In the context of care for cancer patients, printed materials are recognized as a valuable support for information that otherwise would be lost. These booklets are of transcendent importance, far greater than that attributed to them in general health education contexts. Regardless of their effectiveness, measured in various care settings, the brochures are needed as support material for closer interactions, as is implied by studies evaluating this combination of strategies. A mechanistic communication model sees patients as passive individuals, thereby generating a need for anticipating the subjects of their queries and curtailing the need for dialog. Communication prostheses are usually produced to inform without being able to provide comfort, enhance quality of life, or educate.

References

1. Arthur, V. A. (1995). Written patient information: a review of the literature. J Adv Nurs, 21(6), 1081–6.
2. Buki, L. P., Salazar, S. I., & Pitton, V. O. (2009). Design elements for the development of cancer education print materials for a Latina/o audience. Health Promot Pract, 10(4), 564–72.
3. Department of Health. (2004). Better information, better choices, better health: putting information at the centre of health. London: DoH.

4. Doak, L. G., Doak, C. C., & Meade, C. D. (1996). Strategies to improve cancer education materials. Oncol Nurs Forum, 23(8), 1305–12.
5. Entwistle, V. A., & Watt, I. S. (1998). Disseminating information about healthcare effectiveness: a survey of consumer health information services. Qual Health Care, 7(3), 124–9.
6. Farmer AP, Légaré F, Turcot L, Grimshaw J, Harvey E, McGowan JL, et al. Printed educational materials: effects on professional practice and health care outcomes. Cochrane Database Syst Rev. 2008;(3):CD004398.
7. Foltz, A. T., & Sullivan, J. M. (1999). Limited literacy revisited implications for patient education. Cancer Pract, 7(3), 145–50.
8. Freemantle N, Harvey EL, Wolf F, Grimshaw JM, Grilli R, Bero LA. Printed educational materials: effects on professional practice and health care outcomes. Cochrane Database Syst Rev. 2000;(2):CD000172.
9. Freitas, F. V., & Rezende Filho, L. A. (2011). Communication models and use of printed materials in healthcare education: a bibliographic survey. Interface, 15(36), 243–56.
10. Garden, A. L., Merry, A. F., Holland, R. L., et al. (1996). Anaesthesia information—what patients want to know. Anaesth Intensive Care, 24(5), 594–8.
11. Garrud, P., Wood, M., & Stainsby, L. (2001). Impact of risk information in a patient education leaflet. Patient Educ Couns, 43(3), 303–6.
12. Guidry, J. J., & Walker, V. D. (1999). Assessing cultural sensitivity in printed cancer materials. Cancer Pract, 7(6), 291–6.
13. Hunter, J. L. (2005). Cervical cancer educational pamphlets: do they miss the mark for Mexican immigrant women's needs? Cancer Control, 12(Suppl 2), 42–50.
14. Kee, F. (1996). Patients' prerogatives and perceptions of benefit. Br Med J, 312, 958–60.
15. Kreuter, M. (1993). Human behaviour and cancer: forget the magic bullet. Cancer, 72, 996–1001.
16. Kruse, A. Y., Kjaergard, L. L., Krogsgaard, K., et al. (2000). A randomized trial assessing the impact of written information on outpatients' knowledge about and attitude toward randomized clinical trials. The INFO trial group. Control Clin Trials, 21(3), 223–40.
17. Lundberg, G. D. (2008). Passive dissemination of printed educational materials in medicine has no or negligible effect on patient outcomes. Medscape J Med, 10(11), 255.
18. Mann, K. S. (2011). Education and health promotion for new patients with cancer. Clin J Oncol Nurs, 15(1), 55–61.
19. Meredith, P., Emberton, M., & Wood, C. (1995). Comparison of patients' needs for information on prostate surgery with printed materials provided by surgeons. Qual Health Care, 4(1), 18–23.
20. Munir, F., Kalawsky, K., Lawrence, C., Yarker, J., Haslam, C., & Ahmed, S. (2011). Cognitive intervention for breast cancer patients undergoing adjuvant chemotherapy: a needs analysis. Cancer Nurs, 34(5), 385–92.
21. Rozemberg, B., Silva, A. P. P., & Vasconcellos-Silva, P. R. (2002). Hospital leaflets and the dynamics of constructing their meanings: the perspective of health professionals. Public Health Rep, 18(6), 1685–94.
22. Stephens, P. A., Osowski, M., Fidale, M. S., & Spagnoli, C. (2008). Identifying the educational needs and concerns of newly diagnosed patients with breast cancer after surgery. Clin J Oncol Nurs, 12(2), 253–8.
23. Vasconcellos-Silva, P. R., & Castiel, L. D. (2009). New self-care technologies and the risk of self-diagnosis through the Internet. Rev Panam Salud Publica, 26(2), 172–5.
24. Weintraub, D., Maliski, S. L., Fink, A., Choe, S., & Litwin, M. S. (2004). Suitability of prostate cancer education materials: applying a standardized assessment tool to currently available materials. Patient Educ Couns, 55(2), 275–80.
25. Wong, J. J., D'Alimonte, L., Angus, J., Paszat, L., Soren, B., & Szumacher, E. (2011). What do older patients with early breast cancer want to know while undergoing adjuvant radiotherapy? J Cancer Educ, 26(2), 254–61.
26. Pratt, L., Seligmann, A., Reader, G., (1957). Physicians' views on the level of medical information among patients. Am J Public Health Nations Health, 47(10), 1277–83.

Chapter 39
The Benefits and Pitfalls of the Internet in Communication with Cancer Patients

Mirjana Rajer

Abstract The Internet has become a major source of health-related information and support for cancer patients. Information gained through the Internet can enrich patients' knowledge about the disease. Better-informed patients are more involved in the decision-making process and more satisfied with the treatment selected. Unfortunately, some information on the Internet can be of low quality and reliability. In this chapter I explore different aspects of Internet-gained information and doctor–patient communication about it.

Keywords Internet • Cancer • Web-pages • Online support groups • Doctor-patient relationship • Communication

Introduction

The advent of the Internet has had a profound, far-reaching impact on people's lives. It is not surprising that this impact has spread to the field of medicine. Information that was previously available mostly through specialized books and journals is now readily available through specialized websites, online journals, online forums, and other forms. The prerequisite for having access to such information is being able to use the Internet. Despite the spread of Internet usage, it is clearly not yet universal. Research suggests that younger and better-educated people are more likely to use the Internet, while clearly the older are more likely to require health-related information. Of course, access to information can always be by proxy—through the patient's family or friends [1].

Although the advantages of having information within arm's reach seem obvious, there is also a dark side: the quality and veracity of such information varies and

M. Rajer, MD, MSc (✉)
Institute of Oncology Ljubljana, Ljubljana, Slovenia
e-mail: mirjana.rajer@gmail.com

cannot be easily verified. This is especially the case when those seeking information are patients and other nonprofessionals. Distinguishing between accurate information, unconfirmed studies, alternative and complementary methods, and sometimes hearsay or simply misinformation is an open challenge, which can be addressed through communication between the patient and the doctor [1, 2].

Some patients choose to discuss this information with their doctor, seeking feedback regarding its accuracy; others do not. The patient–doctor relationship regarding information sharing needs further exploring, for the following reasons: First, as already mentioned, there is the potential of obtaining inaccurate information. Were the patient to use such information, it could have detrimental effects. Second, if the information is accurate but patients do not understand it properly, they may not use it properly. The doctor can put the information into proper context and relieve the anxiety that it may arouse in patients. Last but not least, the withholding of information obtained from the Internet by the patient due to the fear of offending the doctor must not be ignored [1].

Who Searches for Information on the Internet

In recent decades major changes in the needs of cancer patients and their relatives regarding finding information have occurred. With the development of new treatment options and better treatment results, the word "cancer" is becoming less frightening. Today patients and their relatives need to know more than simply "How much time do I have?" Better-informed cancer patients are more involved in the decision-making process, are more satisfied with treatment choices, and communicate better with their families. Cancer patients search for information from different sources: health professionals, family and friends, cancer survivors, newspapers, books, television, radio, printed educational materials, and the Internet [3].

The Internet has become one of the most important sources of information for cancer patients. It can provide information about their illness, treatment options, and health improvement strategies. Additionally, it can offer support in the form of virtual communities [4, 5]. Advantages of the Internet as an information source are its low costs, convenient and anonymous accessibility, 24-h availability, and its provision of updated, detailed information [5]. The Internet is broadly, though not universally, available in some parts of the world; it is supposed that nearly 80% persons in the so-called developed world have access to it. While data for developing countries show less availability (only about 10% in Africa), trends in achieving Internet access are rising constantly [6].

More than 12 million Internet sites that contain health-related information are used every day worldwide, and cancer is among the top three diseases that patients research on the Internet [7]. The majority of adults (70%) in Western societies use the Internet regularly, and 80% of them seek health information on it. Concerning cancer patients, 31–60% of them and their caregivers use the Internet to search for information on their disease [1].

Patients who search for cancer-related Internet information are more likely to be younger, own a computer, have Internet access at home, and have achieved a higher educational level than cancer patients who do not. Higher education and income were observed among breast and lung cancer patients who use the Internet for information searching, compared to those who do not [1, 5]. While melanoma and prostate carcinoma patients seeking Internet information are of younger age compared to patients who do not, this is not observed for breast cancer patients [1]. Less is known about the psychological characteristics of Internet health-related users. While some trials observed that people who consider themselves as being in very poor health use the Internet frequently, other trials do not support this observation [5].

Internet Health-Related Applications

The Internet offers various health-related applications [5]:

- Informative web pages for searching for health-related information
- Online support groups for sharing thoughts with others who have similar experience
- Communication for searching online advice from health professionals or contacting doctors via e-mail

WebPages

Search engines (e.g., Google, Yahoo) are the most important tool for searching for information. Many more health information seekers start their search with an engine rather than with health-related sites. Even doctors use Google as a first source in finding information about rare diseases. Engine searches, while easily accessible, have some limitations. The broadness of information (in November 2011, there were 276,000,000 hits on the words "cancer disease" in Google) and the lack of quality control can expose the patient to incorrect or out-of-date information and can potentially harm them. Patients may need guidance in finding trustworthy sites and appraising and filtering the information they find [8].

Bylund et al. conducted a trial to address the practice of cancer patients in information search on health-related sites. Half of the patients search for information on cancer organization websites (e.g., American Cancer Society), followed by information services (e.g., WebMD), hospital websites, and foundation and government websites, which are equally represented (20%). About 15% of patients use websites of pharmaceutical companies or a specific drug website, online scientific journal articles, and chat rooms. A minority of patients (<5%) look at individuals' home pages or blogs [1].

McHugh and Corrigan conducted a survey of Internet searches in 2008 and 2010 regarding the four most common cancers (breast, lung, prostate, and colorectal).

In 2 years, searches increased by 183% from 97,531 in 2008 to 179,025 in 2010. Information on breast cancer was the most common (44.1%), followed by lung (23.7%), prostate (19.1%), and colorectal cancer (13.1%). In all but breast cancer, about half of the searches were for general information, followed by diagnosis and screening; most information on breast cancer was about awareness campaigns. About 10% of searches in all cancers were about risk factors and treatment, while less than 1% of searches were about sexual function and legal information. Information on alternative treatments were searched most often for prostate and lung cancers, while less than 1% of breast and colorectal cancer searchers searched for this type of information [9].

The types of information patients seek changes with the different stages of their disease and treatment. Newly diagnosed patients seek general information about their cancer type; they check information provided by their doctors, search for available tests, treatment options, and information on the possibility of getting a second opinion. Patients in active treatment and "survivors" seek information about treatment side effects, long-term outcomes, and complementary and alternative treatments. In addition, they participate in support groups and chat rooms to share experience and purchase medical products via the Internet [4].

Differences may exist even among various cancer types. Nagler et al. reported interesting results regarding this subject. They compared the differences in information seeking for breast, prostate, and colon cancer. Colon cancer patients search for less information compared to the other two groups. Differences are especially evident in early-stage disease. An exact explanation for this phenomenon cannot be made. The authors speculate that the differences are the result of the different quantities of information available on the Internet for different cancers; that the treatment of early-stage colon cancer is more straightforward than the treatments for breast and prostate cancer, and hence there is less need for information; and that late side effects of treatment are less pronounced than in the treatment of early breast or prostate cancer [10].

Online Support Groups

It is very important to make every effort possible to "open communication channels" with the patient—to understand how the patients perceive their condition, their emotional and other nonorganic responses to their organic condition. Such communication channels may ultimately influence the outcome of the therapy, and thus information should flow both ways. Even though some forms of communications necessarily do without nonverbal elements such as gestures, they are still worth the effort [11, 12].

The Internet has been particularly useful in broadening options. New forms of constant, albeit brief, communication have sprung up and are being used by vast numbers of people. Facebook, for example, which allows chatting, among other things, has more than 800 million active users [13]. Twitter, a service enabling the exchange of short message service (SMS)-style messages, has around 100 million users [14]. Skype, a service for online video telephony, already had more than 500 million users in 2009 [15]. Skype is particularly interesting because it at least partly overcomes the aforementioned lack of nonverbal signals—moreover, in a cost-effective way. Since these channels (Facebook, Skype, Twitter, YouTube, etc.) are used more frequently by the younger population, their application in communication with cancer patients should be considered first for younger patients. Twitter and Skype will not be further explored in this chapter as support group tools, since their greatest strengths lie elsewhere [11, 16].

Online support in the form of virtual support groups represents a common mode of social support. During the past few years participation in these groups has quadrupled [16]. This is in accord with the multiplication of online health websites. Besides general health information, these sites often offer support for patients [17].

Online chatting is a form of communication in which two or more people participate in a synchronous exchange of remarks over a computer network. Ripamonti et al. describe a wonderful case of a patient for whom chatting represented a communication bridge. The 22-year-old patient was diagnosed with sarcoma of the retromaxillary region. After treatment with radiation and chemotherapy, he developed painful ulcers in the mouth that made eating and drinking difficult and speaking impossible. The patient was always accompanied by his mother, who spoke on his behalf, while he listened and showed no desire to communicate himself. His mother described him as a shy, taciturn person. The first impression of the caregivers was that the patient experienced psychological withdrawal induced by his physical condition. Despite this, workers in the department providing supportive care did not want to abandon the attempt to communicate directly with the patient. After long conversations with his mother, they found a possible solution in Internet online chatting. The patient agreed immediately. Chatting was extremely successful, as he was now able to express his medical and spiritual needs; this was a source of great satisfaction for him, his family, and the entire medical staff [11].

A blog is a web-based journal, an online diary, that is updated frequently with new content. Blogs are usually maintained by an individual with regular entries of commentary, descriptions of events, or other material such as graphics or video [18]. An illness blog is an online narrative of illness. It can be created by patients themselves or by persons near the patients. In online narratives of the illness experience, patients describe their life during treatment as they live it; they receive responses from family, friends, and even from strangers far away from them. Blogging has several advantages and few disadvantages. Narrative expression can help diminish the psychosocial side effects of illness as well as aid the integration of events into family life. However, if not properly handled, a blog can lead to further isolation [19]. A wonderful personal example is presented by Bach, who describes how he set up such a blog when his wife was ill and ends the article with the thought that "my only regret is that I did not start the blog earlier" [20].

An alternative to blogging that offers more options is posting to video sites, such as YouTube. Whereas blogs are usually written by patients and/or family members and lay out a personal experience, videos on YouTube can provide personal stories, campaigns, or generally informative videos. Chou et al. present an overview of YouTube, focusing on cancer survivor stories. They point out that the diagnosis phase (including reference to medical personnel) and emotional content are strongly present in the videos analyzed [12, 21, 22].

The most complete application falling into the online support group category is nowadays probably Facebook, due to several factors, including its general spread of use and its ability to combine the key features of chatting, blogging, as well as video posting. Bender et al. conducted a content analysis of breast cancer support groups on Facebook. They found 620 groups totaling more than a million members; their analysis was limited to publicly available groups operating in English. Contentwise, the majority were fund-raising groups, followed by awareness and patient/caregiver support. Even though the authors report that more than 85% of the groups had 25 posts or less, a million "connections" is still a dramatic result [16].

Online Communication with Health Professionals

Communication with health professionals either directly (e.g., by e-mail) or via advice seeking on health-related web pages is a reliable mode of obtaining information [4].

Communicating via e-mail with physicians, while in principle easily accessible, is still not commonly practiced. In a trial in the Netherlands reported by Van Unden-Kraan et al., less than 2% of patients used this method of communication. Patients would like to communicate with their doctors via e-mail, though. Singh et al. report similar results for actual usage in southern California (1.3%), while close to half (49.3%) of patients "expressed enthusiasm about the possibility of using it." Authors explain that there are still limited possibilities of communicating with health professionals via e-mail, although patients would like to [23]. Physicians feel that e-consultations would bring them extra workload without adequate reward and that the quality of care would diminish [4, 5].

Positive and Negative Effects of the Internet

The widely available Internet is without a doubt a positive element in the information chain connecting health professionals and patients. The Internet provides ample opportunities to search actively for health and medical information, and doing this helps educate and empower patients [21]. Several authors reported beneficial effects of the Internet: patients who search their disease on the Internet tend to be more actively involved in the decision-making process and consequently show more satisfaction with health services, are more compliant with recommended treatment regimens, and are more likely to follow their doctors' advice about follow-up [21, 24]. Active involvement in decision-making leads to less anxiety and depression during and after cancer treatment and consequently contributes to better quality of life [21].

The relationship of Internet use to active patient involvement may be explained by the fact that the Internet provides cancer patients with information about their disease, possible treatment options, and prognosis. In addition, they can find information about health care delivery options, access to medical care, experience and qualifications of physicians, quality of medical equipment, and options regarding health care systems and research. Patients declare satisfaction with information obtained on the Internet from the time of diagnosis to the survival period [21].

The clearest disadvantage of the Internet as a health information medium is the overwhelming quantity of information and the already-mentioned difficulty of distinguishing good information from hearsay, misinformation, or product sales pitches. It is best that the information be filtered by a trustworthy intermediary, be it a dedicated website, support group, or physician. Of course, this also depends on what information is sought [21, 24].

Doctor–Patient Communication about Internet Information

Health-related Internet information can influence patient–doctor communication. Patients become more active players in the decision-making process. The Internet provides patients and caregivers access to information that was previously either unavailable or difficult to access and lessens the imbalances in the doctor–patient relationship, between the unknowing patient on the one side and the powerful expert on the other. It is estimated that 40% of all cancer patients discuss information found on the Internet with their physician. This percentage is quite similar to the more general population of patients discussing Internet information with their doctors. Discussion of Internet information between doctors and patients can sometimes be challenging for both sides [25].

The Doctor's Negative Perspective

Oncologists report various barriers in communication about Internet information between them and patients/relatives. They think that patients may search for too much information, often of questionable quality; and when patients challenge doctors directly with this information, it may become difficult to continue the consultation [25].

Doctors also think that too much information itself can be harmful: the patient may become overwhelmed, nervous, and confused, especially after reading conflicting medical information [25].

On a practical basis, doctors consider themselves too busy to discuss all Internet information in detail; some find such discussions unnecessary. Furthermore, doctors and patients do not always agree on the accuracy of Internet information. A staggering 91% of doctors consider that the Internet can harm patients with incorrect information. Sixty-two percent of patients consider themselves more optimistic about their disease after reading about it on the Internet, while 38% of doctors think the Internet can give false, unfounded hope to patients. It is thus not surprising that 44% of oncologists report difficulties in discussing cancer-related Internet information with their patients [25].

The Patient's Negative Perspective

Internet anonymity enables patients to seek information about sensitive issues like sexual function during and after treatment and information pertaining to litigation. These issues are unlikely to be discussed with health care professionals directly and are underrepresented in trials addressing doctor–patient communication about the Internet. There is also the possibility that patients will not be disposed to discuss searching for alternative medical treatments with their doctors [9].

How to Find the Right Way

Doctors should be aware of the high use of the Internet by patients and the general population to obtain cancer-related information and should be familiar with the high-quality and high-reliability websites in order to give their patients proper advice [9]. They should also be aware of the importance of their reactions to the subject. A doctor can respond to the patient positively, giving value to the patient's efforts and taking the information seriously; or negatively, warning the patient of the negative effects of the Internet or showing disagreement with the information provided without listening to the patient or showing interest in the discussion. Supporting rather than threatening should be the preferred mode of communication if we want to obtain or preserve a good patient–doctor relationship [25]. Cho et al. report interesting research done in South Korea about the types of questions breast cancer patients posted through a dedicated online Q&A board. They found that 93.5% of the questions pertained to "informational" as opposed to "emotional" support. And that is what the doctors should be focused on anyway—providing informational support for the patient [26].

An Example from My Clinical Practice: A 54-year-old Patient Came to My Office for the First Time...

I started by discussing the history of the illness with the patient. I asked him what his symptoms were and how long he had been observing them. He answered: "I have a small-cell lung cancer with upper vena cava syndrome. I diagnosed the vena cava syndrome by looking at the Internet, and then I visited my family doctor." He knew exactly what the disease was and what therapy should be prescribed to him, even though he was a mechanical engineer, who worked in a far-from-medical environment. Fortunately, the information he got from the Internet was not misleading.

Yet, during the course of his disease the pattern of our communication changed. Knowing that his disease was progressing, we no longer discussed the facts, percentages of success, etc. Our conversations were oriented more to his present symptoms. In this phase of the disease he was no longer seeking information on the Internet, or at least he did not express a desire to discuss such information with me.

Talking to this patient for the first time, I was impressed by the knowledge he had about his disease. Knowing the "literacy" of this patient enabled me to communicate with him in a more "technical" way. Much less time and effort were needed to explain to him and his family the disease, treatment, and likely outcome. Being a busy oncologist, this was a lucky thing for me; I hope more patients will come to my office with the information in their pocket.

Conclusions

In recent decades the Internet has become a widely accessible and broadly accepted medium. All aspects of our lives are today interconnected and influenced by our use of the Internet. Patients and their relatives seek information on the Internet mainly to improve their knowledge about the disease and in some cases to find support in the course of the disease. The hours of research in libraries and newspapers that used to be necessary to find proper information are now being replaced by the mere seconds required by Internet browsers to find multiple answers to the questions posed. In this way patients/relatives become more educated about their disease and consequently achieve a more active role in treatment decisions. From paternalistic doctor–patient relationships, in which patients accepted the presented diagnostic/therapeutic decisions without questioning or discussing them with their clinicians, we are changing to a more open and even-handed relationship, in which patients are allowed to discuss matters, ask questions, and even argue with their doctors. As an education tool, the Internet has an important role in this process.

References

1. Bylund CL, Gueguen JA, D'Agostino TA, D'Agostino TA, Li Y, Sonet E. Doctor-patient communication about cancer-related Internet information. J Psychosoc Oncol. 2010;28:127–42.
2. Briceno AC, Gospodarowicz M, Jadad AR. Fighting cancer with the Internet and social networking. Lancet. 2008;9:1037–8.
3. Cho J, Noh HI, Ha MH, Kang SN, Chou J, Chang YJ. What kind of cancer information do Internet users need? Support Care Cancer. 2011;19:1465–9.

4. Chou WS, Liu B, Post S, Hesse B. Health-related Internet use among cancer survivors: data from the Health Information National Trends Survey 2003–2008. J Cancer Surviv. 2011;5: 263–70.
5. Van Unden-Kraan CF, Drossaert CHC, Taal E, Smit WM, Moens B, Siesling S, et al. Health-related Internet use by patients with somatic diseases: frequency of use and characteristics of users. Inform Health Soc Care. 2009;34:18–29.
6. International Telecommunication Union http://www.itu.int/ITU-D/ict/statistics/ict/index.html. Acessed on 24 October 2011
7. van Weert JCM, van Noort G, Bol N, van Dijk L, Tates K, Jansen J. Tailored information for cancer patients on the Internet: effects of visual cues and language complexity on information recall and satisfaction. Patient Educ Couns. 2011;84:368–78.
8. Place SL, Beck R. Cancer information on the Internet. In: DeVita V, Lawrence TS, Rosenberg SA, editors. Cancer principles and practice of oncology. Philadelphia: Lippincott Williams & Wilkins; 2011. p. 2540–6.
9. McHugh SM, Corrigan M. A quantitative assessment of changing trends in Internet usage for cancer information. World J Surg. 2011;35:253–7.
10. Nagler RH, Gray SW, Romantan A, Kelly BJ, DeMichele A, Armstrong K, et al. Differences in information seeking among breast, prostate and colorectal cancer patients: results from a population-based survey. Patient Educ Couns. 2010;81:S54–62.
11. Ripamonti CI, Picinelli C, Pessi MA, Clerici CA. Modern computer technologies facilitate communication with a young cancer patient. Tumori. 2010;96:609–12.
12. Chou WS, Hunt Y, Folkers A, Augustson E. Cancer survivorship in the age of YouTube and social media a narrative analysis. J Med Internet Res. 2011;17:e7.
13. Facebook statistics http://www.facebook.com/press/info.php?statistics. Accessed on 17 October 2011
14. Time Techlands http://techland.time.com. Accessed on 9 September 2011
15. Wikipedia http://en.wikipedia.org/wiki/Blog. Accessed on 6 October 2011
16. Bender JL, Jimenez-Marroquin MC, Jadaj AR. Seeking support on Facebook: a content analysis of breast cancer groups. J Med Internet Res. 2011;13:e16.
17. Im EO. Online support of patients and survivors of cancer. Semin Oncol Nurs. 2011;27: 229–36.
18. Wikipedia http://en.wikipedia.org/wiki/Skype. Accessed on 7 October 2011
19. Heilferty CM. Toward a theory of online communication in illness: concept analysis of illness blogs. J Adv Nurs. 2009;65:1539–47.
20. Bach LA. Blogging during terminal care: communication, color schemes, and creating a community. J Clin Oncol. 2008;26:4504–6.
21. Lee C, Gray SW, Lewis N. Internet use leads cancer patients to be active health care consumers. Patient Educ Couns. 2010;81(Suppl):S63–9.
22. Heilferry CM. Toward a theory of online communication in illness: concept analysis of illness blogs. J Adv Nurs. 2009;65:1539–47.
23. Singh H, Fox SA, Petersen NJ, Shethia A, Street R. Older patients' enthusiasm to use electronic mail to communicate with their physicians: cross-sectional survey. J Med Internet Res. 2009; 11:e18.
24. Bagott C. Patient education: to the Internet and beyond. Pediatr Blood Cancer. 2011;57:6–7.
25. Bylund C, Gueguen JA, D'Agostino TA, Imes RS, Sonet E. Cancer patients' decisions about discussing Internet information with their doctors. Psychooncology. 2009;18:1139–46.
26. Cho J, Smith KC, Roter D, Guallar E, Young D, Ford DE. Needs of women with breast cancer as communicated to physicians on the Internet. Support Care Cancer. 2011;19:113–21.

Chapter 40
To Tell or Not to Tell: No Longer a Question! Communication with Cancer Patients

Branko Zakotnik

Abstract Although there have been no significant social, religious, or political changes in Slovenia in the last 15 years, a tremendous leap forward has occurred in the field of communication with cancer patients. Among the main reasons for this are probably the Internet, which is globalizing the world in all possible fields and ways; democracy, which came to our country with the fall of the Berlin wall and Yugoslavia; and an increased cancer burden, which has had a huge political impact, since cancer patients with their families represent an important voting bloc, thus affecting political programs, which have to incorporate cancer in their agendas. This has actually happened, since Slovenia, as a new member of the EU, has put cancer as the first health priority during her 6-month presidency of the EU. This had quite a huge impact on cancer care and communication in Slovenia, and I am sure also in other European countries, at least in the new member states. Improved communication in the field of cancer in Slovenia is definitely not a result of a systematic approach in communication skills teaching, which has not yet been introduced, although it is known to have a significant impact on patient–doctor communication. If to tell or not to tell is no longer a question when communicating cancer diagnosis and treatment, this question has moved to the palliative care setting, where communication is of the utmost importance.

Keywords Cancer • Communication • Democracy • Internet • Cancer burden • Palliative care • Slovenia

B. Zakotnik (✉)
Department of Medical Oncology, Institute of Oncology Ljubljana,
Zaloska 2, 61000, Ljubljana, Slovenia
e-mail: bzakotnik@onko-i.si

Introduction

Although there were no significant social, religious, or political changes in Slovenia in the last 15 years, a tremendous leap forward has occurred in the field of communication with cancer patients. It is very speculative and nonscientific to claim that this change in the communication pattern was a factor in the improved survival of our cancer patients that we have registered in this period (Fig. 40.1) [1], but well-informed and motivated patients might better adhere to prescribed evidence-based treatment protocols, leading to better outcomes. What are the reasons for this change in communication? Is it democracy, which came to our country with the fall of the Berlin wall and Yugoslavia? Is it the Internet, which is globalizing the world in all possible fields and ways? Has the problem of the increased cancer burden become so huge that it touches almost every family and does not let our inhabitants put their heads in the sand anymore? For Slovenia the cause is certainly not a systematic approach in communication skills teaching, because this has not yet been introduced, although it is known to have a significant impact on patient–doctor communication [2]. If to tell or not to tell is no longer a question when communicating cancer diagnosis and treatment, this question has moved to the palliative care setting, where communication is of the utmost importance.

In the following lines I would like to speculate on some of the factors that might have changed the communication pattern with our cancer patients and their relatives.

Democracy

Can the political system influence treatment outcome in cancer patients? Is communication an important player in this equation? Survival data support this thesis, since survival in East European countries, at the time with a nondemocratic political system, was significantly lower than in West European countries. Cancer-service infrastructure, prevention and screening programs, access to diagnostic and treatment

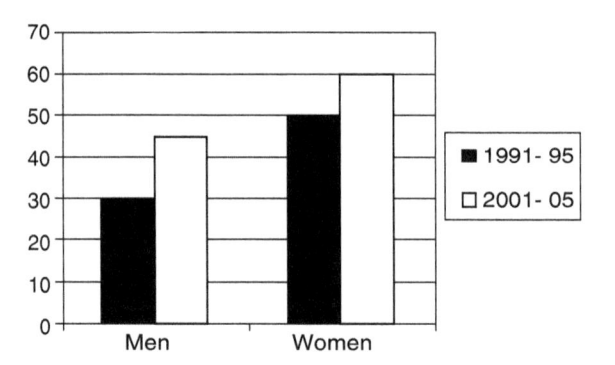

Fig. 40.1 Five-year relative survival rates for all adult cancer patients by sex in the periods 1991–1995 and 2001–2005

facilities, tumor site-specific protocols, multidisciplinary management, application of evidence-based clinical guidelines, and recruitment to clinical trials probably account for most of the differences, as concluded by Verdecchia et al. based on EUROCARE 4 data [3]. Most of these factors can be attributed to more resources spent in healthcare rather than communication with patients, but differences in cancer outcome have also been seen and reported in Western countries [3, 4], and even between different regions in the same countries, such as Norway [5] and Sweden [6], with otherwise the best reported survival outcomes. Obviously some other, probably social, differences, part of which is communication, influence cancer outcome.

Slovenia, as a new member of the EU, has put cancer as first health priority during her 6-month presidency of the EU [7]. This had a huge impact on cancer care and communication in Slovenia, and I am sure also in other European countries, at least in the new member states. In Slovenia screening programs for cervical (ZORA), breast (DORA), and colorectal cancer (SVIT) have started. A high-quality National Cancer Plan and National Palliative Care Program have been adopted by the government, and their implementation is expected in the years to come. Access to cancer treatment has become much better, with new equipment and good access to new cancer drugs. A lot of public debate through mass media has continually been going on during the adoption of all the above changes, and cancer has been almost continually on the agenda. Many times this has been presented in the form of "bad news–good news" in order better to sell newspapers (or radio and TV), but all these have had a big impact on the population's awareness of the problem of cancer and communication about it. In the peaceful socialist times this kind of news was never in the mass media, because everything was always "running really smoothly." Despite the Internet and all possible foreign TV and radio channels, the local (national) mass media have the most important impact on every society, since they are part of the cultural, historical, and political body of the nation and are produced in the native language.

Internet

The Internet obviously has the biggest impact on communication, since by default this is a communication tool. In my paper of the 1997 issue of *Ann. N.Y. Acad. Sci.* the word *Internet* was never mentioned [8]. On the Internet patients today have available free of charge information on all types of cancers, treatments, support groups, journals, etc. Modern search engines enable them to reach all possible URLs worldwide. There is one limitation of equal information to all globally—the English language. But even this problem is being addressed, and the information technology (IT) possibilities will most probably solve it. In Slovenia only older and IT-illiterate people, a minor percent, are not able to access the Internet.

Of course the Internet with its search engines is only a tool to reach the desired databases. A huge effort has been and is being made by those who established and maintain these databases—national cancer institutes and libraries, research institutions, medical associations, journals, cancer leagues and societies, NGOs, and many others. In the future I hope that even more free access to URLs, medical journals, and support groups for patients and health professionals will be available.

So what effect does the Internet have on disclosure of cancer diagnosis, prognosis, and treatment as I experience it in everyday work with my patients? The patients and their families with Internet as their way of life (the majority) in a way have actually skipped the problem of the disclosure to diagnosis, because they really want to type their diagnosis in the search engine as soon as possible for the treatment possibilities, prognosis, and other details that can be found. Due to mass media, Internet, and today's large presence of cancer, patients and their families are already informed that cancer does not mean death. Disclosure of diagnosis in these patients has become a problem when an exact diagnosis cannot be produced as soon as possible in order to start adequate treatment. Many times this phenomenon is driven by the relatives, even more often by the children of the patients, who are usually more IT literate. It works, yes; the Internet is great. Of course, there are still some old-fashioned cases, specially the uneducated patients, without families and without access to the Internet. But even in these patients the disclosure of diagnosis, treatment, and prognosis has probably changed due to mass media.

But as with everything, the Internet has also the other side of the coin—advertising of alternative, unapproved treatments that often can be harmful to the patients. Patients and, even more often, their relatives catch sight of these "promising" treatments on the Internet very quickly. This phenomenon is probably universal [9]. One could speculate that this phenomenon is more prominent in countries with poorer health resources, but Kimby et al. report factors that influence the use of alternative treatments in cancer also in developed countries, such as Denmark, with excellent health resources [10]. How much these treatments are really used is difficult to say, since patients probably do not talk about them with their doctors. But many people do talk and ask all sorts of questions about these treatments, many of which I have never heard before, and quite a lot of communication time is spent on this issue. The popularity of these various complementary treatments, usually plant extracts, comes in waves. At the moment the most popular complementary cancer medicine in Slovenia is a traditionally used Chinese and Japanese mushroom, *Ganoderma lucidum* [11]. Not only patients but also professionals (pharmacologists, doctors, pharmacists) and even some NGOs recommend and advertise *Ganoderma* as a supplement to cancer treatment. Even a phase III randomized trial with *Ganoderma* in one arm and placebo in the other besides standard treatment in patients with prostate cancer is going on in Slovenia, led by urologists. In the era before the Internet, when we did not have a free market, such advertisements did not exist; but today I have to keep pace with these trends in order to communicate with the patient who is at the mercy of this information technology jam. Often it is difficult to find the right answers to all the questions.

Another kind of advertisement through the Internet, also very active (I receive several offers at my e-mail address daily, Fig. 40.2), is the advertisement of all the new drugs for cancer (cytostatics, monoclonal antibodies, tyrosine kinase inhibitors, and other targeted agents), usually produced in Asia and substantially cheaper than the registered, legally marketed substances. Fortunately, this does not affect

```
From:           Euroasia [karanchokhani@reliancemail.net]
Sent:           nedelja, 31. januar 2010 06:20
To:             Zakotnik Branko
Subject:        ANTI-CANCER - API/FP & INT
Importance: High
```

Dear Sir / Madam,

We can offer Anti-Cancer Compounds and New Products for reseach purposes only. Please find below some of the compounds that we sell. We can offer them from miligram to kilogram quality.

Adriamycin
Gemcitabine
Bleomycin
Dasatinib
Sunitinib

Kindly let us have your specific inquiry with quantity you require by return for us to submit our offers.

We also sell intermediates on route to the synthesis of these compounds.

Apart from these products, if you require any other product kindly let us know we can offe at a very competitive price.

THANKS AND REGARDS

Euroasia's

*** EUROASIA'S - An International Sourcing Agent at your Fingertips ***

Fig. 40.2 E-mail offer to purchase new cancer drugs

many patients in Slovenia, since access to cancer drugs is excellent and part of the obligatory insurance policy. This is actually a black drug market through the Internet. Here I see a global ethical paradox between legality and morality. One could speculate that the black market is illegal but moral, while legally marketed drugs are legal but immoral, since the majority of the global population with limited resources cannot afford them [12]. The most often-heard argument against these black market drugs is that they are produced in a garage, not validated, and hence dangerous, if not only ineffective. From the safety standpoint this is true; but a friend of mine, a professor of pharmacology, claimed that the tyrosine kinase inhibitors, for example—the so-called small molecules—are easy to manufacture in immense quantities. In practice this has proved to be true, for example with imatinib (Glivec® or Gleevec®), since the drug is produced in one factory in Cork, Ireland for the whole world.

It would be interesting to know how much of these drugs advertised through the Internet are really sold, who buys them, and what impact they have on global cancer survival. Obviously counterfeit drugs are here and pose a huge problem, not only in developing countries, where an affordable price for a counterfeit drug that is active and safe and saves lives can be morally accepted, but also in developed countries, where they are more often sold by criminal societies, are inactive, and often harmful. More information on this issue is available at http://www.safemedicines.org/counterfeit-drugs-1/. Is a similar situation happening, or might it happen, in the cancer drug market as in the AIDS drugs market? AIDS is a disease that the rich can treat and the poor cannot [13, 14]. We can clearly draw a parallel between the chronic antiretroviral treatments of AIDS and chronic targeted treatments of cancer: both require lifelong treatment. The drug prices are much higher for cancer than for AIDS.

Other parts of this book deal thoroughly with all the possible impacts the Internet has had, has, and will have on cancer patients and their relatives and communication; but for patients and doctors in Slovenia I can say that this impact is enormous.

Cancer Burden

As in other countries of the Western world, the incidence of cancer has doubled in Slovenia in the last 15 years, from 6,000 new cases in 1995 to 12,000 in 2010, in a population of two million that remained almost unchanged through this period. An even bigger change happened in cancer prevalence in this period, from 40,000 to 80,000 [15, 16]. If we multiply this last number by four (cancer patient plus their average number of family members), this is already 320,000 people, which represents a huge potential voting bloc and hence political power in a population of two million. Through democratic election mechanisms, cancer care should therefore become one of the health priorities. This has actually happened in our country, as mentioned above. This enlarged cancer burden has also led to the formation and empowering of cancer patients' organizations, which have had and continue to have a large role in demystifying cancer. Patients and their relatives are communicating continually on different forums through various societies and organizations, and probably nowadays more often through global tools such as YouTube and Twitter.

Palliative Care

The to tell or not to tell question has moved in this period from diagnosis disclosure to the palliative setting. One of the main reasons for not answering this question in a proper way is that death as a natural part of our life course has been hidden from everyday family life. Most people die in institutions, mainly homes for the elderly and hospitals, in part because Slovenia, a rural society in the past, has become a working-class society that has moved to cities and small towns. A palliative care network, which would be of great help to families when one of their members is dying, is not yet in place in our country. Although we have made a lot of effort in organizing educational events in this field, publishing manuals in the Slovene language [17, 18], the palliative care teams that exist in our institution and a few other hospitals have not yet been introduced countrywide. In the last year we, with the help of WHO experts, have put on paper an Action Plan of the National Palliative Care Program. It is an extremely large challenge to implement this program, but it is also extremely rewarding. I hope that in the next overview of communication with cancer patients 15 years from now, most of the paper by the author from Slovenia will deal with communication in a well-organized palliative care network encompassing the whole country. Palliative care will forever remain one of the most important and subtle topics in the field of cancer in which communication has an essential role.

Two Cases

Case #1

Eighteen years ago I was treating a 34-year-old female patient with locally advanced breast cancer. She received neoadjuvant chemotherapy, was operated on, and irradiated to the chest wall. She is without relapse today and otherwise healthy. I still remember the huge psychological problems that I confronted when communicating with her about her disease. She never asked me for any details. At that time not much was known about the *BRCA* gene. Recently her 48-year-old younger sister was operated on and treated with chemotherapy for ovarian cancer. At this occasion both sisters came to me with their daughters (each has two daughters) with very exact data from the Internet concerning the *BRCA* gene and risk for ovarian and breast cancer. They decided to undergo genetic counseling and testing. The younger sister wanted to know everything about her disease, the treatment options, and prognosis. Eighteen years ago when the first sister was treated, the patients and their relatives were not motivated to know much about their disease; although I must admit that the information then available, at least in Slovenia, was very scarce. Most of the cases I see today are similar to this case.

Case #2

I have been treating a lady for metastatic GIST (gastrointestinal stromal tumor) for almost 10 years. She was first admitted to my outpatient clinic in 1997, after she was operated on for a leiomyosarcoma of the small intestine. The tumor was radically dissected; at the sarcoma tumor board we decided that no further treatment was needed. At that time she was 67 years old, was married, and had one adult married daughter. She came again to my outpatient clinic in spring 2001 with metastatic disease in her abdomen and liver, which the surgeon had told her was inoperable.

She was still in quite a good performance status. She told me that since 1997, when I had last seen her, her daughter had gone to live in Australia with her family, her husband had a stroke (in 1999), and since then she has been taking care of him, because he is bedridden. She asked me to tell me all the options she had in order to plan her life. I told her that metastatic leiomyosarcoma cannot be cured, but that perhaps with chemotherapy we could achieve some benefit, though in a limited number of cases. After I explained all the details, she refused chemotherapy and asked me for help and support in palliative treatment; meanwhile she would take care of her personal obligations regarding her husband and daughter. We agreed to meet again in autumn or before if she had problems.

Just at that time a new treatment for the recently discovered new diagnosis GIST was becoming available globally [19, 20]. The first patient in the world treated successfully with STI571 (imatinib-Glivec®) in spring 2000 in Helsinki was reported on in the *New England Journal of Medicine* [21]. Information about this traveled globally very quickly. While I was reading through all these abstracts and papers in Pubmed, my lady patient came to mind. "What if she has GIST?" OK, even if she has it, we won't be able to get STI571 for at least 2–3 years, until its registration and availability in the Slovene market (we became a member of the EU on May 1, 2004). I had to tell her the options, including that she might be able to get the drug through her daughter living in Australia. So I ordered a revision of her histology, which was clearly a c-kit-positive GIST (even to get the staining was story in itself). Somehow we managed to get Glivec® through Novartis and extra financing permission from our institution's committee, since it was just the time of a new financial paradigm of expensive drugs coming into the clinic and real life. She started the treatment in November 2001, among the first in Slovenia. (We also reviewed the histology of some other metastatic leiomyosarcoma patients being treated at our institution at that time, most of which came out as GISTs.) The treatment was successful, and she was very grateful. Her husband died in 2005, but her daughter returned home with her family. She lived happily and was taking care of her grandchildren. Every time she came to my outpatient clinic, she asked me how she could ever repay society, since her monthly therapy was costing seven times her pension and had been effective for so many years.

She came to my outpatient clinic again in May 2006 with an enlarged liver, multiple palpable tumors, and ascites in her abdomen. She said, "I have lived for 5 years more than I thought I would; I took care of my husband; now my daughter is back, and I want to be with my grandchildren for at least 1 year more. What can you do, doctor?" I doubled the dose of Glivec®, but she came back in the beginning of July. She was bedridden for more than half of the day. The CT scan confirmed diffuse progression in her liver and abdomen. Now she was lucky again, as sunitinib [22] had just been registered by EMEA (European Medicines Agency) in July 2006, also for patients with GIST progressing on Glivec; and we were then part of EU. She started sunitinib, and again she had an excellent response and lived a very good quality of life for four more years; she died at home in 2010, 80 years old. Many other patients profited similarly from these new targeted drugs, which can often prolong life and its quality.

Communication is extremely important in these settings. The patients and doctors must be aware of the new possibilities in order to monitor the efficacy and toxicity of new treatments. Patients will have to know much more about drugs and their toxicity. Often they will have to take other drugs to overcome these toxicities (my patient had to take antihypertensive drugs and thyroid hormone replacement drugs during treatment with sunitinib). In our country patients usually say, "I take a yellow pill and a blue pill every morning and evening." Many of them do not know what they are for. Perhaps, as in the case of my patient (Case #2 above), the drug prices will change this old philosophy, when everything was free and nobody, including us doctors, knew what the drugs we were prescribing and taking cost.

Conclusion

Probably the biggest leap forward in the fields of medicine and particularly cancer treatment in the last 15 years has been in the field of communication, with the new communication tools, mainly IT technology and the Internet. Nevertheless, direct, warm, interactive health professional–patient relationships will remain the most important modality of communicating bad news and giving hope to patients and their families in order to cope with cancer and other chronic diseases.

References

1. Primic Zakelj M, Zadnik V, Zagar T, Zakotnik B. Survival of cancer patients from 1991–2005 in Slovenia. Ljubljana: Institute of Oncology Ljubljana; 2009.
2. Fallowfield L, Jenkins V, Farewell V, Saul J, Duffy A, Eves R. Efficacy of a Cancer Research UK communication skills training model for oncologists: a randomized controlled trial. Lancet. 2002;359(9307):650–6.
3. Verdecchia A, Francisci S, Brenner H, Gatta G, Micheli A, Mangone L, Kunkler I; EUROCARE-4 Working Group. Recent cancer survival in Europe: a 2000-02 period analysis of EUROCARE-4 data. Lancet Oncol. 2007;8(9):784–96.
4. Abdel-Rahman M, Stockton D, Rachet B, Hakulinen T, Coleman MP. What if cancer survival in Britain were the same as in Europe: how many deaths are avoidable? Br J Cancer. 2009;101 Suppl 2:S115–24.
5. Kalager M, Kåresen R, Wist E. Survival after breast cancer—differences between Norwegian counties. Tidsskr Nor Laegeforen. 2009;129(24):2595–600.
6. Eaker S, Dickman PW, Hellström V, Zack MM, Ahlgren J, Holmberg L. Regional differences in breast cancer survival despite common guidelines. Cancer Epidemiol Biomarkers Prev. 2005;14(12):2914–8.
7. Watson R. Combating cancer is priority while Slovenia holds presidency of Europe. BMJ. 2008;336(7640):353.
8. Zakotnik B. To tell or not to tell? Communication with cancer patients. Ann N Y Acad Sci. 1997;809:500–7.
9. Richardson MA, Straus SE. Complementary and alternative medicine: opportunities and challenges for cancer management and research. Semin Oncol. 2002;29(6):531–45.

10. Kimby CK, Launsø L, Henningsen I, Langgaard H. Choice of unconventional treatment by patients with cancer. J Altern Complement Med. 2003;9(4):549–61.
11. Olaku O, White JD. Herbal therapy use by cancer patients: a literature review on case reports. Eur J Cancer. 2010;47(4):508–14.
12. Derme AI, Tiono A, Hirsch F, Sirima SB. Pharmaceutical black market in Burkina Faso: an illicit but socially adapted market. Med Trop (Mars). 2009;69(1):103–4.
13. Giuliano M, Vella S. Inequalities in health: access to treatment for HIV/AIDS. Ann Ist Super Sanita. 2007;43(4):313–6.
14. UNAIDS, Report on global AIDS epidemics 2006.
15. Cancer incidence in Slovenia 1994, Ljubljana: Institute of Oncology Ljubljana, Cancer Registry of Republic of Slovenia, 1997.
16. Cancer incidence in Slovenia 2006, Ljubljana: Institute of Oncology Ljubljana, Cancer Registry of Republic of Slovenia, 2009.
17. Červek J, Zakotnik B. Paliativna oskrba. In: Borštnar S, Matos E, Novaković S, et al, editors. Bolniki in strokovnjaki—skupaj uspešnejši pri premagovanju raka: zbornik 21. onkološki vikend; 2008 June 6–7; Laško. Ljubljana: Kancerološko združenje SZD; 2008. p. 92–96.
18. Novaković S, Červek J, Anderluh F, Bešić N, Ebert M, Frković-Grazio S, et al. Paliativna oskrba bolnikov z rakom. Ljubljana: Slovensko zdravniško društvo, Kancerološko združenje; 2005. p. 136.
19. Hirota S, Isozaki K, Moriyama Y, Hashimoto K, Nishida T, Ishiguro S, et al. Gain-of-function mutations of c-kit in human gastrointestinal stromal tumors. Science. 1998;279(5350): 577–80.
20. Miettinen M, Sarlomo-Rikala M, Lasota J. Gastrointestinal stromal tumours. Ann Chir Gynaecol. 1998;87(4):278–81.
21. Joensuu H, Roberts PJ, Sarlomo-Rikala M, Andersson LC, Tervahartiala P, Tuveson D, et al. Effect of the tyrosine kinase inhibitor STI571 in a patient with a metastatic gastrointestinal stromal tumor. N Engl J Med. 2001;344(14):1052–6.
22. Goodman VL, Rock EP, Dagher R, Ramchandani RP, Abraham S, Gobburu JV, et al. Approval summary: Sunitinib for the treatment of imatinib refractory or intolerant gastrointestinal stromal tumors and advanced renal cell carcinoma. Clin Cancer Res. 2007;13(5):1367–73.

Chapter 41
Impact of the Internet and the Economy on Cancer Communication in China

Zhi-gang Zhuang and Jia-Ling Chou

Abstract The rapid development of economy and wide use of Internet over the last 2 decades in China have changed how cancer patients are managed, and how doctors and patients communicate. The traditional paternal pattern is being replaced gradually by a more transparent and two-way communication between doctors and patients. Patients and their relatives are more involved in decision-making. Withholding cancer diagnosis and prognosis by medical staff is no longer considered ethical. Properly managing terminally ill patients is gaining support. Although the above major changes happen more in urban and coastal areas, it is probably a matter of time before the management of cancer patients and concept of information-sharing gain more momentum in inland and rural areas, considering the deep-rooted tradition could change within such a short period.

Keywords Communication • Breast cancer • China

The last 2 decades have witnessed major changes in China. There has been major development in the economy and expansion of exchanges with the outside world in many walks of life. These changes have generated a tremendous impact on every aspect of life, including cancer treatment and communication between physicians and patients. In this article, an attempt has been made to use breast cancer as a model to dissect dynamic changes. As discussed below, the incidence of breast cancer over the last 2–3 decades has increased rapidly, especially among middle-aged

Z. Zhuang (✉)
Department of Breast Surgery, Shanghai First Maternity and Infant Hospital,
Tongji University School of Medicine, Shanghai, China
e-mail: Zhuang-zg@163.com

J.-L. Chou
Southern California Kaiser Permanente Medical Center, Woodland Hills, CA, USA

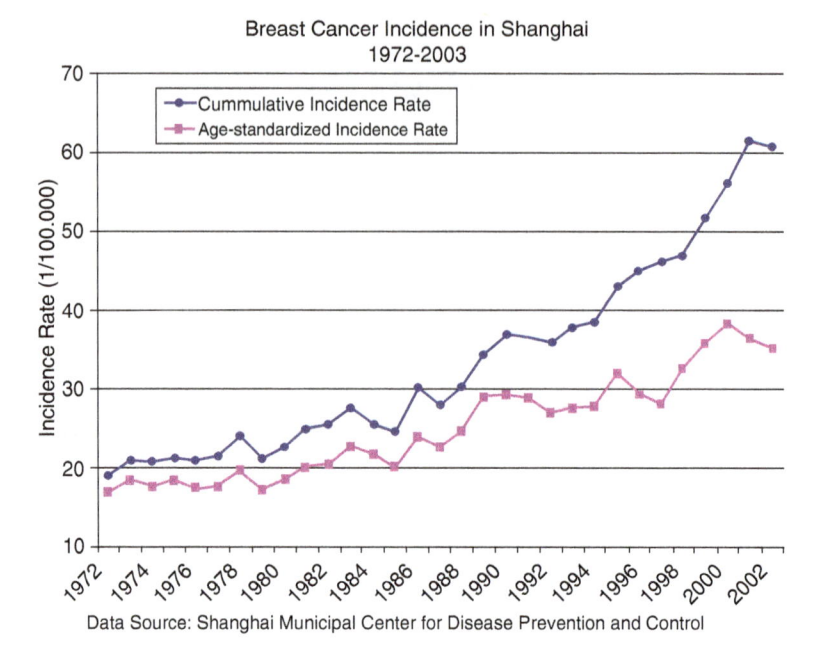

Fig. 41.1 Cumulative and age-standardized breast cancer incidence rate from 1972 to 2003 among women in Shanghai

women, and has topped the female malignancies in Shanghai. This increase has affected many patients, their families, and the workforce. It is therefore an ideal model to explore what has occurred in cancer communication in the last 2 decades.

The incidence of breast cancer started to climb since the mid-1980s of the last century (Fig. 41.1). It can be found, for example, that the incidence of breast cancer in Shanghai before 1982 was below 25 per 100,000 (18.9 per 100,000 in 1972), while it exceeded 60 per 100,000 in this century. The more-than-twofold increase occurred in less than 20 years. In 2003, women affected with breast cancer accounted for 21.6% among all cancers among women and topped other types of cancers (Fig. 41.2), while in 1972 breast cancer accounted for only 9.7% and was ranked the third most common in women (data not shown). It is unlikely that this increase is the result only of improved diagnostic techniques and the increased availability of mammogram screening. It is hypothesized that, with the improved economy, lifestyle changes such as intake of more saturated fat and calories coupled with weight increase might have been contributory. For example, it was found that consumption of animal fat among Shanghainese in the 1990s has increased fivefold compared with that in 1950s [1]. Passive smoking has been found to be a risk factor in studies among breast cancer patients in a few large cities [2].

Another important feature of breast cancer incidence is that more middle-aged women have been diagnosed. The fastest increase, from 1972 to 2008, occurred in the age group between 45 and 59 years (data not shown). The second fastest was among women aged over 60.

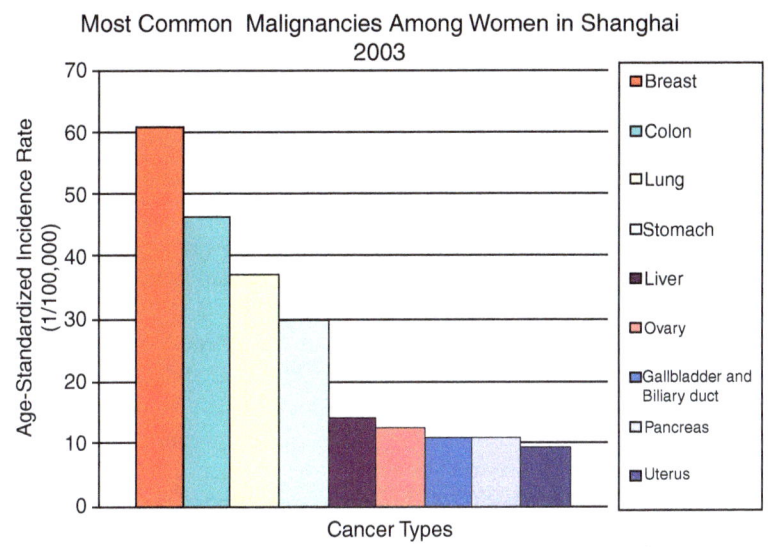

Most Common Malignancies Among Women in Shanghai 2003

Fig. 41.2 Age-standardized incidence rate of the most common female malignancies in Shanghai in 2003

Breast cancer screening starts from age 40, as recommended by the Health Ministry in China. Women aged 40–59 should have an annual mammogram, while those who are 60–69 get a mammogram every 1 or 2 years. Those who are diagnosed with breast cancer are operated on by surgeons, and subsequent adjuvant chemotherapy or hormonal therapy are also administered by surgeons in general, or by medical oncologists if patients are treated in cancer centers or major teaching hospitals.

Prior to 1990, the choice of breast cancer treatment was limited in China just as in the West. Therapy was dictated by treating doctors, and there used to be little discussion. It was essentially paternalistic medicine. Things started to change gradually after the 1990s, thanks to the development of the Internet and the availability and affordability of more drugs throughout the whole country due to the improved economy. Internet service has expanded rapidly. It was reported that in the 6 months from July to December 2008, about 298 million people (older than 6) in China used the Internet. That number represented a 41.9% increase compared with the same period in 2007 [3]. The Internet has changed the practice of cancer medicine. There are a number of web sites that provide a list of hospitals for any specific cancer and details about the treatment to be expected. Some cancer patients have done extensive "homework" after their initial diagnosis in order to choose a hospital and even doctors based on patients' review of individual physicians if available on the web sites. Some patients may be still in self-denial during their first consultation and question whether the diagnosis is correct. That is usually followed by a request for a second opinion, as "suggested" by the Internet.

For second opinions, many patients prefer cancer centers or teaching hospitals in large cities such as Shanghai, Tianjin, and a few others. These hospitals are "recommended" on the Internet. There is only one national insurance system in China, under which patients have the freedom to choose any hospital, where treatment is equally covered. Improvement of economic status has also made this patient migration possible. Consequently, most breast cancer cases are cared for in a small number of hospitals in a few large cities.

While some women who need adjuvant chemotherapy receive treatment as outpatients in a few major centers, many others are still treated as inpatients. Inpatient service actually creates opportunities for interactions between doctors and patients as well as among patients. Questions arise, such as why chemotherapeutic drugs are different between patients, what disease characteristics necessitate targeted drugs, and why some patients need Filgrastrin, etc. Doctors have more time to answer questions that patients may not be able to ask during consultation. Further, the patients themselves provide moral support to one another. Those who do poorly after chemotherapy may be able to get encouragement from those who do better.

So far there is no official social worker service to help patients deal with social or financial issues. However, over the last 2 decades, a form of patient support group has found a place in many hospitals, especially in many cancer hospitals. It goes by the name of Salon. Usually a head nurse is in charge; it is partially sponsored by drug companies. Regular meetings and talks are held between patients and doctors. There is also a Cancer Recuperation Club, established by cancer survivors in Shanghai. The club provides information for cancer patients and is financially supported by donations. In general, these organizations do not provide financial support to patients, nor do they have the means of doing so.

For those patients who do not join patient support groups, the Internet has become increasingly popular for seeking moral support. There is a sharing of experience between patients on the Web. This represents a change from the past. A few decades ago, a cancer diagnosis in China would be known only by treating doctors and patients' close relatives. Although this has become less of an issue in breast cancer lately, as more and more women are diagnosed and survival has improved [4], the availability of Internet information provides a safe haven for many breast cancer patients who seek to discuss their concerns freely and anonymously. Besides, this is a free service and does not involve waiting in the queue to see a specialist.

On the other hand, the Internet has also changed how doctors receive information and interact with patients. It appears that updating one's knowledge by reading books or even journals is being phased out. Many doctors can learn from the Internet, which carries the most up-to-date medical information from overseas. They feel the knowledge gap between medical staff and patients is narrowing as compared with that of a few decades ago. There are a few web sites in China where surgeons and medical oncologists write articles to address issues about cancer treatment and to answer specific questions from patients.

One of the major issues is how to deal with women with metastatic breast cancer. When surgery is no longer an option for recurrent disease, patients are transferred to medical oncologists, who prescribe palliative chemotherapy or hormonal therapy.

For those breast cancer patients, many lines of palliative chemotherapeutic drugs can be administered. The question is whether the patient should be told about the prognosis. Legally, patients have the right to know their own disease status. Doctors wish to tell patients the stage and prognosis if there is no special request from patients or their relatives. In Chinese philosophy, it is believed by many, especially patients' close relatives, that giving patients bad news, such as terminal condition, when they still have a good performance status may compromise their fighting spirit. Under certain circumstances, perhaps only when the disease is very advanced or there are few effective treatment choices available, the prognosis is told to relatives or patients.

For patients in an advanced or terminal stage, it is very common to seek therapy from traditional Chinese medicine. In a few hospitals, doctors trained in Chinese medicine are in charge of palliative care and terminal care units. Patients are referred by medical oncologists. These units dispense treatments such as herbs, pain medications, analgesics, and narcotics infusions. Psychological consultation is also part of this supportive care. Some patients are even admitted to a hospital for terminal care. However, these are nonprofit services and usually available only in a few major centers. There is a great demand for this kind of supportive care, and it has drawn attention that financial support needs to be channeled to create more palliative service.

Overall, there is more open communication between treating doctors and cancer patients compared with only 2 or 3 decades ago, especially in large cities. The Internet certainly is a catalyst for rapid change.

References

1. Qile W, Jiaqi J, Aizheng S. Comparison of three nutritional studies in shanghai. Shanghai J Prev Med. 1995;7(Suppl):2.
2. Qijing W, Ling L, Weixing Z, Xiumei X, Yanrong Z. Study of breast cancer risk factors in six Chinese cites. Chin J Epidemic. 2000;21:216.
3. Xiaoyan H, Yan H. Current status of the role of internet in facilitating recovery of breast cancer survivors. Chin J Mod Nurs. 2009;15:28.
4. Hong L, Pei X, Kexing C, Haixing L, Xishan H. Analyses of pathological features and changes in prognosis among female breast cancer patients in Tienjing over the last 20 years. Natl Med J China. 2007;87:2405.

Chapter 42
Communication with Patients in Clinical Research

Matjaž Zwitter

Abstract Verbal and written information given to patients who are invited to participate in clinical research is the basis for informed consent. Such consent should be based on a full understanding of the nature of the disease and of the procedures used in the trial, including their real benefits and risks. Such consent should also be voluntary, after free consideration of what standard treatment outside the trial would consist of. A critical look at the practice of informing such patients reveals that the information offered to them is often very extensive and not understandable to a substantial proportion of them. Through such overload of information, the process of informed consent has lost its primary role, that of helping the patient; rather, it has been transformed into a legalistic transaction, designed chiefly to protect the sponsor. Three practical proposals to alleviate the present situation are presented. First, the text of information provided to patients should be shorter and written in plainer language than is now the practice, possibly with several versions, adapted to the particular patient's education, literacy, age, and general ability to comprehend the medical situation. Second, every text longer than five pages should begin with a short summary, containing all the essential information. Third, like all diagnostic and therapeutic procedures, the process of informed consent should be subject to quality control. Thus, the sponsors would have the duty to monitor long-term the ability of patients to recall the essential elements of the trial in which they are participating.

Keywords Communication • Cancer • Clinical trials • Informed consent

M. Zwitter, MD, PhD (✉)
Institute of Oncology, Zaloska 2, Ljubljana 1000, Slovenia
e-mail: mzwitter@onko-i.si

Introduction

During the past 50 years, all aspects of clinical research have changed dramatically: its extent; its human, organizational, and financial resources; and its influence upon everyday medical practice. Noninterventional clinical observations have been replaced by prospective clinical trials. To a large extent, individual academic research without financial support has been replaced by a myriad of full- and part-time researchers and dozens of cooperative groups. On the global scene, commercial sponsors alone or in cooperation with contract research organizations are active in the design and organization of clinical trials, in identifying the most suitable pools of patients, in recruitment of researchers, and in monitoring trials. The results are then analyzed and presented to the professional audience and to agencies responsible for registration of pharmaceutical products. Experience from clinical research is the basis for a new paradigm, evidence-based medicine. This, in turn, has had a huge impact not only on medical decisions, but also on the distribution of financial resources.

The lives of millions of people worldwide depend on a continuous flow of medical research projects, from their design to their implementation, analysis, and promotion. Interested parties include not only pharmaceutical companies, but also employees of cooperative oncology research groups, international and national anticancer organizations, research units at academic and private institutions, and companies involved with conduct and monitoring of research. Last, but not least, medical publications and conferences also depend on the fruits of new knowledge from recently completed clinical trials.

It is fashionable to say that the needs of the patient and curiosity for new and more effective treatment of the disease occupy the central position in medical research. This is far from being so. Curiosity is limited by financial interests: no matter how promising an idea might be, projects with no potential financial benefits will not be supported. At any moment on the time scale of medical research, only a minority of new drugs are studied for their possible role in medical treatment. Little or no attention is given to older drugs for which patent protection has expired, to drugs for rare diseases, or to diseases that prevail among the poor, who will not have adequate resources when the need for treatment arises. Photographs of happy patients and sweet words about commitment to the improvement of global health are seen on all Internet presentations by pharmaceutical companies. Yet, not a single company shows a picture of what is really driving their activities—money.

After this critical introduction, we explore the real role of a patient who has been invited to participate in clinical research. Our particular interest here is in the process of informed consent. We conclude with a summary of the weak points in the present situation and with the most important proposals for improvement.

The Process of Informed Consent

Much of the information offered to a patient invited to participate in a clinical trial is communicated informally, in a conversation. Unfortunately, we do not have much data on orally communicated information. We therefore focus on the written information provided to such patients.

Written and signed informed consent is a widely accepted standard. The consent should provide a clear proof that the patient:

1. Understands the medical situation (diagnosis, standard treatment options, prognosis)
2. Understands the proposed procedure (single-arm trial or randomized trial)
3. Understands the benefits of the proposed treatment
4. Understands the risks of the proposed treatment
5. Voluntarily agrees to participate in the trial, understands alternative options of treatment outside the clinical trial, and understands the right to quit the trial at any time

For each of these five requirements, we will review the available evidence regarding how it is respected in the practice of medical research.

Understanding the Diagnosis and Medical Situation

Without adequate understanding of the medical situation, a patient's informed consent is a purely legalistic procedure without any professional or ethical validity. In addition, a patient who remains uninformed will have poor compliance with the protocol and will not provide adequate feed-back information on side effects of the treatment, leading to questionable scientific validity of the trial.

Medical research is becoming global. Many trials recruit several thousands of patients over a very short time. Due to the limited pool of patients in developed countries and to lower costs, sponsors and contract research organizations are moving their research to developing countries [1].

In the developed world, the patient's understanding of the diagnosis and of the medical situation is taken for granted. In most cases, information for patients invited to participate in a clinical trial starts with a brief paragraph or a single sentence such as "As your doctor told you, you have advanced non-small cell lung cancer in progression after first line of chemotherapy." While this sentence may be sufficient for a patient who is educated and well-informed, a different approach is needed for the majority of patients, who have a much lower level of understanding of their disease.

Low educational background, limited literacy, language barriers in multicultural societies, advanced age, emotional stress in the presence of a threatening disease, pain, and other physical symptoms — all these factors limit the patient's understanding of the medical situation and may lead either to exclusion of certain groups of patients from participation in clinical research or to abuse of the patient's consent.

[2–5] This is particularly true for patients from developing countries [6, 7]. Wide-spread prejudices and traditional misbeliefs or modern pseudoscientific theories about the causes and nature of cancer and about its treatment present additional barriers to the rational acceptance of the diagnosis.

Understanding the Research Procedure

Virtually all clinical trials include at least a few procedures that are not common in routine diagnostics and treatment. Here is a list of some of these procedures:

- Additional diagnostics to confirm compliance with the inclusion/exclusion criteria: blood tests, tests for assessment of function of organ systems (lung, cardiac, liver, kidney, bone marrow), imaging studies, test for pregnancy in women of childbearing age. Quite often, some of these additional diagnostics, such as tumor imaging, had been done previously and has to be repeated due to a narrow time window (e.g., "within 2 weeks prior to initiation of treatment"), as specified in the trial protocol.
- Randomization to choose among treatment options. Patients are told that the treatment will be chosen "like tossing a coin." Still, the sentence about randomization is often hidden among many pages of lesser importance, and for many patients the concept of a random decision remains poorly understood [8].
- Additional blood tests to study the pharmacokinetics and toxicity of a new drug. This brings discomfort due to frequent venipunctures (especially problematic for patients with poor veins, a common problem in patients on chemotherapy) and more frequent visits to or longer stays in a hospital.
- Additional and more frequent diagnostics to monitor response to treatment. Most trials now require assessment of response following the RECIST criteria [9]. In accordance with RECIST, clinical assessment of response, ultrasound, or plain X-ray are not accepted methods. Instead, response to treatment has to be monitored by CT or MRI and has to be confirmed after an additional month. This additional diagnostic procedure requires more frequent visits to the medical center and brings some discomfort to the patient. Frequent CT scanning also means radiation exposure and risk of renal damage due to infusion of intravenous contrast.
- More frequent follow-up visits, some additional procedures such as regular monthly pregnancy tests, and filling of questionnaires on quality of life. Some of these questionnaires are quite extensive or include questions that offend the patients' privacy.

When invited to participate in a trial, patients are offered written information that includes a detailed description of all procedures. With respect to communication, the problem is an overload of information. During the last 2 decades written information for patients in clinical trials has more than doubled in length. The text is written from the medical and legal perspectives, not the patient's. Thus, the information of crucial importance to the patient is hidden in medical jargon understandable only by a doctor. As an example, we offer a few paragraphs from the information for patients invited to participate in a trial of a new drug for the treatment of advanced lung cancer:

> Blood samples for determination of CP-751,871 PK will be taken during the 1st cycle no more than 2 h prior to infusion of CP-751,871 on day 1 and 1 h after infusion on day 2. During the next cycles, blood samples will be taken no more than 2 h prior to infusion of CP-751,871 in 2nd, 4th, 5th, and 6th cycle; and 1 h after infusion of CP-751,871 in 5th cycle. In case you were randomized to erlotinib only and were, after progression, treated with CP-751,871 as a supplement to best supportive care (BSC), blood samples will be taken not more than 2 h prior to infusion of CP-751,871 in 1st, 2nd, and 4th cycle.
>
> Serum samples for determination of antibodies against the drug will be taken not more than 2 h prior to infusion of CP-751,871 in 1st, 2nd, and 4th cycle for patients, randomized to treatment with erlotinib and CP-751,871. In patients randomized to erlotinib only who received, after progression, CP-751,871 as a supplement to BSC, samples for determination of antibodies to the drug will be taken not more than 2 h prior to infusion of CP-751,871 in 1st, 2nd, and 4th cycle.
>
> It may be that on day 1 of cycle 1, a non-obligatory blood sample (9 mL, or approximately 2 tea spoons) will be taken, in order to better understand the scientific…
>
> In case you were randomized to the group receiving erlotinib and CP-751,871, additional samples of blood and serum for determination of antibodies to the drug will be taken at the end of treatment and during the 4th follow-up visit. In case you were randomized to erlotinib only, and were, after progression, treated with CP-751,871 as a supplement to BSC, blood samples for determination of antibodies to the drug will be taken at the end of treatment and during the 4th follow-up visit.
>
> During your visit at the end of treatment, blood samples will be taken for testing to IGF-IR positive CTCs.

The information for this particular trial continues in the same style for a total of 35 pages. Few patients will have the skill, patience, and will to read such a long medical text; even fewer will find a clear answer to such simple questions as:

- How many samples of blood will be taken solely for the purpose of the study?
- How many additional visits to the hospital are proposed?

In an American survey, the majority of patients who recently signed consent for participation in a trial did not recognize the nonstandard nature of the treatment (74%), the potential for incremental risk from participation (63%), or the unproved nature of the treatment (70%) [10].

In general, physicians overestimate the efficiency of the process of informed consent. This was confirmed in a recent report on the discrepancy between physicians and patients regarding the contents of the information for participants in a clinical trial [11].

Understanding the Benefits

In routine clinical practice, treatment is based on approved methods. While physicians have the duty to explain the purpose, benefits, and risks of a particular treatment, patients most often trust their doctors and rely on their expertise. In most cases, informed consent for a routine treatment is unproblematic for both physician and patient.

Phase I, II, and III clinical trials are based on research methods that are not easily understood by a layperson. The purpose of a treatment within a clinical trial is not simply to benefit the particular patient. The main objective of Phase I clinical trials is to define the dose-limited toxicity of a new drug, maximal tolerated dose, optimal schedule for application of the drug, and pharmacokinetics. Tumor response is monitored but is not among the primary objectives. Indeed, only about 5% of patients in Phase I clinical trials show an objective response to treatment [12, 13]. This low figure is due to the fact that a single new drug is tested on patients with advanced cancer that is resistant to several standard combinations of drugs. In this setting, the chances for an objective response to a new drug or a new combination of drugs are often very slim. Yet, most patients agree to join such a trial hoping that the new drug will lead to improvement of their disease and overestimate their chances of therapeutic benefit [14]. This therapeutic misestimation undermines the validity of informed consent. Instead of an honest talk with the physician about their true perspective and about the most valuable plan for their limited life span, patients continue with the "battle against cancer."

In addition to written information, computer-based presentation on early-phase clinical trials was tested on patients with advanced cancer [15]. Patients offered information in this way indeed showed better understanding of the main objective of early-phase trials; nevertheless, the majority still believed that they would experience long-term benefit.

In randomized Phase II and Phase III clinical trials, the main objective is comparison with existing therapies to show superiority or noninferiority of the new treatment. When consenting to such a trial, many patients decide to participate because they wish to receive a new, promising treatment and do not understand that they may well get the "old" or standard treatment.

Understanding the Risks

A patient's perception of the risks involved in Phase I, II, and III trials is, again, often clouded by overload of information. Few patients get a balanced impression about the real risks linked to participation in a trial; most of them fall into one of three groups: frightened, confused, or blindly trusting their doctor.

For legal purposes and to avoid claims for compensation for malpractice, the information for patients contains all probable and rare risks and a long list of real or potential side effects of the treatment. Many patients confess that reading such a document is a frightening experience. Indeed, some patients refuse to participate in a trial in spite of their doctor's assurance that the treatment is easily tolerable and in their best interest.

Regarding perception of risk, the second group are patients who read all the information, consent to participate in the trial, but are confused and do not understand the real burden of a particular treatment. Common side effects of anticancer treatment such as "febrile neutropenia," "anorexia," "nausea and vomiting," or "general malaise" are difficult to imagine by a person who has not had such an experience.

Patients who blindly trust their doctor represent the third group. These patients stop reading information offered to them and simply decide to follow the advice of their physician. We should understand that a layperson has the right to refuse responsibility for decisions that depend on deep professional knowledge and experience. In such cases, a physician has the duty to act in the patient's best interests and should continuously inform the patient about all aspects of the disease and treatment, to the extent desired by the patient.

Voluntary Agreement, Alternative Options of Treatment outside the Trial, and the Right to Quit the Trial

The question of voluntary agreement and the need for the individual patient's consent is still open in clinical research that does not directly involve the patient's body. Studies on archived bioptic material serve as an example in which seeking individual consent would present a disproportionate burden to the researchers. In such cases, approval of an institutional protocol review board may replace individual consent.

In all therapeutic clinical trials, individual consent is now widely accepted. Yet, this does not mean that the consent is always voluntary. Part of voluntary agreement to participate in a clinical trial is a real option to get treatment outside the trial. For many patients, treatment outside a trial is not a real possibility. For a large proportion of patients in developing countries and also for nonprivileged patients in the developed world, invitation to participate in a clinical trial comes as the only possibility of treatment.

Even when another option exists, information on alternative treatments is often unsatisfactory. This is especially true for large multicenter trials, where differences in standard treatment for a certain medical condition vary considerably from one center to another [16].

Our survey of published randomized trials for patients with lung cancer revealed more subtle pressures to participate in clinical trials [17]. Analysis of the questionnaire mailed to principal investigators revealed a number of benefits offered to patients in clinical trials, as compared to those in routine treatment: shorter waiting time and easier appointments to out-patient departments; quicker admittance to the hospital; personal treatment by an experienced physician; quicker diagnostics; higher quality of all diagnostic and therapeutic procedures; access to drugs not available outside a trial. It is clear that the patient's real autonomy is compromised if the choice is between immediate treatment within a clinical trial and a waiting list for standard treatment.

Similar comments are applicable also to the patient's right to quit the trial at any time. Many patients have no other alternatives and will remain in the trial regardless of their actual preference.

Discussion and Conclusions

We have stated that current practice does not give adequate information to patients invited to participate in clinical research. Uniform documents, offered to all patients regardless of their literacy, education, and social background, are clearly inadequate. A clear, understandable description of the patient's medical condition is an essential basis for a proposal to join a clinical trial. The diagnostic and therapeutic procedures should be clearly described, with a focus on those that are different from the standard treatment. A balanced presentation of the potential benefits and risks helps the patient towards a reasonable decision.

Overloading of information is a real, yet rarely discussed, weakness of the process of informed consent. For legal purposes, sponsors of clinical trials produce documents that are very difficult to read and understand even by an educated person. This is not to say that sponsors have the intention of diminishing the patient's role as a partner in clinical research; rather, they simply do not have any idea, and perhaps also no interest, in knowing how such documents function in the real world. They have no insight into the reality of cancer medicine, which involves the rich and the poor, the educated and the illiterate, people with a clear idea about the biology of cancer, and people who base their understanding on misbeliefs or magic forces.

To alleviate some of these problems, I would like to offer three practical proposals.

Adaptation of the Text to the Educational Level

Information to the patient should be written in plain language and should be shorter than is now the practice [18]. Additional argument against the extensive text of informed consent comes from the Eastern Cooperative Oncology Group, which randomized patients between the standard consent procedure and an easy-to-read consent statement. A simplified text did not lessen patient's comprehension and resulted in significantly lower consent anxiety and higher satisfaction [19]. When appropriate, a uniform text of information to patients might be replaced by several versions, adapted to different levels of the patient's literacy, education, age, and general understanding of his/her disease. For legal purposes, every patient may receive all versions but will be able to choose the one he/she considers most understandable.

Rather than continuing with what is increasingly obviously a fiction—that fully informed consent has been obtained—we should move to a consent protocol, that is a simple consent in the presence of full information. A summary paragraph to each information sheet would allow the patient to focus on that alone if he/she chooses to do so [20].

Abstract

Any text that is longer than, say, five pages should begin with an abstract of not more than one page, containing all the essential information. As scientists, we know that abstracts are standard parts of any scientific text and greatly help in absorbing the information. The text of information for patients in clinical research is not an exception to this general practice. An abstract gives the reader a general idea about the whole text and greatly improves his/her capacity to remember what is essential.

Quality Control

The whole consent procedure—including written *Information to Patients*—should be subject to quality control. Quality control is an essential component of all diagnostic and therapeutic procedures used in medicine, and, in particular, in clinical research. For any procedure, quality control is necessary to assure that the technique is reproducible and offers reliable results.

There is every reason to perform quality control also for the process of informed consent to clinical trials. The purpose of informed consent for a clinical trial is to make sure that the patient really has understood the essential procedures, and especially those that are different from the standard treatment. Furthermore, patients should be able to recall this essential information for the duration of the trial, which may take several months or even years. This long-lasting understanding by the patient should be monitored by researchers or research nurses and included in the scientific report. Finally, unsatisfactory results of information recalled by patients should lead to appropriate adaptation of the process of informed consent.

References

1. Annas GJ. Globalized clinical trials and informed consent. N Engl J Med. 2009;360:2050–3.
2. Surbone A. Telling the truth to patients with cancer: what is the truth? Lancet Oncol. 2006;7:944–50.
3. Townsley CA, Chan KK, Pond GR, Marquez C, Siu LL, Straus SE. Understanding the attitudes of the elderly towards enrolment into cancer clinical trials. BMC Cancer. 2006;6:34.
4. Jefford M, Mileshkin L, Matthews J, Raunow H, O'Kane C, Cavicchiolo T, et al. Satisfaction with the decision to participate in cancer clinical trials is high, but understanding is a problem. Support Care Cancer. 2011;19:371–9.
5. Surbone A. Cultural aspects of communication in cancer care. Recent Results Cancer Res. 2006;168:91–104.
6. Angell M. Ethics of clinical research in third world. N Engl J Med. 1997;337:847–92.
7. Verástegui EL. Consenting of the vulnerable: the informed consent procedure in advanced cancer patients in Mexico. BMC Med Ethics. 2006;7:13.

8. Williams CJ, Zwitter M. Informed consent in European multicentre randomised clinical trials: are patients really informed? Eur J Cancer. 1994;30A:907–10.
9. Therasse P, Arbuck SG, Eisenhauer EA, Wanders J, Kaplan RS, Rubinstein L, et al. New guidelines to evaluate the response to treatment in solid tumors. European Organization for Research and Treatment of Cancer, National Cancer Institute of the United States, National Cancer Institute of Canada. J Natl Cancer Inst. 2000;92:205–16.
10. Joffe S, Cook EF, Cleary PD, Clark JW, Weeks JC. Quality of informed consent in cancer clinical trials: a cross-sectional survey. Lancet. 2001;358:1772–7.
11. Jenkins V, Solis-Trapala I, Langridge C, Catt S, Talbot DC, Fallowfield LJ. What oncologists believe they said and what patients believe they heard: an analysis of phase I trial discussions. J Clin Oncol. 2011;29:61–8.
12. Rosa DD, Harris J, Jayson GC. The best guess approach to phase I trial design. J Clin Oncol. 2006;24:206–8.
13. Horstmann E, McCabe MS, Grochow L, Yamamoto S, Rubinstein L, Budd T, et al. Risks and benefits of phase 1 oncology trials, 1991 through 2002. N Engl J Med. 2005;352:895–904.
14. Sulmasy DP, Astrow AB, He MK, Seils DM, Meropol NJ, Micco E, et al. The culture of faith and hope: patients' justifications for their high estimations of expected therapeutic benefit when enrolling in early phase oncology trials. Cancer. 2010;116:3702–11.
15. Kass NE, Sugarman J, Medley AM, Fogarty LA, Taylor HA, Daugherty CK, et al. An intervention to improve cancer patients' understanding of early-phase clinical trials. IRB. 2009; 31(3):1–10.
16. Resnik DB, Patrone D, Peddada S. Evaluating the quality of information about alternatives to research participation in oncology consent forms. Contemp Clin Trials. 2010;31:18–21.
17. Zwitter M, Tobias JS. A survey of the ethical considerations in randomised trials for lung cancer. Lung Cancer. 1998;19:197–210.
18. Jefford M, Moore R. Improvement of informed consent and the quality of consent documents. Lancet Oncol. 2008;9:485–93.
19. Coyne CA, Xu R, Raich P, Plomer K, Dignan M, Wenzel LB, et al.; Eastern Cooperative Oncology Group. Randomized, controlled trial of an easy-to-read informed consent statement for clinical trial participation: a study of the Eastern Cooperative Oncology Group. J Clin Oncol. 2003;21:836–42.
20. Jayson G, Harris J. How participants in cancer trials are chosen: ethics and conflicting interests. Nat Rev Cancer. 2006;6:330–6.

About the Authors

Donald I. Abrams, San Francisco, CA, USA, Chief of Hematology-Oncology at San Francisco General Hospital and Professor of Medicine at University of California San Francisco Osher Center for Integrative Medicine, is a clinician and educator. After 25 years of working in the field of HIV malignancies and treatments, he currently focuses on integrative oncology, a patient-centered discipline in which patient and provider work together to combine complementary therapies and conventional cancer care that addresses the needs of the whole person—body, mind, and spirit.

Neil Krishan Aggarwal, New Haven, CT, USA, conducts research on cultural psychiatry and global mental health at Columbia University as a coinvestigator of the DSM-5 cultural formulation field trials and is developing a module with international collaborators in patient–physician communication.

Ali M. Al-Amri, Al-Khobar, Saudi Arabia, is Associate Professor of Internal Medicine and Oncology, treats cancer patients from responsibility for diagnosis, supervising, and ensuring treatment with the best options of therapy, and palliative treatment. He teaches and trains undergraduate and postgraduate medical students and residents.

María Angelica Alizade, Buenos Aires, Argentina, is a psychologist, psychodramatist, and psychooncologist. For 20 years she has been engaged in health care activities guided by the experience of the hospice movement and Dr. Twycross's work at Sobell House in England. She is a founding member and member of the board of the Argentine Association for Palliative Care (AAMyCP). Working with children led Dr. Alizade to integrate psychoanalysis, psychodrama, puppets, and creativity into an alternative model of therapy.

Ali Aljubran, Riyadh, Saudi Arabia, is a medical oncologist, King Faisal Specialist Hospital and Research Center. He completed his training in Saudi Arabia and Toronto, Canada, and has a special interest in gastrointestinal cancers and psychosocial aspects of cancer.

Maria Antonietta Annunziata, Aviano, Italy, is Director of the Unit of Oncological Psychology at Centro di Riferimento Oncologico Aviano, National Cancer Institute and Assistant Professor in Psychooncology at the University of Udine. For more than 10 years she has been training healthcare professionals on communication and relationship courses. She is the author of several articles and book chapters on psychooncology topics.

Fusun Aysin Artiran Igde, MD, Samsun, Turkey, is Associate Professor of Family Medicine at Ondokuzmayis University, School of Medicine, Department of Family Medicine, which focuses on family medicine education in undergraduate and residency programs and continuous professional development in primary care.

Lea Baider, Jerusalem, Israel, Professor of Medical Psychology at the Hebrew University Medical School, is a pioneer in psychooncology, having introduced it in Israel, and in developing new methods of helping cancer patients within the family context cope with the trajectory of the illness. Her eclectic research also includes areas of diagnosis and clinical practice in the treatment of first- and second-generation Holocaust survivor breast cancer patients and their families; and the effects of gender differentiation, religious beliefs, and culture on the cancer family.

Walter F. Baile, Houston, TX, USA, Director of the MD Anderson Cancer Center Program for Interpersonal Communication and Relationship Enhancement (I*CARE), an online repository of video-based material illustrating effective communication (mdanderson.org/icare). He has been honored for his teaching and scholarly work in communication skills with the 2011 Lynn Payer Award for excellence in teaching and research in communication skills by the American Academy of Communication in Healthcare.

Lodovico Balducci, Tampa, FL, USA, Senior Adult Oncology Program at Moffitt Cancer Center, the first geriatric oncology center in the world that has served as an international model. Dr. Balducci is the recipient of many recognitions, including First Paul Calabresi lecture for the International Society of Geriatric Oncology, BJ Kennedy Award for Excellence in Geriatric Oncology by the American Society of Clinical Oncology, Claude Jacquillat Award by the International Society of Anticancer Research, Medih Tavassoli Award from the University of Mississippi, the Award for Excellence in Clinical Research by the Association of Community Cancer Centers, and the Nimmo Professorship award by Adelaide University, Australia.

G.S. Bhattacharyya, Pune, India, medical oncologist, at AMRI HOSPITALS, Salt Lake City, Kolkata; Head, Department of Medical Oncology, Fortis Hospitals, Anandapur; Director, Orchid Nursing Home, Kolkata (Community Cancer Research Center); is associated with several national and international bodies, with principal subjects of interest in drug development, clinical trials, palliative and supportive care, and breast cancer.

Guido Biasco, Bologna, Italy, Professor of Medical Oncology and Scientific Director of the Academy of the Science of Palliative Medicine in cooperation with the University of Bologna in education, training, and research in palliative care as an educator to healthcare professionals on communication and help relationship courses. He is committed to the diffusion of palliative care in Italy.

Anne Brédart, Amsterdam, The Netherlands, is a clinical psychologist and researcher at Institut Curie in Paris. Her activities focus on the psychological care of cancer patients and their families. She coordinates research programs related to the impact of communication skills training in France and to the evaluation of supportive care interventions in oncology. She is actively involved in the development of cancer patient reported outcome measures and was the principal investigator, within the European Organisation for Research and Treatment of Cancer—EORTC Quality of Life Group, of the development and validation of a questionnaire measuring cancer patient satisfaction with care (EORTC IN-PATSAT32).

Itzhak Brook, Washington, DC, USA, is Professor of Pediatrics at Georgetown University, Washington, DC and specializes in pediatrics and infectious diseases. He studied anaerobic and respiratory infections, anthrax, and infections following exposure to ionizing radiation. Dr. Brook was diagnosed with throat cancer in 2006 and received radiation therapy. Two years later he had his larynx removed and currently speaks with a tracheoesophageal prosthesis. He currently lectures about his experiences as a patient with neck cancer. He is the author of the book: *My Voice: A Physician's Personal Experience with Throat Cancer*.

Andre T. Brunetto, Porto Alegre, Brazil, is a medical oncologist at Hospital de Clinicas and Hospital Ernesto Dornelles, Porto Alegre. Most of his oncology training was at the Royal Marsden Hospital and the Institute of Cancer Research at the University of London, with focus on communication in cancer trials. He is now conducting clinical trials in South America in various stages of drug development.

Phyllis Butow, Sydney, Australia, is Chair of the Psycho-Oncology Co-operative Research Group and Co-Director of the Centre for Medical Psychology and Evidence-Based Medicine at the University of Sydney. By virtue of her research over the last 20 years, she has an international reputation for her work on doctor–patient communication and has been instrumental in developing and facilitating many communication skills training courses for cancer health professionals in Australia. With the coauthors of this chapter, she has developed question prompt lists for patients to help them ask difficult questions and get the information they need at the end of life.

Karen J. Carapetyan, New York, USA, is a clinical coordinator at New York University School of Medicine in the Department of Medicine, Division of Pulmonary and Critical Care. She has worked at various centers in Lima, Peru as a psychooncologist. She subsequently worked at Mount Sinai School of Medicine in New York as a research assistant. Since then she has been at the New York University School of Medicine as a Coordinator of The Lynne Cohen Clinic for High-Risk Women. Other positions include member of Latina Share for Breast and Ovarian Cancer, American Association of Cancer Education, American Public Health Association, American Translation Association, and mentor for the High School Fellow Program at NYU.

Rosangela Caruso, MD, Ferrara, Italy, is a psychiatrist at the University Clinic of Ferrara, Psycho-Oncology service, and her research interests focus particularly on psychiatric and psychosocial consequences of cancer and intervention models.

Jia-Ling Chou, Woodland Hills, CA, USA, began focusing on breast cancer management when he started working at the breast service in Memorial Sloan Kettering Cancer Center in the late 1990s. Following his move to California, Dr. Chou has maintained this focus on the disease in addition to other cancers. For more than 10 years, he has witnessed the dynamic changes in the relationship and communication between treating doctors and patients.

Josephine Clayton, Sydney, Australia, is a practicing consultant physician in palliative medicine based at Greenwich and Royal North Shore Hospitals in Sydney, Australia. She is also Associate Professor of Palliative Care at the University of Sydney. She leads a research program on palliative care and communication about end-of-life issues, including the development and evaluation of patient- and clinician-based interventions for improving communication. She is passionate about research that enhances the palliative and supportive care of patients and families, and teaching end-of-life communication skills to health professionals in diverse settings.

Miri Cohen, Mount Carmel, Haifa, is Associate Professor, School of Social Work and Head, Department of Gerontology, Faculty of Social Welfare and Health Sciences at the University of Haifa. Her main research areas are psychooncology; psychoneuroimmunology, especially the effects of stress, coping, and personal resources on endocrine and immune systems in health and illness; psychooncology; and screening behaviors for the early detection of cancer.

Eugeny Demin, St. Petersburg, Russia, is a cofounder of the charitable voluntary organization HOPE, which provides breast cancer patients physical, pyschoemotional, and cosmetic support within the framework of the international Reach to Recovery Program. This organization has received international recognition and has become a good example for similar groups in Russia focusing on education and cancer communication and education to professionals and patients.

Ludovica De Panfilis, Bentivolgio, Italy, researches philosophy and communication aspects in oncology. She is involved in the task force of research programs on communication with cancer patients and family sponsored by the Academy of the Science of Palliative Medicine. The philosophic approach to communication in terminal illness represents a fundamental integration of the point of view of clinicians, oncologists, and psychologists.

Blanca Diez, Buenos Aires, Argentina, Head of the Neuro-Oncology Program of the Institute for Neurological Research Dr. Raul Carrea (FLENI), completed her residency in pediatrics and pediatric surgery at the Children's Hospital Ricardo Gutiérrez, and subsequently at St Jude's Children Research Hospital, USA. Dr. Diez has won several awards for original research.

Mustafa Fevzi Dikici, Samsun, Turkey, Associate Professor of Family Medicine, founder of Ondokuzmayis University School of Medicine, Department of Family Medicine, focuses on family medicine education and clinical skills teaching in undergraduate and family medicine residency programs, assessment and evaluation of teaching programs, curriculum development, care of cancer patients in family medicine, teaching in rational drug use, continuous professional development in primary care. He coordinates first-phase teaching courses for family doctors for the Ministry of Health.

Sylvie Dolbeault, Paris, France, Head of the Interdisciplinary Supportive Care Department, Curie Institute, which integrates psychooncology, palliative care, social work, nutrition, rehabilitation, addiction, and oncogeriatrics. After training with Dr. J.C. Holland at Memorial Sloan Kettering Cancer Center, she was recruited to build a psychooncology unit at the Curie Institute. This department allows better clinical management of patients defined by a high level of complexity, but also a better recognition from the medical community of the importance of global and patient-centered managed care. Her research encompasses fields such as distress, psychoeducational interventions, oncogenetics, quality of life, and communication in cancer care.

Martine Extermann, Tampa, FL, USA, is Professor of Oncology and Medicine at the University of South Florida and Senior Adult Oncology Program at Moffitt Cancer Center. She earned her medical diploma and her medical Ph.D. at the University of Geneva, Switzerland. She has a Swiss Board Certification in internal medicine, specialty oncology-hematology. She also holds ABIM certifications in internal medicine and medical oncology. Her research focuses on cancer in the elderly. Her main areas of investigation are comorbidity, comprehensive assessment, and prediction/prevention of treatment toxicity in older cancer patients. She served as Chair of the Eastern Cooperative Oncology Group's Subcommittee on Aging and is currently involved in the South West Oncology Group. She is also the immediate past president of the International Society of Geriatric Oncology (SIOG). Dr. Extermann was presented at ASCO 2009 with the B.J. Kennedy Award for Scientific Excellence in Geriatric Oncology.

Maiko Fujimori, Tokyo, Japan, Psycho-Oncology Division at the National Cancer Center Hospital, works on communication regarding bad news between patients with cancer and oncologists, particularly encouraging patients' preferred communication. Based on the results of the surveys regarding patient preferences, she and coworkers developed the communication skills training (CST) program for oncologists to learn patient's preferred communication and the train-the-trainer program in Japan. The programs have been adopted by the Health Ministry led by the National Cancer Control Act implemented in April 2007.

David Goldstein, Sydney, Australia, Department of Medical Oncology at Prince of Wales Hospital is a senior staff specialist. He works in a clinical capacity seeing a wide range of malignancies but specializes in gastrointestinal malignancies, lymphoma, and renal cell carcinoma. He has been involved as a senior investigator in numerous therapeutic clinical trials and phase I, II, III, and IV studies. A major research interest has been psychosocial aspects of cancer care, including studies in cross-cultural aspects of cancer, the incidence and natural history of fatigue after adjuvant treatment, and participating in studies of enhancing communication.

Luigi Grassi, Ferrara, Italy, Professor and Chair of Psychiatry, and Chair of the Department of Medical and Surgical Disciplines of Communication and Behavior, University of Ferrara, Chief of the University Clinical and Emergency Psychiatry Unit, Integrated Department of Mental Health and Drug Abuse in Ferrara, Italy. Within this field, his clinical and research activity mainly concerns the psychiatric and psychosocial consequences of cancer, particularly depression, and the efficacy of communication skills training in oncology. He is past president of the International Psycho-Oncology Society (IPOS) (2006–2008), and he currently serves as Chair of the World Psychiatric Association—Section on Psychooncology and Palliative Care and the Federation of the National Societies of Psycho-Oncology within IPOS.

Tolga Güven, Istanbul, Turkey, Department of Medical Ethics and History of Medicine of Marmara University Faculty of Medicine, is a lecturer with particular interest in ethical issues in the patient–physician relationship and research ethics.

Bettina S. Husebø, Bergen, Norway, has had clinical experience in anesthesiology, intensive care, and pain and palliative care at the Malteser University Hospital Bonn, Germany (1988–1997). She was Medical Director of The Red Cross Nursing Home from 1997 to 2011. Her Ph.D. was on Assessment of Pain in Patients with Dementia: 2008. She has numerous scientific publications and national and international awards. Postdoctoral Fellow at the University of Bergen, Norway. Chair of the Norwegian Society for Nursing Home Medicine.

Stein B. Husebø, Bergen, Norway; clinical experience and specialist (1980–1990), head of the Department (1990–1995) of Anesthesiology, Intensive Care, Pain and Palliative Care at the University Hospital Bergen, Norway. He has been the Editor of the *Scandinavian Journal of Palliative Care* since 1988. Cofounder and first president (1988–1994) of the Scandinavian Society of Palliative Care. Cofounder of the European Association of Palliative Care (1989). Head of the National Dignity Center—Care for the Frail Elderly since 1998.

Marjorie Kagawa-Singer, Los Angeles, CA, USA, is Professor, UCLA School of Public Health and Department of Asian American Studies. Her research focuses on the etiology and elimination of disparities in physical and mental healthcare outcomes for communities of color, primarily with the Asian American and Pacific Islander communities. A major focus of her work is testing the cross-cultural validity of health behavior theories and measures and its implications for clinical care cross-culturally.

Johann Klocker, Klagenfurt, Austria, is a consultant for internal medicine and a psychotherapist, also specializing in hematooncology. He studied medicine at the University of Vienna and philosophy at the Universities of Salzburg, Vienna, and Klagenfurt. He studied music at the Mozarteum Salzburg and at the College of

Music and Performing Arts in Vienna. He is head of interdisciplinary oncology at Klagenfurt General Hospital, deputy head of oncological rehabilitation in Althofen/Kärnten, and was Lecturer at the University of St. Gallen, Switzerland from 1990 to 2010. He is a training therapist and Balint group leader for the Austrian Medical Association.

Ursula Klocker-Kaiser, Klagenfurt, Austria, is a consultant for psychiatry and psychotherapy and a psychotherapist. She studied medicine at the Universities of Graz and Vienna. She is qualified in Gestalt therapy, katathym imaginative psychotherapy, and systemic family therapy. She is senior physician in the Department of Psychiatry and Psychotherapy at Klagenfurt General Hospital and Head of Psychooncology in Oncological Rehabilitation in Althofen/Kärnten. Specializations: psychooncology, eating disorders, psychosomatic medicine, supervision. She is a training therapist and Balint group leader for the Austrian Medical Association.

Sonia Krenz, Lausanne, Switzerland, specialized in clinical psychology and psychotherapy, is a senior staff member in the Psychiatric Liaison Service of the University Hospital Lausanne, Switzerland. On a clinical level she works as a psychotherapist with patients suffering from cancer and other somatic diseases and supervises psychologists and psychiatrists working in liaison psychiatry. Over the last years Sonia Krenz has been active as a teacher of communication skills training for oncology clinicians and has contributed to various research projects on topics such as patient–physician communication and psychotherapy in patients with cancer.

Eulalia Lascar, Buenos Aires, Argentina, is a pediatrician, specializing in palliative medicine. After completing her residence in pediatrics Dr. Lascar began training in palliative care with Dr. Blanca Diez, working in the Oncology Unit at the Buenos Aires-based Hospital Ricardo Gutierrez, an institution that pioneered the creation of a pediatric palliative care unit in Argentina. Following a period of training at the Bristol Royal Hospital for Sick Children, Helen House, and Great Ormond Street Hospital (UK), Dr. Lascar undertook to lead the Pediatric Palliative Care Program (1996). This endeavor was to meet the growing demand from different hospital areas and was grounded on a holistic approach from diagnosis through terminal care and bereavement. In addition, she has been developing a continuing education program through the Annual Postgraduate Course of Interdisciplinary Pediatric Palliative Care and Clinical Research.

Jerome Lowenstein, New York, USA, is a professor at the Department of Medicine, New York University School of Medicine, where he is a clinician, educator, and director of the Humanistic Aspects of Medical Education program, which he created 30 years ago. He was director of the Patient Narrative program (First Year) for 15 years.

Bakir Mehić, Sarajevo, Bosnia and Herzegovina, is a professor of respiratory medicine. He has been engaged in thoracic oncology for more than 20 years. He has much experience in working with patients who suffer from lung cancer and is also engaged in researching the effects of cultural and social aspects of patients' relation to their disease.

Ali Montazeri, Tehran, Iran, dedicates his research to the study of health-related quality of life in cancer patients. He is a member of several professional societies, including the International Society for Quality of Life Research (ISOQOL), the International Psycho-Oncology Society (IPOS), and the Multinational Association of Supportive Care in Cancer (MASCC). At present he lives in Iran and is working with the Iranian Center for Breast Cancer and the Iranian Institute for Health Sciences Research.

Matteo Moroni, Bologna, Italy, is a psychologist in communication problems at the end of life and a current Ph.D. student in palliative medicine. He is the director of a hospice and involved in education and research programs in palliative care. Dr. Moroni is leading a research program on language and comprehension in palliative medicine. The clarification and use of an identified and common language represent the challenges to the widespread diffusion of palliative care culture.

Franco Muggia, New York, USA, marks 50 years as a physician, and he is pleased to continue much of what constituted his mainstream work: combining patient care with teaching and research. Dr. Muggia led the Cancer Therapy Evaluation Program at the National Cancer Institute (1975–1979). Currently, Dr. Muggia continues to engage in some government service as Editor-in-Chief of the Adult Treatment Board of the Physician Data Query (cancer.gov). His current contribution is the result of ongoing collaboration with colleagues who have interests in preventive measures and survivorship issues and in reaching out to women at high risk of cancer.

Barbara Muzzatti, Aviano, Italy, is an Assistant Professor of Psychooncology, Health and Clinical Psychology, University of Udine, and a Research Psychologist at Centro di Riferimento Oncologico—National Cancer Institute in Aviano (Italy).

Maria Giulia Nanni, Ferrara, Italy, researcher in the Department of Medical and Surgery Disciplines of Communication and Behavior, University of Ferrara, is a psychiatrist of the Psycho-Oncology Service of the University Clinic, Integrated Department of Mental Health and Drug Abuse, Local Health Agency, Ferrara. Dr. Nanni's research interests include prevalence, diagnosis, and treatment of psychiatric comorbidity in the hospital, with particular interest in psychiatric and psychosocial consequences of cancer (prevalence, risk factors, and intervention models, with specific reference to palliative care), and educational interventions in psychiatry. Dr. Nanni is a teacher of consultation-liaison psychiatry at the University of Ferrara.

Ntokozo Ndlovu, Harare, Zimbabwe, Chairperson of the Radiology Department at the University of Zimbabwe, College of Health Sciences and Head of the Radiotherapy and Oncology Department at Parirenyatwa Hospital, Harare, is a radiation oncologist and clinical epidemiologist. In the African region she is the Project

Scientific Consultant for the IAEA Radiotherapy Project and President of the African Radiation Oncology Group (AFROG).

Lorenzo Norris, Washington, DC, USA, is the director of the Survivorship Center Psychiatric Services (SCPS), which was formed to help treat the mental health needs of cancer patients. Building on the success of SCPS, the psychiatric department helped form the Thriving after Cancer Clinic (TAC). This clinic treats young adult survivors of pediatric cancer. The clinics serve as excellent education sites for staff, and their structure has been presented at multiple meetings.

Purvish M. Parikh, Mumbai, India, member of the Indian Cooperative Oncology Network, the largest cooperative study group in India, is former professor and head of medical oncology at Tata Memorial Hospital, an institution he served as faculty member for 17 years. Dr. Parikh continues as Editor-in-Chief of the *Indian Journal of Cancer*, as well as President of the Indian Society of Medical and Pediatric Oncology.

Victoria Patxot, Buenos Aires, Argentina, has been a psychologist in the Mental Health Section of the Juan A. Fernández Hospital since 1984. Dr. Patxot became a psychologist at Fundaleu in 1992. She has been a consulting psychologist for the Lymphomas Association of Argentina since 2008.

Astrid Pavlovsky, Buenos Aires, Argentina, works as a hematologist with a primary interest in oncology-hematology, at FUNDALEU and Centro de Hematologia. Dr. Pavlovsky and her team aim to use the highest academic standards to support their patients in every way. Through her family experience, Dr. Pavlovsky has records of the great scientific progress in her field; still the most profound gratitude of her group's patients is not for the result of their treatment but for the group's commitment to them as individuals. A proportion of the group's patients will have no cure, and it is part of their daily challenge to treat each case according to the patient's specific needs.

Carolina Pavlovsky, Buenos Aires, Argentina, is head of the Clinical Research Department at FUNDALEU. Her main interest is in chronic leukemias. Since 2003 she has been working in FUNDALEU on multiple chronic leukemia research protocols and is in charge of CML projects. Since 2005, she has been conducting a multicentric Argentinean project in FUNDALEU for serial molecular monitoring by RQ-PCR and adherence to treatment in CML patients.

Christina M. Puchalski, Washington, DC, USA, is the founding director of the George Washington Institute for Spirituality and Health (GWish) and Professor at The George Washington University School of Medicine and Health Sciences in Washington, DC. Her work focuses on the clinical, academic, and pastoral understanding of spiritual care as an essential element of health care. She developed the FICA spiritual assessment tool, which is used around the world.

Mirjana Rajer, Ljubljana, Slovenia, is a medical oncology student at the Institute of Oncology, Ljubljana, specializing in thoracic oncology, responsible for radiotherapy and chemotherapy of lung cancer. As a Ph.D. student she is involved in clinical research in lung cancer and conducts research in cancer–patient communication, with special emphasis on the impact of media and the Internet on patient–physician communication. Her previous experience was as a counselor at the Centre for Medical Health (suicide hotline), and she was a lecturer in the course for counselors. She is also a lecturer in palliative medicine and mentor to medical students.

Michael Rowe, New Haven, CT, USA, is Associate Clinical Professor. His research concerns mental health services and supports the goal of effective citizenship for persons with serious mental illness. He also writes and conducts medical research in the areas of narrative medicine and medical humanities.

Lidia Schapira, Boston, MA, USA, is a medical oncologist with a clinical practice focused on breast cancer based at Massachusetts General Hospital. She is actively engaged in research in breast cancer and psychosocial oncology. She served on the board of directors of the American Society of Psychosocial Oncology and serves as associate editor for ASCO's website for the public, Cancer.Net. Dr. Schapira has championed international efforts to improve training in communication for oncology clinicians and developed innovative curricula to address the needs of this community of professionals and patients. She has an abiding interest in understanding how patients cope with life-limiting illness and how professionals can best support their needs.

Gilberto Schwartsmann, Porto Alegre, Brazil, is Professor of Medical Oncology at the Academic Hospital, Federal University. He completed his postgraduate training in Medical Oncology at Middlesex Hospital, London and received his Ph.D. at the Free University, Amsterdam. He was director of the EORTC New Drug Development Office and a faculty member of ESMO. He was also a member of the ASCO International Affairs Committee. He is a member of the National Academy of Medicine in Brazil. Dr. Schwartzmann is cited as inventor in two patents of new experimental agents.

Allen C. Sherman, Little Rock, AR, USA, is Director of the Behavioral Medicine Division and Associate Professor at the University of Arkansas for Medical Sciences. He completed a B.A. in psychology at Brown University, a Ph.D. in clinical psychology at the University of Kansas, and an internship and postdoctoral fellowship at Harvard Medical School in Cambridge Hospital. He has been principal investigator on numerous research protocols regarding quality-of-life outcomes among patients with chronic medical illnesses, risk/protective factors, and religiousness and health.

Yuki Shirai, Tokyo, Japan, is a project research associate of the Human Resource Development Plan for Cancer at the University of Tokyo. Dr. Shirai has focused her efforts on research in the area of communication between patient and clinician in oncology. Together with her coauthors, Drs. Fujimori and Uchitomi, she has played an active role in the development and spread of communication skills training programs for cancer patients and oncologists in Japan.

Julia Smith, New York, USA, Director of the Breast Cancer Prevention Program at the NYU Clinical Cancer Center and Bellevue Hospital, has had experience as a medical oncologist specializing in breast cancer and evaluates the safety and efficacy of SOM230 on DCIS prevention. Her long-standing clinical work with breast cancer patients, as well as with high-risk patients, gives her the tools to evaluate and talk effectively with candidates and participants in the trial and to inform subjects of the issues involved. In addition, these clinical skills are necessary for proper follow-up and evaluation of risks, issues with side effects and toxicities, and clinical symptoms that may arise during study of the trial drug. In addition, Dr. Smith has worked collaboratively and in a multidisciplinary fashion with the subspecialties involved and is able to coordinate the patient care.

Friedrich Stiefel, Lausanne, Switzerland, is Professor and Chief of the Psychiatric Liaison Service of the University Hospital. On a clinical level he works as a psychotherapist for patients suffering from somatic diseases, and he supervises psychiatrists and psychologists working in liaison psychiatry and healthcare professionals caring for patients with cancer. His research activities focus on psychotherapy in the medically ill, case complexity, patient–physician communication, and defense mechanisms of clinicians. He provides communication skills training for oncologists and teaches on communication in the healthcare setting at the pregraduate level.

Antonella Surbone, New York, USA, is a medical oncologist working in Italy and the United States. Dr. Surbone developed a personal, research, and scholarly interest in cross-cultural communication within the patient–doctor relationship and in the ethical and psychosocial implications of oncology. She obtained a bioethics degree in Rome and a Ph.D. in philosophy from Fordham University in New York. She is Ethics Editor of *NYU Clinical Correlations* and *Critical Reviews in Oncology Haematology*, and Associate Editor of *BMC Medical Ethics* and *Supportive Care in Cancer*. She is a member of the American Society of Clinical Oncology (ASCO) Educational Committee, Ethics Track Team Leader, and on the Board of Directors of the International Psycho-Oncology Society (IPOS) and the Multinational Association for Supportive Cancer Care (MASCC). She chairs the MASCC Psycho-Social Study Group and the Task Force on Cultural Competence in the Elderly of the International Society of Geriatric Oncology (SIOG). Together with Professor Zwitter and Richard Stiefel, she authored and edited the 1997 New York Academy of Sciences volume *Communication with the Cancer Patient: Information and Truth*, which inspired her further work and this present book.

Martin H.N. Tattersall, Sydney, Australia, undertook medical training in Cambridge, London, and at Harvard. He was a medical oncologist at Charing Cross Hospital before moving to Sydney in 1977 to establish a clinical cancer research program at the University of Sydney. He has been Professor of Cancer Medicine and a cancer physician at Royal Prince Alfred Hospital for more than 30 years. His research interests in the recent past have included cancer consultation, means to better inform patients of treatment options, and estimating and talking to patients about prognosis.

Avinash Thombre, Little Rock, AR, USA, is Associate Professor in the Department of Speech Communication at the University of Arkansas. He received his Ph.D. from the University of New Mexico, before which he worked as a journalist specializing in health reporting with *The Times of India* newspaper in India. His scholarship broadly concerns health communication, with a focus on understanding individual responses to traumatic health events that result in transformative experiences. His research also involves use of Web-based technologies, especially the social media, to disseminate public health messages. He has authored articles in the *Journal of Health Communication*. Along with a group of like-minded physicians, he campaigns in India, riding bicycles from village to village, to reduce maternal mortality and promote physical exercise.

Luzia Travado, Lisbon, Portugal, is a clinical psychologist and psychotherapist, specialized in health psychology and psychooncology. She is Chief of Clinical Psychology at Hospital S. José-Central Lisbon Hospital Centre, where she began her career and has pioneered psychosocial programs for chronic patients who have undergone trauma (e.g., severe burns) or disease (including cancer). She teaches psychooncology and communication skills, having been responsible for the implementation of the National Pilot Program on Communication Skills Training launched by the Coordination for Oncological Diseases, Portuguese Ministry of Health.

Maria Die Trill, Madrid, Spain, is coordinator of the Psycho-Oncology Unit of the Hospital Universitario Gregorio Marañón and Assistant Professor at the School of Psychology, Universidad Complutense. She has held appointments at Bellevue Psychiatric Hospital-New York University Medical Center, Memorial Sloan-Kettering Cancer Center, New York, and Dana-Farber Cancer Institute and Harvard Medical School in Boston, MA, USA. During her work with adult and pediatric cancer patients, she has had close collaboration with oncology professionals, teaching communication skills and helping them work through personal and professional issues.

Yosuke Uchitomi, Tokyo, Japan, has been Chairman and Professor of Neuropsychiatry, Okayama University, Japan since 2010 and has led psychooncology development in Japan as Chief of the Psycho-Oncology Division, National Cancer Center since 1995. Since the Cancer Control Act in Japan (2007), Drs. Fujimori, Shirai, and Uchitomi have played an active role in conducting both basic and advanced communication skills workshops for oncologists throughout Asia.

Paulo Roberto Vasconcellos-Silva, Rio de Janeiro, Brazil, has 16 years of experience in production and evaluation of informative and educational products for lay people. For 10 years he was Coordinator of the Educational Material Division of the National Cancer Institute—Brazil. He earned a doctorate degree in health communication (2003) and a postdoctorate on media, Internet, and health communication studies (2101) at the National School of Public Heath/Oswaldo Cruz Foundation. He has been Director of the Research Center of the Longitudinal Study of Adult Health

ELSA (National School of Public Health/Oswaldo Cruz Foundation). Currently he is a researcher on health communication at the Oswaldo Cruz Institute (Laboratory of Therapeutic Innovation, Education, and Bioproducts) and associate professor of bioethics and medical ethics, Federal University of the State of Rio de Janeiro.

Kathryn J. Walseman, Washington, DC, USA, is a resident physician at The George Washington University Department of Psychiatry and Behavioral Sciences in Washington, DC. She has a particular interest in mental and spiritual health for those with chronic medical illnesses. Her other recent publication, *Finding Meaning at the End of Life*, is a case report that explores the concept of demoralization in a patient with terminal cancer.

Fusun Yaris, Samsun, Turkey, is a professor of family medicine, cancer epidemiologist, and Chair of Ondokuzmayis University School of Medicine, Department of Family Medicine. She focuses on family medicine education and clinical skills teaching in undergraduate and family medicine residency programs, cancer prevention, care of cancer patients in primary care, rational drug use, and continuous professional development in primary care. She coordinates first-phase teaching courses of family doctors at the Ministry of Health. She has been a cancer patient (ovarian) over the past 2 years.

Branko Zakotnik's, Ljubljana, Slovenia, communication with patients and ethical dilemmas have been a challenge since his first encounter with cancer patients 30 years ago as a resident at the Institute of Oncology Ljubljana (Specialist from December 1988, President of the Institutional Ethics Committee, 1991–2003)— after which it became more fascinating for him to observe how changes in society (democracy) and new technologies (IT, diagnostic tools, pharmaceutical industry) can dramatically influence and change the traditional doctor–patient–family relationship.

Zhi-gang Zhuang, Shanghai, China, has a long-term research interest in the development of surgery and oncogenes in treating breast cancer. The biological activity of the targeted tumor antigen and its involvement in cancer invasion and metastases is being characterized in his research. He is also working closely with clinician-scientists and basic researchers in studies that characterize breast cancer behavior and develop molecular classifications for advanced breast cancer.

Matjaž Zwitter, Ljubljana, Slovenia, Chief of the Lung Cancer Unit, Institute of Oncology in Ljubljana, is a radiation oncologist with a long-term interest in lung cancer, Hodgkin's disease, and medical ethics. He has designed, conducted, and published several trials on treatment of non-small cell lung cancer and mesothelioma. Among his favorite topics is treatment with low-dose gemcitabine in prolonged infusion, characterized by mild toxicity, good efficacy, and low cost. In addition, he serves as Professor of Medical Ethics at the Medical School, University of Maribor, Slovenia.

Index

A
ACS. *See* American Cancer Society
Aging and cancer
 clinical research, 172–173
 current information, 170–171
 missing information, 171–172
American Association of Retired People (AARP), 85
American Cancer Society (ACS), 431
American Medical Association
 Code of Ethics, 45
American Society of Clinical Oncology (ASCO), 211
Anosognosia, 16

B
Bad news disclosure
 attitudes
  case study, 146–147
  challenges, Saudi Arabia, 147
  paradigm shift, Saudi Arabia, 149–151
  patient autonomy, 149
  patient's basic right, 150
  psychosocial influences, 147
  public and physician preferences, 150–151
  public education, 149
  recommendations, 151–152
  sociocultural background, 148–149
  in the West, 147–148
 ethical issues (*see* Ethical issues, Saudi Arabia)
 French process, 336–337
 history, 40
 individualized approach, 141–142
 Iranian perspective
  anxiety and depression scores, 405–406
  future research, 403–404
  literacy and knowledge of cancer diagnosis, 407–408
  psychological distress study, 405, 408
  quality of life study, 404, 405, 408
  Western literature, 403–404
 training doctors for, 265
 truth telling, Australia
  communication with family members, 382–383
  cultural issues, 383–384
  demographic factors, 378–379
  guidelines and training, 380–381
  level of difficulty, 381–382
  policy factors, 379
  tools for assistance, 384
  work-related stress, oncologists (*see* Work-related stress, oncologists)
BATHE (background, affect, trouble, handling, empathy), 268–269
Beneficence, 46
Bereavement, 70–72
Binary logic
 hope and realistic expectations, 251–252
 medical ethics, 250
 nerve conduction and brain function, 249
 in our lives, 248–249
 truth telling, 250–251
 word processors, 247–248
BRCA mutations
 breast cancer
  embryo cryopreservation, 211
  genetic cancer risk assessment, 211
  intra-abdominal malignancy, 210
  mammographic screening, 210

BRCA mutations (*cont.*)
  ovarian cancer
    bilateral adnexal masses, 208
    CA125 and CA27.29 abnormalities, 210
    carboplatin and paclitaxel, 209
    p53 signatures, 210
    relapse, 208
    stages III and IV, 208
    surveillance *vs.* risk-reducing surgery, 209

C
Cancer Alarm Approach, 431
Cancer diagnosis disclosure
  French disclosure process. (*see* French disclosure process)
Cancer patients
  aging and cancer, 170
  in Argentina, hematological malignancy
    in Buenos Aires, 352–353
    chronic/indolent, 355–357
    chronic myeloid leukemia (*see* Chronic myeloid leukemia)
    communicating to the patient, 354, 357, 359–361
    communication in the interdisciplinary team, 361–362
    cultural variables, 353
    decision-making process, 354
    diagnosis, 355–357
    doctor-patient relationship, 354
    formal education, 353
    FUNDALEU, 354
    healthcare institutions, 352
  in China
    breast cancer, 491–492
    traditional medicine, 495
    treatment, 493–495
    types of malignancy, 492–493
  clinical research, 172–173
  communication
    message content, 169, 173–174
    message delivery, 169, 174–175
  frail and elderly
    case studies, 180–183
    cognitive failure patients, 187–188
    end of life communication, 183–185
    hematological and nonhematological patients, 171
    life perspective, 185–186
    palliative plan, 188–189
    roles of key persons, 186–187
  function and comorbidity, 170
  geriatric assessment, 170–171
  in Israel
    Arab community, 319–320, 326
    beliefs and perceptions, 320–321
    breast cancer, 322
    coping patterns, 323–325
    cultural competence, 326–329
    culture and effecting change, 326–328
    epidemiology, 320
    ethnic and cultural diversity, 317–318
    family context, 322–323
    Jewish community, 319, 326
    population of, 318–319
    psychosocial care, 325–326
  neutropenia and neutropenic infections, 171
  in Russia, 430–432
  screening programs in Slovenia, 483
  survival data, East European countries, 482
  written information, 169
Cancer patients, hereditary factor
  breast cancer and BRCA mutations
    embryo cryopreservation, 211
    genetic cancer risk assessment, 211
    intra-abdominal malignancy, 210
    mammographic screening, 210
  educational material, 212–213
  Lynch syndrome, 212
  ovarian cancer and BRCA mutations
    bilateral adnexal masses, 208
    CA125 and CA27.29 abnormalities, 210
    carboplatin and paclitaxel, 209
    p53 signatures, 210
    relapse, 208
    stages III and IV, 208
    surveillance *vs.* risk-reducing surgery, 209
Cancer Recuperation Club, 494
Chemotherapy Risk Assessment Score in High-Age Patients (CRASH) predicts, 171
Chronic myeloid leukemia (CML)
  adherence to recommendations, 357–359
  causes of, 357
  nonadherence problem, 357
  Pavlovsky, Santiago (case study), 358
Clinical trials
  benefits, 501–502
  current practices
    abstract, 505
    issues, 504
    language of information, 504
    quality control, 505
  diagnosis, understanding of, 499–500
  information to patient, 504
  informed consent process, 499

Index 521

medical situation, 499–500
patient's rights, 503
research procedure, 500–501
risks, 502–503
Code of Ethics, 1847, 420
COH-QOL tool, 101
Communication challenges.
  See also Printed educational
    materials (PEMs)
  Bosnia and Herzegovina
    case study, 412–413
    palliative care, 417
    patients and education, 416–417
    patient's right to know, 415–416
    physician's problems, 414–415
  in Bosnia and Herzegovina
    health system, 415
    physician-patient relationship,
      412–413, 415–416
  in China
    economy's impact, 493–494
    internet's impact, 494
  in clinical research (*see* Clinical trials)
  in everyday life, 354
  impact on survival, 357
  internet information (*see* Internet
    communications)
  paradigm shift in
    authoritarian and asymmetric
      relationship, 7
    connection-based equality, 8
    cross-cultural differences, 8
    degree of ambiguity, 7
    functional rigidity/limitation, 6
    genetic predisposition, 9
    genetic testing, 9
    honest reciprocal communication, 7
    humanistic practice, 10
    medicalization and stigmatization, 9
    paternalism and contractualism, 8
    professional and caregiver stresses, 7
    trust, 8
    truth telling, 6, 8
  refractory patients, 359–361
  in Russia
    cancer awareness, 431
    clinical trial, 435
    current issues, 434
    developments of, 432
    early diagnosis and cancer control,
      430–431
    family and group support, 437–438
    history of development, 432
    informed consent, 435

    mass media support, 436–437
    media's role, 435–437
    physician's role, 434–435
    psychosocial support groups, 437–438
    real and ideal communication, 433–434
  in Slovenia
    cancer incidence, 486
    democracy's influence, 482–483
    importance of, 489
    internet's effect, 483–485
    palliative care, 486–488
  in Turkey
    cultural barrier, 398–399
    cultural difference argument, 393–396
    medical paternalism, 392–393
    minimalist approach, 396–397
    therapeutic privilege, 398
  in Zimbabwe
    chemotheraphy, 449
    compliance with treatment, 449–450
    counseling issues, 447–448
    double diagnosis, 445
    future needs, 451
    HIV patients, 444–446
    language barrier, 448
    radiotheraphy, 448
    relatives and health care workers,
      446–447
    treatment misconceptions, 448–449
Communication skills, teaching
  didactic anchors, 286
  educational principles
    adult learning theory, 278
    conveying information, 277
    elements, 277–278
    learners' confidence, 277
    learning road map, 278, 279
    positive psychology, 278
    reflective practice, 278
  evaluation, 288
  faculty demonstrations, 286
  faculty learners and fellows, 282
  investigators
    experienced learner, 280
    life of the group, 280, 281
    life of the learner, 280, 281
    retreat program, 280
  strategies for promoting learning, 287–288
  teaching format
    cognitive road map, practice session,
      283, 284
    investigator role, 285–286
    retreat day, 283, 285
  verbal and nonverbal behaviors, 276

Communication skills training (CST), 52–53
  in Japan
    aims of, 307
    train-the-trainers program, 308
  in Portugal
    clinical practice, 292
    Department of Medical Psychology of the School of Medicine, 292
    doctor-patient communication program, 292
    general practioner, residency training, 292–293
    initiatives in, 297
    National Program for the Prevention and Control of Oncological Diseases, 295–296
    physician–patient communication, 293
    pilot training group, 294–295
    SEPOS, 294
    SPIKES breaking bad news protocol, 295
Complementary and alternative medicine (CAM), 82
  AARP and NCCAM survey, 85
  antioxidants, 86
  audiotapes, 84
  clinical trial-generated evidence, 87
  communication skill, 89
  cytochrome p450 hepatic enzyme system, 86
  denial system, 87
  drug interactions, 86
  evidence-based information, 84
  patients divulgement, 84–85
  plant-based protocols, 88
  psychooncology, 87
  "refusnik" patients, 87
  treatment algorithms and interventions, 84
Complicated bereavement-triggered depression, 70
Complicated grief therapy (CGT), 74
Conceptualization, 129
Contractualism, 8
Counter-transference, 60
Cross-cultural palliative care, 200–201
Cultural competence
  biopsychosocial ecological system, 368
  cancer sites and rates, immigrants, 370
  and clinical encounters, 367
  defining culture, 366–369
  economic burden
    demographic changes, 370
    health disparities, 369
  functions of, 368
  inequities due to lack of, 366
  JAHCO requirements, 370
  language concordance, 371
  nonverbal communication, 371–372
  practice strategies, 372–373
  triple-negative breast cancers (TNBC), 367
  truth telling, 371

D

Dementia in Norway
  case studies, 180, 183, 184
  and cognitive impairment, 186, 187
  individual pain treatment, 188
  reduced communicative abilities, 188
Demoralization, 66
Denial in Cancer Interview (DCI), 19, 20
Denial, patient-physician communication
  anosognosia, 16
  anxiety, 20
  beneficial/detrimental impacts, 16
  case studies, 16–18
  closure, 15–16
  DCI, 19, 20
  defense mechanism, 19, 21
  disciplinary differences, 19
  entity, 22
  fighting spirit, 19
  framing denial, 23
  guilt and inadequacy feelings, 20
  hysterical personality, 18
  interethnic differences, 20
  maladaptive and adaptive forms, 20
  psychoanalysis, 18
  psychobiological reaction, 18
  self-image and self-esteem, 19
  social and demographic factors, 19
  social-cultural complexities, 22
  time, 16
  truth and facts, 21
  truth telling, 21–23
  unconscious mechanism, 22
Deontology Code, Italian Medical Association, 421
Depression
  assessment and recognition, 65
  cancer patients
    assessment and diagnostic issues, 65–67
    psychological intervention issues, 68–69
  emotional distress, 64–65
  grieving relatives. (*see* Grieving relatives)
  prevalence rates, 64
  psychosocial and psychiatric disorders, 64
  psychotherapy and psychopharmacology, 65
Diagnostic disclosure procedure
  continuation of assessment, 345–346
  coordination, 344–345

Index

definition and aims of, 337–338
distress identification, 341–342
doctor-patient relationship, 343–344
health-care trajectory, extension to, 342–343
procedure evaluation, 338–339
structure of, 339–341
therapeutic education programs, 345
Dynamic communication, 6
division of time-illness, 199, 200
physician and patient relationship, 198
questions and answer, 199
trained physician, 198

E
EMA. *See* European Medicines Agency
Emotional exhaustion, 51, 53
Empathy, 30, 33, 34, 59–60, 68
EORTC QLQ. *See* European Organization for Research and Treatment of Cancer Quality of Life
Ethical imperialism, 390
Ethical issues, Saudi Arabia
principles, 40, 46
religion, 41–42
tradition, 41
truth communication
community, 45
patients, 42–43
physicians, 44–45
policy and law, 46–47
prognosis, 47
relatives, 43–44
Ethnicity, 367
European Medicines Agency (EMA), 488
European Organization for Research and Treatment of Cancer Quality of Life Questionnaire (EORTC QLQ), 404
functioning and global quality of life scores, 404–405

F
Family-focused grief therapy (FFGT), 74
Family physicians (FP), role of
biopsychosocial medicine, 268–269
breaking bad news, 265
cancer care, 264–265
cancer epidemiology, 263–264
oncologist, collaboration with, 265–266
ownership, 269
patient-centered care, 266–267

patient-centered communication, 267
in patient health behavior, 271–272
patient's perspective, 266
in primary palliative care, 272
prognosis, 267–268
shared decision-making, 266
therapeutic advice
behavior, 270
feelings, 270
guidance, 269–270
listening skills, 271
options, 270
reinterpreting situations, 270–271
thoughts, 270
Family's role in cancer, 129–131
FICA tool, 101
Forbidding disclosure, 397
Foundation for the Fight against Leukemia (FUNDALEU), 352, 354
French disclosure process
diagnostic disclosure procedure
continuation of assessment, 345–346
coordination, 344–345
definition and aims of, 337–338
distress identification, 341–342
doctor-patient communication training, 343–344
extension of, 342–343
procedure evaluation, 338–339
structure of, 339–341
therapeutic education programs, 345
historical development, 334–336
Full-disclosure model, 40

G
Ganoderma lucidum, 484
Gastrointestinal stromal tumor (GIST), 487–488
Genetic predisposition, 9
Geriatric syndromes, 170
GIST. *See* Gastrointestinal stromal tumor
Grieving relatives
assessment and diagnostic issues
bereavement, 70–72
complicated (pathological) grief, 70
death, 69–70
distress intensity, 73
mental health services, 72
practical support and counseling, 72
prolonged grief disorder, 70
self-validation and positive feelings, 72
variability and fluidity, 70
psychological intervention issues, 73–74

H

HADS. *See* Hospital Anxiety and Depression Scale
Hedonism, 127
Hermeneutics, 126
Hippocratic writings, 420
Holistic approach, 233
Honest disclosure, 399
Hope *vs.* realistic expectations, 251–252
Hospital Anxiety and Depression Scale (HADS), 404
Hypopharyngeal carcinoma, 254
Hysterical personality, 18

I

Illness appraisals, 114
Independent choice model, 390
Integrative oncology
  body's innate healing response, 82
  CAM (*see* Complementary and alternative medicine)
  integrative medicine, 82–83
  words of Maimonides, 83
International Classification of Childhood Cancer 1996 (ICCC), 155, 157
International Classification of Diseases for Oncology, 155
Internet communications
  cancer patients usage in Slovenia, 483–485
  doctor's negative perspective, 477–478
  doctor's right response, 478–479
  health-related applications
    online communication, 476
    online support groups, 474–476
    positive and negative effects, 476–477
    web pages, 473–474
  information seekers, 472
  patient-doctor communication, 477
  patient's negative perspective, 478
Interpersonal communication, 106
Interpersonal psychotherapy (IPT), 68, 74
Interprofessional spiritual care model, 98

J

Japanese clinical oncology
  CST program, 307–308
  cultural characteristics, patient behavior, 311
  patient preferences in communication
    additional information component, 304
    bad news disclosure, 304, 306
    individualized communication, 303
    patient's perspective, 303
    physician communication, 306–307
    reassurance and emotional support, 304–306
    setting component, 304
  QPS (*see* Question-asking prompt sheet)
  truth telling, 302
Justice, 46

L

Life, meaning of
  categories, 127
  correspondence and disparity, 132
  death, 132
  hermeneutics, 126
  in illness, 129–132
  internal and external permeability, 128
  life review, 126
  patients and families, 133
  psychodynamics, 128
  psychological issues, 131
  religion and spirituality, 132

M

Meaning-centered group psychotherapy (MCGP), 102
Medical Deontology Regulation, Turkey, 398
Medical errors
  breathing difficulties
    otolaryngology ward, 258–259
    surgical intensive care unit, 258
  cancer recurrence, 254–257
  hypopharyngeal carcinoma, 254
  medical and surgical errors, 253
  nursing errors, 259–260
  premature oral feeding, 259
Medicalization, 9

N

National Center for Complementary and Alternative Medicine (NCCAM), 85
National Program for the Prevention and Control of Oncological Diseases, 295–296
Nondisclosure model, 40
Nonmalfeasance, 46

O

Oncology, role of emotion
   patient (*see* Patients' emotions)
   physician, 242–243
   physician-patient relationship, 237–238, 243–244
Oncotalk Teach Model. *See* Communication skills, teaching
Orientalism, 395

P

Palliative care, 486–487
   bioethical paradigm, 196
   concept of pain, 196
   cost, 195
   cultural background, 197
   dynamic process of communication
      division of time-illness, 199, 200
      physician and patient relationship, 198
      questions and answer, 199
      trained physician, 198
   end-of-life care, 200–201
   ethics of the cure, 197–198
   language of communication, 192–193
   patients typology, 194
   perception of terms, 197
   sensible communication, 193
   short and long prognosis, 192
   staging, 195
   too-early intervention, 194
   truth, 193
Paternalism, 8, 29
   communication barrier in cancer care, 392–393
   contemporary bioethics, 390
Patient autonomy, 5, 46
Patient-doctor relationship
   information sharing, 472
   internet, 477
Patient-health care professional communication
   cultural expectations, 396
   in Turkey, 390, 391
Patient-physician communication
   clinical setting
      family members, 232
      nursing staff inclusion, 232
      pretreatment interview, 231
   dimensions of, 233–234
   emotion (*see* Emotion)
   truth
      holistic approach, 233
      patient's comprehension, 232–233
      relevant truth, 233
Patients' emotions
   active to palliative care, 241
   diagnostic phase, 239
   follow-ups, remission, and long-term cancer survival, 240
   genetic counseling, 241
   phase of treatment, 240
   relapse, 241
Patient's personality
   and bad news disclosure, 141–142
   and communication challenges, 139–140
   communication strategies, 138
   potential for miscommunication, 138
   unknown and frightening communication, 139
Pediatric oncology
   Argentina
      ethnic predominance, 155
      ICCC, 155, 157
      oncology day beds, 158
      open communication, 158
      palliative care, 155
      population distribution, 154–156
      reality control, 158–159
      ROHA, 155, 157
      self-sufficiency, 157
      symbiotic union, 157
   communication rules, 160–161
   death, 165–166
   effective communication aspects, 161–162
   emotional and spiritual impact, 154
   honest communication, 160
   intervention time, 154
   medication and injection fantasies, 162–164
   professionals, 159–160
   siblings with sick child, 164–165
PEMs. *See* Printed educational materials (PEMs)
Perspective transformation, Western India
   benefit-finding, 107
   constructs, 107
   cultural context, 115
   cultural influences, 108
   data analysis, 110
   disorienting dilemma, 106
   domains
      altruism, 110
      forgiveness, 112–113
      integrity *vs.* despair, 116
      life review, 112
      life satisfaction, 111–112

Perspective transformation,
    Western India (*cont.*)
        low and high perspective
            transformation, 117
        spirituality, 113
        stress-related changes, 116
    Indian culture, 117
    interpersonal communication, 106
    limitations and future research, 118–119
    participants, 108–109
    pathways, 117–118
    portrayed changes, 110
    positive changes, 110
    posttraumatic growth, 107
    procedures, 109–110
    process dimensions, 114, 116
    sense-making, 107
    themes, 113–114
Physicians' emotions
    anger, 220
    emotional intimacy, 221
    fear, 221
    intrapsychic variables, 219
    omnipotent healer, 220
    professional caretakers, 221
    resiliency, 221
    satisfaction, 227–228
    self-analysis questions (*see* Self-analysis
        questions)
    severely ill and dying patient, 220
Preoperative Assessment of Cancer in the
    Elderly (PACE), 171
Preparatory communication, 188, 189
Printed educational materials (PEMs)
    beneficial effects, 462–463
    in Brazil, 456–457
    as communication prostheses, 465
    disadvantages, 461–463
    efficiency, 460–461
    impact levels, 466
    leaflets
        efficacy in delivering information,
            460–461
        inadequacy of information, 461–463
        and individual needs, 463–466
    review and second-order review, 457–459
    strategic analysis, 456–457
    uses, 456
Professional demotivation, 51
Prognosis, 47
Psychodynamics, 128
Psycho-oncological counselling, 417
Psychosocial care, 325–326
Public education, 149

Q

Qualitative prognosis, 47
Quality of life and disclosure of diagnosis,
    404–405
Quantitative prognosis, 47
Question-asking prompt sheet (QPS)
    advanced cancer patients, 309
    mean usefulness rate, 309–311
Question prompt list (QPL), 384, 385

R

Rationalization, 130
Registro Oncopediátrico Hospitalario
    Argentino (ROHA), 155, 157
Regulation on Patient Rights (RPR), 396
Reification, 4
Relational communication, 6
Relevant truth, 233
Research, importance for the physician, 28
Role of emotion
    patients
        active to palliative care, 241
        diagnostic phase, 239
        follow-ups, remission, and long-term
            cancer survival, 240
        genetic counseling, 241
        phase of treatment, 240
        relapse, 241
    physician, 242–243
    physician-patient relationship, 237–238,
        243–244
RPR. *See* Regulation on Patient Rights

S

Self-actualization, 127–128
Self-analysis questions
    communication skills
        training, 225
    continuity of care, 227
    expectations and awareness, 222–223
    grief-related issues, 223
    helping situations, 227
    helplessness, 224–225
    importance of, 218
    intrapsychic stressors, 225
    mental health professional, 226
    need for, 218
    perception, 227
    personal career choice, 222
    psycho-oncologist staff meeeting, 226
    responsibility sharing, 226
    specific emotions identification, 226

Index 527

staff well-being, 218–219
transference and countertransference, 224
Self-transcendence, 128
Short Term Life Review (STLR), 102
Southern European Psycho-oncology Study (SEPOS), 294
Spirituality
  barriers, 96–97
  biopsychosocialspiritual model, 96
  in clinical setting, 97–98
  clinicians personal views and biases, 99
  COH-QOL tool, 101
  communication style, 99
  definition, 94
  FICA tool, 101
  goal of interaction, 99
  HOPE questions, 101
  interprofessional spiritual care model, 98
  medical history, 102
  open-ended questions, 101
  personal philosophies, 95
  perspective transformation, Western India, 113
  religion, 94, 95
  spiritual assessment, 99–100
  transcendent, 94, 95
  treatment dissatisfaction and noncompliance, 95
  treatment models, 102
Staff helplessness, 224–225
Stigmatization, 9
Suicide assessment, depression
Supportive-expressive psychotherapy, 68

T
Teaching communication
  crosscultural communication
  race and ethnicity
Therapeutic alliance, 68
Train-the-trainers program, 308
Transcendent, 94, 95
Traumatic grief, 70
Treatment-derived somatic symptoms, 65
Truthful disclosure, 390, 391
Truthfullness and honesty, 46
Truth telling, 250–251, 390
  Australia
    communication with family members, 382–383
    cultural issues, 383–384
    demographic factors, 378–379
    guidelines and training, 380–381

    level of difficulty, 381–382
    policy factors, 379
    tools for assistance, 384
  binary logic, 250–251
  and cultural competence, 371
  denial, patient-physician communication, 21–23
  Japanese clinical oncology, 302
  paradigm shift in communication, 6, 8
  in Russia
    conservative attitude, 438
    patients' preference, 433–434
Truth-telling practices
  Brazil and South America
    communication strategies, need for, 421–422
    guidance to communicate for oncologists, 424–426
    illiteracy as a barrier, 422
    Medical Code of Ethics, 423
    oncologists' education, 424
    patients' preferences, 423–424
    prognosis communication, 425
  Code of Ethics of 1847, 420
  Deontology Code, 421
  in the twentieth century, 420–421
Truth telling to truth making, 5
  See also Paradigm shift in communication

U
Uncertainty management
  audiotapes, 30
  avoidance, 29–30
  death conversations, 29
  deceit, 30
  emotions, 33–34
  futile chemotherapy, 29
  iatrogenic complications, 29
  illness threat, 30
  language and framing, 32–33
  medical research, 28, 34–35
  paternalism, 29
  therapeutic value, communication, 27–28
  threat transformation
    cognitive-based coping strategies, 31
    family meetings, 32
    medical culture, 30
    psychoeducation and encouragement, 31
US health disparities, 369–370

W
Work-related stress, oncologists
 anxiety, 52
 archetypical situations, 54
 biographical elements, 53
 CST, 52–53
 curative to palliative care
  transition, 56–58
 death and dying, 59–61
 defense mechanisms, 52
 diagnosis announcement, 54–55
 emotional exhaustion, 51, 53
 intrapsychic echo, 53
 personal achievement, 51
 professional demotivation, 51
 psychiatric morbidity, 51
 relapse, deception, 55–56
 uncertainty, 59